2b. 17

# LATERALIZATION
# IN THE
# NERVOUS SYSTEM

# LATERALIZATION
# IN THE
# NERVOUS SYSTEM

*EDITED BY*

### STEVAN HARNAD

Department of Psychiatry
College of Medicine and Dentistry
of New Jersey
Rutgers Medical School
Piscataway, New Jersey

### ROBERT W. DOTY

Center for Brain Research
University of Rochester
Rochester, New York

### LEONIDE GOLDSTEIN

Department of Psychiatry
College of Medicine and Dentistry
of New Jersey
Rutgers Medical School
Piscataway, New Jersey

### JULIAN JAYNES

Department of Psychology
Princeton University
Princeton, New Jersey

### GEORGE KRAUTHAMER

Department of Anatomy
College of Medicine and Dentistry
of New Jersey
Rutgers Medical School
Piscataway, New Jersey

ACADEMIC PRESS    New York   San Francisco   London   1977
A Subsidiary of Harcourt Brace Jovanovich, Publishers

ACADEMIC PRESS, INC.
111 Fifth Avenue, New York, New York 10003

*United Kingdom Edition published by*
ACADEMIC PRESS, INC. (LONDON) LTD.
24/28 Oval Road, London NW1

Library of Congress Cataloging in Publication Data

Main entry under title:

Lateralization in the nervous system.

    Includes bibliographies and indexes.
    1.   Cerebral dominance.    I.    Harnad, Stevan R.
QP385.5.L37        591.1'88       76-47014
ISBN 0−12−325750−6

# Contents

CONTENTS

# LIST OF CONTRIBUTORS

Numbers in parentheses indicate the pages on which the authors' contributions begin.

*Samuel W. Anderson* (403), Department of Communication Sciences, New York State Psychiatric Institute, New York, New YOrk

*Charles I. Berlin* (303), Department of Otorhinolaryngology, Louisiana State University Medical Center, Kresge Hearing Research Laboratory of the South, New Orleans, Louisiana

*William D. Chapple* (1), Regulatory Biology, Biological Sciences Group, University of Connecticut, Storrs, Connecticut

*Robert L. Collins* (137), The Jackson Laboratory, Bar Harbor, Maine

*Irving S. Cooper* (123), Institute of Neuroscience, St. Barnabas Hospital, Bronx, New York

*James H. Dewson, III* (63), Hearing and Speech Sciences, Stanford University, School of Medicine, Stanford, California

*Emanuel Donchin* (339), Department of Psychology, University of Illinois, Champaign, Illinois

*Robert W. Doty, Sr.* (75, xvii), Center for Brain Research, University of Rochester, Rochester, New York

*Susan E. Folstein** (89), Edward W. Bourne Behavioral Research Laboratory, New York Hospital-Cornell Medical Center, Department of Psychiatry, Westchester Division, White Plains, New York

*Alcides Gadotti†* (385), Department of Psychology, State University of New York, Stony Brook, New York

*Martin F. Gardiner* (481), Seizure Unit, Division of Neurophysiology, Department of Neurology, Children's Hospital Medical Center, and Harvard Medical School, Boston, Massachusetts

*Eric H. Geiger* (89), Edward W. Bourne Behavioral Research Laboratory, New York Hospital-Cornell Medical Center, Department of Psychiatry, Westerchester Division, White Plains, New York

*Stanley D. Glick* (213), Department of Pharmacology, Mount Sinai School of Medicine of the City of New York, New York, New York

*Leonide Goldstein* (451), College of Medicine and Dentistry of New Jersey-Rutgers Medical School, Department of Psychiatry, Piscataway, New Jersey

*Charles G. Gross* (109), Department of Psychology, Princeton University, Princeton, New Jersey

*Raquel Gur* (261), Department of Psychiatry, University of Pennsylvania School of Medicine, Philadelphia, Pennsylvania

*Ruben Gur* (261), Department of Psychiatry, University of Pennsylvania School of Medicine, Philadelphia, Pennsylvania

*Charles R. Hamilton* (45), Division of Biology, California Institute of Technology, Pasadena, California

*Stevan Harnad* (xvii), College of Medicine and Dentistry of New Jersey-Rutgers Medical School, Department of Psychiatry, Piscataway, New Jersey

*Kenneth M. Heilman* (285), Department of Neurology, College of Medicine, University of Florida, Gainesville, Florida

*T. P. Jerussi* (213), Department of Pharmacology, Mount Sinai School of Medicine, of the City of New York, New York, New York

*Marta Kutas* (339), Department of Psychology, University of Illinois, Champaign, Illinois

*Jerre Levy* (195), Department of Psychology, University of Pennsylvania, Philadelphia, Pennsylvania

*Gregory McCarthy* (339), Department of Psychology, University of Illinois, Champaign, Illinois

*Donald F. Mervis* (89), Department of Anatomy, Mount Sinai School of Medicine, of the City University of New York, New York, New York

*Mortimer Mishkin* (109), National Institute of Mental Health, Bethesda, Maryland

*Michael Morgan* (173), The Psychological Laboratory, University of Cambridge, Cambridge, England

*Judith M.Nelsen* (451), College of Medicine and Dentistry of New Jersey-Rutgers Medical School, Department of Psychiatry, Piscataway, New Jersey

*Fernando Nottebohm* (23), The Rockefeller University, New York, New York

*William H. Overman, Jr.* (75), Center for Brain Research, University of Rochester, Rochester, New York

*Ruth Phillips* (451), College of Medicine and Dentistry of New Jersey-Rutgers Medical School, Department of Psychiatry, Piscataway, New Jersey

*Manuel Riklan* (123), Institute of Neuroscience, St. Barnabas, Hospital, Bronx, New York

*Steven C. Rosen* (385), Department of Psychology, State University at Stony Brook, Stony Brook, New York

*Alan B. Rubens* (503), University of Minnesota Medical School, Hennepin County Medical Center, Minneapolis, Minnesota

*Jeri A. Sechzer* (89), Edward W. Bourne Behavioral Research Laboratory, New York Hospital-Cornell Medical Center, Department of Psychiatry, Westchester Division, White Plains, New York

*Sally P. Springer* (325), Department of Psychology, State University of New York, Stony Brook, New York

*John S. Stamm* (385), Department of Psychology, State University of New York, Stony Brook, New York

*Robert W. Thatcher* (429), Brain Research Laboratory, Department of Psychiatry, New York Medical College, New York, New York

*Gerald Turkewitz* (251), Department of Psychology, Hunter College, City University of New York, and Department of Pediatrics, Rose F. Kennedy Center Albert Einstein College of Medicine, New York, New York

*Donald Walter* (481), Department of Physiology, and Anatomy, University of California, Los Angeles, California

*John M. Warren* (151), Animal Behavior Laboratory, The Pennsylvania State University, University Park, Pennsylvania

*Robert T. Watson* (285), Department of Neurology, The College of Medicine, University of Florida and the Veterans Administration Hospital, Gainesville, Florida

*William G. Webster* (471), Department of Psychology, Carleton University, Ottawa, Canada

*B. Zimmerberg* (213), Department of Pharmacology, Mount Sinai School of Medicine, of the City of New York, New York, New York

*Present address: Department of Psychiatry, Johns Hopkins University, Baltimore, Maryland
†Present address: Department of Psicologia, Universidade Federal do Pará Belém-Pará, Brazil

# PREFACE

That research on the many aspects of lateralization has been growing enormously in recent years is evident from the innumerable scientific papers and no less than 20 volumes on the topic prepared since 1962 (see the Bibliography). However, no volume has as yet attempted to provide a thorough current perspective on the entire spectrum of existing approaches to lateralization with the object of bringing out the unifying themes pervading this multidisciplinary research. Review volumes have the disadvantage of being secondary, and often quite dated, sources. Moreover, some of this lateralization research is so recent, and originates from such disparate areas of investigation that no one has yet had a chance to draw it together and digest it.

In the present volume, the most recent original work representing the principal approaches to the investigation of lateralization has been assembled and organized, with copious cross references, and an Introductory Overview to orient the reader.

Certain newer approaches, such as the investigation of turning tendencies and electrocortical indices of hemispheric asymmetry, have been emphasized, while other, more classical approaches, already extensively described in the literature (such as human split-brain studies), have been given less intensive treatment. Throughout the volume, great stress has been placed upon experimental paradigms and outcomes that are applicable to both human and nonhuman species. Several chapters also place brain asymmetry in context with other biological asymmetries in the quest for general mechanisms and principles of lateralization. A variety of different perspectives, environmentalist and nativist, have been brought to bear on the problem of the inheritance, embryology and development of asymmetry. Highly suggestive invertebrate and avian models for lateralization are presented, and the evidence for cerebral dominance and handedness in nonhuman species is examined. Recent work on interhemispheric relations, the functions of the commissures, and on subcortical lateralization is reported.

The important theme of turning tendencies and attentional asymmetries pervades the volume, and is traced from rotation in invertebrates to lateral eye movement correlates of personality and cognition in man. Human clinical neuropsychological findings are presented, such as the effects of unilateral cortical and thalamic lesions and the syndrome of unilateral neglect; more than one model for the "minimal brain damage" syndrome in children is proposed. Cognitive asymmetries in human information-processing are investigated via dichotic listening and tachistoscopic half-field studies.

After an exhaustive review and critique of current research on surface electroencephalographic (EEG) and event-related potential laterality in man, a series of chapters report new findings from the application of these new electrographic techniques to the study of asymmetries during sleep, learning, performance, and information-processing in adults, infants, and animals.

Finally, there is a review of the gross anatomical asymmetries of the brain in human and nonhuman species and their implications for electrophysiological studies and hemispheric specialization.

The volume will be of interest to psychologists (physiological, cognitive, developmental, and clinical), behavioral biologists, neuroscientists, neurologists, and psychiatrists, as well as to scholars and educators from the humanities and social sciences who are concerned with the nature and biological bases of left–right differences in brain, behavior, and thinking.

## BIBLIOGRAPHY

*Volumes on lateralization, cerebral dominance, and interhemispheric relations (chronological order)*

Mountcastle, V.B. (Ed.) *Interhemispheric relations and cerebral dominance*. Baltimore: Johns Hopkins Press, 1962,

Hécaen, H., & de Ajuriaguerra, J. (Eds). *Left-handedness: Manual superiority and cerebral dominance*. New York: Grune & Stratton, 1964

Ettlinger, G. (Ed.). *Functions of the corpus callosum*. London: Churchill, 1965.

Gazzaniga, M.S. *The bisected brain*. New York: Appleton, 1970

Cernacek, J., & Podvinsky, F. (Eds.). *Cerebral interhemispheric relations*. Bratislava: Czechoslovak Academy of Sciences, 1972.

Dimond, S. *The double brain*. Edinburgh: Churchill Livingstone, 1972.

Brain Information Service Conference Report #34: *Cerebral dominance*. Los Angeles: UCLA BIS/BRI, 1974.

Dimond, S. & Beaumont, J.G. (Eds.). *Hemispheric function in the human brain*. Springfield, Illinois: Thomas, 1974.

Kinsbourne, M. & Smith, W.L. (Eds.). *Hemispheric disconnection and cerebral function in the human brain*. London: Elek, 1974.

Schmitt, F.O., & Worden, F.G. (Eds.). Hemispheric Specialization and Interaction. In: *The neurosciences: Third study program*. Cambridge: MIT Press, 1974, Pp. 3–89.

Michel, F., & Schott, B. (Eds.). *Les syndromes de disconnexion calleuses chez l'homme*. Lyon: SPCM/Imprimerie J.J., 1975.

Brain Information Service Conference Report #42: D.O. Walter, L. Rogers & J.F. Finzi-Fried (Eds.). *Conference on human brain function*. Los Angeles: UCLA BIS/BRI, 1976.

Corballis, M., & Beale, I.L. *The psychology of left and right*. New York; Halsted, 1976.

Harnad, S.R., Steklis, H.D., & Lancaster, J.B. (Eds.). Origins and Evolution of Language and Speech. *Annals of the New York Academy of Sciences* 280, 1976.

*In preparation*

Kinsbourne, M. (Ed.). *Asymmetrical functions of the brain*. London and New York: Cambridge University Press (1977)

Desmedt, J.E. *Language and hemispheric specialization in man:* Event-related cerebral potentials. Progress in Clinical Neurophysiology Basel: Karger (1977)

Dimond, S. (Ed.). Evolution and Lateralization of the Brain. *Annals of the New York Academy of Sciences (1977)*.

Segalowitz, S.J. and Gruber, F. (Eds.). *Language development and neurological theory. New York: Academic Press, 1977.*

*Herron, J. (Ed.).* The sinistral mind (in preparation).

Bogen, J.E., & Bogen, G.M. *The other side of the brain* (in preparation).

# ACKNOWLEDGMENTS

This volume has grown out of a symposium on lateralization sponsored by the New Jersey Chapter of The Society for Neuroscience at CMDNJ–Rutgers Medical School on|April|19-21,|1975|and|organized|by|S.|H. Not all chapters are by participants in the symposium, and most were prepared subsequently. However the symposium itself was the occasion for the remarkable convergence from all over the country of most of the authors represented in this volume.

*Notably missing from this volume are contributions from the following symposium participants:*

**Roland Puccetti** (*Dalhousie University*), that watchdog, gadfly, and kindred spirit from a more venerable discipline, whose absence from this volume would, in a less fragmented day and age, have surely been unthinkable. He continues to exercise, across interdisciplinary (and other) boundaries, a salutary effect upon the minds of brain scientists by his many provocative writings and by actively participating in events such as this one (see, e.g., Dimond, 1977; Harnad, Steklis, and Lancaster, 1976).

**Marcel Kinsbourne** (*Toronto Hospital for Sick Children*) whose spirit pervades the book, and about whose ideas many of the contributions turn.

**Daniel Gardner** (*Cornell Medical College*) who, appropriately enough, opened this symposium on *asymmetry* with a stimulating discussion of *symmetry* (in the buccal ganglia of *Aplysia*) and who, owing to our indecorous haste to ready this timely volume, could not submit his paper in time (see Bilateral symmetry and interneuronal organization in the buccal ganglia of Aplysia, *Science* 1971, *173*, 550-553 and *Journal of Neurophysiology*, 1977, in press).

**Morris Bender** (*Mount Sinai School of Medicine*), who graciously chaired the symposium and who, out of self-defense, declined to vouchsafe us the elaborate introduction we endeavored to prevail upon him to write.

*Present in the volume but not at the symposium:*

**Kenneth Heilman** (*University of Florida College of Medicine*, with co-author Robert Watson) who was invited but could not attend at the time.

**Michael Morgan** (*University of Cambridge*) who was located much too far for us to have the temerity to invite him to attend out of pocket, as did all the other participants.

**James H. Dewson** (*Stanford University Medical Center*) whose lateralization results did not yet exist at that time.

We are indebted to the NIMH Interdisciplinary Research Training Program of CMDNJ–Rutgers Medical School (Arthur Kling, Director) for helping to support the symposium. Editorial royalties from this volume will be donated to the Society for Neuroscience (N.J. Chapter) for the purpose of encouraging future symposia.

# Introductory Overview

*STEVAN HARNAD AND ROBERT W. DOTY, SR.*

THE LATERALIZATION PROBLEM

In many respects lateralization constitutes a model problem in the neurosciences: It has its subcellular as well as its fine and gross anatomical aspects; it can be approached by means of electrophysiological, and recently also pharmacological, techniques; it has provided a coherent substrate for the study of important comparative and phylogenetic issues in addition to being uniquely amenable to investigation in man, both clinically and by non-invasive psychophysiological techniques; it poses a well defined problem in terms of its genetics and developmental biology, and is eminently suited to research on plasticity of function; it is rich in its behavioral superstrate, both simple and complex, and has ramifications also in the study of perception and language in man. In short, the lateralization problem impinges upon the entire spectrum of brain-behavioral research from the synapse to the sentence.

And yet in several of its manifestations it has also proved to be singularly refractory, at least to innocent approaches. In genetics, next to IQ, laterality probably presents some of the most frustrating problems: so deceptively simple and seemingly well-defined phenotypically, and yet constantly evading straightforward solutions, and complicated by elusive environmental effects.

The anatomical problem is much the same way. Left-right differences appear, even across species, but they are often highly variable, and invariably small, too small to endow with any *prima facie* function. Functional studies too turn out to be dogged with complexities. No lateralized function, language not excepted, has turned out to be an all-or-none affair. Invariably both sides

xvii

of the brain will exhibit it to some degree. And marked variability, together with astonishing plasticity, make lateralization of function almost as intractable as other classical problem of localization.

The question of origins and evolution is also still an open one. Do animals exhibit cerebral dominance, or even handedness? Some studies have found they do, others have found they do not. At any rate, we are certainly far from being able to construct an intelligible phylogenetic series, particularly as our fellow-primates seem to present some of the most ambiguous cases.

Finally, even the uniquely human and tantalizingly tangible aspects of the lateralization problem have often proved false friends. Despite the seemingly clearcut picture some people feel they have of what constitute left hemisphere or right hemisphere "modes", the new non-invasive approaches have failed to produce dramatic insights. At best they have weakly corroborated some of what was already known on the basis of brain damage studies, but they have not bridged the gap between injured and intact brain function.

So why make so much of this "model" problem which produces such muddled results? We feel that, as is the case with most serious branches of inquiry, the hasty, simplistic approaches had first to be exhausted, gotten out of the way, before any real work could begin. We have had our day in which counting the proportion of left handers was going to tell us how laterality originated or developed; or animals were going to be miniature replicas (or antitheses) of ourselves; or morphology was going to stand up and tell us about function; or the brain was going to behave like a static cognitive map; or a few milliseconds of reaction time, a small percentage difference in error scores or an elusive microvolt or two over the scalp would sustain some Janusian fantasy we had secretly harbored.


FUNCTIONAL LATERALIZATION IN NONHUMAN SPECIES

*NEURAL CONTROL OF VOCALIZATION IN SONGBIRDS*

And serious work *has* begun. Who can fail to be impressed by Nottebohm's (Chapter 2, this volume) dramatic discovery of a possible "animal model" for cerebral dominance in the asymmetric control of vocalization in several species of songbird ? His original finding that song is severely disrupted by section of the left but not the right hypoglossus nerve has been extended in this chapter to nuclei higher up along the ipsilateral pathway controlling vocalization, in particular, to the caudal portion of the ventral hyperstriatum in the telencephalon which is dominant on the left and involved in the learning and memory of the "engrams" for song. This model system also exhibits striking counterparts of both adult functional recovery and early hemispheric

equipotentiality as observed in man. Adult canaries recover partially from left (dominant) hyperstriatal lesions, suggesting
that perhaps contralateral inhibition of the minor side has been
removed by the lesion. Early section of the left tracheosyring-
alis nerve can completely reverse dominance such that subsequent
lesions of the left hyperstriatum in the adult have only the effects normally following a lesion of the minor (right) side.

As suggestive as these outcomes are, Nottebohm cautions against
pressing the analogy too far, partly on the grounds of phylogenetic separation, partly because some highly vocal species such as
the parrot are not lateralized while some relatively inarticulate
domestic fowl appear to be, and partly because it is not yet clear
whether the relevant similarity with the human case is sensory or
motor. Nevertheless, the central control of vocalization in songbirds is unquestionably one of the most robust and promising systems yet discovered for the study of mechanisms of lateralization
in the nervous system.

## ASYMMETRY IN INVERTEBRATES

Other powerful models for lateralization are provided by certain invertebrate systems described by Chapple (Chapter 1). Although most invertebrates are symmetrical, the gastropod molluscs
and the decapod crustaceans are prominent exceptions. Of these,
the gastropods, although of considerable neurobiological interest
currently, provide the more complicated case because their asymmetry is due to a 180° torsion of the viscera during development,
entailing several other major secondary changes, including secondary returns to symmetry.

The decapods provide instances of a simpler process of lateralization. The asymmetries, such as the *heterochely* displayed by
the fiddler crab (whose claws differ in form and function on the
two sides) or the rightward coiling of the abdomen of the hermit
crab (due to occupying the shells of asymmetrical gastropods),
are in these crustaceans superimposed upon a prior bilateral symmetry. Hence that critical developmental stage can be examined
when the structures on the left and right first become uncoupled
and the asymmetry appears. This process, as Chapple reminds us,
can also be investigated in the more general context of the development of anterior-posterior and segmental asymmetries. A
further advantage of studying arthropods is provided by their
large, identifiable motoneurons, allowing reliable homologies to
be made, not only between the right and left sides of the nervous
system and from organism to organism, but even from (symmetrical)
species (such as the crayfish) to (asymmetrical) species (such as
the hermit crab).

Heterochely in the fiddler crab begins to appear at 2 months
and provides a number of analogies with higher forms of lateralization, both in terms of the development of its peripheral
morphology and its central nervous control. As with cerebral do-

minance, there is some left-right equipotentiality, reversibility, and structural and functional regenerability. The process of lateralization itself appears to be mediated by differential growth rate on the two sides (cf. Nottebohm, Chapter 2, and Morgan, chapter 11 and below), a functional decoupling at the motoneuron level, and perhaps also contralateral inhibition.

The hermit crab is symmetrical until the last larval stage. Then homologous motoneurons come to innervate a different number of muscle fibres on the right and the left, differ in size, display different tonic firing rates, and become less tightly couple than in symmetric species such as the crayfish. There is also an asymmetry in the number of motoneurons and the neuropil mass on the two sides, possibly due to differential loss of motoneurons and interneurons during development. The primary function of these asymmetries is to coordinate movement of the rightward coiled abdomen. Perhaps in the interplay of this differential modification of flexors and extensors, their excitors and inhibitors, and perhaps some "command" interneurons, there also lie clues to the mechanisms of some of the functional complementarities displayed by vertebrates.


## VISUAL VERSUS AUDITORY EFFECTS IN RHESUS MONKEYS

Not that these higher functional complementarities are not elusive. In an elegant series of studies, Hamilton (Chapter 3) has eliminated a number of hopeful possibilities that rhesus monkeys may exhibit hemispheric dominance for a variety of visual pattern discriminations, either in terms of learning capacity, performance or memory. Even with training concentrated on one hemisphere, as long as at least the anterior commissure or the splenium were intact, no lateralization was observed.

Hamilton argues that earlier reports of positive results may have been due to artifacts such as (1) insufficient over-training (2) differential post-surgical diaschisis with different partial sections (and possibly also asymmetrical sectioning), (3) inconclusive measures of retention, (4) unbalanced experimental designs with inappropriate surgical controls, and (5) pure chance.

Hamilton did however find an initial decrement (probably due to the surgically induced sensory asymmetry) in the performance of the untrained hemisphere of split-chiasm monkeys when first tested following complete commissurotomy. (There was also some conflicting evidence toward a trend in this direction when precommissurotomy training had been with anterior commissure alone or splenium alone intact.) If the commissures do indeed function as Doty (below and Chapter 5) proposes, it is conceivable that in the intact brain such asymmetries may normally be amplified by some such mechanism as contralateral inhibition (discussed above), thus providing a possible basis for functional lateralization after all. It may also be the case that Hamilton's investigations are addressing the wrong sensory modality (see Dewson, Chapter 4 and below), the wrong task (see Stamm *et al.*, Chapter 20 and below) or the wrong primate (see Rubens, Chapter 26 and below) for successfully demonstrating lateralization. However, as far as visual perception and memory are concerned, the *prima facie* counterparts of human lateralization have certainly been decisively eliminated by this work.

Audition seems to have faired somewhat better. In a preliminary report, to be interpreted cautiously because based on only six monkeys, Dewson (Chapter 4) has shown that removal of the superior temporal gyrus (Brodmann's area 22, construed by the author as the rhesus homologue of Wernicke's area) results in a lasting deficit on a delayed auditory-visual match-to-sample task when the lesion is on the left side, but not when it is on the right. If this outcome proves to be reliable, it focusses attention upon the auditory modality (as also suggested by Nottebohm's work, Chapter 2 and above) as well as the importance of asymmetries in the temporal regions (Rubens, Chapter 26 and below) and perhaps also tasks involving delayed responding (Stamm *et al.*, Chapter 20 and below).

## *SUMMARY*

The research on functional lateralization in nonhuman species may be summarized as having yielded a number of highly suggestive models in species relatively distant from man, such as crustaceans and songbirds, but as becoming increasingly problematic with phylogenetic proximity, with nonhuman primates presenting some of the most equivocal cases. It also appears that presently the likelihood of finding robust homologues and precursors of cerebral dominance in monkeys is greater in the auditory than the visual modality.

THE NEOCORTICAL COMMISSURES AND INTERHEMISPHERIC RELATIONS

*THE UNILATERAL ENGRAM*

Aside from the need for animal models embodying some of the properties of functional asymmetry, the role of the interhemispheric commissures requires elucidation. According to the model of Doty (Doty & Overman, Chapter 5) the anterior commissure and the splenium of the corpus callosum differ with respect to their functions in interhemispheric transfer.

Doty and co-workers devised a two-stage commissurotomy technique whereby one of these commissures could be sectioned and the other ensnared for instant sectioning after the macaque had learned a response to direct unilateral stimulation of the striate cortex. It was found that with either commissure intact during the unilateral training the animals could perform the re-

sponse to initial stimulation of the untrained side, indicating
that either commissure alone could subserve interhemispheric
transfer in this task.  However, when the final stage of the
sectioning was performed, the outcome differed depending upon
which commissure had been intact during training: if the anterior
commissure, then the animal continued to respond to stimulation on
either side; if the splenium, then the animal responded only on
the trained side.

Doty concluded that the anterior commissure effects interhemispheric transfer by establishing a memory for the learning in
both hemispheres, a *bilateral engram,* whereas the splenium effects interhemispheric transfer by establishing a *unilateral engram* (ipsilateral to the side of stimulation) and provides commissural *access* to the other side.  Hence, with complete transection, access is lost.

Since these results directly contradict those of Hamilton
(above, and Chapter 3) both authors attempt to account for the
discrepancies, and to Hamilton's list (above), Doty and Overman
add several factors unique to direct striatal stimulation, such
as (6) absence of denervation effects from chiasm-sectioning, (7)
difference in learning paradigms and (8) by-passing subcortical
pathways; all are resolvable experimentally.  Note also that
only the sensory component of the learning was found to lateralize; the response could be executed by either hemisphere.

The role of the splenium in providing access to contralateral
information is further supported by a study in which the optic
tract was removed on one side and the amygdala on the other. With
vision and the interpretation of fear-provoking visual stimuli
thus lateralized to separate hemispheres, commissural involvement
was necessary to mediate fear responses.  With splenium alone
intact, macaques continued to show normal fear responses to visual
stimuli, but as soon as the transection was completed there was
indifference to visual threat, just as with a bilateral amygdalectomy, indicating that either the splenium had provided access
to visual input for "fear-processing", or vice versa.

The role of the anterior commissure in interhemispheric transfer was further examined by subjecting it to tetanic stimulation.
It was found that this could interfere with learning and prevent
the occurence of learned responses (to striatal stimulation).
Controls for siezure activity and visual effects supported the
interpretation that the tetanization blocked access to memory
rather than generating competing sensory or motor activity.

Although successful in elucidating some of the interhemispheric
mechanisms of lateralization, Doty and Overman have confirmed the
difficulty in finding evidence for hemispheric specialization in
monkeys.  In a test for cerebral dominance in maze-learning, *prima
facie* a visuo-spatial task, results were inconclusive, in part
because monkeys differed in "cognitive style", with some using a
visual strategy and others a proprioceptive strategy in negotiating the maze.

*INFERIOR TEMPORAL CORTEX AND INTERHEMISPHERIC TRANSFER*

Neurons in the inferior temporal cortex (ITC) are prominent for their very large visual receptive fields, which often extend into both half-fields of both eyes. This means that a particular ITC cell will respond similarly to a particular stimulus irrespective of the latter's retinal location within its field. Gross and Mishkin (Chapter 7) propose the bold hypothesis that it is this multiple convergence from large parts of the retina upon ITC neurons which is the basis of *stimulus equivalence across retinal translation* (i.e. why things look the same no matter where they appear in the visual field) and, as a special case, *interhemispheric equivalence* (i.e. why things look the same no matter which hemisphere "sees" them: See Franz, 1933).

With commissures and chiasm intact, binocular equivalence for stimuli on corresponding retinal loci (i.e. why things look the same no matter which eye sees them) is due to binocular convergence upon cells in the striate cortex. These striate fields are, however, still strictly segregated hemispherically in terms of the hemiretinae (i.e. each side receives only contralateral field input see Springer, Chapter 18 and below). Gross and Mishkin point out that further downstream two-thirds of the neurons in ITC have binocular and bi-hemiretinal receptive fields, half receiving their ipsilateral fields via the splenium, and half via both the splenium and the anterior commissure. Section of these commissures (and the optic chiasm) eliminates interhemispheric transfer of visual engrams (as discussed above), a process which is likewise severely disrupted by bilateral ablation of ITC together with chiasm section (but not by ITC ablation alone). The authors therefore conclude that it is the convergence on single neurons in ITC which mediates interhemispheric transfer, a special case of trans-retinal transfer.

Gross and Mishkin's model has the especial virtue of assimilating the particular problem of interhemispheric relations to one of the more general problems of neuroscience, namely the integrative and unifying aspect of higher nervous function. One easily falls prey to split-brain thinking, as if only *two* functions existed to be accounted for, whereas in fact there are a multitude. Hierarchical convergence on single cells appears to be one of the ways the nervous system approaches the problem of unification, and it appears that bihemispheric unification may partake of the same principle.

*NEONATAL COMMISSUROTOMY IN KITTENS*

Both Hamilton (Chapter 3) and Sechzer *et al.* (Chapter 6), the former working with monkeys and the latter with cats, reaffirm that adult split-brain animals learn visual pattern discriminations with much greater difficulty than do normal animals. Given the importance then of the neocortical commissures, as demonstrated in these and the foregoing studies, what consequences are to be expected from early deconnection? The celebrated "early

plasticity" of the brain, whereby early lesions are not as dele-
terious as late ones, would lead one to expect that the effects
of early commissurotomy would be milder than those of the adult
operation, and indeed the remarkable absence of deconnection symptoms in individuals with congenital agenesis of the corpus callosum would tend to support this. However more recent work on
early plasticity has suggested that after early lesions *early*
comparisons with normal performance may not be the relevant ones;
some deficits of early injury may only emerge later, when the
structure or function involved has reached its maturity (Goldman,
1974). Since it is known that mammalian forebrain commissures are
unmyelinated at birth (and in man this myelination is not complete
until the age of 10 years) there are grounds for being unsure what
outcome to expect from early commissurotomy.

The actual outcome in neonatal split-brain kittens as reported
by Sechzer et al. (chapter 6) is very much like the "minimal
brain damage" (MBD) syndrome in children: hyperactivity, learning
and memory disorders and "paradoxical" response to amphetamine
(i.e. calming and improvement, instead of the over-activation
caused by amphetamine in normals). The authors do not propose
that MBD is ordinarily due to callosal damage, but they do point
out that neonatal commissurotomy seems to mimic the disorder,
whether due to neuronal loss, neurotransmitter changes, interruption of specific pathways or disruption of interhemispheric relations, and recommend further research. The topic is further dealt
with by Glick et al. in Chapter 13 and below.


SUBCORTICAL LATERALIZATION

In Chapter 7, Gross and Mishkin were at pains to eliminate the
possibility that the pulvinar (which projects to posterior parietal and temporal cortex and receives fibres from medial and lateral geniculate bodies, superior colliculus and occipital cortex)
was involved in the visual responsiveness of ITC (it was not). In
Chapter 8 Riklan and Cooper examine the involvement of the pulvinar and the ventrolateral nucleus of the thalamus (which receives fibres from the dentate nucleus of the cerebellum as well
as from globus pallidus and substantia nigra, and has reciprocal
somatotopically organized connections with the precentral motor
regions, Area 4 and perhaps 6) in cognitive lateralization.

The authors find that the human thalamus is indeed lateralized,
as determined by deficits on verbal and nonverbal psychometric
tests following unilateral surgery for Parkinsonism, but apparently to a considerably lesser degree than the cerebral cortex.
The most reliable outcome was a more pronounced (but usually
transient) postsurgical decrement in verbal fluency following
left-sided ventrolateral lesions, and to a lesser extent also
left pulvinar lesions. The authors conclude that although there
is evidence for asymmetric effects from thalamic surgery, the
functions of the thalamus seem to be more bilaterally represented,

with differences rather quantitative than qualitative. They suggest that even cortical asymmetries may be better viewed as matters of degree.


*SUMMARY*

The chapters on interhemispheric relations provide evidence that the commissures are involved in providing access to unilateral engrams and allowing for bilateral engrams, with the splenium of the corpus callosum perhaps functioning more along the former lines and the anterior commissure along the latter. Unilateral engrams would obviously have the advantage of doubling storage capacity but conflicting outcomes due to procedural differences prevent the rejection of the possibility that monkeys do *not* form unilateral engrams as long as either commissure is intact.

The basis of interhemispheric transfer in vision may be convergence upon single neurons in inferior temporal cortex which receive input from the visual half-fields of both hemispheres, the ipsilateral one via the splenium and anterior commissure. This equivalence of information from the hemiretinae may be a special case of equivalence of information across all regions of the retina. The mechanism provides a salutary reminder also that the brain functions to unify and integrate experience, not to split it.

Early commissurotomy in kittens gives rise to a condition which resembles the "minimal brain damage syndrome" in children. It is not known, however, to what degree this outcome is specific to hemispheric or commissural dysfunction rather than more general effects of early damage.

Psychometric evaluation of patients after unilateral thalamic surgery reveals evidence of some functional asymmetry in the ventrolateral nucleus and palvinar but also of considerably more bilaterality than in the cortex.


INHERITANCE AND DEVELOPMENT OF LATERALITY

*PAW PREFERENCES IN MICE*

Sechzer et al's neonatal commissurotomy studies (Chapter 6) point to the issue of the development of left-right differences and the relative role of constitutional and experimental factors. The principal questions are: (1) Do stable asymmetric phenotypes exist? With respect to behavioral lateralities this is a crucial question, typified by the problem of handedness. (2) To what extent is laterality inherited and to what extent acquired? (3) If inherited, *how* is it inherited?

The answers to these questions depend partly upon the organism one chooses to investigate. Collins (Chapter 9) has found that

mice do exhibit stable paw preferences (for obtaining food from a
narrow cylinder) but that there are marked individual differences
even among highly inbred  strains, indicating that the variation
is not genetic.  He found also that females were more lateralized
than males, i.e. they exhibited stronger paw preferences.

When the environment was biased to favor one side (by posi-
tioning the cylinder asymmetrically) Collins found that he could
influence the paw preference distribution, but that some mice
consistently resisted the bias, indicating that their prior
(nongenetic) handedness had been quite stable and persistent.  Females tended in general to resist the environmental bias more,
and hence under these conditions males displayed stronger lateralization.

Finally, Collins found that in a subsequent environment with
a bias opposite to the prior one, some mice acquiesced to the
second bias who had resisted the first.  Moreover, earlier
preferences were predictive of whether or not a bias would be
resisted.  Collins  concludes from this evidence that the mice
must have come to the experiment with "native" paw preferences,
albeit nongenetic ones, and, since the only genetic variation was
the male-female difference in *degree* of lateralization, that this
is the only aspect of asymmetry which is subject to genetic variation: the initial *direction* of the asymmetry is due to some
random process which is then coupled with genetic variation in
the degree of asymmetry such that males are less lateralized than
females but more adaptable to an asymmetrical environment.


*HANDEDNESS IN MONKEYS*

It is not clear to what extent Collins' results can be generalized to other species (although he does propose a model which
applies to man) and even to other tasks.  Warren (Chapter 10)
finds that rhesus monkeys tested on a variety of manipulation
tasks may exhibit some relatively stable hand preferences, but
that these are task-specific, and their directions may differ
from task to task.  Unlike Collins, Warren finds that monkeys
come to the experiment with highly unstable initial preferences
which are *not* predictive  of later laterality.  What *is* predictive is prior experience: with repeated practice on a particular
type of task, stable hand preferences develop which tend to generalize to other tasks of the same type.

Warren has also extended Hamilton's (Chapter 3) negative findings regarding cerebral dominance for pattern discrimination
learning, showing that the effects of unilateral temporal or frontal lesions do not differ for surgery ipsilateral of contralateral to the preferred hand.

## ORIGINS AND ONTOGENY OF ASYMMETRY

From a panoramic survey of the ontogeny and heritability of asymmetry, Morgan (Chapter 11) comes to the surprising conclusion that asymmetry is not transmitted genetically but via an inherent asymmetry in the oocyte which favors the left side in terms of developmental rate. He also concurs with Collins that only the degree and not the direction of asymmetry is genetically encoded.

Morgan makes his claims in rather apodictic terms (that *all* organisms have a left-sided developmental advantage and that symmetry *cannot* be encoded in the genome) which, despite the wealth of stimulating and suggestive evidence he adduces on asymmetries in a variety of organs and organisms, renders him vulnerable to counterexamples, and the excellent little essay by Levy (Chapter 12) follows hard on his heels proferring just those. However it does not take a great deal to recast Morgan's argument in more relative terms, and then this lively exchange becomes a highly instructive dialectical excursion through the world of asymmetries, their origins and development.

## SUMMARY

The research on laterality in nonhuman species suggests that there does not exist a reliable counterpart of human handedness. Genetically uniform inbred mice vary in terms of stable paw preferences which cannot be genetic and do not appear to be environmental. Sex differences in the strength of paw preferences suggest that in mice only the degree of lateralization is genetic while its direction is determined randomly.

In monkeys handedness varies in direction from task to task and stable preferences within a task-type are evidently due to repeated practice. There is no difference between the effects of unilateral lesions in the hemisphere ipsilateral or contralateral to the preferred paw.

Much evidence suggests that morphological asymmetries occurring in a variety of species tend to favor the left side in terms of developmental rate and degree of differentiation. There is also evidence that the direction of many asymmetries is determined with reference to developmentally earlier asymmetries, possibly *ab ovo,* with genes only modulating the asymmetry in terms of degree. The existence of some counter-examples to each of these trends, however, speaks against their being universal ones.

## TURNING TENDENCIES

*Turning tendencies* (also called "versive tendencies", "rotatory bias" and "spatial orientation bias") are a variety of motor asymmetry wherein the organism turns all or part of its body toward one side of space. This phenomenon is one of the principal unifying themes of the present volume. Nor is it restricted to the section bearing its name (Part IV): It is also discussed in invertebrates by Chapple (Chapter 1), in monkeys by Warren (Chapter 10) and Stamm *et al.* (Chapter 20), and in man by Anderson (Chapter 21); in its sensory aspect, where it is manifested as an attentional asymmetry, with relative neglect of one side of space and heightened attention to the other, it reappears in all three chapters of the section following the present one (Part V, *Asymmetries in Attention and Perception*).

The reason for the importance of turning tendencies is that they appear to be a phylogenetically old and pervasive lateral synergism with which many other asymmetries of interest may be *coupled*. This means that other lateralized nervous activities may trigger turning (usually contraversive) and conversely (sic), turning may facilitate other asymmetric activities. Moreover the mechanisms underlying gross left-right rotatory synergisms may be revealing models for how the brain coordinates more finely modulated left-right motor activity.

## NEUROPHARMACOLOGICAL BASIS OF ROTATION IN RATS

The thorough and highly-original work of Glick and his co-workers (Chapter 13) represents the deepest and most direct approach to this phenomenon. Their research issues from the often-noted observation that many kinds of unilateral lesions tend to be accompanied by versive effects (usually ipsiversive), and in particular that in rats unilateral lesions in the nigro-striatal region, whose pharmacology is relatively well-known, result in marked ipsiversive rotation which is potentiated by amphetamine. Glick et al. found that normal unlesioned rats also rotated with large doses of amphetamine.

Now the pathological lesion-induced rotation was known to have been caused by depletion of striatal dopamine on the lesioned side, so these investigators sought, and found, underlying the rotation phenomenon in normal rats, a small naturally-occurring asymmetry in dopamine content between the striata on the two sides. Amphetamine enhanced the dopamine asymmetry and rats rotated toward the side with the lower dopamine content. With other pharmacological agents Glick et al were able to unearth what appears to be a delicate interplay of pre- and post-synaptic asymmetries involving more than one neurotransmitter system. Their finding that section of the intercaudate pathway in the ventral callosum also potentiates the dopamine asymmetry suggests that the commissure may be involved in regulating neurotransmitter asymmetries.

The turning tendencies were found to be stable across time and to be in the same direction as the rats' side-preferences in mazes and in bar-pressing (where there was a choice between a bar on the left and the right); the direction was not directly related to paw preference (however see below), At high levels, unilateral electrical stimulation of the caudate nucleus produced contraversive turning, and at low levels reversed side preferences while applied to the "non-dominant" (lower dopamine/ipsiversive turning) side. The effects of unilateral caudate lesions depended upon the side, with twice as much rotation after a lesion on the "nondominant" side.

Strength of side-preference (and hence degree of striatal asymmetry) was also found to be related to the level of proficiency on various operant tasks and interacted with paw preference. Rats with moderately strong side-preference concordant in direction with stable paw preferences were the best overall performers; rats with an absence of striatal symmetry were the worst. The authors conjectured about the possible mechanisms of the "minimal brain damage syndrome" (see Sechzer et al., Chapter 6 and above) in terms of amphetamine inducing a more optimal degree of striatal asymmetry.

It is hardly necessary to point out all the salient respects in which this important and provocative work impinges upon the problem of lateralization. The chapter ought to be read closely by any serious student of the subject.

## ORIENTATION BIAS IN HUMAN INFANTS

Unlike in rats, in which they occur with equal frequency toward the left or the right in the population, turning biases in man are overwhelmingly toward the right from birth. Turkewitz (Chapter 14) has shown that most infants lie in an asymmetrical *posture,* with their heads turned toward the right. They also exhibit asymmetry in *responsiveness* to auditory, visual and tactile stimuli: they make more reliable responses to stimuli on the right, and are more likely to orient and to turn their eyes toward stimulation in that direction.

Turkewitz has shown that the postural asymmetry, which necessarily induces asymmetric adaptation and pre-stimulation of the ears, eyes and cheeks while the child is supine, is thereby partially responsible for the asymmetry in responsiveness. The asymmetry in muscle tonus due to the posture also makes a contribution. But that there is still an independent factor involved in the asymmetric responsiveness is demonstrated by the fact that with head position and pre-stimulation controlled, there is still an asymmetry in responsiveness.

So postural asymmetry interacts with at least one prior asymmetry in mediating responsiveness asymmetry. Turkewitz also suggests that although postural and responsiveness asymmetry are coupled early in development, they may become more independent later on.

Turkewitz reports that postural asymmetry is weaker in neonates, but rapidly strengthens by positive feedback from experience. Its experiential origins, if such they are, are not known, although the possibility that they are due to Left-Occipital-Anterior presentation at birth has been eliminated. Turkewitz holds with nongenetic factors and suggests that the cause may be intrauterine events; however structural asymmetry of the brain (Rubens, Chapter 26, and below) and other organs (Morgan, Chapter 11, and above) at birth provide alternative explanations.

## CORRELATES OF OCULOVERSIVE ASYMMETRIES IN MAN

As mentioned earlier, a good deal of the interest in turning tendencies derives from the possibility that they may be coupled with other lateralization variables. Glick and co-workers have shown that performance in rats may depend upon an interaction between side-preference and paw preference. Turkewitz has shown that postural and responsiveness asymmetries are coupled early in ontogeny, but he suggests that these may become decoupled later. Gur and Gur (Chapter 15) now take up this problem in adults. Their dependent variable is *conjugate lateral eye movement,* a versive response system which is a part of the larger eye-head-body turning synergism. This oculoversive asymmetry is thought to be coupled with asymmetric activation of the cerebral hemispheres in information processing, with the direction of the eye movement being *toward the side of space opposite the more active hemisphere* (contraversive turning: see Anderson, Chapter 21 and below).

The oculoversive asymmetry is usually measured while a subject is reflecting upon the answer to a question which has just been posed. Gur & Gur have resolved some earlier conflicts in the literature by showing that under face-to-face conditions (which presumably entail more anxiety) the measure is sensitive to relatively stable individual biases in cognitive style, and hence, by inference, the subject's hemisphere biases; when the questions are instead posed from behind the subject, the measure tends to co-vary with the nature of the question: rightward for verbal and leftward for nonverbal. Subjects were also found to perform better on those questions for which, according to the eye-movement measure, they had "used" the optimal hemisphere.

Both the "trait" and the "state" variable turned out to be reflected in classroom seating preferences. "Left-movers" reported preferring to sit on the right and "right-movers" on the left. This was superimposed upon a tendency to report preferring to sit on the left for "hard" science subjects and on the right for "soft" arts subjects. Oculoversive bias also correlated with a number of personality variables and yielded an interesting pattern of interactions with handedness, eye-dominance and sex differences.

Clearly in this, their evolutionarily highest manifestation, these ancient turning tendencies are still a valuable resource for understanding lateralization.

*SUMMARY*

Turning tendencies pervade phylogeny. Starting as apparently random, non-functional rotatory asymmetries in invertebrates, they become coupled to progressively more elaborate lateralizations in mammals. In rats their underlying mechanism is a complex network of pre- and post-synaptic asymmetries in dopamine and other neurotransmitter systems in the basal ganglia. These asymmetries appear to be regulated by an inter-caudate pathway in the ventral callosum. They are potentiated by amphetamine and callosal section and interact differentially with unilateral lesions. Behaviorally, they underly spatial preferences and interact with paw preference in influencing learning proficiency.

In human infants turning tendencies are manifested as a postural bias and a multimodal asymmetry in responsiveness to stimulation on the two sides. In adults oculoversive asymmetries are coupled with lateralized hemispheric activity and are correlated with a number of cognitive and personality traits.

## ASYMMETRIES IN ATTENTION AND PERCEPTION

*UNILATERAL NEGLECT*

Neglect is the other side of the orientation bias phenomenon: if one turns *toward* one side of space, one inevitably turns *away from* the other. The result is consequently an asymmetric *sensory* as well as a motor effect, as already noted in the interaction of the postural and responsiveness asymmetry in the findings of Turkewitz (Chapter 14 and above). Glick et al. (Chapter 13 and above) also reported neglect of the contralateral side of space after unilateral dopamine depletion. By extension one might suppose that just as "subliminal" ipsiversive rotation was in normal rats manifested as spatial orientation bias, "subliminal" neglect may also exist, in the form of relative inattention to contralateral space.

Heilman and Watson (Chapter 16) describe the classical clinical picture of unilateral neglect. The patient, in the absence of a primary sensory deficit (an important qualification), appears to be totally unaware of events occurring on one side of space (usually the side opposite his injury). The condition may be restricted to one sense modality, but in the full syndrome, all senses are affected. Recovery passes through two stages: (1) *allesthesia*, when the patient begins to respond to stimuli on the neglected side, but as if they were occurring on the good side, and (2) *simultaneous extinction*, when there is already some appropriate responding to stimuli on the weak side except if there is homologous bilateral input, in which case only the stimulation on the good side is noticed.

There are several hypotheses about unilateral neglect. Some

STEVAN HARNAD AND ROBERT W. DOTY, SR.

feel it is primarily a *higher-order sensory asymmetry,* others
that it is due to *unilateral failure in reciprocal interhemispheric inhibition,* disinhibiting the intact side so it now pre-
dominates. Heilman and Watson propose instead that it is a *unilateral deficit in the orienting response* involving the interruption of a "cortico-limbic-reticular loop which results in a
lack of arousal on one side. Evidence consists of the induction
of multimodal neglect by unilateral lesions in the regions involved in the loop, including the mesencephalic reticular formation, the lateral hypothalamus, the cingulate gyrus, the frontal
arcuate gyrus and the inferior parietal lobule (as well as primary and secondary sensory regions).

Not only the "loop" structures produce neglect, of course: so
do unilateral lesions in the basal ganglia (as already mentioned),
the superior colliculus, and probably a number of other structures.
However the authors concentrate their attention on the "loop" as
one of possibly several parallel systems involved.

Further evidence for an arousal rather than a sensory deficit
comes from unilateral EEG slowing on the lesioned side, as well
as unilateral changes in the late (attentional) but not the early
(sensory) components of the averaged evoked potential (see Parts
VI and VII and below).

It is not clear whether the lesioned side is under-responsive
or the intact side is over-responsive in neglect. Allesthesia
and extinction support the latter view; but the former is supported by evidence of inferior performance on the unlesioned side
relative to controls, and the induction by bilateral lesions of
*akinetic mutism,* a profound bilateral neglect. The interhemispheric inhibition hypothesis is weakened by the fact that
unilateral neglect fails to be abolished by commissorotomy.

Finally, there is some evidence that in man neglect is more
likely to occur with right than with left hemisphere lesions,
although this may be confounded by the masking effects of aphasia
when injury is on the left. If there is a hemispheric asymmetry
in susceptibility to neglect, one possible explanation would be
that Turkewitz' (Chapter 14) endogenous rightward turning bias
perseveres subliminally into adult life and lesion effects are
analogous to Glick *et al.'s* results with the caudate: a more
profound neglect effect with injury to the nondominant side.

*AUDITORY AND VISUAL ASYMMETRIES IN MAN*

And apparently as already shown by Gur and Gur (Chapter 15 and
above), asymmetries in attention and responsiveness *do* persevere
into adulthood, although they may become more labile as a function
of individual cognitive styles. But Gur and Gur have also shown
that turning tendencies can be governed by the particular information processing demands of a task. Underlying this is the
*functional* asymmetry of the cerebral hemispheres, with the left

specialized for activities involving language and the right specialized for nonverbal activities such as visuospatial perception and auditory pattern perception. The principal techniques for investigating this functional asymmetry in normal, neurologically intact humans involve capitalizing upon the partial left-right separation of input in the various sensory modalities.

In vision, information from the left and right hemiretinae is separate until the level of the striate cortex, and even at the inferior temporal level contralateral field information must arrive via the commissures (see Gross and Mishkin, Chapter 7 and above), which may involve some slowing and reduction of information.

The *tachistoscopic hemifield* research takes advantage of this partial separation by presenting stimuli very briefly in the right or left visual fields, before eye movements can re-center them. Performance in the two fields is then compared in terms of error scores or reaction time. The independent variable can be either the nature of the stimulus (e.g. verbal or nonverbal) or the nature of the task. Right-left presentations may be separate or simultaneous, the latter taking advantage of any subliminal "extinction" (see above) which may exist in the normal visual system. The tachistoscopic paradigm is unfortunately complicated by left-right scanning tendencies derived from reading, by the constraints of very brief exposure, by the problem of eye movements and by the fact that despite the partial separation there is nevertheless substantial cross-integration of the two hemispheric half-fields. New techniques involving restricting images to one half-field for more extended periods by means of corneal diffraction or half-opaque contact lenses also exist, but they are, of course, still further "disadvantaged" by the intergrative functions of the intact brain (see Gross and Mishkin, Chapter 7 and above.) and are hence more useful for studying split-brain patients. For first such studies in normals see Franz, 1933.

In audition left-right separation does not exist beyond the cochlear nucleus as all nuclei on both sides receive projections from both the ipsilateral and the contralateral ear; however under conditions of binaural competition there does appear to be a relative "extinction" of the ipsilateral input (by a mechanism which is not yet fully understood: see Berlin, Chapter 17 and below). *Dichotic listening* takes advantage of this by presenting competing material to both ears. Performance of the left and right ears is then compared, with independent and dependent variables as in the visual studies except that here the constraints are those of simultaneous competing presentation, the confounding effects of attentional strategies, and uncertainties in the degree of ipsilateral extinction.

Berlin (Chapter 17) has subjected dichotic listening to unusually close and thorough scrutiny. The dichotic "right ear advantage" is the well-verified superior identification of consonant-vowel (CV) pairs from the right ear (left hemisphere) in dichotic listening. While other investigators have rushed to use the *magnitude* of this advantage as if it were a stable individual difference parameter in order to study the development of lateralization and differences in "degree of lateralization" between groups, Berlin has demonstrated that the magnitude variable is neither stable in individuals nor a reliable developmental or population parameter. Individuals' scores vary radically, and the real factor underlying changes with age is the *total number of correct identifications from both ears,* i.e. the total dichotic channel capacity, which increases with age and is depressed in certain pathological populations.

No one had previously made much of the fact that *both* ears, even the superior right ear, always perform worse under dichotic than under monaural conditions except when *one* of the competing input materials is of a different *type* (e.g. music), in which case the performance of both ears approaches monaural levels. Hence somewhere in the nervous system some sort of *interference* between *acoustically similar* inputs is responsible for the reduction of channel capacity and the depression of each ear's performance. Berlin has accordingly used the degree of dichotic interference with CV stimuli to assess the degree to which acoustic stimuli resemble speech (to the brain) and hence to isolate speech-specific acoustic properties. He has also examined a number of acoustic parameters which can alter the relative balance of the ear asymmetry, such as intensity, frequency, signal/noise ratio and time-lag. Having isolated these acoustic properties, Berlin proposes that auditory input must pass at least one *gate* somewhere in the nervous system where contralateral and ipsilateral information interfere with one another whenever they share (the neural equivalents of) these properties, in which case the ipsilateral information is suppressed.

It remains only to determine the locus of the "gate". One locus has been thought to be the auditory processing region of the temporal lobe. Patients with unilateral temporal lobectomy must rely entirely upon the ipsilateral projections of the ear opposite the injury. Under dichotic conditions, the performance of this weak ear is profoundly depressed, indicating great ipsilateral suppression. Hemispherectomy heightens the effect, with the strong ear performing as well as monaurally. If this is normally what happens on *both* sides, then commissural input may be the source of the competing material from each hemisphere's ipsilateral ear in dichotic listening.

In a patient with a unilateral lesion in the medial geniculate nucleus of the thalamus, dichotic symptoms mimicked effects intermediate between temporal lobectomy and hemispherectomy. Since units which suppress competing ipsilateral information and pass contralateral information have been found in the medial geniculate of the cat, Berlin concludes that this may be the locus of ipsilateral suppression in man as well, and that if other known temporal lobe and thalamic asymmetries (see Riklan and Cooper,

Chapter 8 and above, and Rubens, Chapter 26 and below) extend to
this nucleus, it may also be a substrate of the right ear
advantage.

Springer (Chapter 18) reviews the nature of functional hemispheric asymmetries as investigated in dichotic listening and
tachistoscopic half-field studies in normals and split-brain
patients. She points out more recent emphases upon asymmetries
in the nature of the *processing* rather than the nature of the
input. The former can be influenced by instructions alone. For
example, alphabetic letters normally exhibit a right hemifield
(left hemisphere) advantage. If subjects are instructed to make
a discrimination on the basis of the *name* of the letters, there
is the usual right field advantage; however if they are instructed to discriminate in terms of shape, a left field advantage is
obtained. (Stimulus characteristics are of course still critical
in some cases, as demonstrated by Berlin above, and perhaps
moreso in the auditory than the visual modality.) Failure to control for information processing strategies and cognitive style
options of this sort may lead to conflicting or null results. The
alternatives appear to be either to impose the strategy or to
select tasks which are sufficiently difficult so only one strategy is optimal.

In both visual and auditory paradigms a null result in terms of
error scores may still involve an asymmetry in terms of reaction
time, suggesting that the latter is the more sensitive measure.
Springer has employed this measure with dichotic listening in
order to gather more evidence on the important question of whether
interhemispheric differences are qualitative or quantitative (see
Riklan and Cooper, Chapter 8 and above); i.e. are there functions
which only one hemisphere is able to perform, or is it just that
one is relatively more proficient at some functions than the other?

Split-brain studies indicate that for most functions interhemispheric differences are only a matter of degree, with each hemisphere capable of performing to some extent. This evidence is
compromised by the fact that (1) recovery and reorganization may
be expected to have occurred after surgery in the split-brain
patients, rendering the separated hemispheres less representative
of normal function, (2) the absence of the commissures themselves
is a pathological factor whose perturbing effect on outcomes is
hard to assess, and (3) the patients' epileptic history is a further pathological factor which may have altered their hemispheric
function. On the other hand, with normal intact subjects the
limitations of the perceptual asymmetry techniques and the limited separation of hemispheric pathways prevent null results from
being convincing either. Hence the recourse to the more sensitive
reaction time measure.

Springer used a dichotic CV test in which the task was to
signal by means of either a manual or a verbal response whether
a target CV had occurred in either ear. She first showed that
there was a right ear advantage whether the right or the left

hand was used. Then she reasoned that if the asymmetry in speech perception is only quantitative, with speech successfully processed, but less efficiently, in the right hemisphere, then reaction time to targets in the left ear should be longer with a verbal than a right-hand manual response because the verbal output (which *is, qualitatively, only* a left hemisphere function) would require an extra increment of transfer time. Since there was no such difference, she reasoned that only the left hemisphere could process the input.

Finally, Springer showed that the dichotic listening performance of monozygotic twins is more similar than that of dizygotic twins, indicating a genetic component in lateralization (although on Berlin's interpretation, this could be a channel-capacity rather than a lateralization effect).

*SUMMARY*

Unilateral lesions in any of a number of structures in a "cortico-limbic reticular loop" can produce a unilateral deficit in orienting and arousal in which there is neglect of all stimulation from one side. In some respects, this condition is the *ab*versive counterpart of *ad*versive turning tendencies. The right hemisphere may be more susceptible.

Hemiattentional effects may interact with functional hemispheric asymmetries to produce left-right performance differences in perceptual lateralization experiments which capitalize on the partial separation of hemispheric information in normal subjects.

The magnitude of the "right ear advantage" in dichotic listening is not a measure of degree of lateralization but of channel capacity, which changes with age and pathology. Dichotic competition depresses the performance of *both* ears whenever the input stimuli are similar, and is hence an indication of the degree to which stimuli share speech-like acoustic properties. The locus of this interference, which results in the suppression of ipsilateral information by similar contralateral information, may be the medial geniculate body.

Left-right differences in perception occur not only with different kinds of stimuli, but also with different processing strategies for the same stimuli. Reaction times are more sensitive measures than error scores; they can be used to infer the hemispheric locus of processing in assessing whether functional asymmetries are qualitative or quantitative.

## SURFACE ELECTROCORTICAL INDICATORS OF LATERALIZATION

*METHODOLOGICAL SURVEY AND CRITIQUE*

Donchin *et al.* (Chapter 19) provide an exhaustive and penetrating methodological survey and critique of the recent proliferation of studies which have attempted to use surface electrocortical measures as indicators of laterality during various kinds of activities. The authors review all the existing research on EEG (electoencephalogram) and ERP (averaged event-related potential) asymmetries. This work includes frequency and amplitude analyses of the ongoing EEG, and studies of the *exogenous* or sensory components of the ERP (auditory, visual and somatosensory evoked potentials) as well as the slow, later *endogenous* ERP components which are thought to be sensitive to the information processing demands of the task. Among the latter are the Readiness Potential, which appears in anticipation of a motor response, and the Contingent Negative Variation (CNV) which appears in anticipation of a stimulus which signals an event (usually a response to be performed).

Donchin *et al.*'s survey concludes that although the neurophysiology of the surface electrocortical activity is not yet known, and although interhemispheric differences will be found to be minute, the techniques are promising as means of investigating hemispheric lateralization. The existing literature however is inconsistent, confusing and fraught with methodological inadequacies such as the following:

(1) Insensitive and inadequate experimental designs (insufficient resolving power for detection of minute differences, "type II" statistical errors, artifacts, pooled data instead of repeated-measures/within-group designs, failure to provide non-lateralized control tasks or to demonstrate "double dissociation" between the effects of left and right hemisphere tasks, etc.).

(2) Experimental tasks which have not been validated as addressing lateralized functions or are not sufficiently demanding and unambiguous to display asymmetries (cf. Springer, Chapter 18 and above).

(3) Failure to take subject individual differences into account (e.g. degree of handedness, cognitive style, etc.).

(4) Inappropriate choice of electrocortical dependent variables (e.g. wrong frequency band, too gross a measure, faulty transformations, etc.).

(5) Inadequate measuring techniques (faulty electrode and reference placement, insufficient loci, failure to decompose multivariate components, etc.).

(6) Incorrect quantification and data analysis (spurious multiple univariate comparisons, grand averaging, failure to estimate error variance, etc.).

The authors make very specific proposals for remedying these deficiencies. This material is highly recommended for researchers with a serious interest in studying lateralization by surface electrocortical means.


I:  EVENT-RELATED POTENTIALS (ERPS)

*ASYMMETRIES DURING HAND-USE AND STIMULUS-MATCHING IN MAN*

Donchin *et al.*'s own data (Chapter 19) corroborate the complexity and elusiveness of scalp electrocortical asymmetries, for even their own fastidious approach yields only modest returns. They find that the pre-motor Readiness Potential (RP) is greater over the hemisphere opposite the responding hand, but only when a certain amount of force is involved. The asymmetry reverses after the response and can co-exist super-imposed upon a symmetric Contingent Negative Variation (CNV) in anticipation of another signal.

The CNV can also be asymmetric. With a task involving matching stimuli on either *form* or *function* (already validated with split-brain patients as right and left hemispheric functions respectively) Donchin *et al.* showed first that the alpha band EEG during the task was asymmetrical, indicating relatively greater left-hemisphere activity (lower amplitude) during functional matching, particularly in the parietal region. However since the polarity of the asymmetry was in the *same* direction under both conditions, the effect may have been due simply to task difficulty, with the more difficult task unmasking the amplitude asymmetry as in the RP study above.

There was also a unidirectional asymmetry of the CNV, especially marked when the signal indicating whether to perform a form or a function match varied randomly from trial to trial. But this too could have been due to task difficulty; and there were no CNV differences between form and function matches. Principal Components Analysis of the quantified CNV waveform yielded several factors, of which one displayed right-left asymmetries and another anterior-posterior differences.

Clearly, until a "double dissociation" is demonstrated, with the asymmetry reversing polarity for right and left hemisphere tasks, preferably with a neutral symmetric control task, and with all tasks equated or at least co-varied for difficulty (errors, reaction time, etc.), no strong conclusions concerning the hemispheric lateralization of form and function matching in normal intact man can be drawn.

## ASYMMETRIES DURING HAND-USE AND SPATIAL DELAYED RESPONDING IN MONKEYS

Remarkably enough, similar experiments with monkeys *do* give clear evidence of hemispheric lateralization and, significantly, the effects are observed in spatial tasks, and may be mediated by orientation bias (see Parts IV and V and above). Stamm *et al.* (Chapter 20) recorded electrical activity from the right and left sides in occipital, precentral and prefrontal (principalis) cortex in monkeys during a delayed responding task: a cue light appeared on the right or left side, followed by a delay period, after which the monkey received a reward if it pressed a disc on the same side as the prior cue. Measures were the averaged cue-evoked potential (CEP) in response to the cue light and the averaged Steady Potential Shift (SPS), a slow anticipatory surface-negative wave (analogous to the RP and the CNV above) occurring during the delay period.

It was found that the positive component of the prefrontal CEP was greater over the hemisphere contralateral to the hemifield in which the cue appeared. This was not true of the occipital CEP, suggesting that this asymmetry was not just a primary sensory one, but that it was involved in the visuospatial or oculomotor initiation of a transient spatial memory (for which single units have been found in prefrontal cortex).

It was also found that the *magnitude* of the prefrontal SPS during the delay was predictive of the correctness of the subsequent response, suggesting that it reflected a transient memory process. This magnitude was highly asymmetric in monkeys trained unimanually, being considerably greater over the hemisphere opposite the responding hand. (There was no relation to hand preferences.) If the monkey was forced to switch to the untrained hand, the prefrontal SPS remained dominant over the side opposite the hand used in training, while the precentral SPS asymmetry was reversed, becoming higher now opposite the hand being used. This dissociation suggests that the precentral asymmetry is motor while the prefrontal asymmetry is mnemonic.

Evidence from the electro-oculogram (EOG) also suggested that in most monkeys the prefrontal SPS asymmetry is coupled with a spatial orientation bias: prior to the cue the animals tended to orient toward the side opposite the higher prefrontal SPS (as indicated by an EOG shift toward the non-preferred side whenever the cue appeared there). If monkeys were trained with alternating use of left and right hands, SPS magnitude was high bilaterally, but with a slight asymmetry again corresponding to the animal's orientation bias. Subsequent unimanual practice could still establish the usual asymmetry, with the higher SPS emerging opposite the responding hand.

These results suggest that only one side of the prefrontal cortex is dominant for the performance of delayed spatial responding.
The dominance is a function of unimanual experience and is also
somehow coupled to, and perhaps mediated by, spatial orientation
bias, as indicated by the EOG.


*OCULOVERSIVE AND ELECTROCORTICAL ASYMMETRIES
DURING LISTENING AND SPEAKING*

In most electrocortical studies eye movements (like eye-
blinks) are considered artifacts, and the EOG is only monitored in
order to exclude epochs which have been thus contaminated. The
electrodes most susceptible to oculomotor contamination are in the
frontal region. But the source of the effects is not necessarily
the obvious one (i.e. the nearby massive corneo-retinal potential
which generates the EOG) for the frontal *cortex* is also functionally involved in the control of eye movements, as well as in lateralized cognitive functions which may be coupled with eye movement asymmetry (such as those described by Gur and Gur, Chapter
15 and above).

Anderson (Chapter 21) has examined the relationship between
frontal averaged evoked potential (AEP) asymmetry and EOG asymmetry. He first administered a verbal dichotic listening test
(consonant-vowel pairs: see Berlin, Chapter 17 and above) to
right-handed subjects and selected the three who exhibited the
largest right-ear-advantage and the three with the largest left-
ear-advantage. These subjects then participated in a listening
task (hearing consonant-vowel pairs) and a speaking task (pro-
nouncing words beginning with "p", as well as nonspeech control
vocalizations) while EOG and AEP were recorded.

Both the "right-eared" and the "left-eared" subjects had significant positive correlations between EOG laterality and frontal
AEP laterality during the listening and speech tasks, but only the
"left-eared" subjects exhibited the correlation during the nonspeech task, indicating that EOG and AEP laterality could under
some circumstances be dissociated. A control experiment comparing
EOG and AEP asymmetry during voluntary eye movement in a normal
subject and a subject with a prosthetic eye also suggested that
frontal asymmetries are not passive but active followers of the
corneo-retinal potential.

An examination of the averaged EOG revealed that both experimental groups produced a slow rightward eye movement during the
listening task, but that in the "left-eared" subjects this was
preceded by a rapid leftward movement. Patterns on the speech
task were less systematic, but eye movements also tended to be
toward the right in both groups, while during the nonspeech
vocalization their laterality was random.

Anderson concludes that lateral eye movements during the experimental tasks are a consequence of local overflow from frontal
speech cortex to frontal eye fields (Area 8) and hence to the AEP,

rather than from direct contamination of the AEP by the corneo-
retinal potential.  Hence the correlation arises from a *central
coupling* due to local cross-talk between a lateralized function
and a turning tendency.  The initial leftward shift of the "left-
eared" subjects suggests that the turning tendency and the lateralized function can also be partially dissociated, and even at
odds (as in the orientation bias of Stamm *et al.*'s monkeys, above,
on trials when the cue appeared on their non-preferred side, and
in the inferior performance of Gur and Gur's subjects, Chapter 15
and above, when their eye movements were not in the "appropriate"
direction).


*ASYMMETRIES DURING DELAYED SEMANTIC MATCHING IN A VISUAL MODE*

In a visual delayed matching paradigm Thatcher (Chapter 22) has
also, among other things, confirmed the existence of some dissociation between EOG and AEP asymmetry, finding that in a multivariate analysis they load on different factors and that AEP
asymmetry is greater in the posterior than in the anterior
regions (which are closer to the eye).
Thatcher's paradigm consists of a series of random dot displays
with an information-bearing stimulus at an early point in the
series and a test stimulus (to be indicated by the subject as
*matching* or *mismatching* the prior stimulus by means of a lever-
response) near the end of the series.  The informational and test
stimuli were individual alphabetic letters in one experiment and
words (synonyms, antonyms and neutral words, to be matched in
terms of meaning) in the semantic matching experiment.  The random dot stimuli were equated for size and luminance with the experimental stimuli and served as probes for baseline visual AEP
throughout the trial, and for specific changes during the delay.
Results indicated that AEPs from physically identical stimuli
can differ depending upon whether or not they match the prior information stimulus (suggesting that even "exogenous" ERP components may be more than sensory:  see Donchin *et al.*, Chapter 19
and above).  AEP asymmetry of one polarity (left greater than
right) was observed and was most marked with the test stimulus.
Asymmetry also occurred with random dot stimuli during the delay,
possibly indicating rehearsal or memory processes.  Factor analysis also revealed asymmetries of the wave-form in posterior regions, also of the same polarity as the above.  Since most visual
AEP studies report asymmetry in the opposite direction (right
greater than left), the present result seems promising; but as indicated in Chapter 19 and above, a double dissociation will have
to be shown within the same paradigm before these asymmetries
can be interpreted.

*SUMMARY*

The research on electrocortical laterality suffers from
severe methodological difficulties which require considerable
care and sophistication to overcome.
In man, if sufficient manual force is exerted a Readiness
Potential Asymmetry is unmasked, revealing greater amplitude opposite the responding hand. The CNV can be symmetric, but an
asymmetry (left greater than right) is unmasked in a cognitive
task consisting of matching stimuli in terms of either form or
function. Both the EEG asymmetry during the entire task, which
is more marked during function than form-matching, and the CNV
asymmetry (contingent upon the instruction signal), which is more
marked when the two conditions occur in a random sequence, are
*unidirectional*, and hence difficult to interpret in terms uncon-
founded by task difficulty. Principal components analysis of
the wave-form reveals left-right as well as anterior-posterior
factors.
During delayed spatial responding in monkeys, Prefrontal Cue
Evoked Potentials and Precentral Steady Potential Shifts are
greater contralateral to the input stimulus hemifield and the
responding hand, respectively. Prefrontal Steady Potential
Shifts, however, which seem to reflect spatial memory processes
during the delay, tend to exhibit unilateral dominance. They
remain larger opposite the hand used during training, even when
the responding hand is subsequently switched. There are indications that the effect is accompanied, and perhaps even mediated,
by an orientation bias toward the side opposite the larger
Prefrontal Steady Potential Shift.
EOG and AEP asymmetries during listening to verbal material
and during speaking are highly correlated. This may not be just
because of passive spread of the corneo-retinal potential but
because of a central overflow from speech to eye movement regions
of the frontal cortex. "Right-eared" and "left-eared" subjects
on a verbal dichotic listening task both tend to move their eyes
rightward during linguistic tasks, but the latter make an initial
leftward movement, suggesting some conflict between habitual
turning tendencies and lateralized functions.
In visual delayed responding tasks (matching letters and
matching word-meanings) AEP asymmetries occur in response to the
second stimulus of the pair to be matched, and during the delay.
There are asymmetries in the factor structure of the wave form as
well. Again, unidirectional asymmetries present problems of
interpretation.
With close attention to problems of methodology and experimental design, event-related cortical potentials will perhaps
prove a valuable tool for the study of interhemispheric relations
and lateralization.

SURFACE ELECTROCORTICAL INDICATORS OF LATERALIZATION II:   EEG

*EEG LATERALITY CHANGES WITH DRUGS AND PERFORMANCE IN RABBITS*

The continuous EEG (Electroencephalogram) complements ERPs
(Event-Related Potentials) in several important respects.  It is
a measure of *ongoing* activity rather than being closely locked to
a brief event in time and it is particularly responsive to overall
changes in state such as alertness/relaxation, sleep/wakefulness
and psychoactive drug-effects.

Nelsen *et al.* (Chapter 23) have examined EEG laterality in the
parietal region of the cortex in rabbits under a variety of conditions.  In the normal, relaxed waking state the EEG amplitude
is lower over one hemisphere than the other  -  lower amplitude
indicates greater activation  -  although which side is lower
varies from rabbit to rabbit.  When the rabbit falls into deep
sleep (either normal or pentobarbitol-induced) overall amplitude
rises and there is a reversal of the waking amplitude laterality
relationship, with the formerly lower side now relatively higher.
When the animal passes into REM (Rapid Eye Movement) sleep, the
amplitudes again go down and the laterality once more reverses.
(Similar effects are obtained in cats and man.)  In general the
more labile side during sleep or drug-induced reversals is the
one which is lower during waking, and so the authors have conjectured that this side may normally be "dominant" for consciousness.

On an operant task involving pressing with the nose for water
while a buzzer indicates "on" (reinforced) *vs.* "off" (no reinforcement) periods, one hemisphere (not necessarily the same as
above) again appears to be "dominant" in rabbits, i.e. has relatively lower amplitude during the reinforced performance periods
(an effect reminiscent of Stamm *et al.*'s unilateral prefrontal
dominance in monkeys, Chapter 20 and above).  During the "off"
period neither side appears "dominant" and during the post-task
satiation period the amplitude relations are the reverse of the
"on"-phase (as in Donchin *et al.*'s post-response RP reversal,
Chapter 19 and above).  Drug-induced disruption of performance
by amphetamine or pentobarbitol is reflected by the disappearance
of these orderly lateralities, and their return is predictive
(as with Stamm *et al.*'s Prefrontal SPS asymmetry) of improved
performance.

In general, these observed EEG amplitude laterality changes
were *relative* rather than absolute ones, being calculated as
*deviations* above or below the overall left-right amplitude ratio
averaged across all experimental conditions.  Moreover, as
mentioned, the *direction* of these reversals was not absolute
either, but dependent upon the baseline characteristic of a
particular rabbit in a particular state (and even the particular
anterior/posterior locus of the electrodes; see Webster, Chapter
24 and below).  Finally, the amplitude laterality was found at
most times to be fairly tightly correlated with the concurrent

total (i.e. bilateral) EEG amplitude level, which is itself an (inverse) index of level of arousal. However the fact that the amplitude laterality may still carry some independent information is suggested by the finding that changes in laterality tended to *precede* by several minutes the overall amplitude effects accompanying changes in arousal, as if interhemispheric changes occurred before other arousal-dependent changes. Also, chlorpromazine, a drug which disrupts avoidance but not escape behavior, specifically disrupted the orderly EEG laterality relations, suggesting that its performance effects may have been due to impaired interhemispheric relations rather than sedative effects reducing arousal.

## *EEG AND ANATOMICAL ASYMMETRIES IN CATS*

Webster (Chapter 24) has confirmed in cats the EEG laterality shifts during sleep reported by Goldstein and his co-workers above, but points out some difficulties in interpretation. He found that the shifts do occur in adult cats, and even in four week old kittens, suggesting that any underlying functional asymmetry may be present early in life. However the direction of the shifts appears to bear no relation to individual paw preferences or turning tendencies and the shifts even occur in split-brain cats. Webster also found by recording from electrode pairs in the suprasylvian as well as the marginal gyri that the asymmetries could simultaneously go in opposite directions and that intrahemispheric anterior-posterior shifts seem to have the same magnitude and arousal-dependent characteristics as laterality shifts.

Nor is EEG laterality the only dissociated asymmetry variable. Webster found marked morphologicical asymmetries in the convolutional pattern of the cortex in adult cats as well as in neonate kittens. These tend to occur predominantly in the posterior area, suggesting an association with visual functions. However these anatomic asymmetries vary widely in degree and direction and appear to be unrelated to paw preference. Some earlier data suggesting an association between paw preference and functional asymmetry between the hemispheres on certain visual discrimination tasks in split-brain cats must now be weighed against the negative results of Hamilton (Chapter 3 and above) and others in this regard. It appears that systematic studies examining all these asymmetry variables jointly will have to be undertaken before any clear conclusions can be drawn.

*EEG LATERALITY IN HUMAN INFANTS*

As usual, the most consistent and unambiguous cases of
lateralization are provided by our own species. There has been
some disagreement, however, over the age at which asymmetry first
appears. To a degree this depends upon which asymmetry one has in
mind and how one measures it. Anatomical asymmetries have been
found in fetal brains (see Rubens, Chapter 26 and below) and
postural asymmetry is present within a few hours of birth (Turkewitz, Chapter 14 and above), however functions such as language,
which mature much later, might also be expected to lateralize
later. The dichotic listening approach to this question appears
to be equivocal (Berlin, Chapter 17 and above), but the EEG
approach has yielded interesting results.

Gardiner and Walter (Chapter 25) recorded EEG in six month old
infants during presentations of speech and music. Analyzing the
EEG only during brief quiescent periods (which they took as indicating that the otherwise restless infant was orienting and
attending to the input), they found that all four infants displayed relatively greater left hemisphere activity while listening to speech and relatively greater right hemisphere activity
during music, as indicated by a ratio of the EEG amplitudes. The
effect is particularly marked in a frequency band around 4 hz
(which the authors interpret as the infant homologue of the alpha
band) over Wernicke's area and an adjacent parietal region.
Moreover, unlike similar effects in adults, the asymmetry is not
just unidirectional, with most of the lability exhibited by only
one hemisphere; rather there is a true amplitude drop over the
right for music and over the left for speech. The magnitude of
the asymmetry is also greater than in adults.

These findings suggest that differential processing of verbal
and musical input has already begun in early infancy, prior even
to speech production. The effect is consistent with other recent
studies reporting categorical perception of phoneme boundaries,
"right ear effect", speech-synchronized movement and asymmetrical
event-related potentials in very young infants (see *oper. cit.*
in Chapter 25). The greater magnitude of the EEG asymmetry in
infants than in adults may be due to immaturity of the corpus
callosum, "critical period" effects, or the absence of a cognitive
bias which is to develop later favoring the left (speech)
hemisphere.


ANATOMICAL ASYMMETRIES

*LEFT-RIGHT MORPHOLOGICAL DIFFERENCES IN INFANT, ADULT AND
NONHUMAN PRIMATE BRAINS*

Ultimately functional asymmetries will have to be based upon
structural asymmetries, whether microstructural ones such as
Glick *et al.* have demonstrated in rats (Chapter 13 and above) or

gross morphological ones such as Webster has found in cats
(Chapter 24 and above). But if they are to fit the functional
data in man, these structural asymmetries cannot vary randomly
in direction from individual to individual but must have a fixed
direction, at least in the majority of the members of the species.

Rubens (Chapter 26) reviews the literature on gross asymmetries of the cerebral cortex which have been known since the
nineteenth century. These asymmetries occur chiefly in the
temporo-parietal region in man and have been reported as a longer
sylvian fissure and planum temporale and larger parietal and
posterior temporal operculi on the left. The angle of the sylvian
fissure was also reported to be more horizontal on the left.
These asymmetries all occur around the region of what is called
Wernicke's area on the left, where injury causes severe language
deficits. They are also found in human neonates and foetuses as
well as in the great apes, and perhaps also in some monkeys (cf.
Dewson, Chapter 4 and above).

Due to the difficulty of visualizing these asymmetries jointly,
and because of previous investigators' admitted problems in
establishing reliable landmarks for their measurements, Rubens
superimposed transparencies of the left and right hemiconvexities
to determine the exact relation of the left and right surface
features. He found that the sylvian fissures are congruent until
about two and a half cm. posterior to the central fissure (past
Heschl's gyrus), at which point the right angulates upward
sharply into the inferior parietal region, while the left continues farther posteriorly. Hence the difference is not only
one of length but of abruptness of posterior angulation. The
other effects which have been reported are clearly secondary to
this difference. The more posterior termination of the left
sylvian fissure serves to extend the left parietal operculum
above it and the posterior temporal operculum below, as well as
the planum temporale within the fissure itself. The earlier
planum measurements were partially also an artifact of cutting
along the plane of the straighter anterior portion of the sylvian fissure, thereby eliminating more of the divergent portion
on the right. It must also be noted that the earlier and greater
angulation of the sylvian fissure on the *right* yields a larger
retrosylvian parietal region on that side, including a larger
angular gyrus, which had formerly been thought to be important
for language in mediating cross-modal associations. Clearly, if
these asymmetries are to have a consistent interpretation, the
latter view must be revised.

Asymmetries of the frontal regions in the vicinity of what is
called Broca's area on the left are more ambiguous. The anterior
branch of the sylvian fissure, which subdivides the inferior
frontal gyrus, is more often double on the left than the right,
while the surface area of the *right* frontal operculum is greater
than the left (although deeper convolutional asymmetry may go in
the other direction).

Gross anatomical asymmetries must be interpreted with caution until reliably linked to function. The planum temporale seems to be largely auditory association parakoniocortex, but in general the relative cytoarchitectonics, connectivity and biochemistry of these regions is not known. In addition, the possibility exists that the outcomes of surface electrocortical studies (Parts VI and VII), which rely upon homologous left-right placement of electrodes, are actually being confounded by these underlying anatomical disparities.

*SUMMARY*

Left-right anatomical asymmetries have been found in the temporo-parietal and frontal regions of the brain where injury tends to produce aphasia. Most of these asymmetries seem to favor the left in terms of magnitude in adult man as well as in unborn human foetuses and nonhuman primates, but their interpretation must wait upon microstructural studies. Some surface electrocortical asymmetries may be artifacts of these subjacent anatomical asymmetries.

CONCLUSIONS

In stereochemistry a compound which contains an equal random mixture of enantiomers of both chiralities, dextrorotary and levorotary (referring to the direction in which they rotate light) is called *racemic* (after racemic acid, the grape derivative with which Pasteur did his original painstaking work on molecular asymmetry). *Resolving* racemic compounds so as to yield only isomers of one chirality has been an active stereochemical research pursuit, particularly "abiotic" resolution, i.e. without the intervention of living organisms in the chemical process (although setting up such an "abiotic" experiment by a "biotic" chemist is always a bit self-contradictory).

The resolution of racemic compounds into chiral ones is of interest to us here only by way of suggesting an alalogy which helps to formulate one of the two general questions raised by the research reported in the present volume: We have now encountered a number of random "racemic" asymmetries exhibited by a variety of species: paw preferences, environmental biases, pharmacological asymmetries, turning biases, unilateral engrams, electrocortical lateralities and anatomical asymmetries. Only in two instances (the central motor mechanisms in arthropods and the vocal control system in songbirds) have these been "resolved" by evolution to yield a truly "chiral" population. These two instances are rather far, phylogenetically, from the third prom-

/

inent case of our own strongly chiral population.  The question
therefore remains as to *how. and why some or all of the above
racemic candidates have been resolved into the left-language-
dominant, dextrorotary organization characteristic of the human
species,* including the secondary specialization of the nondominant side and the exceptions in the form of left-handers and
populations with mixed dominance.  Insofar as it is commensurable
with human data, the comparative evidence from "animal models"
of lateralization will have to continue to be studied in order to
advance our understanding on this first question.

The second question raised by the present volume is:  *what is
the nature of hemispheric specialization in the normal intact
human brain, both in terms of physiology and cognition?*  The split-
brain research, formerly so far-removed from data on normals, has
recently done an about-turn, revealing that, at least after
surgical recovery, the right hemisphere is not as different
functionally from the left as originally thought (Zaidel, 1973).
As usual, this may or may not generalize to the intact case.  The
only way to find out is to use the available non-invasive experimental techniques--perceptual, attentional and electro-
cortical--together with rigorous experimental designs and
specific information-processing models, in order to find out.  If
the comparative data from the answers to the first question meet
this second line of research half way, then we are on the road to
solving the problem of lateralization.

REFERENCES

Franz, S. I.  *Studies in Cerebral Function I-IX,* Berkeley, Uni-
versity of California Press 1933.
Goldman, P.S. An alternative to developmental plasticity:
Heterology of CNS structures in infants and adults.  In
*Plasticity and Recovery of Function in the Central Nervous
System* (D.G. Stein, J.J. Rosen, and N. Butlers, eds.).  New
York:  Academic Press, 1974.
Zaidel, E. Linguistic competence and related functions in the
right cerebral hemisphere of man following commissurotomy and
hemispherectomy.  Ph.D. Thesis, California Institute of
Technology, Pasadena, California, 1973.

# LATERALIZATION
# IN THE
# NERVOUS SYSTEM

# Part I

# FUNCTIONAL LATERALIZATION IN NONHUMAN SPECIES

# 1.
# Role of Asymmetry in the Functioning of Invertebrate Nervous Systems

*WILLIAM D. CHAPPLE*

University of Connecticut

*All things counter, original, spare, strange;*
*What ever is fickle, freckled (who knows how?)*
*Gerard Manley Hopkins*

Not all animals have the ability to be asymmetrical. Certain groups of animals show many modifications of structure along one axis of symmetry but few modifications along another. Very little is known about the basis for these differences and the manner in which developmental processes become uncoupled on the two sides so that homologous structures can perform different functions.

Although in the present context *bilateral asymmetry* is of particular interest, it is but one aspect of a larger problem. For example, the segmental organization of annelids, arthropods, and vertebrates results in another mode: *translational symmetry*, in which each segment is primitively a replica of the one before it. Differentiation along the longitudinal axis is extremely common. In crustaceans, appendages along the longitudinal axis may perform many functions: The mouthparts are used for feeding, the chelae for grasping, the walking legs for locomotion, and the pleopods for swimming. All are serial homologues of each other. In contrast, the development of bilateral asymmetry is much rarer. There are only two major groups of invertebrates, the gastropod molluscs and the decapod crustaceans, in which it is at all common. Insects, the most numerous and successful group of invertebrates in terms of number of species, are by and large

*The work on the hermit crabs was supported by NSF Grants GB-12368 and BMS 75-05705 to W. D. C.

3

quite symmetrical. What asymmetries do occur--e.g., in the genitalia of some insects (see Morgan, this volume) or in the mandi-
bles of certain genera of termite soldiers (Wilson, 1971)--are
unusual. It is difficult to produce asymmetrical point mutations
in *Drosophila* (Lindsley & Grell, 1967; see Levy, this volume).
Gynandromorphs and mosaic animals due to nondisjunction of
chromosomes can be produced experimentally, however. In addition, asymmetry in radially symmetrical phyla such as Coelen-
terata, Ctenophora, or Echinodermata, is very rare. Thus there
seems to be a distinction between such groups as crustaceans,
gastropods, and vertebrates, in which lateralization of function
occurs, and groups in which it does not occur.

Most of the cases of asymmetry known in invertebrates are related to asymmetry of peripheral structures. There are exceptions among opisthobranchs such as *Aplysia* in which there has
been a secondary return to symmetry. Since this return to grace
has not been perfect, central asymmetries persist in spite of
the external symmetry. In general, however, there is a close relationship between the periphery and the central nervous system,
and such situations are much more convenient to analyze experimentally. Moreover, if laterality in nervous systems is to be
investigated, another convenient attribute of obvious morphological asymmetry is that it is usually associated with a functional
differentiation of the two sides.

There are, however, asymmetries in behavioral or physiological
properties that do not seem to be associated with any functional
role. For example, in the milkweed bug, *Oncopeltus fasciatus*,
Chapple (1966c) observed an asymmetry in the tonic frequency of
motoneurons to the metathoracic legs on the two sides, and this
asymmetry could be only partially reversed by movement of a
striped drum. Wilson and Hoy (1968) demonstrated that a turning
bias (cf. Glick, Jerussi, & Zimmerberg; Stamm, Turkewitz; Gur &
Gur; Stamm, Rosen, & Gadotti; Turkewitz, this volume) in the intact animal could be demonstrated under conditions in which visual feedback had been effectively excluded. They concluded that
the asymmetry was corrected, not by proprioception as Chapple
had believed, but by visual feedback. Moreover, this turning
bias was complex since it might persist for days or be reversed
in a few minutes.

Further evidence that visual feedback plays a major role in
correcting for errors in motor systems was provided by Wilson
(1968), who showed that flying locusts exhibited a rolling bias
in one direction or the other in the absence of visual feedback.
Removal of a hind wing, which would drastically alter the nature
of proprioceptive information transmitted to the central nervous
system, resulted in instability in flight but did not alter the
activity of the flight motoneurons. This reinforces the belief
that proprioception plays a minor role in correcting for asymmetries in the system. With visual feedback, however, compensa-
tory changes in motor output were observed.

Thus, turning asymmetry seems to be accidental; it may

possibly be caused by developmental variability. Such variability, if it could be shown to be genetically controlled, could represent the raw material upon which the evolutionary process might act. However, the difficulty of obtaining asymmetrical mutants in *Drosophila* suggests that developmental variability is not functional and probably does not represent the germinal stages in the development of laterality.(See Morgan; Levy; Collins, this volume.)

In some closely related species another feature of use in the analysis of asymmetry may be available. Individual cells, recognizable in all members of a species on the basis of (1) connections with other cells, (2) location in the central nervous system, and (3) physiological properties, may be homologous with cells in other species. Wiersma and his co-workers (Wiersma, 1941; Wiersma & Ripley, 1952) showed in decapod crustaceans that the same number of excitor motoneurons innervated the muscles of the walking legs, although the distribution of inhibitor motoneurons was slightly more variable. Homologous central interneurons such as the Mauthner cell in fish or the medial giant fiber in decapod crustaceans (Chapple, 1966b; Turner, 1950; Wiersma, 1952) can be recognized in different species. Because of the vagaries of the evolutionary history of a group and our lack of knowledge of the intervening stages, homologies between cells in different species are inevitably less certain than between cells in different segments, or between left and right sides. Such comparisons can nevertheless provide us with a symmetrical reference for homologous cells in asymmetrical animals. Since homology suggests similar developmental and genetic processes at work in the two organisms, a series of closely related species can be very useful in our attempt to understand how the differentiation of the two sides has taken place.

The most complex kinds of asymmetry occur in gastropod molluscs. During the process of *torsion*, the posteriorly located viscera of the briefly symmetrical veliger larva are swung counterclockwise 180 degrees to face anteriorly, and there is a loss of gills and nephridia on the right side as well as alterations in the circulatory system. As a result, the posterior parts of the nervous system become twisted and there is a progressive tendency for the posterior ganglia to fuse with one another or with the anterior ganglia. The symmetrical stage occurs early in development and the developmental process is complex, because of the independent processes of torsion, ganglionic fusion, and growth of an asymmetric shell. To complicate matters, in the opisthobranchs, a subsequent detorsion occurred, although their larvae still go through an asymmetrical stage.

As a result of this complex asymmetry, using the gastropods as a model system has certain problems. First, no one is quite sure what the functional significance of torsion is. A number of theories (reviewed in Ghiselin, 1966) have been proposed. Some involve locomotor adaptations or protection from predators during the larval stage, but we do not have solid evidence about the functional importance of the various peripheral asymmetries. Second, the complexity of the ontogenetic processes makes it difficult to establish a symmetrical baseline of control, either between segments, left and right sides, or closely related species. Thus, in the cell map of identified neurons in the abdominal ganglion of *Aplysia* (Frazier, Kupfermann, Coggeshall, Kandel, & Waziri, 1967), the numbered pairs, as the Frazier *et al.* are careful to emphasize, are not bilateral homologues. Two cells whose branches and connections are symmetrical but whose cell bodies are located in different ganglia were reported by Hughes (Hughes & Chapple, 1967) but this is an isolated example. Until more is learned about the development of the nervous system in these animals, they will not be very useful in studying the mechanisms by which asymmetries arise. On the other hand, the advantages of gastropod nervous systems are well known: they possess large, identifiable cells that show a variety of interesting electrical and chemical phenomena. The role of single neurons in patterns of behavior has been elegantly studied (Kupfermann, Pinsker, Castellucci, & Kandel, 1971; Kupfermann, Carew, & Kandel, 1974; Willows, Dorsett, & Hoyle, 1973). Undoubtedly, increasing knowledge of development and evolution in gastropods will contribute in a major way to the understanding of the independent differentiation of either side of the plane of symmetry.

In contrast to the gastropods, the decapod crustaceans are fundamentally symmetrical. The most common asymmetry is a difference in size and shape of the first pair of walking legs (heterochely). This asymmetry usually develops early in adult life so that asymmetries in the nervous system can be related to a prior common symmetrical pattern. By observation one can determine the function of the two chelae, which may be used for grasping, crushing, or cutting, and in courtship and agonistic displays. For example, one chela of fiddler crabs, of the genus *Uca*, is greatly enlarged and is used in a waving display (Crane, 1941, 1957, 1966; Salmon & Atsaides, 1968). This display, by which the male courts the female, is species-specific. The major chela is also used for making a rapping sound to attract the female at night, and for agonistic displays with other males. The minor chela is used for feeding. Spirito (1970) showed that the innervation of the major chela conformed to the pattern found in other brachyurans (Wiersma & Ripley, 1952). Ratcliff (cited in Huxley, 1932) showed an asymmetry in the portion of the thoracic ganglion from which the nerves to the chela originated, and believed this to be due to a shift in a population of small cells to the side of the major chela.

How functionally independent are the two chelae? Higher crustaceans can move their chelae independently of each other, but in most cases their displays are symmetrical (Schone, 1968). From the drawings of *Uca* displays (Crane, 1957; Schone, 1968) it appears that the chelae are flexed and extended together. Film of the display of *Uca galapagoensis* (Eibl-Eibesfeldt, Encyclo-

6

pedia Cinematographic E598) was obtained and projected, using
a time-motion analysis projector, onto graph paper.   The
two chelae move in a symmetrical fashion, although the major
chela covers a much greater area than does the minor one.  In the
initial period of the display, the minor chela moves a greater
distance than the major, but the major chela continues to move
after the minor one has ceased its motion.  This independence is
not solely the result of the difference in the inertia of the two
chelae, since in some cases the two move out of phase with each
other.  The display is symmetrical but the coupling between the
chelae is not fixed, which suggests that it may arise from the
activity of symmetrical interneurons, with little coupling at
the motoneuron level.

The development of heterochely involves a greater rate of
growth in the distal segments of the chela of one side (Huxley,
1932).  In the lobster, *Homarus*, this has a profound effect on
the development of the muscles.  Jahromi and Atwood (1971)
showed that the large crusher-claw closer muscle consists of long
sarcomere fibers associated with slow tonic contractions, whereas
the faster cutter-claw closer muscle consists predominantly of
short sarcomere fast fibers.  The two closer muscles are physio-
logically different, as Wiersma (1955) had initially shown.
Closer muscles respond to fast axon stimulation in the cutter
with a twitch to a single stimulus, but paired stimuli are necessary for a twitch in the crusher (Govind & Lang, 1974).  The
asymmetry does not begin to develop until the animal is about 2
months old.  Prior to this time both claws resemble the adult
cutter, consisting primarily of fast muscle fibers, but after
this time there is a progressive development of slow muscle
fibers in the crusher (Goudey & Lang, 1974; Govind, Atwood, &
Lang, 1974).  Since a crusher can develop on either side of the
animal (as can the major chela of *Uca*), such a preparation
should be very useful in analyzing the effects of peripheral
asymmetry on the central nervous system (see Wilson, 1903).

Not all asymmetry in crustacea involves the chelae.  The abdomen of the hermit crab has become decalcified and coiled to
the right, possibly because hermit crabs live in the cast-off
shells of gastropods, which in most cases also curl to the right.
Up until the last larval stage, the hermit crab is symmetrical
(Thompson, 1903); it has a calcified, segmented abdomen and
pleopods on each side.  In the last larval stage (the *megalops*),
a slight asymmetry can be observed in the chelae and uropods.
At the end of the megalops stage the abdomen becomes decalcified
and saclike; it curls to the right, and the pleopods disappear
on the right side.  Little is known about the internal morphology
of the larva beyond the description of the different stages in
1903 by Thompson.  However, the basic organization of the hermit
crab abdomen is very similar to that of macrurans and other
anomurans; it is interesting to compare the hermit crab with the
crayfish, investigated by a number of laboratories over the last
25 years, in describing the change from a symmetrical to an

asymmetrical state.

In the crayfish and the hermit crab there are superficially located flexor and extensor muscles, which are involved in the normal slow postural movements of the abdomen (Figure 1).

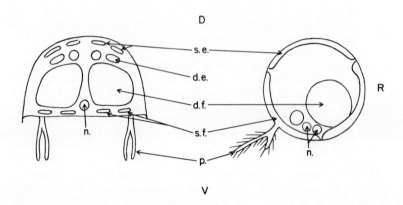

*Fig. 1. Diagram of the major abdominal muscle groups (shown in cross section) of the crayfish (on the left) and hermit crab (on the right). The abdominal nerve cord is paired in the hermit crab but fused in the crayfish. Elements of each major muscle region are identified. Abbreviations: D, dorsal; V, ventral; L, left; R, right; s.e., superficial extensors; d.e., deep extensors; d.f., deep flexors; s.f., superficial flexors; p., pleopod; n., nerve cord.*

Central to these are deep extensor muscles, absent in the hermit crab, and deep flexor muscles, which have become reduced (Marrelli, 1975) and asymmetric in the hermit crab. The crayfish has six abdominal ganglia; the hermit crab has only five, because the first abdominal ganglion moves into the thorax at the end of the megalops stage. Each of the midabdominal ganglia has three pairs of roots. The first pair innervates the pleopods, which are not present on the right side of the hermit crab abdomen; the second innervates the deep and superficial extensor muscles; and the third innervates the deep and superficial flexors (Chapple, 1966a; Hughes & Wiersma, 1960).

In the crayfish (Figure 2) five excitors and one inhibitor innervate the superficial flexors on either side of a segment (Kennedy & Takeda, 1965). In the hermit crab, *Pagurus pollicarus*, there are also five excitors and one inhibitor to these muscles (Chapple, 1969a, b). That this is a pattern common to other decapods can be seen by Kahan's (1971) work on two

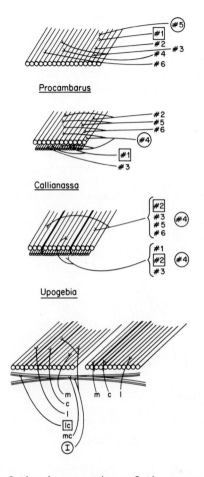

Fig. 2.  Diagram of the innervation of the superficial flexor
muscles in four species of decapod crustaceans.  Procambarus
(the crayfish) from Kennedy and Takeda (1965), Callianassa and
Upogebia from Kahan (1971), and Pagurus (the hermit crab) from
Chapple (1969a).  The muscles of one side only are shown for all
the animals except Pagurus, since only in Pagurus are the motoneurons asymmetrically distributed to the muscle fibers.  The
numbers indicate relative extracellular amplitudes of the units
and do not imply homologies between units in different animals.
For each animal, the circled number indicates the inhibitor, and
the boxed number the excitor, in the next posterior ganglion.  In
Pagurus, because of the division of the root, relative amplitudes
were not used and the motoneurons were identified by the region
of muscle innervated.  Abbreviations:  m, medial; c, central;
l, lateral; lc, lateral circular; mc, medial circular; I, inhibitor.

9

symmetrical anomurans, *Callianassa* and *Upogebia*. In the crayfish, the distribution of the five excitors to the longitudinal
muscle fibers of a segment is random, although there is a slight
tendency for the tonic excitors to innervate the medial, and
phasic excitors the lateral, areas. In *Callianassa* and *Upogebia*,
there is a segregation of the excitors into those innervating a
ventral layer of longitudinal fibers and those innervating a more
dorsal layer. In the hermit crab, in addition to the more centrally located layer of longitudinal muscle fibers innervated by
three of the five excitors, two new layers of circular muscles
innervated by two of the excitors have developed. Each excitor
innervates a longitudinal strip of muscle, so that homologous
motoneurons can be studied by recording EJPs (excitatory junction
potentials) from the appropriate region of muscle. As is the
case in the walking legs, the number of motoneurons remains the
same in these related species.

This pattern is also illustrated in the superficial extensors
(Figure 3) of the crayfish (Fields, Evoy, & Kennedy, 1967) and

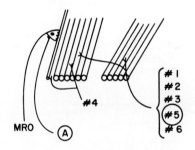

**Procambarus**

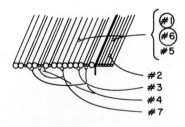

**Pagurus**

*Fig. 3. Diagram of the innervation of the superficial extensor
muscles in the crayfish,* Procambarus, *from Fields, Evoy &
Kennedy (1967) and in the hermit crab,* Pagurus, *from Chapple
(1973c, in prep.). Abbreviations: MRO, muscle receptor organ;
A, accessory fiber (inhibitor).*

10

the hermit crab (Chapple, 1973c, in prep.). In the crayfish
there are five excitors and two inhibitors. One of these excitors innervates the separate muscle of the muscle receptor
organ as well as the main superficial extensors, and one of the
inhibitors innervates the soma of the sensory receptor. In the
midabdominal segments of the hermit crab, *Pagurus pollicarus*, no
muscle receptor organ is found, and five excitors and two inhibitors innervate the muscles. Thus, in terms of number and
physiological properties, we can find homologies between the
asymmetric and the symmetric species. The neurons are very similar, even though the muscles have changed. Even in crayfish,
the number of inhibitors to the stretch receptor may vary (one
in *Procambarus* and three in *Astacus fluviatis*, (Jansen, Nja,
Ormstad, & Walloe, 1971) so that the number of inhibitors in
crayfish and hermit crab, although the same, may not be as significant as the similarity in number of excitors.

In the hermit crab, homologous motoneurons of the superficial
flexors innervate different numbers of muscle fibers on the two
sides (Chapple, 1969a, b). For example, the motoneuron innervating the most ventromedial strips of muscle on the right (the
medial region) innervates two and one-half times the number of
muscle fibers its homologue on the left innervates. In contrast, the most lateral motoneuron on the left innervates about
two and one-half times the number of fibers its homologue on the
right innervates. The two central motoneurons innervate the same
number of muscle fibers on the two sides. The tonic frequency of
all these pairs of homologues is also asymmetrical, but all three
pairs show a higher frequency on the left side. (See Figure 4
and Figure 5, B and C.) During reflex stimulation of the motoneurons a transient decrease in this asymmetry can be observed,
for example in the medial motoneurons of Figure 4. The inhibitors also fire, but at a higher frequency on the right side;
they are not rigidly coupled as they are in crayfish (Evoy,
Kennedy, & Wilson, 1967) and lobster (Otsuka, Kravitz, & Potter,
1967) (Figure 5C).

The superficial extensors are also organized into longitudinal
strips of muscle fibers in the hermit crab, but these are less
rigidly defined, and are symmetrical; homologous motoneurons
appear to innervate the same number of muscle fibers on the two
sides. However, here too there is an asymmetry (Figure 5A) in
the tonic frequency of homologous extensor units, as in the
superficial flexors in which the conduction velocities and fiber
diameters are greater in units on the right side. Thus in both
the superficial flexors and the superficial extensors homologous
motoneurons on the left side fire at a higher frequency than
those on the right, and this seems unrelated to the amount of
muscle tissue innervated.

Three other changes that should be mentioned have occurred in
the periphery. First, there has been a loss of the motoneurons
of the right first roots that innervate the pleopods. Secondly,
the deep flexor muscles have become reduced so that there are

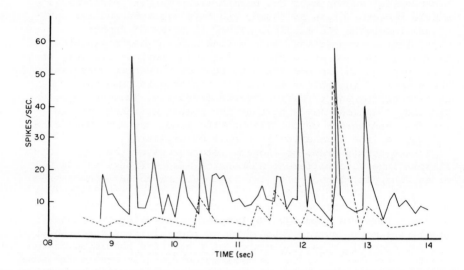

*Fig. 4. Reflex firing of the two homologous motoneurons to left
and right medial regions of the superficial flexor muscles of the
fourth abdominal segment in the hermit crab* Pagurus pollicarus.
*Solid line is the left medial motoneuron, broken line the right.
Note that at different portions of the record, the motoneurons
do not fire in a precise ratio, suggesting that during reflex
activity different factors may contribute to change the underlying asymmetry.*

only 8 motoneurons innervating the muscles on the right side
(Marrelli, 1975) in contrast to 10 in the crayfish (Selverston &
Remler, 1972). There appear to be fewer motoneurons on the left
side (Chapple, 1966b), although this must await confirmation
with techniques involving cobalt injection and electrophysiology.
Finally, there has been a loss of the motoneurons of the absent
deep extensor muscles. In these cases, it may be that differential cell death, so important a mechanism in the development of
vertebrate nervous systems, is playing a role.

What do we know about the function of the abdomen? It is a
hydrostatic skeletal system within which a pressure of about $10^4$
dynes/cm$^2$ is maintained by the normally synergistic activity of
superficial extensors, and the longitudinal and circular layers
of the superficial flexors (Chapple, 1974). The higher frequency of motoneurons on the left side is overridden by the more

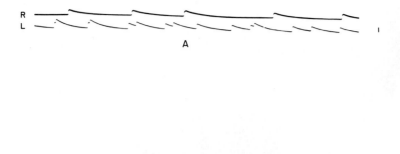

A

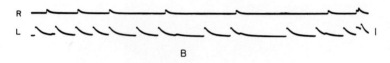

B

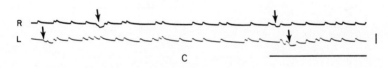

C

*Fig. 5. Intracellular recordings of EJPs (excitatory junction potentials) of homologous pairs of motoneurons innervating three different muscle regions in* P. pollicarus: *(A) lateral region of the superficial extensor muscle; (B) lateral region of the superficial flexor muscle; (C) central region of the superficial flexor muscle. Arrows indicate IJPs (inhibitor junction potentials). The inhibitors are not firing synchronously, but the one on the right is firing at a higher frequency than the one on the left. Horizontal scale: 1 sec; vertical scale: 10 mV.*

massive superficial flexors on the right (Chapple, 1969c) and may be a mechanism for preventing too much of a bending moment to the right in the resting state. The abdomen (Figure 6) carries about a tenth of the weight of the shell (Chapple, 1973a, b), varying its tone with the shell's weight. The changes that have occurred in the deep flexors and extensors seem to be mechanically consistent with the need to make a rapid retreat into the lumen of the gastropod shell (Marrelli, 1975). As a result of this information, we have a fairly clear idea of the functional implications of abdominal asymmetry and the mechanical rationale for the evolution of such a system from a symmetrical ancestor. We do not yet completely understand the reason for the higher firing frequency of homologous motoneurons on the left side, however.

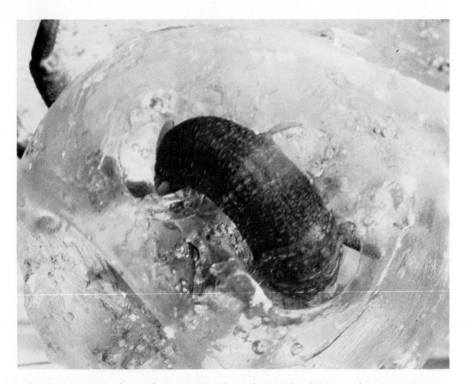

*Fig. 6. Posterior view of the hermit crab abdomen in a transparent shell. The telson and uropods are directly beneath the center of gravity of the shell. As the bending moment to the right increases during reflex activity, the shell is lifted; this asymmetrical bending moment is a result of the asymmetry of the motor units of homologous motoneurons on the two sides.*

The reasons for this asymmetry may be within the central nervous system. The fourth abdominal ganglion of the hermit crab (Chapple & Hearney, 1974) contains about two-thirds the number of cells found in the crayfish (Kendig, 1967). These cells are asymmetrically distributed, with a greater number on the left side. In the crayfish, the position and branching patterns of the six motoneurons of the superficial flexors have been mapped (Wine, Mittenthal, & Kennedy, 1974), and the physiological evidence of Evoy *et al.* (1967) that one of the tonic excitors has its cell body in the next posterior ganglion has been confirmed with cobalt sulfide. The homologous cell in the hermit crab, innervating the lateral circular muscles, is shown in Figure 7, A and B. In addition. Wine *et al.* (1974) have shown that in the anterior ganglion there are five cell bodies, the most contralateral of which is the inhibitor. Figure 7C shows what is most likely the homologue of that cell in the hermit crab. These results have been obtained by centripetal diffusion of cobalt and

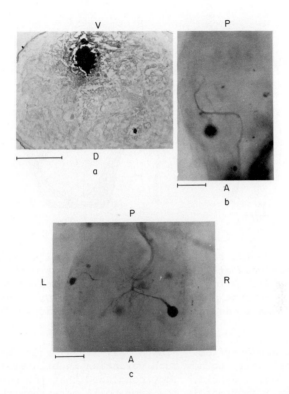

*Fig. 7.* (A) *Motoneuron of the right third root of the fourth ganglion, located in the fifth ganglion, homologous to a cell in the crayfish. Centripetal diffusion of cobalt, sectioned at 10 μm, and stained by the method of Tyrer and Bell (1974).*
(B) *Homologous cell in the fourth ganglion filled by centripetal diffusion of cobalt through the third root of the third ganglion.*
(C) *Two motoneurons filled from the right third root of the fourth ganglion, located in the fourth ganglion. Cell on the left may be homologous to the inhibitor of the superficial flexors of the crayfish.* P. pollicarus. *Scale: 100 μm.*

positive evidence for homologies between the cell bodies in crayfish and hermit crab must await detailed microelectrode recordings from the different cells. By the centripetal diffusion of cobalt a comparison of the sizes of the superficial flexor motoneurons can be made; the results suggest that they are larger on the right side (Figure 8, A and B).

These preliminary results indicate that close homologies may be made between the central structures of homologous cells in

P

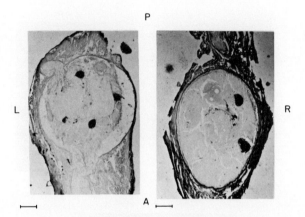

L                                                        R

A

*Fig. 8. Horizontal sections of motoneurons filled with cobalt sulfide, sectioned at 10 μm, and stained by the method of Tyrer and Bell (1974). Motoneurons of the left (b) third root and right (R) third root of the fourth ganglion. Units on the right are larger than those on the left. P. pollicarus. Scale: 100 μm.*

hermit crab and crayfish. Wine *et al.* (1974) addressed themselves specifically to how much variation in bilateral and serial homologues occurs. They concluded that the neuron somas are found in approximately the same position within the ganglion (with some variation within a circumscribed area) but the branching of the dendrites of ipsilateral and contralateral homologues is exact. In the hermit crab, with the considerable rearrangement of the entrances of the ganglionic roots, the cell bodies have clearly been moved around, but there is a similarity between the position of cells filled by centripetal diffusion of cobalt in the superficial third root and the position of those described by Wine, Mittenthal, and Kennedy.

Cell loss probably also plays a role in the central nervous system. Chapple and Hearney (1974) described the hypotrophy of the neuropil on the right side of the ganglion, and suggested that this might be due to the loss of motoneurons in the first roots. Figure 9B shows the results of bilateral filling of the first roots. The neuropil on the left shows many processes filled with cobalt, indicating that at least part of that asymmetry is related to the first roots. This change in cell number may also affect the interneurons; Figure 9A shows the result of diffusing cobalt from the next anterior ganglion up both connectives, thus staining interneurons with axons running anteriorly. The more massive neuropil on the left side indicates

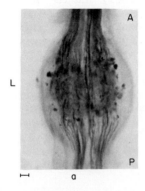
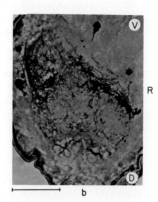

*Fig. 9.* *(A)* *Horizontal view of a whole mount of interneurons of*
*the fourth abdominal ganglion filled from left and right anterior*
*connectives at the posterior margin of the third ganglion.* *Left-*
*side neuropil is slightly more extensive than that on the right.*
*(B)* *Cross section of the fourth abdominal ganglion at the level*
*of the anterior outer commissure.* *Both first roots have been*
*filled.* *The larger fine-fibered neuropil on the left shows ex-*
*tensive cobalt-filled processes, suggesting the anterior fine-*
*fibered neuropil owes some of its greater volume on the left side*
*to the presence of motoneurons on that side.* P. pollicarus.
*Scale:* *100* µm..

that the asymmetry probably involves interneurons as well.

A number of processes thus seem to be at work in this asymmetrical abdomen: (1) loss of motoneurons, and possibly of
interneurons, correlated with loss or reduction of peripheral
structures; (2) increase in the size of motoneurons on the right
side in the superficial flexor system; and (3) an uncoupling of
the giant fibers (Chapple, 1966b) and the inhibitor to the superficial flexors. We need to know much more about the branching
structure of the motoneurons and the interneurons that connect to
them. The hermit crab abdomen can twist in a number of directions
during extension, suggesting that premotor interneurons may exist
that can excite motoneurons of one side but not the other. This
would be very interesting because in the crayfish, Evoy and
Kennedy (1967) found only symmetrical "command fibers" acti-
vating the postural system.

In a more general context, the kinds of questions for which
answers have been sought are related to how a system is altered
in the course of evolution to perform new functions. In the

evolution of asymmetry, it appears that left and right sides must first be uncoupled from a rigid pattern of symmetrical activation before different functions can evolve on each side. For this reason, perhaps the ability to move appendages independently represents a first step toward heterochely and the development of an asymmetrical abdomen. Ultimately, we must learn more about the underlying genetic and developmental processes that can lead first to independent movement of the appendages and then to their functional differentiation. Systems having a fairly well-defined transition from a symmetrical to an asymmetrical state, resulting in a defined change in function, will be very useful; a particular advantage of some invertebrate preparations is that we can begin to answer these questions at the level of the single cell.


SUMMARY

Bilateral asymmetry in animals is relatively uncommon. Crustaceans, gastropods, and vertebrates are the major groups in which examples of independent functional differentiation of the two sides is found. Other groups, such as insects, may show random asymmetries but these appear unrelated to the functional requirements of a particular adaptation. The asymmetry of gastropods is related to the torsion of the viscera during development, the function of which is not well understood, so that gastropod nervous systems are at present less useful in understanding the ways in which laterality arises. In contrast, decapod crustaceans have a number of advantages. Their nervous systems are composed of relatively few neurons, they have striated muscles that are amenable to various experimental manipulations, and in a number of genera functional asymmetries are found superimposed upon a basic bilateral symmetry. Two examples are discussed: (1) heterochely, the independent differentiation of the chelipeds of the two sides, and (2) abdominal asymmetry in hermit crabs. The latter case illustrates some of the processes that may be involved at the level of single neurons. Motoneurons and muscles homologous with those of symmetrical macrurans were studied. Homologous motoneurons on the two sides differ in size and tonic frequencies, apparently independently of the number of muscle fibers innervated (which also differs on the two sides). In several cases there are different numbers of motoneurons (possibly as a result of differential cell death) on the two sides. Systems in which identifiable pairs of homologous neurons can be studied from preparation to preparation may be very useful in elucidating the cellular mechanisms involved in the development of bilateral asymmetry.

REFERENCES

Chapple, W. D. Sensory modalities and receptive fields in the abdominal nervous system of the hermit crab, *Pagurus granosimanus* (Stimson). *Journal of Experimental Biology*, 1966, *44*, 209-223. (a)

Chapple, W. D. Asymmetry of the motor system in the hermit crab *Pagurus granosimanus* (Stimpson). *Journal of Experimental Biology*, 1966, *45*, 65-81. (b)

Chapple, W.D. Motoneuron responses to visual stimuli in *Oncopeltus fasciatus*, (Dallas). *Journal of Experimental Biology*, 1966, *45*, 401-410. (c)

Chapple, W. D. Postural control of shell position by the abdomen of the hermit crab, *Pagurus pollicarus* I. Morphology of the superficial muscles and their nerves. *Journal of Experimental Zoology*, 1969, *171*, 397-408. (a)

Chapple, W. D. Postural control of shell position by the abdomen of the hermit crab, *Pagurus pollicarus* II. Reflex control of the ventral superficial muscles. *Journal of Experimental Zoology*, 1969, *171*, 409-416. (b)

Chapple, W. D. Postural control of shell position by the abdomen of the hermit crab, *Pagurus pollicarus* III. Analysis of movements and calculations of forces exerted by the muscles. *Journal of Experimental Zoology*, 1969, *171*, 417-424. (c)

Chapple, W. D. Role of the abdomen in the regulation of shell position in the hermit crab, *Pagurus pollicarus*. *Journal of Comparative Physiology*, 1973, *82*, 317-332.

Chapple, W. D. Changes in abdominal motoneuron frequency correlated with changes of shell position in the hermit crab, *Pagurus pollicarus*. *Journal of Comparative Physiology*, 1973, *87*, 49-61. (b)

Chapple, W. D. Innervation and reflex activity of the dorsal superficial muscles of the hermit crab, *Pagurus pollicarus*. *Society of Neurosciences*, 1973, *3*, (abstract). (c)

Chapple, W. D. Hydrostatic pressure changes in the abdomen of the hermit crab, *Pagurus pollicarus* during movement. *Journal of Comparative Physiology*, 1974, *88*, 399-412.

Chapple, W. D., & Hearney, E. S. The morphology of the fourth abdominal ganglion of the hermit crab: A light microscope study. *Journal of Morphology*, 1974, *144*, 407-420.

Crane, J. Crabs of the genus *Uca* from the west coast of Central America. *Zoologica*, 1941, *26*, 145-208.

Crane, J. Basic patterns of display in fiddler crabs (Ocypodidae (Ocypodidae, genus *Uca*). *Zoologica*, 1957, *42*, 69-82.

Crane, J. Combat, display and ritualization in fiddler crabs (Ocypodidae, genus *Uca*). *Philosophical Transactions of the Royal Society of London, Series B*, 1966, *251*, 459-472.

Evoy, W. H., & Kennedy, D.  The central nervous organization underlying control of antagonistic muscles in the crayfish. I.  Types of command fibers.  *Journal of Experimental Zoology*, 1967, *165*, 223-228.

Evoy, W. H., Kennedy, D., & Wilson, D. M.  Discharge patterns of neurons supplying tonic abdominal flexor muscles in the crayfish.  *Journal of Experimental Biology*, 1967, *46*, 393-411.

Fields, H. L., Evoy, W. H., & Kennedy, D.  Reflex role played by efferent control of an invertebrate stretch receptor. *Journal of Neurophysiology*, 1967, *30*, 859-874.

Frazier, W. T., Kupfermann, I., Coggeshall, R. E., Kandel, E. R., & Waziri, R.  Morphological and functional properties of identified neurons in the abdominal ganglion of *Aplysia californica*.  *Journal of Neurophysiology*, 1967, *30*, 1352-1376.

Ghiselin, M. T.  The adaptive significance of gastropod torsion. *Evolution*, 1966, *20*, 337-348.

Goudey, R., & Lang, F.  Growth of crustacean muscle; asymmetric development of the claw closer muscles in the lobster, *Homarus americanus*.  *Journal of Experimental Zoology*, 1974, *189*, 421-427.

Govind, C. K., & Lang, F.  Neuromuscular analysis of closing in the dimorphic claws of the lobster *Homarus americanus*. *Journal of Experimental Zoology*, 1974, *190*, 281-288.

Govind, C. K., Atwood, H. L., & Lang, F.  Sarcomere length increases in developing crustacean muscle.  *Journal of Experimental Zoology*, 1974, *189*, 395-400.

Hughes, G. M., & Chapple, W. D.  The organization of nervous systems.  In C. A. G. Wiersma (Ed.), *Invertebrate nervous systems*.  Chicago:  Univ. of Chicago Press, 1967.  Pp. 177-195.

Hughes, G. M., & Wiersma, C. A. G.  Neuronal pathways and synaptic connections in the abdominal cord of the crayfish. *Journal of Experimental Biology*, 1960, *37*, 291-307.

Huxley, J. S. *Problems of relative growth*.  New York:  Dial Press, 1932.

Jahromi, S. S., & Atwood, H. L.  Structural and contractile properties of lobster leg-muscle fibers. *Journal of Experimental Zoology*, 1971, *176*, 475-486.

Jansen, J. K. S., Nja, A., Ormstad, K., & Walloe, L.  On the innervation of the slowly adapting stretch receptor of the crayfish abdomen.  An electrophysiological approach. *Acta Physiologica Scandinavica*, 1971, *81*, 273-285.

Kahan, L. B.  Neural control of postural muscles in *Callianassa californiensis* and three other species of decapod crustaceans.  *Comparative Biochemistry and Physiology*, 1971, *40A*, 1-18.

Kendig, J. J.  Structure and function in the third abdominal ganglion of the crayfish, *Procambarus clarkii* (Girard). *Journal of Experimental Zoology*, 1967, *164*, 1-20.

Kennedy, D., & Tadeka, K.  Reflex control of abdominal flexor muscles in the crayfish. II. The tonic system. *Journal of Experimental Zoology*, 1965,  , 229-246.

Kupfermann, I., Carew, T. J., & Kandel, E. R.  Local, reflex, and central commands controlling gill and siphon movements in *Aplysia*. *Journal of Neurophysiology*, 1974, *37*, 996-1019.

Kupfermann, I., Pinsker, H., Castellucci, V., & Kandel, E. R.  Central and peripheral control of gill movements. *Aplysia Science*, 1971, *174*, 1252-1255.

Lindsley, D. L., & Grell, E. H.  Genetic variations of *Drosphila melanogaster*. Carnegie Institute of Washington, Publication No. 627, 1967.

Marrelli, J.D.  The morphology and activation of the deep abdominal motor system of the hermit crab, *Pagurus pollicarus* (Say), and the homologous relationship to the crayfish deep abdominal motor system. Unpublished Ph.D. dissertation. Univ. of Connecticut, 1975.

Otsuka, M., Kravitz, E. A., & Potter, D. D.  Physiological and chemical architecture of a lobster ganglion with particular reference to gamma-aminobutyrate and glutamate. *Journal of Neurophysiology*, 1967, *30*, 725-752.

Salmon, M., & Atsaides, S.  Visual and acoustical signalling during courtship by fiddler crabs (Genus *Uca*). *American Zoologist*, 1968, *8*, 623-639.

Selverston, A. I., & Remler, M. P.  Neural geometry and activation of crayfish fast flexor motoneurons. *Journal of Nuerophysiology*, 1972, *35*, 797-814.

Schone, H.  Agonistic and sexual display in aquatic and semiterrestrial brachyuran crabs. *American Zoologist*, 1968, *8*, 641-654.

Spirito, C. P.  Reflex control of the opener and stretcher muscles in the cheliped of the fiddler crab, *Uca pugnax*. *Zietschrift für Vergleichende Physiologie*, 1970, *68*, 211-228.

Thompson, M. T.  The metamorphosis of the hermit crab. *Proceedings of the Boston Society of Natural History*, 1903, *31*, 147-209.

Turner, R. S.  Functional anatomy of the giant fiber system of *Callianassa californiensis*. *Physiological Zoology*, 1950, *23*, 35-41.

Tyrer, N. M., & Bell, E. M.  The intensification of cobalt-filled neurone probiles using a modification of Timm's sulphide-silver method. *Brain Research*, 1974, *73*, 151-155.

Wiersma, C. A. G.  The inhibitory nerve supply of the leg muscles of different decapod crustaceans. *Journal of Comparative Neurology*, 1941, *74*, 63-79.

Wiersma, C. A. G.  Neurons of arthopods. *Cold Spring Harbor Sumposium on Quantitative Biology*, 1952, *17*, 155-153.

Wiersma, C. A. G.   An analysis of the functional differences between the contractions of the adductor muscles in the
   thoracic legs of the lobster *Homarus vulgarus L. Archives
   Neerlandica Zoologie*, 1955, *11*, 1-13
Wiersma, C. A. G., & Ripley, S. H.   Innervation patterns of crustacean limbs. *Physiologica Comparata et Oecologia*, 1952, *2*,
   391-405.
Willows, A. O. D., Dorsett, D. A., & Hoyle, G.   The neuronal
   basis of behavior in Tritonia.   III.   Neuronal mechanism of
   a bixed action pattern. *Journal of Neurobiology*, 1973, *4*,
   255-285.
Wilson, D. M.   Inherent asymmetry and reflex modulation of the
   locust flight motor pattern. *Journal of Experimental
   Biology*, 1968, *48*, 631-641.
Wilson, D. M., & Hoy, R. R.   Optomotor reaction, locomotory
   bias, and reactive inhibition in the milkweed bug
   *Oncopeltus* and the bettle *Zophobas*. *Zeitschrift fur
   vergleichende Physiology*, 1968, *58*, 136-152.
Wilson, E. B.   Notes on the renewal of asymmetry in the re-
   generation of the chelae in *Alpheus heterochelis*.
   *Biological Bulletin*, 1903, *4*, 197-210.
Wilson, E. O.   *The insect societies*.   Cambridge, Massachusetts:
   Harvard Univ. Press, 1971.
Wine, J. J., Mittenthal, J. E., & Kennedy, D.   The structure of
   tonic flexor motoneurons in crayfish abdominal ganglia.
   *Journal of Comparative Physiology*, 1974, *93*, 315-335.

# 2.
# Asymmetries in Neural Control of Vocalization in the Canary

*F. NOTTEBOHM*

The Rockefeller University

The investigation of neural control of song in the canary permits us to explore problems of localization and lateralization of function in the vertebrate brain. It also permits the study of neural plasticity following brain lesions.

This chapter will discuss (1) the anatomy and innervation of the syrinx, the avian vocal organ; (2) the adult canary's song, and what is known about its ontogeny; (3) innervation of the left half of the syrinx and how it subserves the vast majority of the canary's song components; (4) brain areas involved in vocal control in the canary, and the pathways connecting these areas; (5) left hemispheric dominance for song control; and (6) song recovery following brain lesion.

## SYRINGEAL ANATOMY, FUNCTION, AND INNERVATION

The physics, anatomy, and physiology of avian vocalization have drawn much recent attention (e.g. Chamberlain, Gross, Cornwell, & Mosby, 1968; Dürrwang, 1974; Gaunt & Wells, 1973; Greenewalt, 1968; Hersch, 1966; Klatt & Stefanski, 1974; Miskimen, 1951; Nottebohm, 1971; Youngren, Peek, & Phillips, 1974). Though many of the details remain speculative and controversial, basically the vocal system of birds can be thought of as consisting of a set of bellows acting on an air-driven sound source. The major air sacs (abdominal and thoracic) are the bellows controlled by the respiratory masculature and inducing vocalization during expiration. The sound source is in

the syrinx, a specialized avian structure surrounded by the air
of the interclavicular air sac.  Flow of air and onset and termination of sounds are also regulated by the opening and closing of
the larynx, a phenomenon revealed externally as the gular pulsa-
tion of singing birds.

The typical songbird syrinx, as exemplified in the canary
(Figure 1), has two sound sources, the two internal tympaniform
membranes, which form the thin, modified medial walls of the
rostral end of each bronchus.  Two connective tissue folds, the

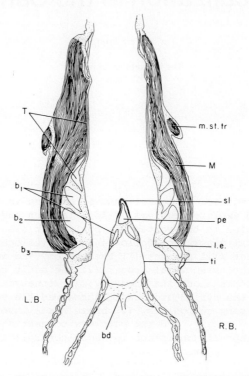

*Fig. 1.  Longitudinal section of syrinx of adult male canary.
Abbreviations:  R. B. and L.B., right and left bronchi; M, section through lateral mass of intrinsic syringeal muscles; T,
tympanum; $b_1$, $b_2$, and $b_3$, bronchial half-rings; bd, bronchi-
desmus; pe, pessulus; sl, semilunar membrane; l.e., labium ex-
ternum; ti, internal tympaniform membrane; m.st.tr., sterno-
trachealis muscle.  Notice that the muscle mass serving the left
syringeal half is heavier than its right counterpart (from
Nottebohm & Nottebohm, 1976).*

external labia, can protrude varyingly into the bronchial bore,
altering the shape and the dimensions of the bronchotracheal
connection and influencing air speed and turbulence.  Because of
the Bernoulli effect, when air flows past the internal tympani-

24

form membranes, they are drawn into the lumen of each bronchus. Presumably an interplay of the Bernoulli effect, interclavicular air sac pressure, position of the external labia, membrane tension and elasticity, and turbulence patterns formed as the air passes by these membranes and into the tracheal bore set the pattern of membrane oscillation and thus determine the amplitude and frequency of the sounds produced. Intrinsic and extrinsic syringeal muscles can influence the tension of the internal tympaniform membranes and the position of the external labia. As a result of (1) the position of the internal tympaniform membranes, (2) their independent air supply, (3) the points of insertion of the internal and external syringeal muscles, and (4) the independent innervation of the right and left syringeal halves, the canary syrinx can and does act as two functionally separate sound sources.

Details of syringeal innervation in the canary are shown in Figure 2. Motor innervation of the synringeal muscles is provided by the tracheosyringealis branch of the hypoglossus nerve (Conrad, 1915; Nottebohm, 1971; Nottebohm & Nottebohm, 1976). Vagal fibers may reach the syrinx via the recurrens branch of the vagus (Conrad, 1915), though according to other authors these fibers innervate the crop, not the syrinx (Youngren et al., 1974). Section of either the right or the left vagus nerve rostral or caudal to its anastomosis with the hypoglossus has no effect on song (Nottebohm and Nottebohm, 1976).


CANARY SONG AND ITS ONTOGENY

*ONTOGENY*

Canaries develop adult song during their first year of life. In subsequent years this song can change to varying degrees. Some sounds do not change at all, others are modified or abandoned, and still others are new (unpublished observations). Though the basic pattern of canary song emerges even in the absence of conspecific auditory models (Metfessle, 1935; Poulsen, 1959), young canaries imitate the song of adult canaries they can hear (Waser & Marler, in press); when reared as a group they develop song patterns that they all share (Poulsen, 1959). Young canaries deprived of auditory feedback, on the other hand, develop abnormally small song repertoires (Marler, Konishi, Lutjen, & Waser, 1973; Marler & Waser, in press), which include normal sounds as well as screeches, hisses, and clicks that would not normally occur in a bird having intact hearing (unpublished observations). Similarly, if an adult canary is deafened its song will regress in quality, eventually resembling that of a bird that has never had access to its own auditory feedback (Nottebohm, Stokes, & Leonard, 1976). For the purposes of this chapter, *vocal learning,* such as found in the canary, refers to vocal ontogeny guided by access to auditory information, including access to the bird's own auditory feedback.

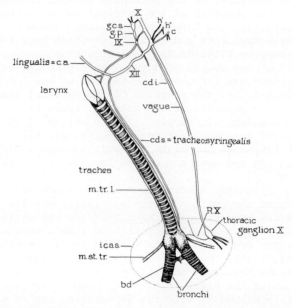

*Fig. 2. Ventral view of syrinx, trachea, and attendant muscula-
ture and innervation as observed under dissecting microscope;
these organs are not appreciably different in the canary and in
the chaffinch, and are illustrated with a drawing of the equivalent areas in the latter species (Nottebohm, 1971, p. 232).
Nerves are shown at an exaggerated diameter to allow for a clearer representation of detail. The IX cranial nerve is included to
show its relation to XII. The tracheosyringealis (cervicalis
descendens superior, c.d.s.) branch of XII runs caudally attached
to trachea and tracheolateralis muscle (m.tr.l.). The sternotra-
chealis muscle (m.st.tr.) attaches caudally to the anterior process of the sternum (not shown). Mass of intrinsic syringeal
muscles shows no detail of individual muscles. Bronchi and bron-
chidesmus membrane (bd) attach dorsally to the wall of the interclavicular air sac (i.c.a.s.). Space between bronchi and bron-
chidesmus opens ventrally to the interclavicular air sac. Three
hypoglossal roots are indicated (h', h", and c), one of which
corresponds to first cervical nerve (c). Other abbreviations:
R.X, recurrens branch of vagus; c.a., cervicalis ascendens
branch of XII, or lingualis; c.d.i., cervicalis descendens inferior branch of XII; g.c.s. and g.p., cervical superior and
petrosum ganglia of IX. Latin nomenclature of nerves and ganglia
follows Conrad, 1915 (from Nottebohm and Nottebohm, 1976).*

*THE SONG OF ADULT CANARIES*

The work described in this chapter was done with Rockefeller University inbred Belgian Wasserschlager canaries. Only male birds were used; female canaries sing little or not at all. In normal adult intact birds the song fundamental falls between .75 kHz and 5.5 kHz. Individual uninterrupted sounds measured on continuous sound spectrographic traces have a duration of from 5 to 400 msec. Typically, the briefer sounds consist of a very fast rising or falling frequency modulation subtending 1 or 2 kHz; the longer sounds consist of sustained whistles with relatively little frequency modulation. Sounds in the middle ranges of these two durations consist of relatively simple frequency modulations that on sound spectrographic display look like a stylized *S, L,* hyphen, or chevron shape. At times, one to three sounds occur as a unit, in a stereotyped, recurring association, separated by minimal temporal intervals or even showing temporal overlap. I shall call the individual sounds *elements* and the groupings they form *syllables,* but syllables can also consist of just one element. Repetitions of the same syllable constitute a *phrase.* These characteristics of canary song and the terminology just described are presented in Figure 3.

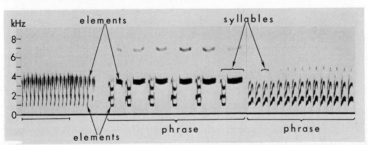

*Fig. 3. Fragment of song of an intact adult male canary. This example includes three different phases; each of the syllables in the first and second phrase is composed of two elements; syllables in the third phrase consist of a single element. Vertical and horizontal axes correspond, respectively, to frequency in kHz and time in seconds; horizontal bar indicates .5 sec. Second and third harmonics occur at twice and thrice the frequency of the fundamental and should not be counted as different elements.*

The complexity of a canary's song repertoire is measured in terms of numbers of different syllables included in its song. Whereas some syllables recur frequently in the song of a particular bird, others may be sung much more rarely. These differences in frequency of occurrence have not been tabulated.

Unlike birds such as the European chaffinch, *Fringilla coelebs,* and the New World's white-crowned sparrow, *Zonotrichia leucophrys,* in which each song is a stereotyped unit of fairly constant duration, successive songs of a particular canary may have grossly

varying lengths, e.g., from 2 to 30 sec. A half-minute song may
include as many as 15 different phrases. The complete song repertoire of adult canaries reared in aviary sound includes 19-37
different syllable types ($n$ = 23; mean = 25.8; SD = 7.5).


LEFT-HYPOGLOSSAL DOMINANCE

   Section of the tracheosyringealis branch of the right or left
hypoglossus nerve has grossly different effects, as measured by
the number of syllables remaining intact after the operation.
Sound spectrographic examples of this are shown in Figure 4.

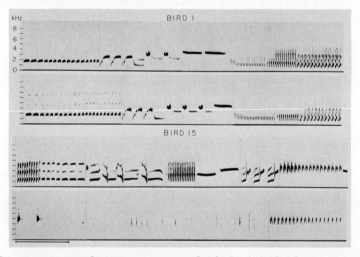

*Fig. 4.  Upper sound-spectrograms of birds 1 and 15 show samples
of their songs prior to surgery.  Lower sound-spectrograms show,
in each case, effects of cutting right (bird 1) or left (bird 15)
tracheosyringealis nerve.  Tables 2 and 4 quantify the losses
undergone by each bird after the operation.  Notice surviving
element at end of bird 15's postoperative song (from Nottebohm &
Nottebohm, 1976).*

In birds tested 5, 10, and 20 days after section of the right
tracheosyringealis nerve, an average of one-tenth of the syllables
disappear or are modified.  Sometimes just one element from a two-
element syllable disappears, to be replaced by a silent gap.
Sometimes the entire repertoire remains intact.  Five representative results of this type of effect are shown in Table 1.  To the
ear these birds sound perfectly normal and sing as well as before the operation.
   Section of the left tracheosyringealis nerve has a much more
dramatic effect.  In the extreme case all syllables disappear and
are replaced by silent gaps, faint clicking sounds, or distorted

28

TABLE 1

*Effects on song after section of right tracheosyringealis nerve*

| | No. of syllables | |
|---|---|---|
| Bird no. | Preoperative | Postoperative[a] |
| 1 | 33 | 31 + 1/2 |
| 2 | 33 | 31 |
| 3 | 29 | 25 |
| 4 | 22 | 19 |
| 34 | 25 | 25 |

[a]Number of preoperative syllables that survived intact after section of the right tracheosyringealis nerve; 1/2 refers to one of the two elements that composed a preoperative syllable.

modulations. Such birds sing vigorously, as judged by their posture and motion, yet look like actors in a silent cinema film. The bird holds its bill slightly open; its throat and chest pulsate in a quick, emphatic manner; the carpal-metacarpal joint (the wing's "wrist") is slightly raised above otherwise sleeked contour feathers; the bird flexes its tarsal-metatarsal joints ("heels") in a quick pumping motion, pivots on its perch, and tries to direct its song to a male or female canary placed in an adjoining cage. Yet no sound is heard, except some extremely faint clicks of undetermined syringeal or laryngeal origin. Then, unexpectedly, the bird breaks into loud song, delivering the one or two phrases that may have survived intact. It is common for such birds to produce, as before the operation, a few single elements of two- or three-element syllables, although the remainder of the syllable disappears or is grossly modified. Preoperative and postoperative scores of five birds with the left tracheosyringealis cut are shown in Table 2.

The simplest interpretation of these results is that syllables or elements controlled by the right tracheosyringealis disappear after section of this nerve, but remain intact after section of the left tracheosyringealis. Conversely, elements controlled by the left tracheosyringealis disappear or are grossly altered after section of this nerve, but remain intact after section of the right tracheosyringealis. These deficits persist at least over a period of a few months. From the scores presented here and elsewhere (Nottebohm & Nottebohm, 1976), it is clear that the tracheosyringealis branch of the left hypoglossus is dominant for song control. This dominance actually extends to the entire vocal repertoire of canaries. After section of the left tracheosyringe-

TABLE 2

*Effects on song after section of left tracheosyringealis nerve*

| Bird no. | No. of syllables | |
| --- | --- | --- |
| | Preoperative | Postoperative[a] |
| 12 | 32 | $\frac{1}{2}+\frac{1}{2}+\frac{1}{2}+\frac{1}{2}+\frac{1}{2}+\frac{1}{2}$ |
| 13 | 35 | $\frac{1}{3}+\frac{1}{3}$ |
| 14 | 37 | $\frac{1}{2}+\frac{1}{2}$ |
| 15 | 36 | $\frac{1}{2}+\frac{1}{2}+\frac{1}{2}$ |
| 25 | 24 | 0 |

[a] Number of preoperative syllables that survived intact after section of the left tracheosyringealis nerve; 1/2 and 1/3 refer, respectively, to one of the two or three elements that composed a preoperative syllable.

alis, virtually all sounds produced by these birds are faint and hoarse.

The different roles of the right and left hypoglossus are not due to the left tracheosyringealis innervating both syringeal halves and the right tracheosyringealis innervating only the ipsilateral syringeal musculature. Such a situation, however, has been described in domestic fowl (Youngren et al., 1974). A canary's song, not affected by section of the right tracheosyringealis nerve, remains unaffected after section of the musculature of the right syringeal half (Nottebohm & Nottebohm, 1976).

Examination of two- or three-element complex syllables (n = eight birds and 19 syllables) revealed that elements controlled by the right tracheosyringealis have higher frequency ranges (median 2.50-4.20 kHz) than those controlled by the left tracheosyringealis (median 1.25-2.40 kHz) (Nottebohm & Nottebohm, 1976). This observation suggests that the two syringeal halves may differ in certain physical characteristics, which are in turn reflected in the sounds they produce. This is only partly true. The left syringeal muscles are heavier (Figure 1), but this is probably a reflection of their greater use. Canaries that have

their left tracheosyringealis cut during their first two posthatching weeks develop normal repertoires, which are under the
sole control of the right tracheosyringealis nerve (unpublished
observation). It seems fair to conclude that either tracheosyringealis nerve and its corresponding syringeal half has the
potential to assume a dominant role in song control, yet this
role is normally bestowed on the left side.

The results of testing left-hypoglossal dominance in 37 adult
canaries have already been published (Notteboem & Nottebohm,
1976), and comparable data on 12 additional adult canaries are
now available. All 49 of the 49 adult male canaries tested so
far have shown left-hypoglossal dominance. The group of 37 birds
mentioned includes 2 individuals that were kept in 100 dB white
noise during their first month, followed by removal of both
cochleas. These 2 chronically deaf birds never had access to
their own auditory feedback. The same group also includes 5
birds that had the right cochlea removed when they were approximately 1 month old, and another 5 birds that had the left cochlea
removed at the same age. All bilaterally and unilaterally
deafened birds showed, when tested as adults, normal left-
hypoglossal dominance. To this extent, left-hypoglossal dominance
seems to emerge in the individual as a motor phenomenon, rather
than as a result of an underlying asymmetry in the processing of
auditory inputs.


CENTRAL CONTROL OF CANARY SONG

The results described thus far refer to the efferent, distal
manifestation of a lateralization phenomenon, whose ontogeny and
control, it was felt, must surely be sought in the central nervous system. A stereotaxic atlas of the canary brain was produced (Stokes, Leonard, & Nottebohm, 1974). It was then possible
to explore the occurrence of brain vocal areas.

The motor neurons innervating the syrinx were identified by
noting retrograde degenerative changes that followed section of
one tracheosyringealis nerve. The large cells of the caudal two-
thirds of what was at the time called *nucleus intermedius*, IM
(Karten & Hodos, 1967), underwent chromatolytic changes and eventually disappeared after section of the ipsilateral tracheosyringealis nerve. This and other tests indicated that IM was a
misnomer for the avian hypoglossal nucleus, and it was decided to
label its posterior two-thirds *pars tracheosyringealis*, abbrevi-
ated nXIIts. The anterior one-third became *pars lingualis*
(Nottebohm *et al.*, 1976). It seemed likely that any song control
system regulating syringeal function would ultimately project to
nXIIts. Since canaries learn their song by reference to auditory
information, it was expected that the highest station of a vocal
control system would be close to field L, the telencephalic auditory projection (Biederman-Thorson, 1970; Karten, 1968; Leppelsack, 1974; Leppelsack & Schwartzkopff, 1972; Rose, 1914). This

speculation proved correct. Large unilateral lesions that included field L had dramatic effects on song. Next, the size of
the lesion was reduced until the full effect ceased to be obtained. In this manner a superficial, discrete, large-celled
area, lying dorsal and slightly caudal to field L, was identified.
This rather novel area, not previously described in other birds,
was named the *hyperstriatum ventrale, pars caudale*, or *HVc*. Unilateral lesions there greatly disturbed the quality of song. Bilateral lesions of HVc resulted in "silent song," described
earlier as characterizing the song of canaries after section of
the left tracheosyringealis nerve. Unilateral lesions of field L
itself had no immediate effects on song.

The relation of HVc, nXIIts, and field L to the rest of the
canary brain can be seen in Figure 5. Lesions of HVc induce

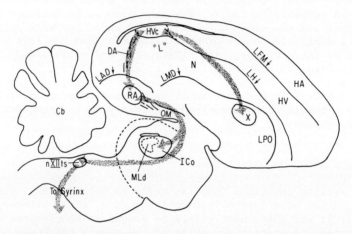

*Fig. 5. Schematic sagittal section of the canary brain on which
brain structures and pathways implicated in song control have
been outlined. Unilateral lesions restricted to hyperstriatum
ventrale, pars caudale (HVc) result in major song disruptions.
Degenerating fibers traced from such lesions end in area X and
nucleus robustus archistriatalis (RA). Unilateral lesions of RA
also disrupt song. A direct pathway links RA to nXIIts, the
motor nucleus innvervating the syrinx (from Nottebohm et al.,
1976).*

degeneration in a pathway that terminates in another hitherto un-
described structure, the nucleus robustus archistriatalis, RA,
which in turn projects to nXIIts. Lesions of RA also have profound effects on the quality of song. Thus, at least three stations, HVc, RA, and nXIIts, that are part of a direct, ipsilateral, efferent pathway controlling song have been identified. A
fourth, cytoarchitectonically discrete area, X of the lobus parol-
factorious (Figure 5), receives a heavy projection from the ipsilateral HVc; its function remains unknown. Similarly, no role has

yet been assigned to the nucleus intercollicularis of the midbrain, ICo, which receives a heavy ipsilateral projection from RA.
Other investigators report that electrical stimulation of ICo in
a variety of birds elicits calls, but no song (Brown, 1965, 1971;
Delius, 1971; Maley, 1969; Murphey & Phillips, 1967; Newman, 1970;
Potash, 1970a, b; Putkonen, 1967). In the canary, unilateral
lesions of ICo have little, if any, effect on song. Because ICo
sends no direct projection to nXIIts it does not seem to be part
of a direct efferent pathway. Perhaps ICo affects vocal behavior
by altering its probability of occurrence, or to put it more
grossly, by setting the "mood" (see also de Lanerolle and Andrew,
1974). Further projections from RA, X, and ICo are described in
Nottebohm et al. (1976).

Efforts to obtain a more complete picture of the connectivity
of the various brain areas that are part of the vocal control
system are still in progress. A pathway linking field L and HVc
has not yet been found; in fact there is no information on projections from field L to anywhere in the telencephalon. The ipsi-

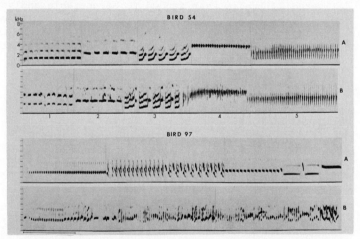

*Fig. 6. Bird 54: (A) Segment of song recorded 5 July 1973.
This bird's right HVc was destroyed on the following day. (B)
Canary 54 was recorded again on 17 July 1973. Notice that good
phrase structure is retained; syllables 1, 2, 3, and 5 closely
resemble their preoperative versions. In this example syllable 2
is accompanied at times by a second, unrelated sound. Syllable 4
did not occur before the operation, though it may be a distortion
of the intact syllable shown above it. Bird 97. (A) Segment of
song recorded 18 April 1974. This bird's left HVc was destroyed
on the following day. (B) Bird 97 recorded 24 April 1974.
Phrase structure is almost absent, most of the sounds produced
are highly variable, and two unrelated sounds occur frequently.
Opening part of this segment of song is the closest match this
bird ever produced to syllables that resembled a preoperative
counterpart (from Nottebohm et al., 1976).*

lateral nature of the projections mapped so far is similarly intriguing. Since lesions of either right or left HVc and RA have
effects on song (see the following section), but virtually all
singing is controlled by the left tracheosyringealis, there would
seem to be a need for pathways integrating the influence of both
halves of the brain on song.

HEMISPHERIC DOMINANCE FOR SONG CONTROL

There were dramatic differences between the postoperative song
of birds lesioned in the right or left hemisphere. Electrolytic
lesions of the right or left HVc were produced in 10 aviary-
reared, adult male canaries by means of two or three electrode
penetrations, each delivering 80-90  µA for 60 sec.

Following lesions of the right HVc, birds reproduced one-third
to three-fifths or more of their preoperative syllable repertoires. Some birds sang as well as before the operation, but
others delivered syllables that tended to be unstable and variable. Some syllables were at times accompanied by simultaneous
and harmonically unrelated frequencies, presumably because the
right and left syringeal sound sources were poorly coordinated

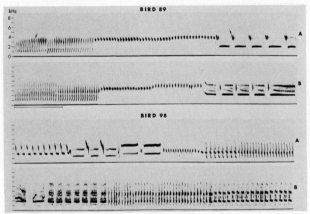

*Fig. 7. Bird 89. (A) Fragment of song recorded 13 March 1974,
while the bird was intact. RA of right hemisphere destroyed on
the following day. (B) Recording of 20 March 1974. Phrase
structure remains unaltered. The first and last syllables, which
before the operation consisted of more than one element, after
the operation lost one element each, indicated by arrows. Last
syllable of the postoperative recording shows a second, poorly
modulated sound. Bird 98. (A) Fragment of song recorded 8 May
1974, while the bird was intact. RA of the left hemisphere destroyed on the following day. (B) Recording of 20 May 1974.
Phrase structure is preserved, but syllable structure is drastically altered. Most of the time the bird produced two unrelated
sounds (from Nottebohm et al., 1976).*

and generated unrelated sounds. Otherwise, these birds sang vigorously and their song was organized in clear-cut phrases, much as had been the case before the operation. To the ear, these songs approached the performance of intact birds.

Following lesions of the left HVc, none, or at most one, of the syllables could be produced as they were preoperatively (see Figure 6 and Table 3). The song of these birds was very monotonous. They sang an unstable, simple succession of notes, rising and falling in pitch. There was also a sporadic incidence of two simultaneous and unrelated sounds. When phrase structure did occur, it was restricted to the one syllable that had been least upset by the operation.

Smaller, unilateral lesions of RA also affected song, and in this case too lesions to the left side induced the greater deficit (Figure 7). Whereas lesions to either right or left RA resulted in a drastic reduction in the number of preoperative syllables produced after the operation (canary 89, right RA lesion had a preoperative repertoire of 28 syllables, a postoperative

TABLE 3

*Syllable count of birds with left HVc lesion*

| Bird no. | Preoperative | Postoperative | | |
|---|---|---|---|---|
| | | 10 days (1974)[a] | 7 months (1975)[b] | Postsection[c] |
| 97 | 20 | 0 | e | |
| 1 | 25 | 1 | 23 | 0 |
| 2 | 28 | 1 | 22 | 0 |
| 3 | 33 | d | 31 | 1½ |
| 4 | 23 | 1 | 10 | 8 |

[a]Preoperative syllables that persisted intact when bird was recorded 7-10 days after operation.

[b]The 1975 syllable repertoire overlaps only partly with the 1974 preoperative repertoire; many of the 1975 syllables are new (see Table 5).

[c]Syllables from 1975 repertoire that survived intact section of the right tracheosyringealis nerve; recorded during the 7 days following the operation.

[d]This bird was not recorded during this period.

[e]Not recorded in 1975.

35

repertoire of 9, 1/2, 1/3, 1/3; canary 98, left RA lesion, had a
preoperative repertoire of 26, a postoperative repertoire of 3),
only a lesion to the left RA resulted in a marked reduction in the
frequency range of the song fundamental. The fundamental frequency of canary 98's preoperativ  recordings ranged between 1 and 4
kHz, but after the operation most of the fundamental frequencies
had a very narrow spread (between 1.7 and 2.1 kHz). Since our
knowledge about the effects of right or left RA lesions is at the
present restricted to two birds (described in greater detail in
Nottebohm et al., 1976), these results should be considered as
preliminary and susceptible to modification as the size of the
sample grows. However, they do confirm a greater involvement of
the left hemisphere in song control.


SONG RECOVERY FOLLOWING BRAIN LESION

Seven of the 10 birds with unilateral HVc lesions (Tables 3
and 4) were recorded during the first 10 days after the operation


TABLE 4

*Syllable count of birds with right HVc lesion*

| | | Postoperative | | |
|---|---|---|---|---|
| Bird no. | Preoperative | 10 days (1974)[a] | 7 months (1975)[b] | Post section[c] |
| 46 | 28 | 8 | d | |
| 54 | 25 | 19 | d | |
| 5 | 24 | 8½ | 24 | 22 |
| 6 | 23 | 14 | 30 | 30 |
| 7 | 21 | 18 | 30 | 30 |

[a]Preoperative syllables that persisted intact when bird was
recorded 7-10 days after operation.

[b]The 1975 syllable repertoire overlaps only partly with the
1974 preoperative repertoire; many of the 1975 syllables are new
(see Table 5).

[c]Syllables from 1975 repertoire that survived intact section
of the right tracheosyringealis nerve; recorded during the 7 days
following the latter operation.

[d]Not recorded in 1975.

and again 7 months later as they came into breeding condition and song for a second time. These birds had been 12 months old at the time of their brain operation. It was expected that the behavioral differences between birds having right HVc lesions and birds having left HVc lesions would become accentuated over the 7-month postoperative period. It was a great surprise to find that, with one exception, by the following year the song of birds in both groups had undergone remarkable recovery. The two groups differed in that whereas the song of right-lesioned birds was as good as it was preoperatively, some syllables of the left-lesioned birds were unstable, and as a group these syllables tended to be simpler than those produced by the right-lesioned birds (see Figures 8 and 9). (The latter impression has not yet been

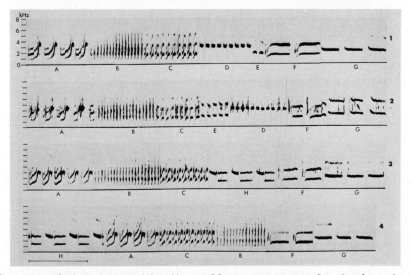

*Fig. 8. Bird 6 (see Table 4). Effects on song of a lesion that totally destroyed the right HVc. (1) Fragment of preoperative song. (2) Song recorded 7 days after lesion of right HVc. (3) Song recorded 7 months after right HVc lesion. (4) Song recorded 4 days after section of right tracheosyringealis. Letters A, B, C, D, E, F, and G identify preoperative syllables. Following recovery from brain lesion these syllables were produced first in a rather unstable and noisy manner; the background noise in (2) is attributable to a poorly controlled second sound source. Seven months after the original operation, this bird's song was much better. Section of the right tracheosyringealis nerve had, if anything, a beneficial effect on song, since after the operation some of the unwanted background sounds disappeared. Syllable H appeared for the first time 7 months after brain lesion.*

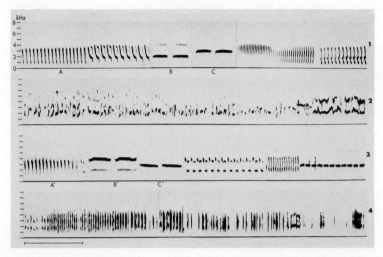

Fig. 9. Bird 2 (Table 3). Effects on song of a lesion that
totally destroyed the left HVc. (1) Fragment of preoperative
song. (2) Song recorded 7 days after lesion of left HVc.
(3) Song recorded 7 months after left HVc lesion. (4) Song recorded 4 days after section of right tracheosyringealis. Letters
A, B, and C identify preoperative syllables; A', B', and C' identify the somewhat altered postoperative version of these same
syllables. No syllable survived section of the right tracheosyringealis (see text).

quantified.) Also, whereas right-HVc-operated birds redeveloped
a repertoire as great as or greater than that of the previous
year, the repertoire developed by left-HVc-operated birds was in
all cases smaller than it had been before the operation.

Much as in intact birds, some of the syllables of our operated
birds were carry-overs from the previous year, but others were
new. Some of the syllables that had been recorded soon after the
operation were now absent; others, absent during the first 10
postoperative days, were now present. Interestingly, whereas the
new repertoire of the right-HVc-operated birds included about
half the previous year's preoperative syllables, that of left-
HVc-operated birds included from none to one-fourth of the preoperative syllables (Table 5). This suggests that under normal
conditions memory of the song repertoire acquired during the
bird's first year of life is strongly associated with the left
HVc, and less so or not at all with the right HVc.

There is as yet no clear picture of the involvement of HVc in
song control, or of the relation between right and left HVc.
However, one possible interpretation of these observations is as
follows: Normally, the left HVc plays a dominant role in song
learning and in storage or retrieval of efferent song memories.
This dominant role is achieved, at least in part, by inhibiting

TABLE 5

*Occurrence of preoperative syllables seven months after unilateral HVc lesion*

| | No. of syllables | |
| --- | --- | --- |
| Bird no. | Preoperative | Postoperative[a] |
| 5 | 24 | 11 (R) |
| 6 | 23 | 11 (R) |
| 7 | 21 | 15 (R) |
| 1 | 25 | $7+\frac{1}{2}+\frac{1}{2}$ (L) |
| 2 | 28 | 6 (L) |
| 3 | 33 | 5 (L) |
| 4 | 23 | 0 (L) |

[a]R, right HVc lesion; L, left HVc lesion.

the involvement of the right HVc. This inhibition is lifted by destruction of the left HVc, and the right HVc can then get more involved in song learning.

If this interpretation is correct, then after a total lesion of the left HVc, both the right HVc and the right hypoglossus (i.e. the right HVc's ipsilateral efferent system) should become dominant, whereas destruction of the right HVc should be followed by no change in left-hypoglossal dominance. These predictions are borne out by the results presented in Tables 4 and 5. The only exception, bird 4 (Table 3), redeveloped a small, 10-syllable repertoire and retained left-hypoglossal dominance. We do not yet know why this bird differed from others in its group. It may have to do with the detailed nature of the lesion, and this is a problem that is currently being explored.

Ongoing experiments indicate that left-hemispheric (HVc) dominance can also be turned into right-hemispheric dominance by cutting the left tracheosyringealis during the first 2 posthatching weeks. In such birds the left tracheosyringealis nerve does not regrow and the left nXIIts disappears. Subsequent destruction of the left HVc in these same birds as adults has the same effect as destruction of the right HVc in an otherwise intact bird!

OVERVIEW

The vocal control system described here is appealing because

it is relatively simple, compared with the human system, and because it is so amenable to manipulation. It is also attractive
in that the lateralization of function seems to be robust and pre-
dictable. A total of 16 chaffinches (Nottebohm, 1971), 49
canaries, and 2 white-crowned sparrows have been tested so far in
our laboratory. Each of these 67 birds was left-hypoglossus dominant. Fifteen white-throated sparrows were tested by Lemon
(1973). Whereas 14 of these birds showed clear-cut left-hypoglossal dominance, the 15th bird seemed to control half of the song
elements with the right hypoglossus, and half with the left hypoglossus. The latter bird's age at the time of the operation was
not known, so part of the ambiguity of this result may reflect
quick relearning by a young bird. It is impressive that out of
81 songbirds of four different species tested, only one bird
failed to give clear-cut evidence of lef-thypoglossal dominance.
Thus, the occurrence of this phenomenon is much more homogeneous
and reliable than handedness or hemispheric dominance in man.

Hemispheric dominance in man and hypoglossal dominance in
songbirds are associated with vocal learning. Thus, when left-
hypoglossal dominance in the chaffinch was first encountered, we
were tempted to conclude that dominance phenomena of this type
may be related to complex learned behaviors (Nottebohm, 1970).
More recent findings raise doubts as to the correctness of this
interpretation. For example, parrots are a group notorious for
their vocal talents and the ability with which they learn new
sounds. Yet, the right and left hypoglossus of the orange-winged
Amazon parrot, *Amazona amazonica*, partake equally in vocal control and each nerve innervates both syringeal halves (n = 7;
Nottebohm, 1976). In the light of this finding it was particularly surprising to learn that in domestic fowl the left hypoglossus innervates both syringeal halves, but the right one only
innervates the right half (Youngren et al., 1974). However, these
authors do not report on whether or not the left hypoglossus
normally has a greater involvement in song control. We do not
know what advantages a species might derive by evolving hypoglossal or hemispheric dominance, and as a result cannot yet predict
what types of behavior may have led to such asymmetric neural
control. If hemispheric dominance in birds such as the canary is
comparable to the human phenomenon, then we might expect to find
the right hemisphere, in turn, specialized or superior in some
other kind of task.

Left-hypoglossal and left-hemispheric dominance, as described
so far in canaries, is a motor phenomenon. Differences in auditory processing, as reported by Kimura (1963, 1967) and Teuber
(1975) could be the primary cause for the observed lateralization. (See Anderson; Berlin; Springer; cf. Dewson, this volume.)
The present experiments with unilaterally and bilaterally-
deafened canaries do not lend substance to this supposition.
However, these experiments do not by themselves negate possible
right-left asymmetries in the processing of auditory signals,

particularly because each cochlea sends information to both halves of the brain (Karten, 1968). Intriguingly, Stanley Cobb (1964) noted that the left midbrain auditory projection (the torus) of an owl (*Aegolius acadicus*) and the oilbird (*Steatornis caripensis*) is larger than the right auditory projection. However, Cobb based these observations on very small samples and it would seem worthwhile to see them repeated.

It seems clear that the left-hemispheric or left-hypoglossal dominance system described for vocal control in songbirds is a useful model for studying localization and lateralization of function, and neural plasticity and recovery of function following brain lesion. Also, because birds are such a diverse phylogenetic group, and because song is such a convenient behavior to study, avian material of the kind described here may be helpful in unraveling the evolution and ontogeny of localization and lateralization of a well-defined function.

SUMMARY

Adult Wasserschlager canaries that are reared in an aviary room where they can hear many other conspecifics develop songs of from 19 to 37 different syllable types. These songs are developed by reference to auditory information and maintained by reference to auditory feedback from each bird's own vocalizations. A majority of song syllables are produced by the left half of the syrinx, under the control of the tracheosyringealis branch of the left hypoglossus nerve. This phenomenon of left-hypoglossal dominance occurs in aviary-reared birds with intact hearing, in canaries unilaterally deafened as juveniles, and in canaries kept in 100 dB of white noise during their first posthatching month, then deafened. To this extent, left-hypoglossal dominance is a motor phenomenon. Left-hypoglossal dominance also occurs in three other songbird species, the chaffinch, white-crowned sparrow, and white-throated sparrow.

Three sites in the brain have been identified and shown to be involved in vocal control: the hyperstriatum ventrale, pars caudale (HVc), the robust nucleus of the archistriatum (RA), and the caudal, tracheosyringealis part of the hypoglossal nucleus (nXIIts). The latter nucleus includes the motor neurons innervating the syringeal muscles. Only ipsilateral connections between these systems have been described. Unilateral lesions of HVc and RA in adult, aviary-reared birds have immediate and dramatic effects on song, and these effects are more marked when lesions are placed in the left hemisphere. Recordings 7 months after lesion of the right or left HVc show a remarkable degree of recovery, so that the song of birds in either group resembles that of intact adult birds. However, even after recovery, the song of left-lesioned birds remains more unstable and less structured, and includes far fewer of its own preoperative elements.

In these latter birds the right hypoglossus is now dominant, and section of this nerve results in the loss of a majority of song syllables.
HVc dominance can also be reversed by early section of the left tracheosyringealis nerve. These birds develop their entire song under the control of the right tracheosyringealis. Subsequent lesion of the left HVc in adulthood results in song deficits of the kind normally following lesion of the right HVc in an otherwise intact adult canary.
The lateralization phenomenon described refers to a complex, learned, behavior controlled by anatomically discrete brain areas. It might prove to be a convenient system for studying the ontogeny of lateralization of function and the nature of processes permitting recovery of function following brain lesion.

## ACKNOWLEDGMENTS

I am greatly indebted to the following people:  Christiana M. Leonard and Harvey J. Karten for advice in neuroanatomy and neurohistology; Tegner M. Stokes and Yvonne Holland for their impeccable processing of histological material; Betsy Manning for her patience in recording my birds.  Marta E. Seeber de Nottebohm did the sound spectrographic analysis of these recordings; I want to thank her for that, but also more particularly for her constant support and enthusiasm.  This work was conducted under the auspices of NIMH Grant 18343.

## REFERENCES

Biederman-Thorsen, M.  Auditory evoked responses in the cerebrum (field L) and ovoid nucleus of the ring dove. *Brain Research*, 1970, *24*, 235–245.
Brown, J. L.  Loss of vocalizations caused by lesions in the nucleus mesencephalicus lateralis of the Redwinged Blackbird. *American Zoologist*, 1965, *5*, 693.
Brown, J. L.  An exploratory study of vocalization areas in the brain of the Redwinged Blackbird (*Agelaius phoeniceus*). *Behaviour*, 1971, *39*, 91–127.
Chamberlain, D. R., Gross, W. B., Cornwell, G. W., & Mosby, H. S. Syringeal anatomy in the common crow. *Auk*, 1968, *85*, 244–252.
Cobb, S.  A comparison of the size of an Auditory Nucleus (n. mesencephalicus lateralis, pars dorsalis) with the size of the optic lobe in twenty-seven species of birds. *Journal of Comparative Neurology*, 1964, *122*, 271–280.
Conrad, R.  Untersuchungen über den unteren Kehlkopf der Vögel. I. Zur Kenntnis der Innervierung. *Zeitschrift für Wissenschaftliche Zoologie*, 1915, *114*, 532–576.
de Lanerolle, N., & Andrew, R. J.  Midbrain structures controlling

vocalization in the domestic chick. *Brain, Behaviour &
Evolution*, 1974, *10*, 354-376.
Delius, J. D.   Neural substrates of vocalization in gulls and
pigeons. *Experimental Brain Research*, 1971, *12*, 64-80.
Dürrwang, R.   Funktionelle Biologie, Anatomie und Physiologie
der Vogelstimme. Unpublished Ph.D. dissertation, Univ. of
Basel, 1974.
Gaunt, A. S., & Wells, M. K.   Models of syringeal mechanisms.
*American Zoologist*, 1973, *13*, 1227-1247.
Greenewalt, C. H.   *Bird song, acoustics and physiology*.
Washington, D.C.:   Smithsonian Institution Press, 1968.
Hersch, G. L.   Bird voices and resonant tuning in helium-air
mixtures. Unpublished Ph.D. dissertation, Univ. of
California, Berkeley, 1966.
Karten, H.J.   The ascending auditory pathways in the pigeon
(*Columba livia*).  II.  Telencephalic projections of the nu-
cleus ovoidalis thalami. *Brain Research*, 1968, *11*, 134-153.
Karten, H.J., & Hodos, W.   *A stereotaxic atlas of the brain of
the pigeon* (Columba livia). Baltimore:  Johns Hopkins
Press, 1967.
Kimura, D.   Speech lateralization in young children as determined
by an auditory test. *Journal of Comparative and Physio-
logical Psychology*, 1963, *56*, 899-902.
Kimura, D.   Functional asymmetry of the brain in dichotic listen-
ing.  *Cortex*, 1967, *III*, 163-178.
Klatt, D. H., & Stefanski, R. A.   How does a mynah bird imitate
human speech. *Journal of the Acoustical Society of
America*, 1974, *55*, 822-832.
Lemon, R. E.   Nervous control of the syrinx in White-throated
sparrows (*Zonotrichia albicollis*).  *Journal of Zoology,
London*, 1973, *71*, 131-140.
Leppelsack, H-J.   Funktionelle Eigenschaften der Hörbahn im Feld
L des Neostriatum caudale des Staren (*Sturnus vulgaris L.,
Aves*).  *Journal of Comparative Physiology*, 1974, *88*, 271-320.
Leppelsack, H-J., & Schwartzkopff, J.   Eigenschaften von
akustischen Neuronen im kaudalen Neostriatum von Vögeln.
*Journal of Comparative Physiology*, 1972, *80*, 137-140.
Maley, M. J.   Electrical stimulation of agonistic behaviour in
the mallard. *Behaviour*, 1969, *34*, 138-160.
Marler, P., Konishi, M., Lutjen, A., & Waser, M. S.   Effects of
continuous noise on avian hearing and vocal development.
*Proceedings of the National Academy of Sciences of the U.S.*,
1973, *70*, 1393-1396.
Metfessel, M.   Roller canary song produced without learning from
external source. *Science*, 1935, *81*, 470.
Miskimen, M.   Sound production in passerine birds. *Auk*, 1951,
*68*, 493-504.
Murphey, R. K., & Phillips, R. E.   Central patterning of a
vocalization in fowl. *Nature*, 1967, *216*, 1125-1126.
Newman, J. D.   Midbrain regions relevant to auditory communication in songbirds. *Brain Research*, 1970, *22*, 259-261.

Nottebohm, F. Ontogeny of bird song. *Science*, 1970, *167*, 950-956.

Nottebohm, F. Neural lateralization of vocal control in a passerine bird. I. Song. *Journal of Experimental Zoology*, 1971, *177*, 229-262.

Nottebohm, F. Phonation in the orange-winged Amazon parrot. *Amazona amazonica*. *Journal of Comparative Physiology, Series A*, 1976 (in galley stage, pages not yet available).

Nottebohm, F., & Nottebohm, M. E. Left hypoglossal dominance in the control of canary and white-crowned sparrow song. *Journal of Comparative Physiology, Series A*, 1976, (in galley stage; no page numbers yet available).

Nottebohm, F., Stokes, T. M., & Leonard, C. M. Central control of song in the canary, *Serinus canaria*. *Journal of Comparative Neurology*, 1976, *165*, 457-486.

Potash, L. M. Vocalizations elicited by electrical brain stimulation in *Coturnix coturnix japonica*. *Behavior*, 1970, *36*, 149-167. (a)

Potash, L. M. Neuroanatomical regions relevant to production and analysis of vocalization within the avian *Torus semicircularis*. *Experientia*, 1970, *26*, 1104-1105. (b)

Poulsen, H. Song learning in the domestic canary. *Zeitschrift für Tierpsychologie*, 1959, *16*, 173-178.

Putkonen, P. T. S. Electrical stimulation of the avian brain. *Annales Academiae Scientarum Fennicae*, 1967, *130*, Series A, 1-95.

Rose, M. Über die cytoarchitectonische Gliederung des Vorherhirns der Vogel. *Journal für Psychologische Neurologie*, 1914, *21*, 278-352.

Stokes, T. M., Leonard, C. M., & Nottebohm, F. The telencephalon, diencephalon, and mesencephalon of the canary, *Serinus canaria*, in the stereotaxic coordinates. *Journal of Comparative Neurology*, 1974, *156*, 337-374.

Teuber, H-L. Effects of focal brain injury on human behavior. In D. B. Tower (Ed.), *The Nervous System*, Vol. 2: *The Clinical Neurosciences*. New York: Raven Press, 1975. Pp. 457-480.

Youngren, O. M., Peek, F. W., & Phillips, R. E. Repetitive vocalizations evoked by local electrical stimulation of avian brains. *Brain, Behavior, and Evolution*, 1974, *9*, 393-421.

# 3.
# Investigations of Perceptual and Mnemonic Lateralization in Monkeys

*CHARLES R. HAMILTON*

California Institute of Technology

The existence of hemispheric specialization in infrahuman animals is frequently denied, although it has seldom been looked for systematically. The extent to which hemispheric specialization exists in animals is of course crucial for understanding the phylogenetic basis of cerebral dominance in man and for evaluating philosophical positions concerning the uniqueness of human consciousness. Furthermore, if hemispheric specialization were found in some animals, it would be singularly useful for studying mechanisms of ontogenetic development and modification of cortical asymmetries. For these reasons I will take for granted the importance of establishing the degree of hemispheric specialization in different animals, and concentrate on presenting the results of some systematic behavioral studies of dominance in rhesus monkeys. Despite my opinion that hemispheric specialization evolved independently of human language as a means for simultaneously and differentially analyzing sensory information by sequential and holistic processes, I shall take the position, perhaps at odds with other chapters in this volume (see Dewson; Doty & Overman; Rubens; Stamm, Rosen, & Gadotti; Webster, this volume), that the cerebral hemispheres of monkeys are not differentially organized for perceptual processing or for storage of memories, but instead that they are essentially equipotential for these abilities.

All the results reported are from experiments with juvenile rhesus monkeys that learned or remembered visual discriminations following varying degrees of forebrain bisection. Two principal questions were asked: (1) Will split-brain monkeys remember with

both hemispheres or just one the problems taught monocularly
while their brains were either still intact or only partially
split?  (2) After brain bisection, will the ability of each
hemisphere to learn or perform discriminations be quantitatively
different, and if so, will it vary qualitatively with the type of
stimuli to be discriminated, as is found with human beings?

Answering these questions adequately requires a large number
of naive animals, trained under similar conditions on several
identical problems in experimental designs balanced for variables
that might correlate with hemispheric asymmetries.  This is
necessary to minimize the effects of previous experience, of
asymmetric procedures for training or testing, and of possible
asymmetries induced by surgery.  It is usually not feasible to
study large numbers of split-brain monkeys under such stringent
conditions, but I had to replace my entire colony because of a
suspected tuberculosis infection, and it was thus possible to
fulfill the conditions.

Thirty-six monkeys were first adapted to the laboratory environment and then tested for several days to determine hand
preferences in reaching for food placed on a tray or in a bottle
(Warren, Abplanalp, & Warren, 1967; Warren, this volume).  Next,
they each learned 3 two-choice visual discriminations (Set I) in
an automated apparatus (Sperry, 1968) to familiarize them with
the training procedures and to ensure that they could use all
eye-hand combinations.  Then the brains of 16 of these monkeys
were split or partially split; the rest remained  unoperated
until after additional training.  All structures were sectioned
from above using standard procedures (Sperry, 1968; Sullivan &
Hamilton, 1973).  The surgical preparations included split-chiasm
monkeys (SC); split-brain monkeys (SB)  with section of the optic
chiasm, corpus callosum, hippocampal commissure, and anterior
commissure; intact splenium monkeys (IS), which were similar to
SB monkeys except that the posterior 1 cm of the corpus callosum
was left intact; and intact anterior commissure monkeys (IAC),
split except for the anterior commissure.  In monkeys with
split chiasms, between .5 and 1 cm of the body of the corpus
callosum was also sectioned to allow a dorsal approach to the
chiasm through the part of the third ventricle lying anterior to
the massa intermedia.  After 1 week of recovery, training was
started on the basic discriminations (Set II).  All experimental
designs were balanced with respect to the hemisphere retracted
during surgery, the eye and hand trained on the different discriminations, and, as far as practical, hand preferences of the
monkeys.


LEARNING ABILITY OF OPERATED MONKEYS

It was necessary first to determine how split-brain surgery
affects the learning and performance of visual problems during
the immediate postoperative period  in order to form a base

level against which performance by the SB monkeys tested for retention could be compared. Groups of partially split monkeys
(SC, IS, IAC) were also included as part of a larger study of the
effects of brain bisection on discriminative abilities. Each of
the monkeys learned four problems comprising Set II, two with the
right eye and left hand and two with the left eye and right hand,
to a criterion of 36 correct out of 40 trials.
    The results are summarized in Figure 1. It is obvious that

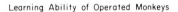

Learning Ability of Operated Monkeys

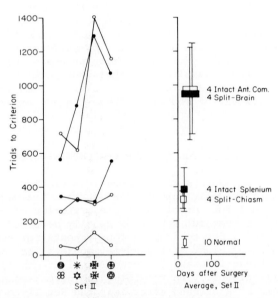

*Fig. 1. On the left are graphed the mean trials to criterion
required for each problem of Set II for the five groups of
monkeys described on the right. The patterns are pictured in the
order presented. On the right is shown the average performance
of each group on these problems. The width of the bars indicates the days after surgery over which the training took place
and the flags indicate the standard deviation of the means of
each monkey's trials averaged for the four problems.*

the SB and IAC monkeys took longer to reach criterion (about 1000
trials) than did the IS or SC monkeys (about 350 trials), which
in turn took longer than the normal (N) monkeys (about 75 trials).
That the large, persistent deficit shown by the SB and IAC
groups was not caused by incidental damage during surgery is
shown by the results from the IS group. This group had essentially the same surgical treatment as the SB and IAC groups, yet
learned no more slowly than the SC group. Therefore, this
large deficit must result from specific disconnection of
posterior cortex interconnected by the splenium; analogous

47

disconnection of inferotemporal areas interconnected by the anterior commissure (IS group) did not produce this severe deficit
(cf. Gross & Mishkin, this volume). Presumably, neural mechanisms needed for learning the problems of Set II are primarily
located in posterior neocortex, and they are depressed by the
denervation caused by splenial section. The smaller deficit seen
in the IS and SC groups could result either from the hemianopia
that follows section of the optic chiasm or from incidental
damage associated with the dorsal approach to the chiasm.

All these deficits diminished over the months following
surgery, although 1 or 2 years later the SB monkeys still required about twice as many trials as N monkeys to reach criterion. The retarded learning could result from deficits in attention, perception, learning, memory, or performance; they are
termed learning deficits for descriptive purposes only. Whatever the cause, these results show that postoperative performance
is depressed, and that surgical controls are needed to evaluate
accurately the extent of memories present in the experimental
groups.

MEMORY ESTABLISHMENT IN THE TWO CEREBRAL HEMISPHERES

Eighteen of the monkeys that learned the problem of Set II as
intact or partially split animals were further trained until they
could remember all four problems at the criterion of 36/40 after
a 1-week rest. Successful retention usually occurred on the
first delayed test, but took up to four retests for some monkeys.
Next, the brains of eight of the normal monkeys were split, and
the forebrain bisection was completed for eight monkeys from the
partially split groups. The remaining two normal monkeys had
only their chiasms sectioned after learning Set II to assess retention deficits arising from this part of the surgery. After a
1-week recuperation period the monkeys were tested for retention
of each problem with each eye and contralateral hand. The design
was balanced for which eye was tested first on the different
problems and in different monkeys. As additional controls, four
naive monkeys were taught Set I followed by a set of four additional problems. The optic chiasm and forebrain commissures were
then split, and 1 week later they were trained on Set II. These
monkeys thus had an equivalent amount of learning experience before surgery, but they had no memories for Set II. Therefore
they provide an estimate of how badly the 16 SB monkeys should
have performed had they no memories for Set II in either of
their hemispheres.

Data for the eight monkeys trained with intact brains will be
described first, followed by analogous data for the eight monkeys
trained with partially split brains, and finally the average results for all experimental and control groups will be presented.

## MONKEYS TRAINED AS NORMALS

If cerebral asymmetries exist for establishing memories preferentially in one hemisphere, then training animals having
normal brains and then testing each hemisphere for retention
after split-brain surgery should reveal which hemisphere has the
memory. Both Gazzaniga (1963) and Webster (1972; this volume)
have reported lateralized memories in animals trained and tested
in this fashion. Since their results seem surprising in view of
the predominantly bilateral memories reported for animals trained
with unilateral sensory input, as summarized in the next section
of this chapter, additional evidence was sought.

Results for the eight monkeys trained with their brains intact are shown in Figure 2. Two measures of retention are given

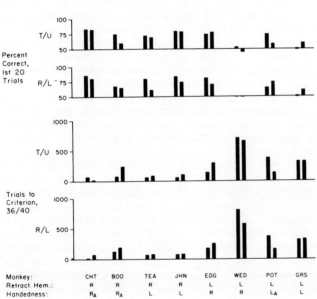

Fig. 2. *Below each monkey's code are indicated the hemisphere
retracted during surgery and the preferred hand. Subscript A
signifies an ambidextrous monkey, defined as making less than 2/3
of its reaches with the preferred hand. Abbreviations: T,
trained; U, untrained; R, right; L, left. In the rows the
monkeys' performances are plotted as pairs of bars with the T eye
placed to the left of the U eye, and the R eye to the left of the
L eye.*

for each hemisphere: (1) initial performance on the first 20
trials, shown in the upper two rows, and (2) trials to criterion,
shown in the lower two rows. For each measure the data are

arranged in two ways: by trained and untrained eyes (T/U) and by right and left eyes (R/L). A comparison of performance between the hemispheres contra and ipsilateral to the preferred hand, or between the retracted and nonretracted hemispheres, can be obtained by rearranging the R/L data according to the designations at the bottom of the figure.

The data in Figure 2 are averaged for the four problems of Set II, but are representative of individual problems. Most monkeys initially performed above chance and took fewer trials to reattain criterion than did the control monkeys that learned the problems after split-brain surgery (Figure 5). It is apparent from both measures of retention that individual monkeys formed bilateral memories of approximately equal strength in the right and left hemispheres. This disagrees with Gazzaniga's (1963) finding of a right-hemisphere advantage in initial postoperative performance of a discrimination taught preoperatively to three monkeys. Furthermore, there is no significant difference between postoperative performance with the hemisphere ipsilateral to the preferred hand and that with the hemisphere contralateral. This differs from Webster's (1972; this volume) finding in a similar experiment with cats that three of eight discriminations were performed significantly better by the hemisphere ipsilateral to the preferred paw than by the one contralateral to that paw. Finally, the average difference between memories in the retracted and nonretracted hemispheres was not significant for either measure, although this difference was the largest found, which at least suggests that surgical damage may mimic cerebral dominance in this type of study.

These data clearly support the hypothesis that normal animals store memories bilaterally. As far as can be judged from the various studies, the amount of overtraining does not account for the differences between these results and those of Gazzaniga or Webster. Gazzaniga's (1963) results may reflect chance variations in the initial performance tests or unilateral cortical damage during surgery. Webster's (1972; this volume) results were significant for just three of eight discriminations and might have occurred because of asymmetries in testing, as he noted. In any event, I conclude from my data from eight animals trained on four problems each that a dominance for laying down memories of visual pattern discriminations in one hemisphere is unlikely to exist for monkeys.

## MONKEYS TRAINED AS PARTIAL SPLITS

In the experiment just described, we asked whether intact monkeys preferentially store memories in one hemisphere even though sensory information is directly available to each hemisphere. In the experiment to be discussed now, we asked whether memories will be duplicated in the untrained hemisphere via the cerebral commissures if the sensory input is lateralized to one hemisphere. A priori, the prospect of finding unilateral engrams seems more likely in this type of experiment because a distinct, although unnatural, bias exists in the distribution of sensory input to the hemispheres during training.

Most of the published data indicate that the cerebral commissures enable a duplicate memory to be formed in the untrained hemisphere (Butler, 1968; Ebner & Myers, 1962a; Myers, 1961; Noble, 1968; Sullivan & Hamilton, 1973). On the other hand, Doty and Negrao (1973; see Doty & Overman, this volume) reported that only unilateral memories were found after training monkeys with section of all the forebrain commissures except the splenium of the corpus callosum; Downer (1962) found rather poor memories in the untrained hemisphere of monkeys that learned with callosum intact; and Myers (1961) did not find memories in the untrained hemisphere of cats if the discrimination was difficult. In the experiments in which good bilateral memories were found, it does appear that the memory in the untrained hemisphere was somewhat weaker than the one in the trained hemisphere (Butler, 1968; Ebner & Myers, 1962a; Sullivan & Hamilton, 1973), but in these experiments the untrained side was always tested first, which makes quantitative conclusions somewhat questionable. Because many variables may explain the discrepancies in the literature, it seemed worthwhile to reinvestigate the degree to which bilateral memories may be established by the anterior commissure, the splenium, or both, under well-controlled conditions similar to those of the previously discussed experiment.

The data for each of the eight monkeys trained monocularly on Set II as partial splits and tested for retention after completion of the brain bisection are presented in Figure 3. The results are essentially the same as in the preceding experiment. Both measures of retention indicate the formation of bilateral memories of approximately equal strength in the two hemispheres. The trained hemisphere, however, did perform significantly better than the untrained hemisphere when initial performance was tested for the group trained with split chiasms ($p < .05$, $t(3) = 3.5$). A similar comparison was not significant for the four monkeys trained with anterior commissure or splenium intact, nor were any of the trained-untrained comparisons using trials to criterion significant. There were also no reliable differences for either measure of retention between the memories in the right and left hemispheres, between the hemispheres ipsi and contralateral to the preferred hand, or between the order of hemispheric retraction for the first and second operations.

Data from an earlier study (Sullivan & Hamilton, 1973) were reanalyzed and plotted in the same way (Figure 4). These data also show that either the anterior commissure or the splenium can establish bilateral memories. Numerous procedural differences preclude quantitative comparisons between these experiments, but the data indicate that the results are qualitatively similar to those of the present study. For both measures of retention the trained hemisphere of the group that learned with

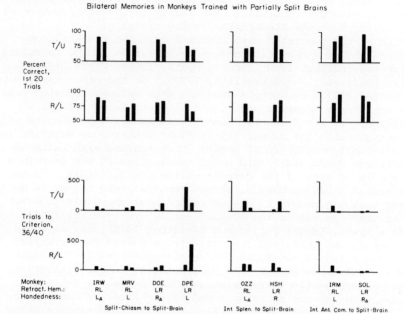

Fig. 3. *Notation is similar to that of Figure 2, except that each hemisphere was retracted in a separate operation.*

anterior commissure intact was significantly better than the un-trained hemisphere, although this result may be biased because the untrained hemisphere was tested first. Both these experi-ments support the hypothesis that with lateralized input bi-lateral memories are formed when either the anterior commissure or the splenium or both are intact during training. It also appears that in these experiments memories were somewhat stronger in the trained than in the untrained hemisphere.

These results agree well with those of Butler (1968), who found good duplicate memories established in the untrained hemisphere of monkeys trained after section of the optic chiasm and anterior commissure and tested with their brains split. They also agree with results of Ebner and Myers (1962a) showing the existence of bilateral memories for tactile discriminations trained through one hand, and with most of Myers' (1961) ori-ginal results with cats.

The present results do not agree with the findings of Doty and Negrao (1973; see Doty & Overman, this volume) that the splenium does not allow memory formation in the untrained hemisphere. Several possible explanations may be offered for the discrepancy between the results of Doty and Negrao and those obtained by other investigators. (1) The amount of over-training may determine the strength of memories established in

Bilateral Memories in Monkeys Trained with Partially Split Brains
From Sullivan and Hamilton, 1973

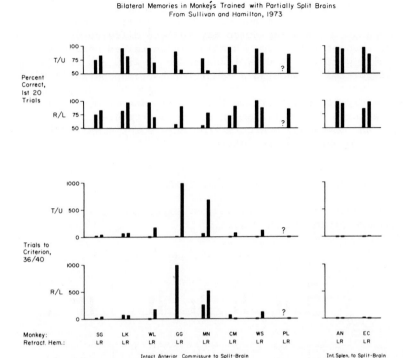

Fig. 4. *Notation is the same as that of the preceding figures.*

the untrained hemisphere. It is hard to estimate overtraining
in various experiments reported in the literature, but some
tendency to produce stronger memories in the untrained hemisphere
following more extensive overtraining has been noted (Sullivan &
Hamilton, 1973). (2) The fact that Doty and Negrao tested their
monkeys immediately after severing the remaining commissural
connections whereas other experimenters waited a week or more may
be crucial. Section of the cerebral commissures partially denervates a large number of cortical neurons, which may seriously
alter the functioning of the associated neural circuitry. If
the memories in the untrained hemisphere were weaker, and therefore possibly more sensitive to the effects of sudden denervation, they might not be observable immediately after surgery.
Partial restoration of neural function over the succeeding weeks
might then allow delayed expression of the duplicate memory, as
found in the present experiments and those of Butler and of
Ebner and Myers. This interpretation, when coupled with the
finding that section of the splenium retards learning more than
section of the anterior commissure (Figure 1), has the further
advantage of accounting for the differential effects of commissural section found by Doty and Negrao. It need only be

assumed that performance of preoperatively learned discriminations is also adversely affected by the denervation accompanying
section of the splenium but not of the anterior commissure.
(3) Some of the discrepancies may reflect differences of emphasis
rather than of fact. For example, an untrained hemisphere that
initially performs at 60-70% and relearns with 30% savings might
be interpreted as showing a memory or not, depending on the experimenter's preference. Memories may have been demonstrable
immediately after surgery in the experiments of Doty and Negrao
if relearning curves for an untrained hemisphere had been obtained and compared to acquisition curves for a naive hemisphere
in the same physiological state.

*SUMMARY OF RETENTION BY EACH HEMISPHERE*

The average results for the four experimental and two control
groups are presented in Figure 5.

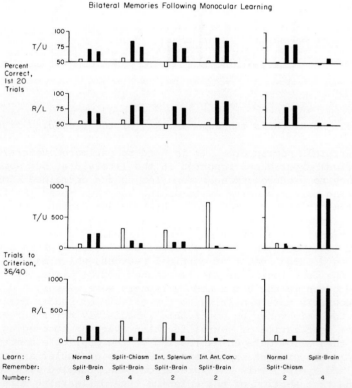

*Fig. 5. Open bars represent trials before the final surgery,
filled bars represent trials after the final surgery. Otherwise
notation is as in preceding figures.*

54

The initial performance levels following surgery are above chance for each hemisphere for all the experimental groups, again showing that, on the average, memories were present bilaterally. In general the level of initial performance was similar for the two hemispheres. Although initial performance was not perfect, it is comparable to that of the SC controls measured for the eye that was tested first, and it contrasts with the chance performance of the SB controls that were learning these problems for the first time.

The data for trials to criterion, when compared to the performance of the SB controls, also show that the experimental groups had memories established bilaterally. Because of the differences in learning and performance ability for the different groups (Figure 1, and open bars of Figure 5), savings relative to the preoperative learning are not seen for the group trained with intact brains, but are found for the groups trained with partially split brains. This demonstrates the necessity of using SB controls to assess the presence of memories by this measure.

Although bilateral memories are present in all the experimental groups, they are not equally strong. It is apparent from both measures of retention that the monkeys trained with intact brains do not perform the discriminations as well when split as do the monkeys trained with their brains partially split. The good performance by the control monkeys trained with intact brains and tested with split chiasms shows that neither the sudden appearance of the hemianopia between training and testing nor incidental damage during the approach to the chiasm is responsible for the depressed performance of the split-brain group trained with intact brains. Perhaps the more extensive surgery performed on the normal group only a week before testing for retention affects performance more than the less extensive surgery required to complete the split in the other groups. Alternatively, the extra effort or overtraining associated with the longer original learning by the partially split monkeys may lead to better memory formation in those groups.

In summary, normal monkeys form bilateral memories for moderately difficult as well as for simple pattern discriminations. Monkeys with input lateralized to one hemisphere and with cerebral commissures intact also form bilateral memories, but the less effective commissural input appears to form a weaker duplicate trace. These experiments with lateralized input, however, are less natural and therefore less useful for assessing the distribution of engrams in normal monkeys. It seems probable that unilateral damage to the hemispheres, chance variations in performance, and testing in unbalanced designs may have mimicked cerebral dominance in earlier experiments. Overall, there is much convincing evidence for and little evidence against the hypothesis that intact monkeys establish memories bilaterally.

HEMISPHERIC EQUIVALENCE IN DISCRIMINATION

The split-brain preparation provides the ideal approach for
studying hemispheric specialization because the two hemispheres
of the same animal can be compared directly on the ability to
learn and perform the same tasks without the complicating effects
of unilateral lesions. In addition, both hemispheres should
have similar genetic, physiological, and experiential back-
grounds, differing only with respect to the hemispheric specialization in question.

The prevailing opinion has been that the two hemispheres of
animals are equally proficient in learning discriminations. The
early studies with cats (Sperry, Stamm, & Miner, 1956; Stamm &
Sperry, 1957) showed dramatically how similar are the learning
curves of the two hemispheres. Analogous results have been
found for monkeys learning tactile discriminations (Ebner &
Myers, 1962b). In those visual discriminations for which individual data are available, the trials to criterion appear approximately equal for the two hemispheres of monkeys (Butler,
1968; Downer, 1962; Hamilton & Gazzaniga, 1964). However, none
of these studies used stimuli that would be expected on the
basis of studies with human subjects to show lateralization.

A few studies have reported differences in postoperative
acquisition or performance by the two hemispheres. It has been
claimed that the left hemisphere of split-brain monkeys shows a
marginally significant advantage in learning to discriminate
(1) direction of movement of a field of dots (Hamilton & Lund,
1970) and (2) orientation of lines (Hamilton, Tieman, & Farrell,
1974). Robinson and Voneida (1973) reported that four split-
brain cats achieved different levels of performance with the two
hemispheres if the tasks were difficult; two did better with the
left and two with the right. Unfortunately, these experiments
were either unbalanced with respect to which hemisphere was retracted during surgery, or else the side of retraction was not
stated. Preliminary data from a more thorough study of the
abilities of the separated hemispheres of monkeys to learn to
discriminate between different types of visual stimuli will now
be reported.

Twenty SB monkeys from the preceding experiments were taught,
in a balanced design, six sets of visual discriminations through
each eye to compare learning and performance abilities of the
two separated hemispheres. Two sets of 6 pattern discriminations, thought unlikely on the basis of previous experience and
results with human subjects to be affected by hemispheric specialization, were trained at widely separated times. These served
as a basis for estimating the amount of any cerebral dominance
or cortical damage that would affect visual learning in general,
and against which the other specific tasks could be compared.
At various times during a 2-year period following surgery, sets
of problems thought likely to show dominance (Hamilton et al.,
1974) were taught to these monkeys. The problems were presented

as symmetrically rewarded go/no-go discriminations with the stimuli presented for up to 5 sec. The monkeys were rewarded with a pellet of food for either responding to the positive stimulus when it appeared or withholding a response to the negative stimulus for 5 sec. The first type of problem involved discriminating between *oriented lines*, paired $0°$ versus $45°$ and $135°$ vs. $90°$. The second type required the monkeys to differentiate the *direction of movement* of a large spiral that rotated either clockwise or counterclockwise (Tieman, 1974). The third type of discrimination consisted of four sets of photographs of monkeys' *faces*, each set composed of five different pictures of one monkey (positive stimuli) and five pictures of another monkey (negative stimuli), intermingled in an 80-trial repeating sequence. The fourth type of problem, presented in the same manner as the faces, used two-dimensional *perspective* drawings of textured surfaces that appeared to human subjects to recede into the distance, sloping either upward or downward.

Average dominance indices, defined as $100(R - L)/(R + L)$ where $R$ represents trials to criterion with the right eye and $L$ represents tirals with the left eye, are given for each monkey for these 6 sets of problems in Figure 6. Although these data are not yet complete, it appears that no trend is present to suggest any form of hemispheric specialization. The average dominance indices are small, showing no advantage for the right or left hemisphere. In addition, there is no obvious correlation between the dominance indices and the hand preferences of the monkeys (see also Warren, this volume), nor was the sex of the monkeys critical. Finally, the indices show no particular consistency among the different types of problems taught to the individual monkeys. There is a suggestion that soon after surgery the sign and magnitude of the dominance indices may be related to which hemisphere was retracted, but this tendency gradually wanes over the succeeding months.

The maintained performance levels on the 80 trials immediately following the attainment of criterion are given in Table 1 for the 6 monkeys that completed the design. No differences in performance are present between the two hemispheres, in contrast to the results of Robinson and Voneida (1972). This is true for all problem sets, even though they vary widely in difficulty as estimated from the trials taken to reach criterion, which ranged from about 1500 for the movement discrimination to about 90 for the second set of 6 patterns.

Thus no evidence that the two hemispheres are differentially specialized for processing pattern, spatial, or facial information was found. Our previous reports, as well as those of Robinson and Voneida (1972), might best be treated cautiously unless replicated under carefully controlled conditions.

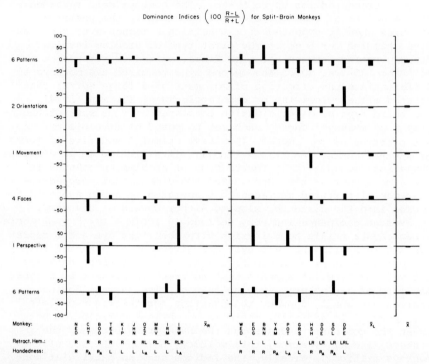

Dominance Indices $\left( 100\ \dfrac{R-L}{R+L} \right)$ for Split-Brain Monkeys

*Fig. 6. Notation is the same as in the preceding figures. The dominance indices are derived from the trials to criterion taken by the right (R) and left (L) hemispheres; positive indices indicate a left-hemispheric preference, with 33% representing a twofold advantage. The discriminations are described in the text.*

COMMENT

It is disappointing to find no evidence for hemispheric spe-cialization in monkeys, and therefore to be forced indirectly to support the opinion that cerebral asymmetries appeared during the later evolution of our human ancestors. Since the null hypothe-sis can never be proven, the key question about these experi-ments centers on the adequacy of the tests used for hemispheric specialization. Although by no means exhaustive or perfect, these tests, particularly those with faces, should have detected asymmetries of the magnitude found with human patients. For example, Levy, Trevarthen, & Sperry (1972), using roughly comparable stimuli, have found clear hemispheric differences in perception of faces by human split-brain patients. Furthermore, discrimination of faces seems as likely an ability as any for

TABLE 1

*Percentage of correct responses by each hemisphere on the eighty trials immediately following criterion* [a]

| Monkey | Retracted Hemisphere | Hand | 6 patterns | | 2 orientations | | 1 movement | | 4 faces | | 5 patterns | |
|---|---|---|---|---|---|---|---|---|---|---|---|---|
| | | | R | L | R | L | R | L | R | L | R | L |
| CHT | R | R$_A$ | 85.4 | 91.4 | 84.4 | 84.3 | 83.8 | 90.0 | 92.5 | 92.8 | 91.5 | 90.4 |
| BOO | R | R$_A$ | 92.1 | 93.5 | 96.2 | 94.4 | 95.0 | 77.5 | 84.5 | 84.7 | 98.1 | 92.3 |
| TEA | R | L | 93.4 | 89.2 | 92.1 | 93.9 | 86.2 | 92.5 | 88.3 | 92.1 | 94.0 | 93.0 |
| EDG | L | R | 94.6 | 90.5 | 93.8 | 96.9 | 88.8 | 85.0 | 88.2 | 88.4 | 98.5 | 97.5 |
| HSH | LR | R | 89.0 | 87.5 | 94.6 | 92.5 | 86.2 | 76.2 | 91.6 | 91.2 | 90.7 | 92.7 |
| DOE | LR | R$_A$ | 88.3 | 90.0 | 91.9 | 98.1 | 62.5 | 85.0 | 82.2 | 86.2 | 91.2 | 93.2 |
| Mean | | | 90.5 | 90.4 | 92.2 | 93.4 | 83.8 | 84.4 | 87.9 | 89.2 | 94.0 | 93.2 |

[a]R, right; L, left; A, ambidextrous.

natural selection to have favored during the evolution of a social primate. It remains possible, of course, that the two hemispheres solved the discriminations according to different strategies, as human subjects sometimes do (Levy *et al.*, 1972), or that the tests simply are inappropriate or otherwise insensitive to simian hemispheric specialization.

In the future, studies of dominance may prove more rewarding if conducted with apes. Alternatively, different types of tests, perhaps involving sequential processing of information or using stimuli differing in number or containing hidden figures, may yet reveal hemispheric differences in monkeys. Finally, tests based on preferences for stimuli, rather than ones based on measures of learning or retention as used in the experiments discussed in this chapter, may detect differences in perceptual processing. At present, though, it appears that demonstrating differential abilities for the two hemispheres of monkeys, even if possible, will not be easy.

## SUMMARY

Two types of experiments were performed to test for hemispheric specialization in monkeys. First, monkeys with their brains intact or only partially split were taught 4 visual discriminations; their brains were then split and each hemisphere was tested for retention of the problems. A series of control experiments showed that immediate postoperative learning by split-brain monkeys was severely depressed; therefore split-brain controls that learned these problems postoperatively were necessary to correctly evaluate retention in the experimental animals. Second, split-brain monkeys were taught with each hemisphere several types of visual discriminations thought likely to reveal hemispheric specialization. Neither formation of unilateral memories nor differential abilities in learning or performance with the separated hemispheres could be found, which suggests that hemispheric specialization in monkeys, if present, will not be easily detected.

## ACKNOWLEDGEMENTS

This research was supported by USPHS Grants NS-06501 (C.R.H.) and MH-03372 (R. W. Sperry). I thank Michael V. Sullivan and Suzannah B. Tieman, who participated in some of the work reported here, for comments on the manuscript, and Eef Goedemans, Lois MacBird, and Josephine Macenka for their help in performing these experiments.

## Note added in proof

The chapter written by Dewson and part of the one written by Rubens were added sometime after the conference. Although cross-referenced, the chapters were not made available to me, and therefore my lack of comment does not reflect my opinion of their contents.

REFERENCES

Butler, C. R. A memory-record for visual discrimination habits produced in both cerebral hemispheres of monkey when only one hemisphere has received direct visual information. *Brain Research*, 1968, *10*, 152-167.

Doty, R. W., & Negrao, N. Forebrain commissures and vision. In R. Jung (Ed.), *Handbook of sensory physiology*. Vol. 7. Berlin: Springer-Verlag, 1973. Part 3.

Downer, J. L. de C. Interhemispheric integration in the visual system. In V. B. Mountcastle (Ed.), *Interhemispheric relations and cerebral dominance*. Baltimore: Johns Hopkins Press, 1962. Pp. 87-100.

Ebner, F. F., & Myers, R. E. Direct and transcallosal induction of touch memories in the monkey. *Science*, 1962, *138*, 51-52. (a)

Ebner, F. F., & Myers, R. E. Corpus callosum and the inter-hemispheric transmission of tactual learning. *Journal of Neurophysiology*, 1962, *25*, 380-391. (b)

Gazzaniga, M. S. Effects of commissurotomy on a preoperatively learned visual discrimination. *Experimental Neurology*, 1963, *8*, 14-19.

Hamilton, C. R., & Gazzaniga, M. S. Lateralization of learning of colour and brightness discriminations following brain bisection. *Nature*, 1964, *201*, 220.

Hamilton, C. R., & Lund, J. S. Visual discrimination of movement: midbrain or forebrain? *Science*, 1970, *170*, 1428-1430.

Hamilton, C. R., Tieman, S. B., & Farrell, W. S. Cerebral dominance in monkeys? *Neuropsychologia*, 1974, *12*, 193-197.

Levy, J., Trevarthen, C., & Sperry, R. W. Perception of bilateral chimeric figures following hemispheric deconnexion. *Brain*, 1972, *95*, 61-78.

Myers, R. E. Corpus callosum and visual gnosis. In A. Fessard, R. W. Gerard, and J. Konorski (Eds.), *Brain mechanisms and learning*. Oxford: Blackwell, 1961. Pp. 481-505

Noble, J. Paradoxical interocular transfer of mirror-image discriminations in the optic chiasm sectioned monkey. *Brain Research*, 1968, *10*, 127-151.

Robinson, J. S., & Voneida, T. J. Hemisphere differences in cognitive capacity in the split-brain cat. *Experimental Neurology*, 1973, *38*, 123-134.

Sperry, R. W. Mental unity following surgical disconnection of the cerebral hemispheres. In *The Harvey Lectures, Series 62*. New York: Academic Press, 1968. Pp. 293-323.

Sperry, R. W., Stamm, J. S., & Miner, N. Relearning tests for interocular transfer following division of optic chiasm and corpus callosum in cats. *Journal of Comparative and Physiological Psychology*, 1956, *49*, 529-533.

Stamm, J. S., & Sperry, R. W. Function of corpus callosum in contralateral transfer of somesthetic discrimination in cats. *Journal of Comparative and Physiological Psychology*, 1957, *50*, 138-143.

Sullivan, M. V., & Hamilton, C. R. Memory establishment via the anterior commissure of monkeys. *Physiology and Behavior*, 1973, *11*, 873-879.

Tieman, S. B. Interhemispheric transfer of visual information in partially split-brain monkeys. Unpublished Ph.D. dissertation, Stanford Univ., 1974.

Warren, J. M., Abplanalp, J. M., & Warren, H. B. The development of handedness in cats and rhesus monkeys. In H. W. Stevenson, E. H. Hess, and H. L. Rheingold (Eds.), *Early behavior: Comparative and developmental approaches*. New York: Wiley, 1967. Pp. 73-101.

Webster, W. G. Functional asymmetry between the cerebral hemispheres of the cat. *Neuropsychologia*, 1972, *10*, 75-87.

# 4.

# Preliminary Evidence of Hemispheric Asymmetry of Auditory Function in Monkeys

*JAMES H. DEWSON, III*

Stanford University School of Medicine

For more than 100 years, clinical evidence has shown that damage to the superior lateral aspect of the left temporal lobe of man (Wernicke's area) leads to severe disturbance of auditory cognitive function, particularly that concerned with the comprehension of spoken language. Since the superior temporal gyrus of the monkey (Brodmann's area 22) is known by anatomical, physiological, and behavioral criteria to be specifically a part of the central auditory system, it is reasonable to believe that this cortical field might be homologous to Wernicke's area (see Rubens, this volume). For the past 12 years, therefore, my colleagues and I have sought to develop a nonhuman primate behavioral preparation that would provide clues to the involvement of the superior temporal gyrus in auditory-governed cognitive activities.

Interpretation of the functional similarities between the superior temporal gyrus of nonhuman primates and Wernicke's area in man traditionally has been frustrated by two critical and related issues: First, severe and enduring behavioral deficits in nonhuman mammals have been thought to require symmetrical bilateral damage; second, the presence of hemispheric asymmetry of function has been thought to be demonstrable only for man (Milner, 1974). Unless both views are invalid, inferences about the functional role of Wernicke's area drawn from studies of the superior temporal gyrus in higher nonhuman primates must have dubious status.

My own research suggests that both of these earlier notions may have been overstated. Most important, we established that *unilateral* damage (via cortical ablation) to the superior temporal gyrus in the monkey results in significant and persistent deficits in auditory-governed behavioral tasks (Cowey & Dewson, 1972; Dewson, Cowey, & Weiskrantz, 1970). Moreover, preliminary evidence indicates that for the successful mastery of a certain task, the *left* cerebral hemisphere of the monkey plays a disproportionate role. These two findings, running counter to prevailing views (e.g., Hamilton; Warren, this volume), derive from the use of (1) auditory behavioral tests deliverately selected for their possession of critical temporal factors (Dewson, 1975; Dewson & Cowey, 1969), and (2) psychophysical techniques (methods of titration) that allow the level of difficulty of a given test to be manipulated independently of the effects of treatments (Dewson, 1968; Weiskrantz, 1968).

To explore the nature of the basic unilateral deficit (nonspecific as to hemisphere), we have, during the past 4 years, developed a test that probably reveals aspects of auditory recall capacity in nonverbal animals (Dewson & Burlingame, 1975). Figure 1 illustrates the testing array presented to our monkeys as

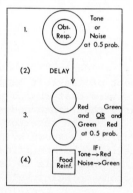

Fig. 1. Testing array and paradigm.

well as the primary contingencies of the task, which, at its final stage, is a response-adjusted delayed symbolic match-to-sample (cf. Stamm, Rosen, & Gadotti, *et al.*, this volume). All monkeys must be trained initially to make a conditional (auditory (auditory-visual) match between two acoustic stimuli--either a .5 sec burst of 1 KHz tone or a .5-sec burst of white noise--and two color-dependent responses. For example, if, after pressing the observing response panel, the monkey hears the *tone* stimulus, the task is to press, after the illumination of the two lower response panels, whichever of them is *red*. Similarly, the correct response to the *noise* stimulus is a press at whichever of the two panels is lit *green*. We have successfully taught 18 monkeys--in 18 attempts--to perform this task to a long-term criterion of 90%-correct response.

To measure auditory recent memory capacity, a delay is inserted between the termination of the acoustic stimulus and the

arming and illumination of the two response panels. The duration of the delay for any given trial is automatically determined by response-adjusted schedules of control by which we are
able to force an animal's performance progressively from the
level of greatest ease (i.e., 0-sec delay) to levels of maximum
difficulty (i.e., longest attainable delays). These schedules
of control allow precise estimates of the location of four points
on a delayed-response performance function that extends from
50%-correct (chance) to 89%-correct response (Wetherill & Levitt,
1965). Additionally, all subjects are checked periodically in
full daily sessions (100 or 200 self-paced trials) under 0-sec
delay conditions; their performance in these control sessions
rarely falls below 94%-correct response once the basic conditional matching problem has been learned.

The ability of these animals to discriminate between very
brief presentations of tone and noise bursts is also routinely
assessed. In this instance, the duration of the acoustic stimuli
is titrated progressively downward to four separate and prede-
termined levels of performance, which thus yield a psychometric
function. Typically, the monkeys' abilities mirror those of
human subjects on the identical task: A tone burst can be identified (and discriminated from a noise burst) when its duration
is as short as 1-2 msec, but no shorter (Dewson & Burlingame,
1975).

The remainder of this chapter presents postoperative results
obtained from five monkeys (evaluated preoperatively for at
least 2 years) following surgical removal of the cortex of the
superior temporal gyrus. The intended extent of each of the
ablations involves the cortex of the lateral aspect of the
approximate middle one-third of this gyrus including the tissue
of the superior bank of the superior temporal sulcus. The cortex
of the supratemporal plane lying dorsally, and of the inferior
bank of the superior temporal sulcus lying ventrally, is apared
(Dewson, Pribram, & Lynch, 1969; Dewson, et al., 1970). No
histological verification of these lesions is yet available, but
since the chief surgeon, Dr. K. H. Pribram, has successfully performed more than 800 similar ablations of various cortical fields
of the temporal lobe, it is not unreasonable to be highly confident of the placement of the present lesions.

Figure 2 and Table 1 present the findings for each of the
five subjects. In Figure 2, the six frames show the five monkeys
and summarize the effects upon delayed symbolic match-to-sample
performance as a function of the hemisphere in which the ablation
was made. One monkey, He, has had a bilateral ablation: stage 1
in the right hemisphere and stage 2, five months later, in the
left hemisphere. Unilateral cochlear destruction by means of
encocochlear labyrinthectomy was performed on four of the animals before any behavioral training, that is, 2-3 years prior to
the cortical ablations.

Table 1 lists the five subjects, the basic anatomical relationships existing between cochlear and cortical lesions, and

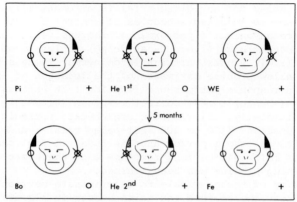

*Fig. 2. Pictorial representation of experimental findings. The darkened areas indicate the side of cortical ablation; the X's mark the side of cochlear destruction. Symbols: +, presence, and O, absence, of postoperative deficit.*

the primary experimental results. Note that the major combinations of location and type of surgical lesion have been balanced and that the deficit is present in one monkey whose cochleas are presumably undamaged and normal. The results suggest that the observed deficit is not correlated with the disruption, specifically of either the crossed or the uncrossed primary ascending auditory pathway. Monkey W.E. provided the single instance in which initial postoperative performance of the conditional matching task at 0-sec delay—a control, or baseline, condition—was deficient. Though the decrement was minor, this animal remained consistently below criterion level for some 2 months following unilateral cortical ablation. After reaching criterion (90%-correct response at 0-sec delay for three consecutive 100-trial daily sessions), the monkey demonstrated, as had the other three left-hemisphere operates, a defect in auditory recent memory.

Each animal (with the exception of W.E.) immediately attained criterion-level scores on the 0-sec delay test despite unilateral cortical ablation and the 2-week inactive recovery period following it. This situation obtained as well following the second operation on monkey He. Further, no animal showed any deficit whatever on the task demanding discrimination between brief acoustic stimuli: Postoperative performance functions all fell easily within the ranges determined prior to surgery for each monkey.

The general nature of the deficit is depicted in Figure 3, which shows the initial postoperative delays attained by the five monkeys after six separate ablations. Preoperative variability of the subjects is indicated by the barred lines, and the curve passes through the means yielding a psychometric function.

TABLE 1

*Lesions and Their Behavioral Effects*

| Subject | Intact Cochlea | Cortical Ablation | Anatomical Relationship | Postoperative Deficit |
|---------|---------------|-------------------|------------------------|----------------------|
| Pi | Right | Left | Opposite good ear | Yes |
| He (1) | Left | Right | Opposite good ear | No |
| W.E. | Right | Left | Opposite good ear | Yes[a] |
| Bo | Right | Right | Opposite good ear | No |
| He (2) | Left | Left | Opposite good ear | Yes |
| Fe | Both | Left | Opposite good ear | Yes |

[a]Monkey W.E. provided the only instance of deficient initial postoperative performance of the conditional matching task at 0-sec delay (control or baseline condition).

67

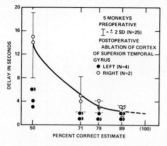

*Figure 3. Graph of auditory memory defect.*

The four postoperative left-hemisphere values shown on the 50%-correct response ordinate are spuriously high, reflecting the occasional coincidence of stimulus runs and response bias during testing sessions in which the delay adjustment increment is set for its longest duration, namely, 1.0 sec. This increment, the titration basic unit (TBU), in large measure determines the delays attainable by the subjects in any given testing session. Our standard preoperative evaluations involve not only repeated assessments of performance at the four levels (i.e., 50%-, 71%-, 79%- and 89%-correct response) dictated by the control schedules in force during the particular session, but also multiple determinations of performance at each level as a function of four distinct TBU durations: .2, .3, .5, and 1.0 sec. The fact that greatest delays are achieved at the longest TBU duration can easily be appreciated by considering the following example: Suppose the 50%-correct response level is fought; the control schedule specifies that after each correct trial the delay in the next trial is increased by one step, and after each incorrect trial the delay is decreased by one step. Starting from the level of greatest ease, i.e., 0-sec delay, and progressing incrementally toward increased difficulty, i.e., increasingly greater delays, a subject can attain any given delay in fewer correct trials the longer the duration of the TBU. Thus, a consecutive strong of 15 correct trials at a TBU of 1.0 sec gains a delay interval of 25.0 sec, whereas at a TBU of .2 sec, such a delay interval can be achieved (via a string of consecutive correct responses) only after 75 trials. The animals' motivation and the experimenters' available time both tend to dictate testing sessions containing no more than 50 trials, especially under these maximally burdensome conditions.

In seeking to ascertain more precisely the nature of the deficit following left-hemisphere damage, we observed that the deficient animals either responded randomly or adopted strong response biases whenever they apparently detected a change in the delay interval from the previous trial. This was most noticeable at a TBU of 1.0 sec where the initial trial of a session (at 0-sec delay) was invariably responded to correctly, and the next trial (at 1.0-sec delay) was responded to in a disorganized (frustrated) manner by the subjects. Figure 4 shows pre- and postoperative performance for a single monkey, Pi (subsequently

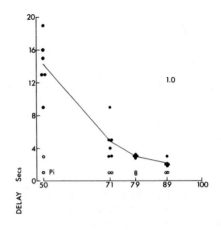

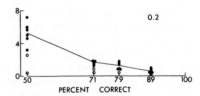

Fig. 4. Preoperative (filled circles) and postoperative (open circles) delays attained by monkey Pi under titration conditions of ].0-sec increments (upper graph) and .2-sec increments (lower graph). The curves connect the preoperative means of the four assessed levels.

studied in greater detail), who sustained a lesion of the left hemisphere. Values are plotted for the TBUs of longest duration (1.0 sec, upper graph) and shortest duration (.2 sec, lower graph) assessed prior to surgery. The effect of TBU duration upon delays attained is plainly seen in the preoperative functions. Also to be noted in this figure, as in the preceding one, are two relatively high postoperative delays attained on a 50%-correct titration schedule; we are confident that the magnitude of these values reflects an artifact of the particular titration schedule used.

We next decided to investigate this monkey's performance during sessions in which the TBU was lowered to durations which one might expect to be below the animal's jnd for detection of delay interval increase. Figure 5 gives results for 50%-correct response titrations at four TBUs; the original pre- and postoperative values at a TBU of .2 sec are now recapitulated at the extreme right-hand end of the abscissa. The delay values obtained from seven daily sessions wherein very short-duration TBUs were used are plotted and numbered according to their order of presentation. What seems most noteworthy about this result is the normal trend toward increased delays (hence better memory) with increased TBU duration, so long as this duration is held close to or below some apparently critical value (approximately .2 sec). The animal's performance shows, in effect, a release from the deficit, and the records of that performance indicate

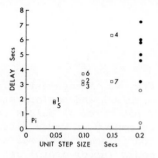

Fig. 5. Postoperative release from deficit in monkey Pi. Values from the 50% ordinate of the lower graph of Figure 4 are recapitulated at the extreme right-hand end of the abscissa (titration increment). For further details, see text.

that neither random responding nor response bias contributed in any way to the delays attained. This suggests that self-generated interference at the time of retrieval is a major component of the defect. Investigations of this tentative interpretation are in process with the other deficient monkeys.

In summary, at this early stage of the research I am strongly forced to conclude that the *left* hemisphere of the monkey plays a disproportionate role in the mediation of certain complex auditory-dependent activities. It must be stressed that these results are preliminary and that numerous controls are yet demanded. Nonetheless, the deficit described here is reliable and readily demonstrated in four monkeys even 10 months after its initial appearance.

## ACKNOWLEDGMENTS

This research was supported by grants from the National Science Foundation, Stanford University, and the Stanford University School of Medicine. The initial report of these findings was presented at the 90th meeting of the Acoustical Society of America, San Francisco, November 1975. I thank Ken Kizer, Sue Dewson, Patti Kenney, and Dr. Karl Pribram for their assistance during various stages of these experiments. I am particularly grateful to Allen Burlingame, whose continued and dedicated help made this work possible.

## REFERENCES

Cowey, A., & Dewson, J. H. III  Effects of unilateral ablation of superior temporal cortex on auditory discrimination in *Macaca mulatta*. *Neuropsychologia*, 1972, *10*, 279-289.
Dewson, J. H. III  Efferent olivocochlear bundle: Some relationships to stimulus discrimination in noise. *Journal of Neurophysiology*, 1968, *31*, 122-130.

Dewson, J. H. III  Recall of auditory patterns by monkeys. *Journal of the Acoustical Society of America*, 1975, *57*, S 11.

Dewson, J. H. III, & Burlingame, A.  Auditory discrimination and recall in monkeys. *Science*, 1975, *187*, 267-268.

Dewson, J. H. III, Burlingame, A., Kizer, K., Dewson, S., Kenney, P., & Pribram, K. H.  Hemispheric asymmetry of auditory function in monkeys. *Journal of the Acoustical Society of America*, 1975, *58*, S 66.

Dewson, J. H. III & Cowey, A.  Discrimination of auditory sequences by monkeys. *Nature (Lond.)*, 1969, *222*, 695-697.

Dewson, J. H. III, Cowey, A., & Weiskrantz, L.  Disruptions of auditory sequence discrimination by unilateral and bilateral cortical ablations of superior temporal gyrus in the monkey. *Experimental Neurology*, 1970, *28*, 529-548.

Dewson, J. H. III, Pribram, K. H., & Lynch, J. C.  Effects of ablations of temporal cortex upon speech sound discrimination in the monkey. *Experimental Neurology*, 1969, *24*, 579-591.

Milner, B.  Hemispheric specialization: Scope and limts.  In F. O. Schmitt & F. G. Worden (Eds.), *The neurosciences third study program*. Cambridge, Massachusetts: M.I.T. Press, 1974. Pp. 75-89.

Weiskrantz, L.  Some traps and pontifications.  In L. Weiskrantz (Ed.), *Analysis of behavioral change*. New York: Harper, 1968. Pp. 415-429.

Wetherill, G. B., & H. Levitt  Sequential estimation of points on a psychometric function. *British Journal of Mathematical and Statistical Psychology*, 1965, *18*, 1-10.

71

**Part II**

# THE NEOCORTICAL COMMISSURES AND INTERHEMISPHERIC RELATIONS

# 5.

# Mnemonic Role of Forebrain Commissures in Macaques

*ROBERT W. DOTY, SR. AND WILLIAM H. OVERMAN, JR.*

Center for Brain Research
University of Rochester

More fragmented than Gaul, this paper is divided into five
parts: one of theory and four of experimentation, perhaps an
appropriate balance. The common theme that brings these pieces
together is the forebrain commissures and their role in interhemispheric mnemonic transfer. The first four of these pieces
have repeatedly appeared in extensive summary (Doty, 1969, 1974,
1975; Doty & Negrão, 1973; Doty, Negrão, & Yamaga, 1973, 1974;
Negrão & Doty, 1969), as here, but will eventually receive detailed exposition. Readers familiar with previous accounts may
wish to concentrate on the fifth section, on the electrical
stimulation of the anterior commissure, which presents new work
in progress.

## A THEORY OF CALLOSAL MNEMONIC FUNCTION--THE UNILATERAL ENGRAM

Negrão and Doty have proposed that the callosal system (1)
enables each hemisphere to have access to memory traces stored
in the other and (2) controls the formation of engrams in such
a way that they are laid down only in a single hemisphere. This
prevention of redundancy, coupled with ready access, would effectively double the mnemonic storage capacity of the brain.
Evidence adduced in favor of this hypothesis is, first, as
outlined in the next section, the finding that an engram for
interpreting the significance of direct electrical excitation
of the striate cortex in macaques can be "read out" by stimulation in the hemisphere contralateral to that used initially but

*Supported by Grant NS 03606 from the National Institute of
Neurological and Communicative Disorders and Stroke, National
Institutes of Health.

is not transferred into this hemisphere by the splenium.    In
man there is, of course, strong evidence for the existence of
unilateral engrams, not only for language in the left hemisphere,
but for spatial analysis in the right.  That the unilaterality
of the engrams for language arises as a result of a callosal
mechanism is attested to by the fact that linguistic engrams
were found to be bilateral in a case of agenesis of the callosum,
where only the anterior commissure was present (Sperry, 1974).

The brilliant work of Nottebohm (e.g., this volume) demonstrates that unilaterality for the engrams of learned vocal behavior also exists in canaries.  Since there is no callosal system in birds, this can scarcely be offered as evidence in favor
of the Negrão-Doty hypothesis, but it does clearly demonstrate
the principle that unilateral engrams can arise despite seemingly symmetrical afferent mechanisms (see also Dewson; Stamm,
Rosen, & Gadotti, this volume).

More germane in showing that the callosal mechanism can suppress the formation of engrams in one hemisphere while establishing them in the other are the experiments of Kaas, Axelrod, and
Diamond (1967).  They found that cats acquired bilateral auditory engrams after the callosum was transected, whereas the engram was normally unilateral.  A further example is probably
seen in the finding of Burešová and Bureš (1973) that, with
monocular visual training, rats initially establish an engram
in both hemispheres which, upon further training, becomes limited
to the single hemisphere receiving the  preponderance of the
sensory information.  Although the callosal system was not
proven to be responsible for this ultimate suppression of the
engram in the visually limited hemisphere, this is certainly
the most straightforward inference.  This also suggests that the
mechanism for producing unilateral engrams may not be as efficient as that yielding a perhaps less sophisticated but more
certain bilateral memory trace.

The thorough work of Hamilton and his colleagues (this volume), which poses a severe challenge and contradiction to the
natural occurrence of unilateral engrams in animals, will be
discussed in the next section.


INTERHEMISPHERIC GENERALIZATION OF REFLEXES CONDITIONED TO
ELECTRICAL EXCITATION OF THE STRIATE CORTEX

To receive food or juice as a reward, macaques can learn to
press a lever upon the signal given by electrical excitation of
the striate cortex (Doty, 1965).  With this procedure the conditional stimulus (CS) is readily confined to one hemisphere.
However, if either the anterior commissure or splenium (but not
body or genu) of the corpos callosum is intact during training
and testing, the monkey responds immediately upon stimulation
of the striate cortex, but not other cortical areas, in the

hemisphere contralateral to that to which the training CS was applied (Doty, 1965, 1969, 1970; Doty & Negrão, 1973; Doty et al., 1973). If both forebrain commissures are cut prior to training, there is no response to stimulation of the striate cortex in the "untrained" hemisphere.

The question is whether, when one of these commissures is intact during training, the animal subsequently responds to the CS in the "untrained" hemisphere because the engram has been laid down in that hemisphere as well as in the "trained" hemisphere (i.e., a bilateral engram), or because the engram is "read out" from the "trained" hemisphere (unilateral engram) upon command via the commissural connections. Surprisingly, in this paradigm the anterior commissure operates in the former mode, the splenium in the latter (Negrão, & Doty, 1973; Doty et al., 1973; Negrão, & Doty, 1969). In other words, with callosum cut and anterior commissure intact during training, the monkey continues to respond to the CS in the "untrained" hemisphere even after the anterior commissure is transected (under local anesthesia by pulling a previously placed snare encircling the commissure). With the same procedure but with anterior commissure cut and the splenium of the callsoum ensnared, the monkey responds to the CS in the "untrained" hemisphere only so long as the splenium is present. In both cases, comprising six to nine animals each, the learned responses are still obtained for stimulation of previously "untrained" points in the striate cortex of the "trained" hemisphere. This demonstrates that failure to respond in the latter instance is not attributable merely to some general condition of the animal.

All tests were run "on extinction" so that the monkey was neither punished nor rewarded for its response or absence thereof for stimulation of the test loci. This procedure limits the number of tests that can be given, because the response to stimulation at the test points is ultimately extinguished. It does, however, assay directly whether the animal finds the stimuli equivalent in significance and thus does not rely upon less direct measures such as "savings" in learning to respond to stimulation at a new point. It seems unlikely, however, that this could contribute significantly to the difference between these results with the splenium and those of Hamilton (this volume), since Hamilton tested for both stimulus generalization and transfer of training.

Although cutting the splenium to complete the loss of forebrain commissures eliminates the response to a CS applied to the "untrained" hemisphere, it does not in the least affect the animal's ability to respond with the arm controlled primarily by the hemisphere contralateral to the still effective CS in the "trained" hemisphere. For example, an animal that responds to stimulation of the left striate cortex by pressing the lever with its left hand continues to do so after the transection of forebrain commissures is completed, even though it stops respond-

ing to stimulation of the right striate cortex. Thus, although
the engram for analyzing the significance of the CS is unilateral
when controlled by the splenium, and in the present circumstances
accessible from the other hemisphere only via the splenium, the
engram for the organization of the conditioned response (CR) per
se passes readily from one hemisphere to the other in the complete absence of forebrain commissures.

These experiments using electrical excitation of the striate
cortex as CS have shown that the engram for interpreting the significance of such a CS remains unilateral when the splenial system alone is present during training, but that it is bilateral if
the anterior commissure is intact either with or without the
splenium during training. In the latter respect the results are
completely concordant with those of Hamilton and his colleagues
(this volume; Sullivan & Hamilton, 1973; see also Gross & Mishkin,
this volume) using natural visual stimuli; but for the splenium
they stand in apparent contradiction. The two bodies of data are
equally consistent, and it must thus be supposed that some procedural difference is significant in achieving a bilateral versus
unilateral engram via the splenium. It is obviously important to
identify this difference since it should elucidate some presently
unsuspected feature of mnemonic processing. Five possibilities
come readily to mind:

1. The degree of training or overtraining at the time of testing may be a critical factor, as already noted in reference to the
experiments of Burešová and Bureš (1973).

2. With direct excitation of the striate cortex as CS the
visual system remains intact, whereas when the optic chiasm is
cut, more than half the visual afferents are lost. If all optic
tract fibers are severed, the striate cortex in monkeys undergoes
profound changes in its electrophysiology (Sakakura & Doty, 1976).
However, it is by no means clear that the partial denervation
from cutting the optic chiasm would produce such drastic effects;
the experiments of Hamilton are largely controlled for this
factor.

3. Hamilton raises the possibility that testing within an
hour to several days after transecting the splenium with the
snare technique is not comparable to testing after several weeks
has been allowed for recovery and reorganization following this
trauma. This point can certainly be checked by using the
splenial snare on animals trained with normal visual stimuli.

4. Probably more important is the difference in the learning
paradigm, a discrimination in the case of Hamilton's experiments,
a simple "go" response in the presence of the CS and withholding
the response in its absence in the Negrão and Doty experiments.
Again, the matter is readily determined by experiment, particularly by training a monkey with split chiasm to respond monocularly to a point source of light. From extensive data on man
(see, Dobelle & Mladejovsky, 1974), it can be inferred that

electrical excitation of the striate cortex in the macaque should produce a punctate phosphene that could be imitated to a considerable degree (except for its absolute fixity) by a small point of light.

5. Finally, it is possible that the significant difference lies in the abnormal entry into the visual system with the electrical excitation at the striate cortex, bypassing the subcortical elaboration normally occurring via the optic tract. Perhaps these subcortical paths reinforce a bilateral engram even though alone they are inadequate to establish it. Again, the possibility is subject to direct test, by applying the electrical CS to the optic tract rather than to the striate cortex.


MAZE BEHAVIOR

As it became apparent that functions other than language are lateralized in the cerebral hemispheres of man (e.g., Bogen & Bogen, 1969; Dimond & Beaumont, 1974; Gazzaniga, 1970; see Gur & Gur; Riklan & Cooper; Springer, this volume), it seemed reasonable to seek evidence for hemispheric specialization in other mammals. All mammals must to some degree orient themselves in relation to external objects, i.e., analyze spatial relations. Since such analysis is a prominent function of the right hemisphere in man, it might conceivably be so in his Old World relatives, the macaques, as well. A maze was thus constructed with five choice points, five blind alleys, and a total length of 5.5 m for the correct path (Doty & Yamaga, 1973; Doty et al., 1973; Yamaga & Doty, 1971). Nineteen macaques were trained to traverse the maze to a criterion of 10 consecutive passages without error. For nine normal animals this required an average of 79 trials (range 13-207). Seven of these macaques had the optic chiasm, anterior commissure, corpus callosum, and psalterium transected after attaining this criterion, and three were subjected to this surgery prior to learning. In six others the chiasm, anterior commissure, and rostral callosum were transected and an ensnaring ligature placed around the splenium and psalterium, which were subsequently transected by pulling the snare after training of one hemisphere was complete. The monkeys wore an opaque contact lens over the pharmacologically constricted pupil of one eye while running through the maze, thus limiting the direct visual experience to a single hemisphere.

In a few instances there was clear-cut evidence for hemispheric dominance (Doty et al., 1973; Yamaga & Doty, 1971). However, the condition was largely transitory and could not be convincingly demonstrated in most monkeys.

Part of the reason for this apparent lack or ephemeral nature of hemispheric dominance probably lies in the potentiality for subcortical transfer of sensory information relevant to the animal's orientation. In the initial testing of the maze it was

found that several fully trained monkeys became hopelessly confused and could not negotiate the maze when both eyes were
covered. It was thus reasoned that only visual input was relevant to the monkey's solution of the maze problem. It subsequently developed, however, that some of the "split-brain"
macaques could run the maze without the slightest hesitation when
both eyes were covered! This, of course, demolished the logical
structure of the experiments. Apparently, different monkeys have
different styles in negotiating the maze (cf. Donchin, Kutas, &
McCarthy; Gur & Gur; Springer, this volume); some rely almost exclusively on vision whereas others obtain their cues from proprioceptive input. Obviously, an animal that relied on vision under
certain conditions might switch to the proprioceptive mode when
visual input became confusing or inadequate for its purpose. This
might occur when visual input was switched from a "trained" to an
"untrained" hemisphere by changing the eye covered by the opaque
lens, the monkey then quickly learning to rely on the interhemispheric transfer provided by proprioceptive cues. Such a change
in the animal's modus operandi would account for the transitory
nature of the disruption of its maze behavior in such a situation.
    That bilateral influences are operative in the maze situation
is seen more directly when a lesion is placed in one hemisphere.
This was done in nine animals, six in the circumstriate cortex
and four along the principal sulcus and in the prefrontal area
(one animal had a lesion in each hemisphere). In every case the
unilateral lesion in the "split-brain" macaque produced confusion
initially in running the maze using either eye. Furthermore, all
but one animal subsequently became able to run the maze perfectly
with either eye open. The exception was an animal in which the
tissue along the left principal sulcus had been removed. In 22
sessions over a 3-month postoperative period it was unable to relearn to negotiate the maze using the left eye, although it was
always able to run the maze perfectly using the right eye. Significantly, this animal could not find its way through the maze
when both eyes were covered, i.e., it did not readily use the
proprioceptive mode.
    In sum, these experiments on maze behavior were inconclusive
on the question of possible hemispheric dominance in macaques.


COMMUNICATION BETWEEN THE VISUAL SYSTEM AND THE AMYGDALA VIA THE
SPLENIUM

    If the amygdala is removed bilaterally, a macaque no longer
flees when it sees its enemy, man. However, its general visual
behavior, such as estimating distances in jumping, is undisturbed.
Downer (1961), Horel and Keating (1969), and Mishkin (1972) have
shown in various ways that the striate cortex of one hemisphere
can interact with the temporal cortex or the amygdala in the
other hemisphere via the splenium of the corpus callosum. Use of

the splenial snare technique provides a useful adjunct to such experiments, and the following paradigm was developed (Doty *et al.*, 1973).

The optic tract was cut on one side to render one hemisphere blind. The amygdala was removed on the other side, making it incapable of evaluating the threatening nature of the human presence. The anterior commissure and rostral callosum were also cut; but so long as the ensnared splenium remained intact, the monkey responded normally by fleeing as far from man as the enclosure (3 x 4 x 3 m) would allow. As soon as the splenium was transected by pulling the snare, the monkey became completely oblivious to such visual threat, although it continued to watch the movements of the experimenter, and would blink upon the rapid approach of an object (cf. Heilman & Watson, this volume).

It is thus apparent that the visual cortex of one hemisphere, which sees but lacks the amygdala to interpret the significance of this input, can somehow communicate with the contralateral amygdala on the blind side via the splenium. Even the direction, let alone the nature, of this interchange between visual and motivational systems is unknown. A priori, it would seem reasonable that the visual system should encode and abstract patterns from the input and transmit them continually across the splenium into the contralateral temporal lobe. How the amygdala "recognizes" a pattern as significant, or instructs the visual system to do so, goes directly to the heart of one of the most difficult and important problems of neurophysiology.

In any event, this surgical preparation creates a very dramatic lateralization of function, and it should in the future be instructive to determine how, in the face of this hemispheric specialization, the macaque achieves a normally unified and adaptive behavioral output. The still deeper question as to which hemisphere, or both, experiences the fear probably cannot be answered, at least in monkeys.

TETANIZATION OF THE ANTERIOR COMMISSURE

Since the anterior commissure can establish a memory trace or engram in the hemisphere contralateral to that receiving the sensorial cue or conditional stimulus (see under Interhemispheric Generalization of Reflexes Conditioned to Electrical Excitation of the Striate Cortex, this chapter), it should provide an opportunity for studying the electrophysiological concomitants of this mnemonic processing.

However, before undertaking what will undoubtedly be an arduous series of experiments along these lines, it would be wise to know when this mnemonic transfer occurs in relation to the time of training. Though not considered likely, it is nevertheless conceivable that the transfer might occur at times remote from the episodes of training. This possibility could be assayed if commissural transmission could be eliminated during the training periods and remain normal at other times. This might be achieved by cooling the commissure to the point where axonal conduction is blocked. It is not known how reversible such a conduction block may be, especially when repeated many times. Since, in addition, the adjacent preoptic area contains temperature sensitive neurons, it seemed prudent to try a simpler approach initially. Thus, we hoped that effective transmission within the commissural system might be reversibly curtailed by tetanizing the commissure.

The corpus callosum was transected and "bipolar" stimulating electrodes, made from .2-mm platinum-iridium wire with 1-mm tip separation, were placed in the anterior commissure under direct vision in three *M. nemestrina* (Figure 1). Several days later, under secobarbital anesthesia, single pulses, .1 msec, 15 V, were applied to the electrodes in the anterior commissure while recording electrodes were lowered into the radiation of the anterior commissure. The latter electrodes, four on each side in each monkey (Figure 1) were implanted at loci where potentials exceeding 100 μV were evoked by the commissural stimuli.

In the alert animal a pulse to the anterior commissure produced a sharp spike, after a latency of about 4 msec, 10 mm lateral along the fiber path of its lateral radiation, as well as a simple, almost monophasic response, focused primarily in the lower bank of the superior temporal gyrus (Figure 1), after a latency of about 8 msec. For stimulation in one superior temporal gyrus and recording in a corresponding point contralaterally, the latency was usually about 18 msec, although for some loci it was shorter. Precise alignment of stimulating and recording electrodes seemed to be required for eliciting interhemispheric responses, since only a few examples were found despite the fact that all loci had responded to stimulation of the commissure. Commissural stimulation evoked no responses in the striate cortex of the lateral posterior surface of the operculum and, with the one exception of "foveal" cortex projecting into the inferior temporal gyrus, stimulation at none of the striate loci elicited any response at the temporal loci shown in Figure 1. There was no relation between the characteristics of the evoked potentials and the ability of a given locus to effect the inhibition of conditioned responses.

At the conclusion of these tests, training was begun to teach the monkey to respond by pressing a lever to receive fruit juice when electrical stimulation was applied to the striate cortex (50-Hz, .2-msec pulses, .6 to 1.5 mA for training). For two of the monkeys the unusual feature was added that all presentations of the striate cortex stimulation were applied while the anterior commissure was being tetanized, with randomized interpulse intervals in the range corresponding to pulses of 81-154 Hz (average 117.6 Hz) and 2.0-mA. As noted above, this procedure was designed to prevent meaningful transmission across the commissure during training. The commissural stimulation commenced at randomly

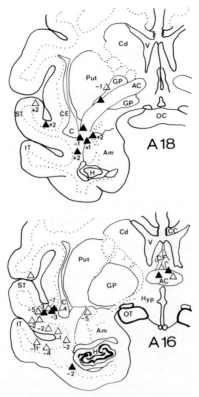

Fig. 1.   Locations of deep tip of electrode pair with 1-2 mm tip
separation at which potentials could be evoked by electrical
pulses applied to anterior commissure in three macaques at the
positions shown at A16 for each of them.   Solid triangles indicate those loci the stimulation of which eliminated conditioned
responses if applied concurrently with onset of the conditional
stimulus; open triangles, loci from which this suppressive effect was lacking.   Numbers next to the symbols specify level
anterior (+) or posterior (-) that fits the actual electrode
location more accurately than this composite.   Loci on the right
have been consolidated with those on the left.   Note that suppression is obtained from loci within the commissure and its
radiation, and at the junction of the superior temporal gyrus
and insula, provided that the point is not too far posterior.
Drawings and levels adapted from the atlas of Winters, Kado and
Adey (1969).   Abbreviations:   AC, anterior commissure; Am,
amygdala; C, claustrum; CC, corpus callosum; Cd, caudate nucleus;
CE, external capsule; CF, columns of the fornix; GP, globus
pallidus; H, hippocampus; Hyp, hypothalamus; IT, inferior
temporal gyrus; OC, optic chiasm; OT, optic tract; Put, putamen;
ST, superior temporal gyrus; V, lateral ventricle.

selected times from 5 to 20 sec prior to onset of the 4-sec stimulation of the striate cortex and continued for 5 sec after its cessation.

The unexpected result was that the two monkeys were unable to learn under these conditions. Each received over 1600 trials without showing any sign of learning. One learned within 350 trials (50 trials per day), once tetanization of a second striate locus was substituted for the concurrent tetanization of the anterior commissure. The other monkey never did learn the task. It did learn to respond to stimulation of the inferior temporal cortex when trained without the interfering commissural stimulus.

It was soon discovered, and tested in all three macaques, that concurrent stimulation of the anterior commissure or its radiation (Figure 1) at 50 Hz, with .5-1.0 mA (.25-.6 mA for "radiation" loci), .2-msec pulses, eliminated all conditioned responses. In other words, the monkeys could not respond to a CS if its onset coincided with the stimulation of the anterior commissural system.

This inhibition of the conditioned response was not limited to cases where electrical excitation of the striate or temporal cortex was used as the CS. It occurred as well for an auditory CS (clicks) and for a natural visual CS (red light). To test whether the effect was general or applied only to reward-motivated performance, one of the macaques was taught to press the lever to avoid application of an electric shock to its limbs. This it did with particular vigor and skill, lashing out angrily at the lever whenever the warning red light appeared. Yet if the red light was turned on concurrently with tetanization of the anterior commissure at .6-mA, 50-Hz, .2-msec pulses, the monkey looked calmly at the light when it came on, definitely turning toward it or "noticing" it. Aside from this mild alerting or curiosity, the monkey displayed no reaction to it. There was no sign of fear nor was any effort made to reach the lever.

Prima facie, the effect seems to reflect an inability of the monkey to appreciate the significance of the stimulus, much as in the absence of the amygdala, even though the monkey obviously "perceives" it (in that it is visually fixated in the case of the red light). In other words, the stimulation of the anterior commissural system appears to block access to memory.

There are, of course, a number of alternative explanations, but some of them seem rather unlikely, given the information at hand. For instance, it might be argued that stimulation of the anterior commissure or its radiation gives such an overwhelming visual effect that the minimal input from the visual CS is simply obscured. Visual effects have been reported from commissural stimulation in man (Adams & Rutkin, 1970) and the anterior commissure transmits visual information in macaques (Gross and Mishkin, this volume). In the present study the monkeys frequently peered about as though they were seeing something when the commissure was stimulated at intensities above 1 mA. There was, however, no response to stimulation of the commissure or any of the temporal lobe points after two of the monkeys had learned to respond to stimulation of the striate cortex. There is thus no evidence that the striate stimulation and commissural stimulation give equivalent visual sensations. An additional control for this possibility is provided by the monkey that had initially failed to learn while the commissure was tetanized. In this case intense tetanization of a locus in the striate cortex was substituted for the tetanization of the commissure while training was continued for the initial, adjacent striate locus. The animal readily learned (seven sessions) in this condition despite the possible confusion of applying the CS against a background condition (tetanization of an adjacent point), which can be inferred to yield a comparable, though more intense, visual effect. Finally, of course, the commissural stimulation eliminated responses to an auditory as well as to a visual CS.

With intensities considerably above those required for suppression of response to the CS, stimulation in the temporal lobe could produce evidence of seizure activity, especially electrically recorded afterdischarges. Such seizure activity was clearly not a necessary concomitant of the behavioral suppression. In addition, the animals displayed no confusion when the commissural or temporal area stimulation ceased and, indeed, could respond to the CS if its onset occurred at that time. Although the commissural stimulation could produce visual searching behavior that tended to become stereotyped upon repetition, there was nothing of a "driven" nature or "capture" phenomenon to this evoked activity, since the animal could and often did interrupt it with some other movement. There was no evidence that the commissural or temporal lobe stimulation was itself rewarding.

Although the fornix is near the site of the commissural electrodes, and one electrode close to the hippocampus (Figure 1) was effective in eliciting this behavioral suppression, there is no reason to suppose that the hippocampus rather than the anterior commissural-temporal-insular system is the primary focus for this deletion of mnemonically guided behavior.

It is of interest that the effective points at the base of the rostral insula (Figure 1) lie directly adjacent to fibers passing from the temporal lobe into the orbitofrontal cortex via the uncinate fasciculus (Mishkin, personal communication; and Kuypers, Szwarcbart, Mishkin, & Rosvold, 1965). Future experiments must, naturally, directly examine the hippocampus and the caudate nucleus in this regard, as well as the possibility that cutting the corpus callosum is necessary to obtain the suppression effect. The most straightforward interpretation of the present data, however, is that the anterior commissural system, known to effect interhemispheric mnemonic transfer (Hamilton, this volume, and under Interhemispheric Generalization of Reflexes Conditioned to Electrical Excitation of the Striate Cortex, this chapter), will, when abnormally activated, interfere with access to memory. There were no effects of laterality, i.e., the CS applied to the

striate cortex and the insular or commissural stimulation that
deleted the response thereto could be either ipsi- or contralateral to each other--as would be expected in a commissural
system.

SUMMARY

1.  It is proposed that the corpus callosum provides access by
one hemisphere to memory traces stored in the other, and that it
operates to preclude the formation of redundant, bilateral engrams, i.e., it organizes memory so that engrams are unilateral.
2.  In support of this hypothesis it is found that macaques
trained to respond to electrical excitation of the striate cortex
in one hemisphere respond immediately to comparable stimulation
in the other only so long as the splenium, as the surviving forebrain commissure, is intact.  The anterior commissure, on the
other hand, while intact transfers the engram into the "untrained"
hemisphere, so that the monkey continues responding to stimulation
there even after both forebrain commissures are completely
transected.
3.  Efforts to extend this analysis to the unihemispheric
learning of spatial relations by macaques were frustrated by the
animals' ability to use bilaterally available proprioceptive cues
in negotiating a maze.
4.  The splenium can provide adequate communication between the
visual system in one hemisphere and the amygdala in the other
hemisphere to effect proper evaluation of a fear-eliciting
stimulus.
5.  During tetanization of (a) the anterior commissure, (b) its
lateral radiation, or (c) the rostral junction of insular and
superior temporal cortex (Figure 1), macaques (with corpus callosum transected) do not respond to conditional stimuli (clicks,
light, or electrical excitation of the striate cortex) that signal either the availability of fruit juice or the imminence of
electrical shock.  They can respond immediately upon cessation of
the tetanization, and the EEG seems free of seizure activity.
Since the anterior commissural system, as noted above, can effect
interhemispheric mnemonic transfer, it is tentatively inferred
that the tetanization of this system interferes with access to
memory.

REFERENCES

Adams, J. E., & Rutkin, B. B.  Visual responses to subcortical
    stimulation in the visual and limbic systems.  *Confina
    Neurologica*, 1970, *32*, 158-164.
Bogen, J. E., & Bogen, G. M.  The other side of the brain.  III.
    The corpus callosum and creativity.  *Bulletin of the Los*

*Angeles Neurological Society*, 1969, *34*, 191-220.

Burešová, O., & Bureš, J.   Mechanisms of interhemispheric transfer of visual information in rats.   *Acta Neurobiologige Experimentalis (Warsaw)*, 1973, *33*, 673-688.

Dimond, S. J., & Beaumont, J. G.   *Hemisphere function in the human brain.*   New York:   Halsted Press, 1974.

Dobelle, W.H., & Mladejovsky, M. G.   Phosphenes produced by eletrical stimulation of human occipital cortex, and their application to the development of a prosthesis for the blind.   *Journal of Physiology,(London)*, 1974, *243*, 553-576.

Doty, R. W.   Conditioned reflexes elicited by electrical stimulation of the brain in macaques.   *Journal of Neurophysiology*, 1965, *28*, 623-640.

Doty, R. W.   Electrical stimulation of the brain in behavioral context.   *Annual Review of Psychology*, 1969, *20*, 289-320.

Doty, R. W.   On butterflies in the brain.   In V. S. Rusinov (Ed.), *Electrophysiology of the central nervous system.*   New York:   Plenum, 1970.   Pp. 97-106.

Doty, R. W.   Interhemispheric transfer and manipulation of engrams.   In C. D. Woody, K. A. Brown, T. J. Crow, Jr., & J. D. Knispel (Eds.), *Cellular mechanisms subserving changes in neuronal activity.*   Los Angeles:   Brain Information Service, 1974.   Pp. 153-159.

Doty, R. W.   "Ionic" versus "molecular" memory - are there mnemonic neurons?   In R. B. Livingston (Ed.), *Brain and behavior.*   Amsterdam:   Elsevier (in press).

Doty, R. W., & Negrão, N.   Forebrain commissures and vision.   In R. Jung (Ed.), *Handbook of sensory physiology.*   Berlin:   Springer-Verlag, 1973.   Pp. 543-582.

Doty, R. W., Negrão, N., & Yamaga, K.   The unilateral engram.   *Acta Neurobiologiae Experimentalis (Warsaw)*, 1973, *33*, 711-728.

Doty, R. W., Negrão, N., & Yamaga, K.   Odnostoronyaya engramma.   In *Osnovniye Problemi Elektrofiziologii Golovnovo Mozga.*   Moscow:   Nauka Press, 1974.   Pp. 171-178.

Doty, R. W., & Yamaga, K.   Maze behavior in macaques.   *American Journal of Physical Anthropology*, 1973, *38*, 403-406.

Downer, J. D. deC.   Changes in visual gnostic functions and emotional behavior following unilateral temporal pole damage in the "split-brain" monkey.   *Nature*, 1961, *191*, 50-51.

Gazzaniga, M. S.   *The bisected brain.*   New York:   Appleton, 1970.

Horel, J. A., & Keating, E. G.   Partial Klüver-Bucy syndrome produced by cortical disconnection.   *Brain Research*, 1969, *16*, 281-284.

Kaas, J., Axelrod, S., & Diamond, I. T.   An ablation study of the auditory cortex in the cat using binaural tonal patterns.   *Journal of Neurophysiology*, 1967, *30*, 710-724.

Kuypers, H. G. J. M., Szwarcbart, Maria K., Mishkin, M., & Rosvold, H. E.   Occipitotemporal corticocortical connections in the rhesus monkey.   *Experimental Neurology*, 1965, *11*, 245-

262.

Mishkin, M.   Cortical visual areas and their interactions.   In
A. G. Karczmar & J.C. Eccles (Eds.), *Brain and human behavior*.   New York:   Springer-Verlag, 1972.   Pp. 187-208.

Negrão, N., & Doty, R. W.   Laterality of engram in macaques trained to respond to local electrical excitation of area striata.   *Federation Proceedings*, 1969, *28*, 647.

Sakakura, H., & Doty, R. W., Sr.   EEG of striate cortex in blind monkeys:   Effects of eye movements and sleep. *Archives Italiennes de Biologie*, 1976, *114*, 23-48.

Sperry, R. W.   Lateral specialization in the surgically separated hemispheres.   In (F. O. Schmitt & F. G. Worden (Eds.), *The neurosciences: Third study program*.   Cambridge, Massachusetts:   MIT Press, 1974.   Pp. 5-20.

Sullivan, M. V., & Hamilton, C. R.   Memory establishment via the anterior commissure of monkeys.   *Physiology and Behavior*, 1973, *11*, 873-879.

Winters, W. D., Kado, R. T., & Adey, W. R.   *A stereotaxic brain atlas for Macaca nemestrina*.   Los Angeles:   Univ. of California Press, 1969.

Yamaga, K., & Doty, R. W.   Maze learning in split-brain macaques. *Physiologist*, 1971, *14*, 255.

# 6.

# Effects of Neonatal Hemispheric Disconnection in Kittens

*JERI A. SECHZER, SUSAN E. FOLSTEIN, ERIC H. GEIGER,*

New York Hospital-Cornell Medical Center

*AND DONALD F. MERVIS*

City University of New York,
Mount Sinai School of Medicine

Almost 20 years have passed since Myers and Sperry first demonstrated in their now classic experiments with split-brain animals the crucial role of the corpus callosum in the inter-hemispheric transfer of learning and memory (Myers, 1955, 1956, 1957; Myers & Sperry, 1958; Sperry, 1964, 1967).  These investigators concluded that although the transfer of learning and memory between the hemispheres is dependent upon an intact corpus callosum, these processes continue independently and normally in each hemisphere after the callosum is sectioned. However, subsequent experiments have shown that although these functions may proceed independently under such conditions, they do not do so normally in each hemisphere.  When interaction and cooperation cannot occur between the two brain halves, learning is markedly prolonged and retention is impaired (Berlucchi, Sprague, Levy, & Berardino, 1972; Meikle, 1964; Meikle & Sechzer, 1960; Meikle, Sechzer, & Stellar, 1962; Nakamura & Gazzaniga, 1974; Robinson & Voneida, 1970; Sechzer, 1964, 1965, 1968, 1970; Sechzer, Meikle, & Stellar, 1961; Teitelbaum, 1971; Voneida, 1967; see also Hamilton, this volume).

The learning curves shown in Figure 1 (*a* and *b*) and Figure 2 depict these findings.  Figure 1 shows the typical learning curves for *adult*, normal control animals, in this case an adult normal cat prior to commissurotomy.  The animals learn the discrimination (brightness and pattern) quickly, reach the 90% criterion of performance with one eye and show interocular (inter-hemispheric) transfer to the opposite, untrained eye at criterion levels.  This normal learning curve has been described as a

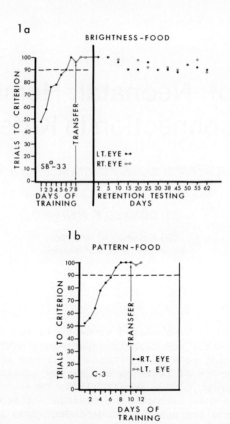

Fig. 1. (a) *Bilateral hemispheric learning curve of a normal adult cat;* brightness *discrimination for food reward. Solid circles represent training with the left eye; open circles, the right eye. Half-solid, half-open circle on day of transfer indicates level of performance with both eyes. Interocular (inter-hemispheric) transfer occurs at criterion levels. Retention testing with the left eye was started as soon as criterion was reached with that eye and proceeded concurrently with training of the right eye. Retention testing with the right eye was started as soon as criterion was reached with that eye.*
(b) *Bilateral hemispheric learning curve of a normal adult cat;* pattern *discrimination for food reward. Solid circles represent training with the right eye; open circles, the left eye. Half-solid, half-open circle on day of transfer indicates level of performance with both eyes. Interocular (interhemispheric) transfer occurs at criterion levels.*

*bilateral hemispheric learning curve,* or a learning curve of an animal that learns with two hemispheres (Sechzer, 1970). Tests

of retention were also normal, remaining at or above 90% for 62
days. There were 2 no-test days prior to retention test day 2
and 5 no-test days prior to retention test day 5. This sequence
was repeated for each retention test day indicated, and ended
with 62 no-test days prior to the final test of retention.

Figure 2 shows a typical learning curve of a split-brain cat
in which both the corpus callosum and optic chiasm were sectioned
in the adult animal. This cat took 32 days to reach the 90% criterion of learning with the first eye (the right). This acquisition time is nearly five times longer than that of its normal
control shown in Figure 1b. When the left eye was tested for the
first time, performance was at a chance level, transfer was absent, and learning with the second eye and hemisphere (the left)
took just as long as with the first. Retention was very poor,
falling below criterion after only 10 days.

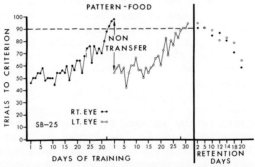

*Fig. 2.  Unilateral hemispheric learning curve of a typical
adult split-brain cat in a visual* pattern *discrimination for
food reward.  Solid circles represent training with the right
eye; open circles, the left eye.  Retention testing with the
right eye started as soon as criterion was reached with that eye
and proceeded concurrently with training of the left eye.  Retention testing with the left eye was started as soon as criterion was reached with that eye.*

The shape of the learning curve in Figure 2 differs markedly
from the bilateral hemispheric learning curve in Figure 1.
This has been described as a *unilateral hemispheric learning
curve* or a learning curve of an animal that learns with only one
hemisphere (Sechzer, 1970). The curves in Figures 1 and 2 are
typical of results obtained with adult normal and split-brain
cats. These results cannot be attributed to visual field loss
from optic chiasm section since it has been shown that acquisition and transfer of a pattern discrimination is normal in cats
after division of the crossed optic fibers (Myers, 1955).
Inspection of the learning curve in Figure 2 shows that acquisition time is the same for each hemisphere. In many cases,
learning curves for each hemisphere in split-brain cats are virtually superimposable (Meikle & Sechzer, 1960; Meikle, *et al*.,

1962; Sperry, 1961; Stamm & Speery, 1957). Such data, obtained
for visual and tactile discrimination tasks, do not support a
concept of lateralization in the cat brain. This concept has,
however, been reexamined recently by Gulliksen and Voneida
(1975) and by Webster (this volume).

The main conclusions derived from these findings were that:

1.   Both cerebral hemispheres usually participate equally
     during learning.
2.   The normal learning curve (thus the normal rate of learn-
     ing) appears to be a function of bihemispheric processing
     of information.
3.   Memory during and after acquisition is also dependent on
     the functional relationships between the hemispheres.

Most knowledge about hemispheric interaction and the mediation
of normal learning and memory via the corpus callosum is limited
to observations of animals in which split-brain surgery was performed during adult life. This is long after maturation of the
central nervous system (CNS), myelination of forebrain commissures, development of adaptive behaviors, and development of
intellectual processes.

These investigations have added to the understanding of interhemispheric mechanisms, as well as of the autonomous capabilities
of each hemisphere in the absence of the normal participation of
its opposite brain half through the corpus callosum. Unfortunately, experiments with adult split-brain animals do not contribute information about the age at which the corpus callosum
assumes functional significance in the transfer of information
from one hemisphere to the other. Studies on adult split-brain
animals tell nothing of a possible role for the corpus callosum
in the normal development of brain function.

However, some observations about the functional development of
the corpus callosum are available from the history of commissurotomy in epileptic patients. Based on a demonstration by
Erickson (1940) in laboratory animals, which showed that the
corpus callosum was the major pathway of interhemispheric
seizure propagation, surgical disconnection of human cerebral
hemispheres was first attempted in 1940 by Van Wagenen and
Herren (1940). Either partial or complete section of the corpus
callosum was carried out on eight adults and two adolescents
who had intractable epilepsy. Observations of these patients
indicated that callosal surgery prevented the spread of an epileptic seizure to the opposite hemisphere.

In 1962, Bogen, Fisher, and Vogel sectioned the corpus callosum and anterior commissure in a second series of adult and
adolescent patients having intractable epilepsy. Their patients
generally showed excellent results with regard to seizure control. Little change was observed in ordinary behavior and tem-
perament except for some compensation for lack of interhemispheric transfer (Bogen, Fisher, & Vogel, 1965; Gazzaniga,

Bogen, & Sperry, 1965; Gazzaniga & Sperry, 1967).

Most recently, Leussenhop, de la Cruz, and Fenichel (1970) reported the results of hemispheric disconnection in three young children (one 7-year-old and two 3-year-olds) and in one infant, 4 months old, whose seizures spread interhemispherically and were refractory to medical treatment. Complete midsagittal section of the corpus callosum and anterior commissure was performed on all patients, and two of them had additional excision of the fornix. Commissurotomy in the 7-year-old child resulted in a dramatic and continued reduction of seizure activity during a 17-month follow-up period. The 3-year-old children showed a decrease in their seizures, but were being managed on medication with only fair success. However, hemispheric division failed to alter the seizure pattern in the 4-month-old infant. These results, after comparison with the excellent results achieved in adult and adolescent patients, indicate that the amount of seizure control achieved by surgical hemispheric disconnection appears to increase gradually with the age of the patient. This clinical evidence suggests that at birth and for a period thereafter the corpus callosum and anterior commissure are not fully functional and are not responsible for the spread of an epileptic discharge from one hemisphere to the other.

Some histological data also support this hypothesis. The corpus callosum and other forebrain commissures are unmyelinated at birth in all mammals including man (Hewitt, 1962; Rorke & Riggs, 1969). In man, the cycle of myelinogenesis of the corpus callosum becomes complete at about 10 years of age (Yakovlev & Lecours, 1967). The corpus callosum would presumably achieve its total functional effectiveness by that time. Therefore, at birth and for a time thereafter, the interhemispheric propagation of seizure activity would necessarily involve other pathways. Early commissurotomy would have little or no effect on seizure transmission in man.

These data in animals and man suggest the following:

1. The development of hemispheric interaction may proceed along a course concurrently with the myelination of the corpus callosum.
2. The development of normal intellectual processes may be dependent upon the development of hemispheric interaction via the corpus callosum.
3. Neonatal corpus callosum section may interfere with normal intellectual development.

One way to investigate these possibilities is to disconnect surgically the hemispheres in kittens during the neonatal period before myelination of the callosum, which begins at approximately 28 days of age (Grafstein, 1963), and before a mature transcallosal response appears. In this way, each hemisphere will develop without callosally mediated interaction.

In order to study such a preparation, we developed a simple

procedure for midsagittal section of the corpus callosum in the
newborn kitten between 36 and 72 hr of age. We also designed
a commissurotomy knife which eliminates retraction of the hemispheres, thus preventing damage to the delicate neonatal brain.
In addition to complete midsagittal section of the callosum, this
operative procedure also severs the psalterium. Details of this
procedure and dimensions of the commissurotomy knife are reported elsewhere (Sechzer, Folstein, Geiger, & Mervis, 1976).

OBSERVATIONS AND BEHAVIORAL TESTS

Observations and tests were conducted only on those animals
that were healthy and gained weight within the same range. At
least three observers participated in every session.

*HOME ORIENTATION*

We used a procedure similar to that described by Rosenblatt,
Turkewitz, and Schneirla (1969) in order to observe how infant
kittens orient toward, or find their way back to, their mothers
and home area, i.e., that area of the cage where the kitten is
nursed. For some test sessions, the mother remained alone in
the home area after the littermates were removed; for other test
sessions, the mother and littermates were removed. Testing
started at 5 days of age and continued three times a week until
the kittens were 1 month old. At the beginning of each trial
the kitten to be tested was placed in the corner of the cage
diagonal to the home area (see Figure 3). By 10 days of age,
the normal kittens and sham-operated kittens were observed to
take a direct path back to the home area and their mother
(Figure 3, *A* and *C*). On the other hand, at the same age, split-
brain kittens took a circuitous path that involved a greater
distance and required more time (Figure 3, *B* and *D*). It is not
known whether disruption of the normal home orientation pattern
is a consequence of cutting the corpus callosum (in which the
transcollosal response is still immature), the psalterium, or
both.

*HYPERACTIVITY*

Birth to Six Weeks of Age

Within a few days after surgery the split-brain kittens showed
increased activity. While normal kittens remained huddled together and sleeping, the split-brain kittens roamed around the
cage and over their mother's body. This behavior persisted even
after their eyes opened at about the end of the first week. By
6 weeks of age the split-brain animals appeared hyperactive.
When they were exercised in our animal quarters, hyperactivity
was expressed by constant, random, and focusless behavior rather

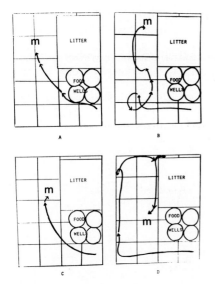

Fig. 3. Orientation of displaced kittens toward home area and mother. A and C show the direct path taken by six normal kittens and two sham-operated kittens, at 10 days of age, to return to mother, m, in the home quadrant. B and D show the circuitous path taken by five neonatal split-brain kittens, also 10 days old. Each arrow represents the location of the animal after 20 sec.

than the excessive bursts of activity so typical of normal kittens. The animals were easily distracted and hurried from one object to the next. This was in contrast to the sham-surgery and normal control groups, which attended to fewer objects but remained with each one for a longer time. These observations were quantified when the kittens were 6 months old.

## Six Months of Age

We wanted to determine whether amphetamine would diminish hyperactivity in the split-brain group, as it does in hyperactive children. This effect is referred to as the *paradoxical response*. Amphetamine and amphetamine-like drugs have a stimulating effect on normal adults and children (Snyder & Myerhoff, 1973), but paradoxically produce a quieting effect on children with Minimal Brain Dysfunction (MBD). When the animals were 5-6 months old, we measured their activity and tested them with *d*-amphetamine.*

The kinds of activity we used included the following:

1. alertness
2. ease of handling
3. locomotion
4. exploration

Each behavior was rated from -4 to +4 and the average score was

*d-Amphetamine was supplied through the courtesy of Smith, Kline, & French Laboratories, Inc., Philadelphia, Pa.

plotted (e.g., locomotion: -4 = lying quietly; 0 = walking about and exploring objects; +4 = constant, random, and focusless behavior).

Activity before and after amphetamine administration is shown in Figure 4. With increasing dosage, the normal kittens became

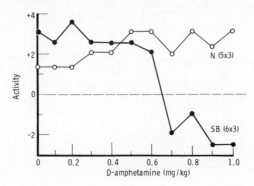

*Fig. 4. Effect of increasing doses of* d-*amphetamine on activity of normal (open circles) and of neonatal split-brain (solid circles) kittens. Five normal kittens were tested three times on each dose ( 5 x 3) and six split-brain kittens were tested three times on each dose (6 x 3) at 48 hr intervals. Saline injections in normal and split-brain kittens did not alter behavior.*

more active. In contrast, with increasing dosage, the split-brain kittens became less active and at an average dose of 0.7 mg/kg hyperactivity was dramatically diminished. Split-brain kittens curled up or sat quietly in their cages, a behavior not previously observed. When removed from their cages, they either stayed in one place or walked about slowly. They were less distracted by sudden sounds or movements and seemed to attend to various objects about them for longer periods. Within 2 hr after amphetamine administration they began to return to their usual hyperactive state.

## Open Field

Open field tests were conducted when the animals were 6 months of age. The open field apparatus consisted of a 150 x 150 cm wood floor with a wood fence 90 cm high. The wood floor was marked into 25 square divisions of 30 $cm^2$ each. In the first test, the number of squares traversed and the pattern of activity shown by each kitten were recorded during several 3-min test sessions. In the second test, toys were introduced and the kittens' attention to them was recorded for 10 min. All observations were made from a 1 m distance using a convex mirror so that the kittens could not see the observers. Figures 5, 6a, and

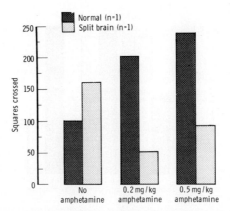

*Fig. 5.* *Effect of amphetamine administration on open field activity for a 5-month-old neonatal split-brain kitten and its control littermate. Ordinate indicates number of squares crossed during a 3-min test session.*

6b depict the results for one split-brain kitten and its normal littermate. A summary of the results follows:

1. *Squares Crossed.* Without amphetamine, the normal kitten crossed 106 squares during the 3-min test period in the open field and the split-brain kitten crossed 161 squares. After receiving 0.2 mg/kg of amphetamine, the normal kitten crossed 200 squares. After receiving 0.5 mg/kg, it crossed 239 squares, more than double its preamphetamine score. The split-brain kitten, however, crossed only 55 squares after receiving 0.2 mg/kg amphetamine; after receiving 0.5 mg/kg, it crossed 92 squares, a decrease of 66% and 43% respectively.* The activity of the split-brain kitten under the effect of amphetamine is comparable to the activity of the normal kitten without amphetamine.

2. *Objects Attended.* Figure 6 summarizes the number of objects attended and the number of seconds spent with each object before and after amphetamine. A paper ball, a plastic cup, and hanging paper streamers were placed in the open field. During a 10-min test period without amphetamine the normal kitten transferred its attention from toy to toy an average of 7.7 times (Figure 6a), spending 16.9 sec (Figure 6b) with each object or a total of 130 sec of playing time. For the remainder of the 10 min the normal kitten walked, ran, or groomed. The split-brain

---

*Repeated dosage with amphetamine results in tolerance. The greater number of squares crossed at 0.5 mg/kg amphetamine than at 0.2 mg/kg amphetamine reflects the tolerance this animal developed following closely repeated doses of the higher dose of amphetamine.

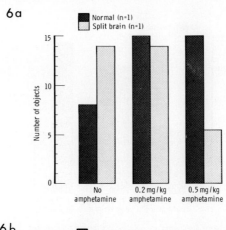

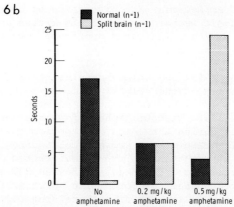

*Fig. 6. Effect of amphetamine administration on open field activity with play objects: (a) number of objects attended, and (b) number of seconds spent with each object, in the open field during a 10-min observation period.*

kitten transferred its attention from toy to toy an average of 14.2 times (Figure 6a), spending only .65 sec with each one (Figure 6b). The split-brain kitten played for a total of only 9 sec and spent most of the remaining time running about and leaping at the sides of the box.

After either 0.2 or 0.5 mg/kg of amphetamine, the normal kitten actually transferred its attention more (15 times), played with each toy for shorter periods (6.5 and 4.3 sec), and had a total playtime of only 67.5 and 97.5 sec. In contrast to the performance of the normal kitten with amphetamine, the split-brain kitten spent more time with each object. At a dose of 0.5 mg/kg the kitten transferred its attention from toy to toy only six times during the 10-min test period spending 24 sec with each object. Its total playtime was 144 sec.

*LEARNING AND MEMORY*

## Procedure

When the animals were 1 year old, their learning and retention were tested. Each animal was trained to make a visual pattern discrimination in order to obtain food. The animals were adapted to and then trained in a visual discrimination apparatus which consisted of (1) a start box and (2) a runway 168 x 53 x 43 cm. At the end of the runway two translucent plastic doors hung side by side. A small compartment behind each door held a food cup and served as a goal box. The pairs of visual stimuli to be discriminated by the animals were identical in shape, differing only in orientation: either upright or inverted triangles, or horizontal or vertical stripes. One out of the pair of stimuli was affixed to each plastic door. One patterned door represented the positive or correct stimulus and was unlocked. The other patterned door was the negative or incorrect stimulus and was locked. Each animal learned to leave the start box, proceed down the runway to the patterned doors, select one of them and push it back to obtain the food in the goal box. When the cat pushed on the correct, unlocked door, it gained immediate access to the food cup. A push on the incorrect, locked door proved to be ineffective and subsequently the cat learned to correct its response to the opposite side. Training was continued until each animal's performance reached a level of 90% or better for 3 consecutive days. The experiments were conducted every other day in a semi-darkened room and with the animals deprived of food for approximately 23 hr. They were rewarded with small pieces of raw spleen for pushing back the correctly patterned door. The same procedure was used when training was carried out with amphetamine.* During this part of the experiment, training started 55

---

*The animals were maintained at 80% of their body weight. On this feeding schedule, animals are very hungry and so develop anorexia in response to amphetamine at much higher doses than when on a 100% feeding schedule. On the other hand, lower doses of amphetamine result in increased activity and increased arousal (normal cats) or decreased activity and decreased arousal (split-brain cats). Thus, without producing anorexia it is possible to obtain an effect on activity with amphetamine and still train the cats to learn a discrimination on the basis of motivation for food. We give our cats the remainder of their daily food portions immediately after each test session and have never found them to be satiated. Because we wanted to minimize any residual effect of amphetamine, the cats were tested every other day.

min after amphetamine was administered.*

Training was carried out first without amphetamine. Two
months later, the cats were trained with amphetamine on a
second and different pattern discrimination. Another group of
cats was trained in the reverse order.

## Results

Regardless of the order of testing, the results were the same.
Neonatal split-brain cats took longer than normal cats to learn
without amphetamine but with amphetamine learning time was shorter. Figure 7 presents these differences. Split-brain cats

PATTERN DISCRIMINATION LEARNING

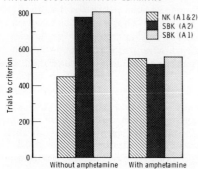

*Fig. 7. Effect of amphetamine
administration on learning a
pattern discrimination to a 90%
criterion in 1-year-old neonatal
split-brain cats (SBK) and their
normal littermates (NK).*

trained first without amphetamine took an average of 780 trials
to reach the 90% criterion of learning for 3 consecutive days.
With amphetamine they learned the second task, which was equal
to the first in difficulty, in only 520 trials, an improvement
of 33%. In the reversed condition, split-brain cats trained
first with amphetamine needed only 560 trials to reach the 90%
criterion of learning but needed 810 trials to reach the same
criterion without amphetamine. This represents a 31% improvement in learning when amphetamine is used. Normal cats took only
450 trials without amphetamine and 550 trials with amphetamine to
reach criterion.

The every-other-day performance of normal and split-brain cats
revealed two different patterns of behavior. The performance of
normal cats on each training session improved. Forty-eight hours
later, when next tested, their initial performance indicated
little or no loss of retention from the previous test session.
However, the responses of split-brain cats suggest a time-
dependent memory deficit. Although performance improved by the
end of a day's session, the initial performance on the next test
day decreased markedly, sometimes to a chance level. This

*Because we wanted to minimize any residual effect of ampheta-
mine, the cats were tested every other day.

pattern of behavior was repeated throughout a large segment of the test. Thus, prolonged training was necessary for the animals to reach the criterion of learning.

Without amphetamine, habituation to the test apparatus was prolonged, and, during training, it was extremely difficult to persuade the split-brain cats to work throughout the 30 trials of a day's session. The animals were easily distracted by the slightest noise and would frequently jump out of the testing apparatus after about 15 trials.

When training with amphetamine was started, the animals' behavior changed. It became relatively easy to complete a 30-trial session and the cats no longer jumped out of the test apparatus. Day-to-day retention increased and learning was faster. These improvements in learning and retention are apparently a result of amphetamine treatment.

## HISTOLOGY

When these experiments were completed, the brains of the animals were perfused with 8.5% sucrose followed by 7.5% sucrose/ 10% formalin and then removed from the skull. After embedding in celloidin, alternate sections of 30 μm were stained with thionine and by Weil's method. Figure 8 shows thionine-stained coronal sections through the hippocampal area of the brains of two neonatal split-brain cats and their normal littermates. The sections of the normal cats show an intact corpus callosum connecting the two cerebral hemispheres. In the sections of the split-brain cats the corpus callosum is completely absent in the midline. There is no evidence of surgical damage to the cortex along the medial aspects of the hemispheres or to subjacent structures. In one of six split-brain animals approximately 2 mm of callosum remained intact at the extreme anterior tip. This animal's performance did not differ from that of the others in the experiment.

## DISCUSSION

Although we have observed only a small number of neonatal split-brain animals, they consistently showed abnormal home orientation, hyperactivity, decreased attention span, deficits in learning and memory, and a paradoxical response to amphetamine.

These behavioral alterations are distinctive and in many ways mimic those presented by children with the Minimal Brain Dysfunction (MBD) syndrome. Because of these similarities, we would like to speculate that the neonatal split-brain kitten may prove to be an analogue or model for this clinical disorder.

At least 5% of school-aged children are afflicted with MBD, and it has become one of the most common disturbances reported by child psychiatrists. The symptoms presented by MBD children

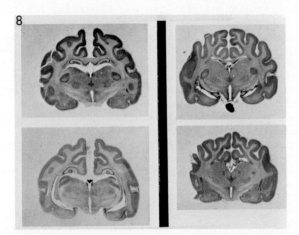

*Fig. 8.  The brains of one group of cats were perfused at 6
months of age, after activity and open field tests.  The brains
of a second group of cats were perfused at 2 years of age, after
learning tests.  Left:  Brain sections of 2-year-old cats.
Upper section, the brain of a normal animal; lower section, that
of a split-brain cat with corpus callosum sectioned 36 hr after
birth.  Right:  Brain sections of 6-month-old cats.  Upper section, from normal control; lower section, from a split-brain cat
with corpus callosum sectioned 60 hr after birth.*

include

1. hyperactivity;
2. incoordination;
3. decreased attention span;
4. deficits in learning and memory;
5. lack of impulse control;
6. anhedonia (the decreased ability to respond to positive
   and negative reinforcement); and
7. the paradoxical response to amphetamine.

The fact that no animal model yet exists for this syndrome has
been a tremendous obstacle to our understanding its nature, cau-
sation, and treatment.  However, the following criteria have been
selected for an appropriate animal model for MBD (Sechzer, Faro,
& Windle, 1973):

1. Symptoms should be evident, in part, from birth.
2. Other symptoms should appear at ages comparable to when
   they appear in children.
3. The symptoms should be ameliorated by amphetamine or
   amphetamine-like drugs and the animals should respond (as
   children do) with a decrease in activity and an improve-

ment in attention, learning, and memory.

4. The opportunity should be available to analyze the brains of the animals for pathological changes using classical histological techniques, histo-fluorescent methods, and biochemical assays.

Our observations demonstrate that neonatal split-brain kittens satisfy many of these criteria. Hyperactivity, decreased attention span, deficits in learning and memory, and the paradoxical response to amphetamine are the salient attributes analogous to those of MBD children.

We do not wish to imply that children with MBD have callosal deficits. It is uncertain how callosal section in the neonatal kitten leads to these symptoms, but it does appear to be a way of producing a syndrome of mild brain dysfunction in this species without any gross neurological abnormalities.

Neonatal commissurotomy in kittens is one way of reducing the number of neurons and/or synaptic connections that would usually participate in organized behavior. This reduction can come about in two ways: (1) by the division of the corpus callosum, which generally isolates the cortical neuronal processes of the two hemispheres from each other, and (2) by the degeneration of callosal fibers and perhaps of the cells from which they are derived.

In addition, a possible physiological consequence of neonatal commissurotomy in kittens is that it may disrupt and limit the interplay of excitatory and inhibitory processes, which, according to Purpura (1973), are so important for normal development.

Some support for conceptualizing a reduction in functional neuronal processes comes from results of amphetamine treatment of MBD children. In addition to the amelioration of hyperactivity, the treated children show improvements in attention, learning, and memory (Stewart, Ferris, & Pitts, 1966; Wender, 1971). Stewart *et al.* have hypothesized a deficit in CNS norepinephrine release to account for the effects of amphetamine in MBD children. Amphetamine facilitates the release of norepinephrine by neurons in the CNS (Schildkraut & Kety, 1967) and increases synaptic transmission; these effects are thought to increase the number of functional neuronal processes. The observation that both children and neonatal split-brain animals respond to amphetamine suggests that the primary sensory and/or perceptual pathways involved in these behaviors may be impaired but they are not permanently damaged. Restoration to their functional level may be accomplished temporarily by amphetamine.

An alternative to a concept of neuronal reduction is the interruption of a specific pathway(s), which results in some or all of these behavioral alterations. In addition to the widespread neocortical interconnections via callosal axons, two other pathways have been reported to cross among the anterior fibers of the corpus callosum. The first, a cortico-striatal pathway, projects from the sensori-motor cortex of one hemisphere to the caudate nucleus of the opposite hemisphere in the rat, rabbit, and cat (Carman, Cowan, Powell, & Webster, 1965; Webster, 1965) and from the cingulum of one hemisphere to the caudate nucleus of the opposite hemisphere in monkey and man (Locke, Kruper, & Yakovlev, 1964; Locke & Yakovlev, 1965). The second, the striate-striate pathway, is a monosynaptic projection from the caudate nucleus of one hemisphere to the caudate nucleus of the opposite hemisphere (Mensah & Deadwyler, 1974). Although no specific function has been associated with the cortico-striatal pathway, Glick, Crane, Jerussi, Fleisher, and Green (1975) have demonstrated a 10% decrease in the dopamine content of the caudate nucleus of each hemisphere after striate-striate transection in adult rats. Associated with this decrement was a change in the amphetamine-induced rotatory bias during locomotion.

Shaywitz, Yager, and Klopper (1976) have proposed an animal model for MBD based on depletion of brain dopamine in neonatal rat pups by intracisternal administration of 6-hydroxydopamine.

To help distinguish between a generalized reduction in functional neuronal processes by corpus callosum section as opposed to the interruption of a specific pathway(s) within the callosum, further investigation is necessary. One avenue of approach would be to section only the anterior portion of the corpus callosum (which includes the cortico-striate and the striate-striate pathways) as well as producing localized lesions in the sensorimotor cortex and caudate nucleus. Subsequent behavioral observations would determine whether one or both of these pathways are responsible for the behavioral alterations observed. Another approach would be to investigate the behavioral effects of neo-cortical and subcortical lesions of various sizes as controls for the reduction hypothesis.

## SUMMARY

Neonatal split-brain kittens show behavioral alterations like those observed in children with Minimal Brain Dysfunction. The similarities of these alterations are striking. Since we have shown that the symptoms in the animals can be ameliorated by amphetamine, as they are in MBD children, we suggest that the neonatal split-brain kitten may prove to be a valuable analogue for the investigation of this clinical disorder.

## ADKNOWLEDGMENTS

Research supported by NSF Grant GB33469 to J. A. S. We thank Ms. Elaine Rossinoff for the preparation of the histological sections.
Some of the data reported here have been presented previously (Sechzer, 1973).

REFERENCES

Berlucchi, G., Sprague, J. M., Levy, J., & Berardino, A. C. Pretectum and superior colliculus in visually guided behavior and in flux and form discrimination in the cat. *Journal of Comparative & Physiological Psychology*, 1972, *78*, 123-172.

Bogen, S. E., Fisher, E. P., & Vogel, P. S. Cerebral commissurotomy: A second case report. *Journal of the American Medical Association*, 1965, *174*, 1328-1329.

Carman, J. B., Cowan, W. M., Powell, T. P. S., & Webster, K. E. A bilateral cortico-striate projection. *Journal of Neurology, Neurosurgery and Psychiatry*, 1965, *28*, 71-77.

Erickson, T. C. Spread of the epileptic discharge. *Archives of Neurology and Psychiatry*, 1940, *43*, 429-452.

Gazzaniga, M. S., Bogen, J. E., & Sperry, R. W. Observations on visual perception after disconnection of the cerebral hemispheres in man. *Brain*, 1965, *88*, 221-230.

Gazzaniga, M.S., & Sperry, R. W. Language after section of the cerebral commissures. *Brain*, 1967, *90*, 131-148.

Glick, S. D., Crane, A. M., Jerussi, T. P., Fleisher, L. N., & Green, J. Functional and neurochemical correlates of potentiation of striatal asymmetry by callosal section. *Nature*, 1975, *254*, 616-617.

Grafstein, B. Postnatal development of the transcallosal evoked response in the cerebral cortex of the cat. *Journal of Neurophysiology*, 1963, *26*, 79-99.

Gulliksen, H., & Voneida, T. An attempt to obtain replicate learning curves in the split-brain cat. *Physiological Psychology*, 1975, *3*, 77-85.

Hewitt, W. The development of the corpus callosum. *Journal of Anatomy*, 1962, *96*, 355-358.

Leussenhop, A. J., de la Cruz, T. C., & Fenichel, G. M. Surgical disconnection of the cerebral hemispheres for intractable seizures: Results in infancy and childhood. *Journal of the American Medical Association*, 1970, *213*, 1630-1636.

Locke, S., Kruper, D. C., & Yakovlev, P. I. Limbic nuclei of thalamus and connections of limbic cortex. *Archives of Neurology*, 1964, *11*, 571-582.

Locke, S., & Yakovlev, P. I. Transcallosal connections of the cingulum of man. *Archives of Neurology*, 1965, *13*, 471-476.

Meikle, T. H. Failure of interocular transfer of brightness discrimination. *Nature*, 1964, *202*, 1243-1244.

Meikle, T. H., & Sechzer, J. A. Interocular transfer of brightness discrimination in split-brain cats. *Science*, 1960, *132*, 734-735.

Meikle, T. H., Sechzer, J. A., & Stellar, E. Interhemispheric transfer of tactile conditioned responses in corpus callosum-sectioned cats. *Journal of Neurophysiology*, 1962, *25*, 530-543.

Mensah, P., & Deadwyler, S.   The caudate nucleus of the rat:
    Cell types and the demonstration of a commissural system.
    *Journal of Anatomy*, 1974, *117*, 281-293.
Myers, R. E.   Interocular transfer of pattern discrimination in
    cats following section of crossed optic fibers.   *Journal
    of Comparative and Physiological Psychology*, 1955, *48*, 470-
    473.
Myers, R. E.   Function of corpus callosum in interocular trans-
    fer.   *Brain*, 1956, *79*, 358-363.
Myers, R. E.   Corpus callosum and interhemispheric communica-
    tion:  Enduring memory effects.   *Federation Proceedings*,
    1957, *16*, 92.
Myers, R. E., & Sperry, R. W.   Interhemispheric communication
    through the corpus callosum:  Mnemonic carryover between
    the hemispheres.   *Archives of Neurology and Psychiatry*,
    1958, *80*, 298-303.
Nakamura, R. K., & Gazzaniga, M. S.   Reduced information process-
    ing capabilities following commissurotomy in the monkey.
    *The Physiologist*, 1974, *17*, 294.
Purpura, D. P.   Analysis of morphophysiological developmental
    processes in mammalian brain.   In *Biological and environ-
    mental determinants of early development*.   Research Publi-
    cations Association for Research in Nervous and Mental
    Disease.   Vol. 51.   Baltimore:  Williams & Wilkins, 1973.
    Pp. 79-112.
Robinson, J. S., & Voneida, T. S.   Quantitative differences in
    performance on abstract discriminations using one or both
    hemispheres.   *Experimental Neurology*, 1970, *26*, 72-83.
Rorke, L. B., & Riggs, H. E.   *Myelination of the brain in the
    newborn*.   Philadelphia:  Lippincott, 1969.
Rosenblatt, J. S., Turkewitz, G., & Schneirla, T. C.   Develop-
    ment of home orientation in newly born kittens.   *Transac-
    tions of the New York Academy of Sciences*, 1969, *31*, 231-
    250.
Schildkraut, J. J., & Kety, S. S.   Pharmacological studies sug-
    gest a relationship between brain biogenic amines and
    affective state.   *Science*, 1967, *156*, 3771, 21-30.
Sechzer, J. A.   Successful interocular transfer of pattern dis-
    crimination in split-brain cats with shock-avoidance
    motivation.   *Journal of Comparative and Physiological
    Psychology*, 1964, *58*, 70-83.
Sechzer, J. A.   Interhemispheric transfer of brightness dis-
    crimination in split-brain cats with unilateral striate
    ablation.   *The Physiologist*, 1965, *8*, 270.
Sechzer, J. A.   Interhemispheric integration and prolonged learn-
    ing in split-brain cats.   *Proceedings of the International
    Union of Physiological Sciences*, 1968, VII, 395.
Sechzer, J. A.   Prolonged learning and split-brain cats.
    *Science*, 1970, *169*, 889-892.
Sechzer, J. A.   The neonatal split-brain kitten as an animal
    model for minimal brain dysfunction.   *Program of the*

*Society of Neurosciences*, 1973, abstract *15.11*.

Sechzer, J. A., Faro, M. D., & Windle, W. F. Studies of monkeys asphyxiated at birth: Implications for minimal cerebral dysfunction. *Seminars in Psychiatry*, 1973, *5*, (1), 19-34.

Sechzer, J. A., Folstein, S. E., Geiger, E. H., & Mervis, R. F. The split-brain neonate: A surgical method for corpus callosum section in new-born kittens. *Developmental Psychobiology*, 1976, in press.

Sechzer, J. A., Meikle, T. H., & Stellar, E. Interhemispheric transfer of tactile and respiratory conditioned responses in corpus callosum-sectioned cats. *Program of the Eastern Psychological Association*, 1961.

Shaywitz, B. A., Yager, R. D., & Klopper, J. H. Selective brain dopamine depletion in developing rats: An experimental model of minimal brain dysfunction. *Science*, 1976, *191*, 305-307.

Snyder, S. H., & Myerhoff, J. L. How amphetamine acts in minimal brain dysfunction. In Minimal brain dysfunction. *Annals of the New York Academy of Sciences*, 1973, *205*, 310-320.

Sperry, R. W. Cerebral organization and behavior. *Science*, 1961, *133*, 1749-1757.

Sperry, R. W. The great cerebral commissure. *Scientific American*, 1964, *210*, 42-54.

Sperry, R. W. Split-brain approach to learning problems. In G. C. Quarton, T. Melnechuk, & F. O. Schmitt (Eds.), *The Neurosciences*. New York: Rockefeller Univ. Press, 1967. Pp. 714-723.

Stamm, J. S., & Sperry, R. W. Function of corpus callosum in contralateral transfer of somesthetic discriminations in cats. *Journal of Comparative and Physiological Psychology*, 1957, *50*, 138-143.

Stewart, M., Ferris, A., & Pitts, N. The hyperkinetic child syndrome. *American Journal of Orthopsychiatry*, 1966, *36*, 861-867.

Teitelbaum, H. Lateralization of olfactory memory in the split-brain rat. *Journal of Comparative and Physiological Psychology*, 1971, *76*, 51-56.

Van Wagenen, W. P., & Herren, R. Y. Surgical division of commissural pathways in the corpus callosum: Relationship to spread of an epileptic attack. *Archives of Neurological Psychiatry*, 1940, *44*, 740-759.

Voneida, T. J. The effect of pyramidal lesions on the performance of a conditioned avoidance response in cats. *Experimental Neurology*, 1967, *19*, 483-493.

Webster, K. E. The corticostriatal projection in the cat. *Journal of Anatomy*, 1965, *99*, 329-337.

Wender, P. H. *Minimal brain dysfunction in children*. New York: Wiley, 1971.

Yakovlev, P. E., & Lecours, A. R. The myelogenetic cycles of regional maturation of the brain. In A. Minkowski (Ed.),

*Regional development of the brain in early life.* Philadelphia: Davis, 1967.

# 7.
# The Neural Basis of Stimulus Equivalence Across Retinal Translation

*CHARLES G. GROSS*

Princeton University

*MORTIMER MISHKIN*

National Institute of Mental Health

How do we recognize an object as being the same no matter what part of the retina it stimulates?  What are the neural mechanisms underlying this *stimulus equivalence across retinal translation*? A particularly puzzling example of such equivalence is the recognition of an object as the same whether it is in the left or right visual half-field, since the neural signals evoked by the object in these two locations travel to opposite hemispheres. How do neural events in the separate hemispheres result in the same perceptual experience?

We know that communications between the hemispheres depends on the forebrain commissures (Sperry, 1961; Doty & Negrão, 1973). Only if these commissures are intact can there be interhemispheric transfer of a visual habit.  That is, if the output from each eye is restricted to one hemisphere (as by midsagittal section of the optic chiasm), interocular transfer of a learned pattern discrimination will occur if the forebrain commissures are preserved, but not if they are cut.  Why are these fibers crucial? What structures are they connecting, and what information are they carrying?

In this chapter we propose that interhemispheric transfer of visual habits is a special case of stimulus equivalence across retinal translation, and that both the transfer and the equivalance are mediated by neurons located in the inferior cortex of the temporal lobe.  In the first section of the chapter we review the properties of inferior temporal neurons.  The second section discusses the intrahemispheric and commissural pathways that contribute to these properties. In the third section, we present some evidence on the role of inferior temporal neurons in inter-hemispheric transfer. And, in the final section, we consider the implications of this evidence for understanding the neural basis of stimulus equivalence.

INFERIOR TEMPORAL NEURONS

In the rhesus monkey the cortex of the inferior convexity of the temporal lobe (Figure 1) is critical for visual discrimination learning. The bilateral removal of inferior temporal cortex

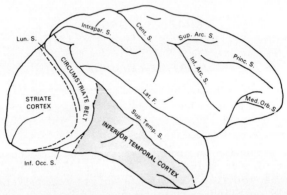

*Fig. 1. Diagram of lateral view of right cerebral hemisphere of Macaca mulatta. The dashed lines show the approximate borders between striate cortex, the circumstriate belt and inferior temporal cortex. Abbreviations: Cent. S., central sulcus; Inf. Arc. S., inferior arcuate sulcus; Inf. Occ. S., inferior occipital sulcus; Intrapar. S., intraparietal sulcus; Lat. F., lateral fissure; Lun. S., lunate sulcus; Med. Orb. S., medial orbital sulcus; Princ. S., principal sulcus; Sup. Arc. S., superior arcuate sulcus; Sup. Temp. S., superior temporal sulcus.*

produces a severe deficit in visual discrimination learning, al-though it does not impair either discrimination learning in other modalities or basic visuosensory functions such as visual acuity, visual thresholds, and the visual fields (see reviews by Gross, 1973a, b, and Mishkin, 1972). In man, removal of the temporal cortex of the minor hemisphere is followed by higher-order visual deficits (see review by Milner, 1973).

In parallel with the exclusively visual effects of inferior temporal lesions, single neurons in inferior temporal cortex respond only to visual stimuli. Their receptive fields almost always include the fovea and are relatively large, the majority being larger than $20^\circ$ x $20^\circ$. About 60% of the receptive fields extend across the vertical meridian and many of them include more than $10^0$ of both visual half-fields; the remaining receptive fields are confined either to the contralateral or to the ipsilateral visual field (see Figure 4A). Most inferior temporal neurons are sensitive to several stimulus parameters such as contrast, wavelength, size, shape, orientation, and direction of movement. The optimal stimulus for a given cell is almost always optimal throughout the entire receptive field of that cell, even when the receptive field extends across the midline into both halves of visual space. Finally, most neurons can be driven by visual stimuli presented to either eye. Thus, many neurons in inferior temporal cortex respond to specific stimuli independent of their location over a wide expanse of both halves of both eyes (Gross, Bender, & Rocha-Miranda, 1973; Gross, Rocha-Miranda, & Bender, 1972).

## VISUAL PATHWAYS AND INFERIOR TEMPORAL CORTEX

How do neurons in inferior temporal cortex receive information from both halves of visual space? Each visual half-field is represented in the contralateral striate cortex, and each striate cortex projects to the surrounding extrastriate visual areas known collectively as *prestriate*, or *circumstriate*, *cortex*. In turn, neurons in circumstriate cortex project to inferior temporal neurons. Furthermore, there are interhemispheric connections between portions of the two circumstriate belts through the splenium and between the two inferior temporal cortices through both the splenium and the anterior commissure. Therefore, each inferior temporal area could receive visual information about the contralateral visual field from the striate cortex in the same hemisphere by way of the circumstriate belt, and about the ipsilateral field from the opposite striate cortex by way of the circumstriate belt and the forebrain commissures. These connections are diagramed in Figure 2 (Cowey, 1973; Jones, 1973: Kuypers, Szwarcbart, Mishkin, & Rosvold, 1965; Pandya, Karol, & Heilbronn, 1971; Zeki, 1974).

In addition to this possible cortico-cortical route from striate cortex, inferior temporal neurons could also receive visual information from the pulvinar. Portions of the pulvinar receive afferents from striate cortex and from the superior colliculus (Campos-Ortega & Hayhow, 1972; Mishkin, 1972; Rezak and Benevento, 1975). Thus, inferior temporal neurons could receive visual information by way of the pulvinar from either the striate cortex or the superior colliculus, as diagramed in Figure 3. However, none of these pulvino-cortical routes could account for the responsiveness of inferior temporal neurons to stimuli in the ipsilateral visual field because there is no evidence of any representation of this field in the pulvinar (Bender, 1975). Information from the ipsilateral field would still have to be

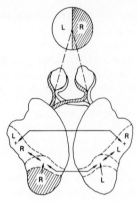

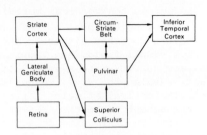

Fig. 3. Afferent routes to
inferior temporal cortex.
The arrows are not intended
to indicate monosynaptic projections. Note the pivotal
position of the pulvinar for
the subcortical routes.

Fig. 2. Diagram showing how
information from the left (L)
and right (R) visual half-
fields might reach inferior
temporal cortex along a
cortico-cortical pathway. The
arrows indicate general routes
of information transmission,
not monosynaptic projections.

carried to inferior temporal cortex by a route that included the
forebrain commissures.

To assess the relative contributions of the cortico-cortical
and the pulvino-cortical pathways, we have disrupted portions of
each and looked for changes in the visual properties of inferior
temporal neurons. In one experiment we interrupted the cortico-
cortical route to the inferior temporal cortex by either ablating
striate cortex or sectioning the forebrain commissures (Rocha-
Miranda, Bender, Gross, and Mishkin, 1975). As shown in Figure 4,
there were three major findings. First, bilateral removal of
striate cortex completely eliminated the visual responsiveness of
inferior temporal neurons (Figure 4B). Second, unilateral striate
lesions eliminated their responsiveness to stimuli in the visual
field opposite the striate lesions; i.e., inferior temporal
neurons in the intact hemisphere had only contralateral receptive
fields (Figure 4C) and those in the hemisphere with the striate
lesion had only ipsilateral receptive fields (Figure 4D). Third,
section of the forebrain commissures eliminated responsiveness to
stimuli in the field ipsilateral to the recording site (Figure
4E). These results indicate that neurons in each inferior temporal cortex receive visual information about one half-field from
the striate cortex in their own hemisphere and that they receive
information about the other half-field from the opposite striate
cortex through the forebrain commissures.

In a second experiment we attempted to interrupt the pulvinar
input to the inferior temporal cortex. Lesions of the portions

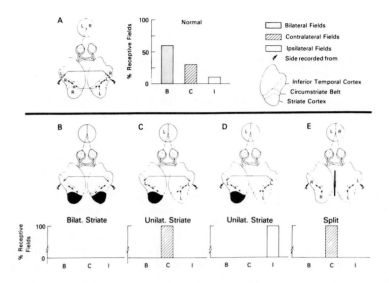

Fig. 4. *The bar graphs show the proportion of inferior temporal neurons that had bilateral, contralateral, or ipsilateral receptive fields in (A) normal monkeys, (B) monkeys with bilateral removal of striate cortex, (C) and (D) monkeys with unilateral removal of striate cortex, and (E) monkeys with section of the forebrain commissures. The brain diagrams show how information from the right (R) and left (L) visual half-fields could reach inferior temporal cortex along a cortico-cortical route and how each lesion (black) interferes with this pathway.*

of the pulvinar complex that project to inferior temporal cortex failed to eliminate the visual responsiveness of inferior temporal neurons. Thus under our experimental conditions it appears that a cortico-cortical pathway from striate cortex by a route that includes the forebrain commissures is responsible for visual activation of inferior temporal neurons.

The same occipito-temporal pathway that underlies the visual properties of inferior temporal neurons is also critical for visual discrimination learning. That is, interrupting this pathway reproduces the visual deficit that follows bilateral inferior temporal lesions. The interruption can be achieved by combining an inferior temporal lesion in one hemisphere, a striate lesion in the other, and section of the forebrain commissures. The commissural section presumably disconnects the remaining inferior temporal and striate cortices (Mishkin, 1966). Moreover, just as pulvinar lesions fail to eliminate the visual responses of inferior temporal neurons, such lesions also fail to reproduce the impairment in visual learning that follows inferior temporal lesions (Mishkin, 1972). Thus, the cortico-cortical pathway from striate to inferior temporal cortex by a route that includes the commissures appears to be both necessary and sufficient not only for the visual properties of inferior temporal neurons but also for visual discrimination learning.

As noted earlier, complete transection of the forebrain commissures eliminates the input to each inferior temporal cortex from the ipsilateral visual field. In a further series of experiments we attempted to determine which parts of the forebrain commissures provide this input (Gross, Bender, Curcio, & Mishkin, 1974). We found that combined section of the splenium and anterior commissure, but not section of either pathway alone, also completely eliminated the ipsilateral responsiveness of inferior temporal neurons. Cutting the splenium alone or cutting the entire corpus callosum reduced the proportion of neurons with bilateral fields by about one-half, suggesting that half the neurons receive ipsilateral information over the splenium. In contrast, cutting the anterior commissure alone did not alter the normal incidence of bilateral and ipsilateral fields; similarly, section of both the anterior commissure and all the corpus callosum except for the splenium also left the distribution of receptive fields unchanged. Since the anterior commissure must be sectioned in addition to the splenium in order to eliminate ipsilateral input completely, the absence of effects from cutting the anterior commissure alone indicates that the neurons this commissure provides with ipsilateral input can also receive such input by way of the splenium. In summary, these results suggest that about half the neurons in inferior temporal cortex that receive information from the ipsilateral field do so through the splenium, and that the other half can do so either through the splenium or through the anterior commissure. Apparently neither the genu nor the body of the corpus callosum carries such information. This interpretation is diagramed in Figure 5. Al though the anterior commissure lies deep in the ventral telencephalon and is hardly a traditional visual structure, our results show that it does in fact carry visual information.

The finding that both the splenium and the anterior commissure contribute to the visual properties of inferior temporal neurons is in striking parallel with results from behavioral studies of hemispheric disconnection. The splenium and anterior commissure are also the specific pathways that participate in interhemispheric transfer of visual habits: Section of both commissures, but not of either alone, will eliminate interhemispheric transfer of visual pattern discriminations (Sullivan & Hamilton, 1973). The fact that these pathways are necessary both for the visual properties of inferior temporal neurons and for interhemispheric transfer of visual habits suggests a functional relation between the neuronal properties and the behavioral transfer. This possibility was examined in the experiment described in the following section.

114

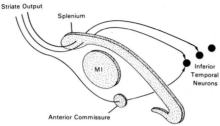

*Fig. 5. Commissural pathways providing information to inferior temporal neurons about the ipsilateral visual field. Approximately two-thirds of inferior temporal neurons receive such information; half of these seem to do so by way of the splenium, and half by way of both the splenium and the anterior commissure. The diagramed pathways are multisynaptic. MI, massa intermedia.*

INFERIOR TEMPORAL CORTEX AND INTERHEMISPHERIC TRANSFER

If a monkey learns a visual discrimination with one eye, it will show good transfer of the habit when tested with the other eye. The basis of this transfer is the convergence of projections from corresponding hemiretinae in the two eyes onto single neurons in the striate cortex, as diagramed in Figure 6A. In this situation the forebrain commissures are not needed for interocular transfer.

However, when the binocular convergence onto striate neurons is eliminated by section of the optic chiasm, interocular transfer becomes critically dependent on the splenium and anterior commissure. As we have shown, these commissures provide a converging input from the two visual fields of both eyes onto inferior temporal neurons. Thus, the basis of interocular transfer after chiasm section may be the converging input received by inferior temporal neurons from the left hemiretina of the left eye and right hemiretina of the right eye by way of the forebrain commissures (Figure 6B). Correspondingly, the loss of interocular transfer after section of both the chiasm and the commissures may be due to the loss of both sources of converging input. If this were true, then removal of inferior temporal cortex should have the same effect on interocular transfer as cutting the splenium and anterior commissure. Specifically, after inferior temporal lesions interocular transfer should be normal if the chiasm is intact (Figure 6C), whereas it should be severely impaired if the chiasm is cut (Figure 6D).

As a test of these predictions, monkeys were prepared with lesions like those shown in Figure 6 (Seacord, Gross, & Mishkin, 1975). In the experimental group, inferior temporal cortex was removed bilaterally, and, in order to restrict input to each hemisphere, the optic chiasm was sectioned. There were three control groups. One control group received bilateral inferior temporal lesions alone, a second received optic chiasm section alone, and a third was left unoperated. Following surgery the groups were trained with one eye and then tested for transfer with the other eye on a series of pattern discrimination problems. According to

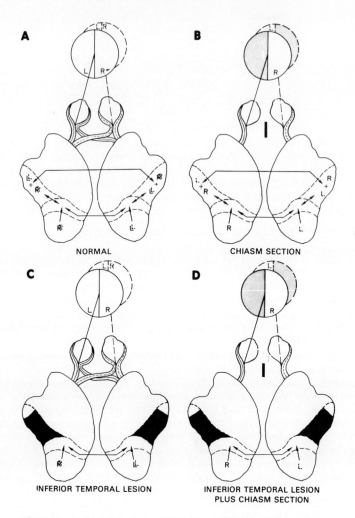

*Fig. 6. Diagrams showing how information from the left and right halves of space converge onto single neurons in striate and inferior temporal cortex (A) in normal animals, (B) after chiasm section, (C) after inferior temporal lesions, and (D) after combined inferior temporal lesions and chiasm section. Information from the left and right visual fields is shown by the letters L and R. The fields of the left and right eye are shown by solid and dashed circles, respectively and information from the left and right eye is shown by solid letters and dashed letters, respectively. The overlapping pairs of identical letters represent convergence from corresponding hemiretinae. The letters joined by a plus sign represent convergence from noncorresponding hemiretinae. Note that convergence from the two eyes is absent only after combined inferior temporal lesion and chiasm section.*

our hypothesis, only the experimental group should show impaired interocular transfer, since only they lack binocular convergence onto single neurons (Figure 6D). In the group with inferior temporal lesions alone, binocular convergence is provided by striate neurons (Figure 6C), and in the group with chiasm section alone, binocular convergence is provided by inferior temporal neurons (Figure 6B). Of course, both groups with inferior temporal lesions were expected to show markedly impaired learning with the initial eye. But once they learned the problem, only the group that had the chiasm section in addition to the inferior temporal lesion should have any difficulty in transfer to the other eye.

As expected, the two groups with inferior temporal lesions learned the discrimination with the initial eye much more slowly than either the normal animals or the ones with only sectioned chiasms (Seacord et al., 1975). But more important, on the transfer test only the animals with the combined inferior temporal le lesion and chiasm section were impaired. They performed much more poorly on the initial transfer trials, took many more trials and errors to relearn the transfer problems, and showed far less savings in doing so than did the control animals (Figure 7).

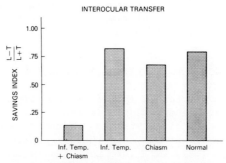

Fig. 7. Interocular transfer of pattern discriminations by monkeys with inferior temporal lesions and section of the optic chiasm (Inf. Temp. + Chiasm), only inferior temporal lesions (Inf. Temp.), only chiasm section (Chiasm), and by normal monkeys. There were three to five animals in each group. Each bar is the mean savings for each group on a series of six pattern-discrimination problems. The monkeys learned each problem with one eye and were then tested for transfer with the other eye before proceeding to the next problem. In the savings index, L is the number of errors made in learning with the first eye, and T is the number of errors made in transfer with the second eye.

The three control groups did not differ on any of these measures.
These results demonstrate that inferior temporal cortex is necessary for interocular transfer when input is restricted to a single hemisphere. Furthermore, the results support our suggestion that it is the binocular convergence onto inferior temporal neurons that sustains interocular transfer when the optic chiasm is cut, and that the splenium and anterior commissure are critical for interocular transfer because they provide this

converging input.

There are other cortical visual areas besides inferior temporal cortex that receive commissural projections, but in view of our results none of these areas appears capable of mediating inter-hemispheric transfer of visual habits. For example, the border between areas 17 and 18 receives a converging input from both sides of the immediate vicinity of the vertical meridian (Brooks and Jung, 1973). However this overlap between the left and right fields was not sufficient to mediate interhemispheric transfer in the experimental animals, probably because the overlap is so small. Other areas located in the circumstriate belt do receive commissural afferents from larger representations of the ipsi-lateral visual field (Zeki, 1974). However, these commissural fibers were also insufficient to mediate transfer in the experi-mental group, perhaps because they do not project to the same neurons that receive information from the contralateral visual field. Neurons with large receptive fields extending well into both visual half-fields have not been reported in circumstriate areas (Zeki, 1974).

In summary, we have found that inferior temporal cortex is crucial for interhemispheric transfer of pattern discrimination habits. In the absence of inferior temporal cortex, no other visual areas appear to perform this role.


PERCEPTUAL CONSTANCY ACROSS RETINAL TRANSLATION

The response properties of inferior temporal neurons suggest how they may mediate interhemispheric transfer. These neurons respond similarly to a given stimulus no matter where it falls within their receptive fields, and their receptive fields are usually large and extend well into both hemiretinae of both eyes. Thus, interocular transfer of a visual habit in a chiasm-sectioned monkey may occur because inferior temporal neurons respond simi-larly to a given discriminandum whether it falls on the left retina of the left eye or the right retina of the right eye. As a result, we suggest, the animal sees the discriminandum as the same through either eye. This proposed mechanism for interocular transfer in the chiasm-sectioned monkey is analogous to that for interocular transfer in normal monkeys. In the normal case, the transfer is due to the equivalence provided by binocular striate neurons for a stimulus falling on corresponding retinal areas in the two eyes. In both cases the animal performs similarly with either eye open because it perceives stimuli as the same with either eye.

Inferior temporal cortex presumably has many functions other than providing for convergence from disparate retinal areas in the two eyes, just as striate cortex has functions other than pro-viding for convergence from corresponding retinal areas. For example, inferior temporal cortex is probably involved in mech-anisms of visual recognition and visual associative memory (Cowey

& Gross, 1970; Iwai & Mishkin, 1968). But the explanation for the interocular transfer of a visual habit in a chiasm-sectioned monkey, just as in the normal monkey, need not invoke any such mechanisms. The known visual properties of striate and inferior temporal cells and the converging pathways that underlie them are sufficient to account for interocular transfer in each case.

Our interpretation of interocular transfer in the chiasm-sectioned monkey also provides a possible explanation for the more general phenomenon of the equivalence of a stimulus across changes in retinal locus in the normal monkey. Inferior temporal neurons respond similarly to a particular stimulus not only when it falls in the opposite hemiretinae of the two eyes, but also wherever it falls within their large receptive fields. Thus, these neurons could mediate stimulus equivalence not only between the opposite halves of the two eyes, but also between the right and left halves of one eye and between the upper and lower quadrants of one hemiretina, or indeed across any retinal translation. That is, the stimulus equivalence shown by inferior temporal cells within their receptive fields may be the basis of the perceptual constancy across retinal translation experienced by the animal.

The hypothesis that inferior temporal cortex mediates stimulus equivalence across changes in stimulus locus may help to explain why removal of this area impairs visual discrimination. In the usual visual discrimination training situation, the discriminanda fall on somewhat different retinal points from trial to trial. For the normal animal, stimulus equivalence across these variations in the site of retinal stimulation presumably greatly facilitates learning, since it obviates the necessity of learning a different discrimination for each retinal site. We suggest that an absence or reduction of such stimulus equivalence in monkeys without inferior temporal cortex is one major reason why they are so impaired in visual discrimination learning.

SUMMARY

We propose an explanation of the interhemispheric transfer of visual habits based on the following four sets of findings from experiments on rhesus monkeys.

*a.* Neurons in inferior temporal cortex usually have large receptive fields that extend across the midline into both visual half-fields. These neurons respond similarly to a given stimulus anywhere within their receptive fields, and most can be activated through either eye.
*b.* Combined section of the splenium of the corpus callosum and the anterior commissure eliminates the responsiveness of inferior temporal neurons in their ipsilateral half-field. Thus, these commissures provide converging visual input from both hemiretinae

of both eyes onto inferior temporal neurons.

   *c.* Combined section of the splenium and anterior commissure also eliminates interhemispheric transfer of visual habits, that is, it eliminates interocular transfer when the optic chiasm has been sectioned.

   *d.* Interhemispheric transfer of visual habits depends on inferior temporal cortex as well as on the forebrain commissures. When the commissures are intact and the chiasm cut, removal of inferior temporal cortex also severely impairs interocular transfer.

We interpret these sets of results as indicating that interhemispheric transfer of visual habits is mediated by the converging visual input onto single inferior temporal neurons provided by the forebrain commissures: These neurons enable the chiasm-sectioned monkey to perceive a stimulus as equivalent with either eye. We suggest further that inferior temporal neurons provide the basis of stimulus equivalence not only across the two temporal retinae in a chiasm-sectioned animal but also across any retinal translation in normal animals and man.

ACKNOWLEDGMENTS

   We thank David B. Bender and Lynne Seacord for use of unpublished data and Christine Curcio for experimental assistance. This research was supported, in part, by NIH Grant MH-19420 and NSF Grant GB 27612X.

REFERENCES

Bender, D. B.   Retinotopic organization in the inferior pulvinar of the rhesus monkey. *Assoc. Res. Vis. Opthalmal.*, 1975, p. 16.
Brooks, B., & Jung, R.   Neuronal physiology of the visual cortex. In R. Jung (Ed.), *Handbook of sensory physiology*. Berlin: Springer-Verlag, 1973. Vol. VII/3B.
Campos-Ortega, J. A., & Hayhow, W. R.   On the organization of the visual cortical projection to the pulvinar in *Macaca mulatta*. *Brain, Behavior and Evolution*, 1972, *6*, 394-423.
Cowey, A.   Brain damage and seeing: A new look at some old problems. *Transactions of the Ophthamological Societies of the United Kingdom*, 1973, *93*, 409-416.
Cowey, A., & Gross, C. G.   Effects of foveal prestriate and inferotemporal lesions on visual discriminations by rhesus monkeys. *Experimental Brain Research*, 1970, *11*, 128-144.
Doty, R. W., & Negrão, N.   Forebrain commissures and vision. In R. Jung (Ed.), *Handbook of sensory physiology*. Berlin: Springer-Verlag, 1973. Vol. VII/3B.
Gross, C. G.   Visual functions of inferotemporal cortex. In

R. Jung (Ed.), *Handbook of sensory physíology.* Berlin: Springer-Verlag, 1973. Vol. VII/3B. (a)

Gross, C. G. Inferotemporal cortex and vision. In *Progress in physiological psychology.* Vol. 5. New York: Academic Press, 1973. (b)

Gross, C. G., Bender, D. B., Curcio, C. A., & Mishkin, M. Role of forebrain commissures in integration of visual half-fields by inferotemporal neurons. *Federation Proceedings,* 1974, *33*, 433.

Gross, C. G., Bender, D. B., & Rocha-Miranda, C. E. Inferotemporal cortex: A single unit analysis. In F. O. Schmitt & F. G. Warden (Eds.), *The neurosciences: Third study program.* Cambridge, Massachusetts: M.I.T. Press, 1973.

Gross, C. G., Rocha-Miranda, C. E., & Bender, D. B. Visual properties of neurons in inferotemporal cortex of the macaque. *Journal of Neurophysiology,* 1972, *35*, 96-111.

Iwai, E., & Mishkin, M. Two visual foci in the temporal lobe of monkeys. In N. Yoshii & N. A. Buckwald (Eds.), *Neuropsychological basis of learning and behavior.* Osaka: Osaka Univ. Press, 1968.

Jones, E. G. The anatomy of extrageniculostriate visual mechanisms. In F. O. Schmitt & F. G. Warden (Eds.), *The neurosciences: Third study program.* Cambridge, Massachusetts: M.I.T. Press, 1973.

Kuypers, H. G., Szwarcbart, M. K., Mishkin, M., & Rosvold, H. E. Occipito-temporal cortico-cortical connections in the rhesus monkey. *Experimental Neurology,* 1965, *11*, 245-262.

Milner, B. Hemispheric specialization--scope and limits. In F. O. Schmitt & F. G. Warden (Eds.), *The neurosciences: Third study program.* Cambridge, Massachusetts: M.I.T. Press, 1973.

Mishkin, M. Visual mechanisms beyond the striate cortex. In R. Russell (Ed.), *Frontiers of physiological psychology.* New York: Academic Press, 1966.

Mishkin, M. Cortical visual areas and their interaction. In A. G. Karczmar & J. C. Eccles (Eds.), *The brain and human behavior.* Berlin: Springer-Verlag, 1972.

Pandya, D. N., Karol, E. A., & Heilbronn, D. The topographical distribution of interhemispheric projections in the corpus callosum of the rhesus monkey. *Brain research,* 1971, *32*, 31-43.

Rezak, M., & Benevento, L. A. Cortical projections of corticorecipient and tectorecipient zones of the pulvinar in the macaque monkey. *Neuroscience Abstracts,* 1975, *1*, 63.

Rocha-Miranda, C. E., Bender, D. B., Gross, C. G., & Mishkin, M. Visual activation of neurons in inferotemporal cortex depends on striate cortex and forebrain commissures. *Journal of Neurophysiology,* 1975, *37*, 475-491.

Seacord, L., Gross, C. G., & Mishkin, M. Role of inferior temporal cortex in perceptual equivalence of stimuli in the left and right visual fields. *Neuroscience Abstracts*, 1975, *1*, 73.

Sperry, R. W. Cerebral organization and behavior. *Science*, 1961, *133*, 1749-1757.

Sullivan, M. V., & Hamilton, C. R. Memory establishment via the anterior commissure of monkeys. *Physiology and behavior*, 1973, *11*, 873-879.

Zeki, S. M. The mosaic organization of the visual cortex in the monkey. In R. Bellairs & E. G. Gray (Eds.), *Essays on the nervous system*. Oxford: Clarendon Press, 1974.

# 8.

# Thalamic Lateralization of Psychological Functions: Psychometric Studies

*MANUEL RIKLAN AND IRVING S. COOPER*

Institute of Neuroscience
St. Barnabas Hospital

Most psychometrically based concepts of hemispheric lateral-ization and dominance emphasize a language-spatial dichotomy, tend to be clinical in nature, and in many instances use the convenient Wechsler-Bellevue Intelligence Scale (WBIS) as the primary method of assessment. In an early study in this area, Anderson (1951) administered the WBIS to a group of individuals with damage to their dominant hemispheres and to an equivalent group of patients with nondominant-hemisphere injury. Signifi-cantly greater loss on verbal tests was reported for the dominant-hemisphere group and a correspondingly greater loss on performance and spatial tasks for the population with damage to the nondominant hemisphere. A number of confirmatory studies have since appeared (Bauer & Becka, 1954; Benton & Van Allen, 1968; Costa & Vaughan, 1962; Heilbrun, 1956; Lansdell, 1968; McFie, 1960; Morrow & Mark, 1955; Reitan, 1955; Reitan & Fitz-hugh, 1971; Start, 1961).

The prevailing belief concerning the effect of brain lesions on language is exemplified by Bauer and Wepman (1955) and Boone (1959), who agree that cerebral dominance seems unique to the left hemisphere. In contrast, Heilbrun (1956) failed to find any significant differences in spatial performance in assessing the effects of right-hemisphere lesions. This result is compatible with other studies (Battersby, Bender, Pollack, & Kahn, 1956; Piercy & Smyth, 1962), in which spatial representa-tion was found to be bilateral but unequal, with differences in degree rather than in kind. For this particular function, the evidence tends to be against strict unilateral representation

(Osgood & Myron, 1963, p. 53).

In the area of cerebral dominance and language, a similar recent changing emphasis is also apparent. Instances of spontaneous recovery of language following brain injury indicate that there must be some replication of function "either between the two hemispheres or between regions of the dominant hemisphere (Osgood & Myron, 1963, p. 49)." Cerebral dominance may thus be a graded characteristic, according to Zangwill (1962, p. 27), Eisenson (1962), and Critchley (1962, pp. 208-214). Critchley conceived of speech function as involving a spectrum ranging from the "normal" subject, at one extreme, through the linguistic pattern of nondominant hemisphere defect, to a full-fledged aphasia from disease of the dominant half of the brain. Reviews by Meyer (1961), Reitan (1962), and Piercy (1964) also emphasize a lack of clear-cut hemisphere distinctions in psychological functions.

Contemporary psychological concepts of functional laterality in man have been derived predominantly from studies of patients with insults to the cerebral cortex, including epileptics, hemiplegics, and brain-operated or traumatically injured patients. In many reported cases subcortical lesions were also present along with cortical damage. Recent evidence, moreover, suggests a possible unwarranted equating of differences in degree with differences in kind in lateralization concepts (cf. Gur & Gur; Springer, this volume), along with a failure to account for the role of subcortical structures in psychological behavior. The purpose of this chapter is to review data derived from psychological studies of patients subjected to thalamic surgery for the alleviation of neurological symptoms.

## LATERALIZED EFFECTS OF THALAMIC SURGERY

### THE VENTROLATERAL LESION

A series of psychological investigations were undertaken with individuals undergoing chemothalamectomy (Cooper, 1961), or cryothalamectomy (Cooper, 1964), for the relief of tremor and rigidity in Parkinson's disease. Such operations involve unilateral surgical production of a lesion aimed at the ventrolateral nucleus (VL) of the thalamus. Neuroanatomical studies have confirmed the site of lesion placement (Caracalos, Levita, & Cooper, 1962; Cooper, Bergmann, & Caracalos, 1963; Dierssen, Bergmann, Gioino, & Cooper, 1962).

In an initial study by Riklan, Diller, Weiner, and Cooper (1960), using the WBIS, both left- and right-hemisphere groups demonstrated significant decreases in verbal scores; only right-brain operates showed a decrease in performance tests during the immediate postoperative period. No significant differences in postoperative intellectual effects were found between specific lesion sites within the VL nucleus. A return to preoperative status for the total group was observed on follow-up assessment, approximately 9 months postoperatively. These results appeared compatible with Sheer's (1956) study involving surgically produced cortical lesions. Moreover, an association between left-hemisphere cortical lesions and deficits in language seemed to be verified. It was later found (Riklan & Diller, 1961) that immediately postoperatively, patients who had surgery on the right thalamus regressed in visual-motor performance, but the left-hemisphere group showed no such change. However, results of the Human Figure Drawing Test administered before and after chemosurgery (Riklan, Zahn, & Diller, 1962) suggested that body-image perception underwent postoperative modification irrespective of side of subcortical surgery. It was suggested then that both hemispheres may contribute to body-image integration. This finding also questioned earlier studies relating body-image function primarily to the right hemisphere (Critchley, 1953; Kolb, 1959).

Further exploration into the nature of presumed lateralized differences following thalamic lesions was achieved through a factor analysis of change scores for 35 variables from the WBIS, the Bender-Gestalt test, Human Figure Drawing Test, and the Rorschach Psychodiagnostic Test (Riklan & Levita, 1964). Observed lateralized differences occurred primarily in factor loadings, with greater verbal loadings for the left-brain operates and greater nonverbal loadings for the right-brain operates. However, the apparent qualitative similarity factors led to the hypothesis that certain psychological functions might be subserved by systems available to both subcortical regions. These findings opened to further consideration earlier reports that either failed to weigh thalamic laterality (Freed & Pastor, 1951; Gillingham, 1961; Krayenbuehl & Yasargil, 1961; Orchinik, 1960; Orchinik, Koch, Wycis, Freed, & Spiegel, 1950), or ascribed more definitive differences in functions to the left and right subcortical structures (McFie, 1960).

Verbally and nonverbally mediated cognitive tasks were later administered to unoperated parkinsonian patients for further elaboration and clarification of the nature of subcortical laterality. No significant differences were obtained as a function of lateralized involvement for groups of predominantly right-handed subjects (92% right-handed). No differences were found in unoperated patients with predominant left- or right-sided neurological symptoms, i.e., presumably right- or left-sided basal ganglia damage (Levita, Riklan, & Cooper, 1964). Moreover, in a partial cross-validation and extension of Riklan and Levita's (1964) original factorial study, a battery of cognitive-perceptual tests was administered to another group of unoperated parkinsonian patients and also subjected to factor analysis (Levita & Riklan, 1965). The major, almost identical factors, specifically a visual-spatial and verbal discrimination factor for each hemisphere group, were found. In the case of surgery, no significant immediate postoperative differences were found between left- and right-thalamic lesions as a function of symbolization, whether verbally or nonverbally mediated (Levita, Riklan, & Cooper, 1964b). Finally, laterality and site of surgery did not significantly differentiate verbal or perceptual changes. In the light of the foregoing findings, the conclusion seemed warranted that laterality of predominantly subcortical impairment does not result in the kinds of differences reported for cortical lesions with or without some subcortical involvement. It follows that reassessment of lateralized aspects of neural organization as it pertains to integrative behavior is indicated.

Further psychometric testing of verbal and nonverbal effects of left- and right-VL thalamic lesions, respectively, was later undertaken using still another battery of verbal and nonverbal tests (Riklan & Levita, 1970). The tests included the Stroop Word Color Interference Test (Stroop, 1935), the Graham-Kendall Memory for Designs Test (Graham & Kendall, 1947, 1960), the Odd Words Test (Holzinger & Crowder, 1955), the Minnesota Paper Form Board (Patterson, Elliott, Anderson, Toops, & Heidbreder, 1930; Quasha & Likert, 1937), and tests involving object naming and word fluence. These were administered to a series of parkinsonian patients before and after left and right cryothalamectomy. Lateralized differences were noted. These were most pronounced in tests of manipulation, creative retrieval, and categorization of symbols, particularly in tests of word fluency and object naming. For such functions, left-hemisphere operates revealed a significant decrease in performance immediately after surgery, whereas right-brain operates did not. Bilateral operates also tended to perform less well than unoperated control patients during the immediate postoperative situation. In tasks of verbal fluency or verbal flexibility, left-brain surgery affects performance, as does a second, opposite hemisphere operation, regardless of laterality. However, a unilateral right-brain operation does not have any such effects. Thus, tasks of verbal fluency or flexibility yield a pattern of changes clearly associated with lesion laterality where standard clinical tests do not (cf. Riklan & Levita, 1964, 1969). Of further interest was the finding that a number of spatial-perceptual tests did not seem to differentiate between the groups to any degree.

## THE PULVINAR LESION

In a psychometric study of pulvinar lesions in man (Riklan, Weissman, & Cooper, 1973), a battery of psychological tests including the Wechsler Adult Intelligence Scale (WAIS), Wechsler Memory Scale, and Bender Visual-Motor Gestalt test were administered to 32 consecutively tested patients who underwent surgery involving the pulvinar or VL thalamus. Data concerning the surgical technique and pathological confirmation of lesion placement have been presented elsewhere (Cooper, Amin, Chandra, & Waltz, 1973; Cooper, Waltz, Amin, & Fujita, 1971). With respect to the WAIS subtest scores, the question of verbal versus non-verbal effects of left- and right-pulvinar lesions was of particular relevance; data were tabulated comparing both pulvinar and VL thalamic subjects, to demonstrate the effects of left- and right-thalamic surgery on verbal and performance portions of the psychometric tests respectively.

Following right-hemisphere lesions of either pulvinar or VL, no significant pre- to immediate postoperative changes occurred in either verbal or performance tests of cognitive or perceptual functions. However, left-hemisphere operates, both pulvinar and VL, showed a differential effect with respect to verbal and performance scores. Specifically, decrements in scores were noted for verbal functions following left-hemisphere surgery for both the pulvinar and VL operates. For the VL lesion the pre- to postoperative changes were significant ($p = .05$), based upon a one-tailed test of significance. Such data suggest a differential effect of pulvinar and VL lesions on verbal functions.

## DISCUSSION

Numerous psychometric studies are in substantial agreement that surgically induced thalamic lesions tend to alter psychological functions during the immediate postoperative period. This pattern has been confirmed by neurosurgical reports and assessments by speech pathologists. In the longer range status, most aspects of "integrative" psychological functions, including verbal performance, return to their preoperative level. Thus, concepts of thalamic lateralization derived from assessment of surgically induced thalamic lesions are based largely upon the acute postoperative status.

Within the overall pattern of immediate postoperative decrements in a variety of psychological and behavioral functions, one special differentiation obtains: Different degrees of postoperative alterations appear to result from left- and right-sided lesions, whether the pulvinar or VL is involved. Patients undergoing left-thalamic surgery decline more significantly in verbally mediated cognitive performance than those undergoing right-sided surgery. In contrast, very few statistically significant changes, either in verbal or nonverbal tests, occur in patients having undergone right-hemisphere surgery. This finding would seem to confirm a number of suggestions concerning a thalamic role either in language per se or in verbal test performance, and a tendency toward lateralization of this function to the left hemisphere (cf. Penfield & Roberts, 1959; Riklan & Levita, 1969).

The immediate postoperative decrement in patients undergoing left-side operation is in a function best described as verbal fluency. Assessments by speech therapists also suggest that some aspects of fluency are correlated with left-thalamic functions, confirming that the thalamus, either the ventrolateral nucleus or nuclei functionally related to it, plays a decisive role in some aspects of verbal formulation and expression. Data on the pulvinar lesions are similar, but more tentative because of limitations in numbers of patients studied.

Some other standardized psychological tests of verbal behavior tend to show relatively little differentiation between the effects of left- and right-thalamic surgery. The verbal functions tapped by these psychological tests thus may be somewhat different from those involved in fluency, which may require a creative, flexible approach to searching and sorting. The fact that patients operated upon bilaterally--who in most cases underwent right-hemisphere operation for the second side--showed changes in word fluency similar to those undergoing left-hemisphere surgery makes it apparent that the right thalamus also participates in this function, at least in the presence of a previous lesion of the left thalamus.

We have previously questioned the implied qualitative dichotomy between the left- and right-hemisphere functions (Riklan & Levita, 1964, 1965, 1969). A number of other investigators have proposed quantitative gradations between the hemispheres, i.e., differences in emphasis along a single continuum in the case of both hemispheres (Critchley, 1962; Eisenson, 1962; Hecaen, 1959; Zangwill, 1962). Recent studies on split-brain preparations (Gazzaniga, Bogen, & Sperry, 1965; Gazzaniga & Sperry, 1967; Sperry, 1961) have further underlined the importance of interhemispheric relations. The assumed bilaterality of hypothetical *engrams* or memory traces would also stress the role of interhemispheric relations of the integration and elaboration of information (Ebner & Myers, 1962, cf. Doty & Overman, this volume). Greater similarity may obtain between the hemispheres than has been thought previously. Future studies of interactions may be more relevant than attempts to seek exclusive functions for each hemisphere.

During recovery the mean verbal and nonverbal scores for patients following either pulvinar or VL lesions return eventually to their approximate preoperative status, as has been described for other series of VL and globus pallidus lesions (Riklan & Levita, 1969). This finding seems related to the fact that such surgical lesions ordinarily involve only portions of larger zones of functional activity, and that sufficient mechanisms of neural duplication and replication are available so that no continuing functional deficit is manifest. As an example, in postmortem studies of three patients previously subjected to pulvinectomy, lesions were typically described as including no more than half the nucleus. Current standardized psychological tests also may not be sufficiently refined to discern subtle continuing changes that might result from such lesions. Possible neural mechanisms include duplication of function within the thalamus or the hemisphere which permit the reestablishment of integrated behavioral patterns. Finally, the particular functions usually assessed may not be directly related to VL or pulvinar zones.

With regard to neural concepts underlying thalamic interactions, it has been generally established that the thalamus plays a critical role in the relay of sensorimotor information, participates widely in both specific and diffuse afferent and efferent integration, and is involved in the elaboration of physiological data. Penfield and Roberts (1959, pp. 207-208) proposed that a bilaterally-distributed subcortical zone is responsible for the integration of speech. Changes in behavioral arousal, manifested by body movements and vocalization, have been observed in parkinsonian patients after repetitive unilateral stimulation in the ventrolateral area of the thalamus (Schaltenbrand, 1965). Therefore, stimulation or destruction of various points within the basal ganglia and thalamus seems related to bilateral cortical responses and general behavioral reactions involving the entire organism.

Alerting or arousal of the central nervous system is not just a function of the reticular formation (Moruzzi & Magoun, 1949; Magoun, 1963). The functionally related nonspecific thalamo-cortical projections also modulate bilaterally the sensorimotor functions of a wide area of cortex (Jasper, 1949, 1960; cf. Heilman & Watson, this volume). The basal ganglia may exert a bilateral influence upon ascending nonspecific activity and may be considered integrative centers as well (Krauthamer & Albe-Fessard, 1965; Martin, 1959; cf. Glick, Jerussi, & Zimmerberg, this volume). At the thalamic level, diffuse and specific neural systems intimately interact in the elaboration of cognitive information, verbal and nonverbal. Diffuse bilateral processes might contribute alerting or attention components while concurrent specific processes would contribute more content-oriented information. At the thalamic level, the less completely organized data may require greater diffuse activity to achieve elaboration.

SUMMARY

An assessment was made of psychometric studies undertaken before and after placement of lateralized thalamic lesions in parkinsonian patients and other neurologically impaired groups. Lateralized effects of thalamic lesions were noted. In particular, the ventrolateral nucleus and pulvinar play a role in verbal function fluency. The left thalamus tends to be dominant in this respect. The right thalamic nuclei are less specific in this regard. Differences between thalamic and cortical lateralization were noted. Subcortical systems involve a higher degree of bilateral action and are more intimately involved with arousal functions than are cortical systems.

REFERENCES

Anderson, A. L.   The effect of laterality localization of focal
    brain lesions on the Wechsler-Bellevue subtests.  *Journal
    of Clinical Psychology*, 1951, *7*, 149-153.
Battersby, W. W., Bender, M. B., Pollack, M., & Kahn, R. L.
    Unilateral "spatial agnosia" ("inattention") in patients
    with cerebral lesions. *Brain*, 1956, *79*, 68-93.
Bauer, R. W., & Becka, D. M.   Intellect after cerebral vascular
    accident. *Journal of Nervous and Mental Disease*, 1954, *120*,
    379-384.
Bauer, R. W., & Wepman, J. M.   Lateralization of cerebral func-
    tions. *Journal of Speech and Hearing Disorders*, 1955, *20*,
    181-177.
Benton, A. L., & Van Allen, M. W.   Impairment in facial recogni-
    tion in patients with cerebral disease. *Cortex*, 1958, *4*,
    344-358.
Boone, D. R.   Communication skills and intelligence in right and
    left hemiplegics. *Journal of Speech and Hearing Disorders*,
    1959, *24*, 241-248.
Caracalos, A., Levita, E., & Cooper, I. S.   A study of roentgeno-
    anatomic lesion location and results in cryosurgery of the
    basal ganglia. *St. Barnabas Hospital Medical Bulletin*,
    1962, *1*, 24-31.
Cooper, I. S.   *Parkinsonism: Its medical and surgical therapy*.
    Springfield, Illinois:  Thomas, 1961.
Cooper, I. S.   Cryogenic surgery in the geriatric patient.
    *Journal of the American Geriatric Society*, 1964, *12*, 813-
    855.
Cooper, I. S., Amin, I., Chandra, R., & Waltz, J. M.   A surgical
    investigation of the clinical physiology of the LP-Pulvinar
    complex in man. *Journal of Neurological Science*, 1973, *18*,
    89-110.
Cooper, I. S., Bergmann, L., & Caracalos, A.   Anatomic verifica-
    tion of the lesion which abolishes parkinsonian tremor and
    rigidity. *Neurology*, 1963, *13*, 779-787.
Cooper, I. S., Waltz, J. M., Amin, I., & Fujita, S.   Pulvinec-
    tomy:  A preliminary report. *Journal of the American
    Geriatric Society*, 1971, *19*, 553-554.
Costa, L. D., & Vaughan, H. G. Performance of patients with
    lateralized cerebral lesions.  I.  Verbal and perceptual
    tests. *Journal of Nervous and Mental Disease*, 1962, *134*,
    162-168.
Critchley, M.  *The parietal lobes*.  London: Arnold, 1953.
Critchley, M.   Speech and speech loss in relation to the quality
    of the brain.  In V. B. Mountcastle (Ed.), *Interhemispheric
    relations and cerebral dominance*.  Baltimore:  Johns
    Hopkins Press, 1962.  Pp. 208-214.
Dierssen, G., Bergmann, L., Gioino, G., & Cooper, I. S.  Surgi-
    cal lesions affecting parkinson symptomatology. *Acta
    Neurochirurgica*, 1962, *10*, 125-133.
Ebner, F. F., & Meyers, R. E.   Corpus callosum and the inter-

hemispheric transmission of tactual learning. *Journal of Neurophysiology*, 1962, *25*, 380-391.

Eisenson, J.   Language and intellectual modifications associated with right cerebral damage. *Language and Speech*, 1962, *5*, 47-53.

Freed, H., & Pastor, J. T.   Evaluation of the "Draw-A-Person Test" (modified) in thalamotomy with particular reference to the body image. *Journal of Nervous and Mental Disease*, 1951, *114*, 106-120.

Gazzaniga, M. S., Bogen, J. E., & Sperry, R. W.   Observations in visual perception after disconnexion of the cerebral hemispheres in man. *Brain*, 1965, *88*, 221-236.

Gazzaniga, M. S., & Sperry, R. W.   Language after section of the cerebral commisures. *Brain*, 1967, *90*, 131-148.

Gillingham, J.   Surgical treatment of parkinsonism. *Transactions of the Medical Society of London*, 1961, *77*, 52-56.

Graham, F. K., & Kendall, B. S.   Note on the scoring of the Memory-for-Designs test. *Journal of Abnormal and Social Psychology*, 1947, *42*, 253.

Graham, F. K., & Kendall, B. S.   Memory-For-Designs test: Revised general manual. *Perceptual and Motor Skills*, 1960, *11*, 147-188.

Hecaen, H.   Dominance hemispherique et preference manuelle. *Evolutionary Psychiatry*, 1959, *1*, 1-50.

Heilbrun, A. B.   Psychological test performance as a function of lateral localization of cerebral lesion. *Journal of Comparative and Physiological Psychology*, 1956, *49*, 10-14.

Holzinger, K. J., & Crowder, N. A.   *Manual for the Holzinger-Crowder-Unifactor Tests*. New York: Harcourt, 1955.

Jasper, H.   Diffuse projection systems: The integrative action of the thalamic reticular system. *Electroencephalography and Clinical Neurophysiology*, 1949, *1*, 405-420.

Jasper, H.   Unspecific thalamo-cortical relations. In J. Field (Ed.), *Handbook of Physiology*. Vol. 2. Washington, D.C.: American Physiological Society, 1960. Pp. 1307-1322.

Kolb, L.   Disturbances of the body image. In S. Arieti (Ed.), *American handbook of psychiatry*. New York: Basic Books, 1959. Pp. 749-769.

Krauthamer, G., & Albe-Fessard, D.   Inhibition of nonspecific activities following striopallidal and capsular stimulation. *Journal of Neurophysiology*, 1965, *28*, 100-124.

Krayenbuhl, H., & Yasargil, M. G.   Ergebnisse der stereotakitschen Operationen beim Parkinsonismus, insbesondere der doppelseitigen Eingriffe. *Deutsche Zeitschrift fur Nervenheilkunde*, 1961, *182*, 530-541.

Lansdell, H.   The use of factor scores from the Wechsler-Bellevue Scale of Intelligence in assessing patients with temporal lobe removals. *Cortex*, 1968, *4*, 357-268.

Levita, E., & Riklan, M.   Laterality of subcortical involvement and cognitive performance: A factor analysis. *Perceptual and Motor Skills*, 1965, *20*, 151-157.

Levita, E., Riklan, M., & Cooper, I. S.  Cognitive and perceptual performance in parkinsonism as a function of age and neurological impairment. *Journal of Nervous and Mental Disease*, 1964, *139*, 516-520. (a)

Levita, E., Riklan, M., & Cooper, I. S.  Verbal and perceptual functions after surgery of subcortical structures. *Perceptual and Motor Skills*, 1964, *18*, 195-202. (b)

Magoun, H. W.  *The waking brain.* (2nd ed.). Springfield, Illinois:  Thomas, 1963.

Martin, J. P. Remarks on the function of the basal ganglia. *Lancet*, 1959, *1*, 999-1005.

McFie, J.  Psychological effects of stereotaxic operations for the relief of parkinsonian symptoms. *Journal of Mental Science*, 1960, *106*, 1512-1517.

Meyer, V.  Psychological effects of brain damage.  In H. J. Eysenck, (Ed.), *Handbook of abnormal psychology.*  New York: Basic Books, 1961. Pp. 529-565.

Morrow, R. S., & Mark, J. C.  The correlation of intelligence and neurological findings on twenty-two patients autopsied for brain damage. *Journal of Consulting Psychology*, 1955, *19*, 282-289.

Moruzzi, G., & Magoun, H. W.  Brain stem reticular formation and activation of the EEG. *Electroencephalography and Clinical Neurophysiology*, 1949, *1*, 455-473.

Orchinik, C. W.  Some psychological aspects of circumscribed lesions of the diencephalon. *Confina Neurologica*, 1960, *20*, 292-310.

Orchinik, C. W., Koch, R., Wycis, H. T., Freed, H., & Spiegel, E. A.  The effect of thalamic lesions on emotional reactivity (Rorschach and behavior studies). *Proceedings of the Association for Research in Nervous and Mental Disease*, 1950, *29*, 172-207.

Osgood, C., & Myron, M.  *Approaches to the study of aphasia.* Urbana:  Univ. of Illinois Press, 1963.

Patterson, D. G., Elliott, R. M., Anderson, L. D., Toops, H. A., & Heidbreder, E.  *Minnesota mechanical ability tests.* Minneapolis:  Univ. of Minnesota Press, 1930.

Penfield, W., & Roberts, L.  *Speech and brain mechanisms.* Princeton, New Jersey:  Princeton Univ. Press, 1959.

Piercy, M.  The effects of cerebral lesions on intellectual functions.  A review of current research trends. *British Journal of Psychology*, 1964, *110*, 310-352.

Piercy, M., & Smyth, V. O.  Right hemisphere dominance for certain nonverbal intellectual skills. *Brain*, 1952, *85*, 755-790.

Quasha, W. H., & Likert, R.  The Revised Minnesota Paper Form Board Test. *Journal of Educational Psychology*, 1937, *28*, 197-204.

Reitan, R. M.  Certain differential effects of left and right cerebral lesions in human adults. *Journal of Comparative and Physiological Psychology*, 1955, *48*, 474-477.

Reitan, R. M.  Psychological deficit. *Annual Review of Psychology*, 1962, *13*, 415-444.

Reitan, R. M., & Fitzhugh, K.  Behavioral deficits in groups with cerebral vascular lesions. *Journal of Consulting and Clinical Psychology* 1971, *37*, 215-223.

Riklan, M., & Diller, L.  Visual motor performance before and after chemosurgery of the basal ganglia in parsinsonism. *Journal of Nervous and Mental Disease*, 1961, *132*, 307-313.

Riklan, M., Diller, L., Weiner, H., & Cooper, I. S.  Psychological studies on effects of chemosurgery of the basal ganglia in parkinsonism.  I.  Intellectual functioning. *A.M.A. Archives of General Psychiatry*, 1960, *2*, 22-31

Riklan, M., Zahn, T., & Diller, L.  Human figure drawings before and after chemosurgery of the basal ganglia in parkinsonism. *Journal of Nervous and Mental Disease*, 1962, *6*, 500-506.

Riklan, M., & Levita, E.  Psychological effects of lateralized basal ganglia lesions: A factorial study. *Journal of Nervous and Mental Disease*, 1964, *138*, 233-240.

Riklan, M., & Levita, E.  Laterality of subcortical involvement and psychological functions. *Psychological Bulletin*, 1965, *64*, 217-224.

Riklan, M., & Levita, E.  *Subcortical correlates of human behavior: A psychological study of basal ganglia and thalamic surgery.*  Baltimore:  Williams & Wilkins, 1969.

Riklan, M., & Levita, E.  Psychological studies of thalamic lesions in humans. *Journal of Nervous and Mental Disease*, 1970, *150*, 251-265.

Riklan, M., D. Weissman, & Cooper, I. S.  Psychological functions following pulvinectomy in man.  In I. S. Cooper, M. Riklan, & R. Rakic (Eds.), *The pulvinar-LP complex.*  Springfield, Illinois:  Thomas, 1973.  Pp. 138-171.

Schaltenbrand, G.  The effects of stereotactic electrical stimulation in the depth of the brain. *Brain*, 1965, *88*, 835-840.

Sheer, D. W.  Psychometric studies.  In N. Lewis, C. Landis, & H. E. King (Eds.), *Studies in topectomy.*  New York:  Grune & Stratton, 1956.  Pp. 56-74.

Sperry, R. W.  Cerebral organization and behavior. *Science,* 1961, *133*, 1749-1757.

Stark, R.  An investigation of unilateral cerebral pathology with equated verbal and visual-spatial tasks. *Journal of Abnormal and Social Psychology*, 1961, *62*, 282-287.

Stroop, J. R.  Studies of interference in serial verbal reactions. *Journal of Experimental Psychology*, 1935, *18*, 643-661.

Zangwill, O. L.  *Cerebral dominance and its relation to psychological function.*  Springfield, Illinois:  Thomas, 1962.

# Part III

# INHERITANCE AND DEVELOPMENT OF LATERALITY

# 9.
# Toward An Admissible Genetic Model for the Inheritance of the Degree and Direction of Asymmetry

*ROBERT L. COLLINS*

The Jackson Laboratory

Asymmetries may be likened to mathematical vectors, quantities completely specified by a direction or sense, such as *left* and *right,* and a magnitude, such as the degree of lateral specialization.  Most of the experimental research, model building, and controversy associated with the question of hereditary influences on the expression of lateralized form or function has centered on whether or not the directions of asymmetry are encoded in the individual's own genetic material.  Are the alternative sense descriptions of left and right (for the case of bilateral asymmetries), or of clockwise and counterclockwise (for the case of radial asymmetries), themselves inherent properties of alternative genetic alleles?  Experimental studies of the handedness of mice defined genetically by inbreeding as well as continuing analyses of published data on human handedness and hair whorl have led me to conclude, with some reluctance, that genes are quite indifferent to the sense of asymmetry.

However, I believe that hereditary influences do play important roles in the maintenance of asymmetries.  These roles may be discerned if we temporarily set aside the notion that the directed senses are coded genetically, and if we focus our attention on the problem of the magnitude or degree of lateral specialization.  By attending to the problem of magnitude first, we will return easily and unexpectedly to the problem of the inheritance of sense of asymmetry.  I propose to develop here an admissible genetic model for the inheritance of the magnitude ‘ and sense of asymmetry--a genetic model for the asymmetry vector that is compatible with Morgan's view (this volume) that "genes are left-right agnosic."

Because my proposal may initially appear counterintuitive, I ask each reader to join me in carefully considering without prejudice the problem of genetics and asymmetry. I believe we will see that, although genes do not appear to specify the sense of asymmetry, they can influence the degree of lateralization. We will see that when organisms exist in biased worlds (i.e., environments that differentially favor the expression of one or the other sense of an asymmetry), then genetic effects on lateralization may be translated into differences in the proportion of individuals exhibiting a given sense of asymmetry. Under these conditions genetic differences in lateralization will mimic an inheritance of left and right. We will see that the genes that increase the proportion of individuals possessing one sense are the same genes that increase the proportion of individuals possessing the alternative sense, and those that decrease the proportion of individuals possessing one sense are the same that decrease the proportion of individuals possessing the alternative sense. Even more simply, I believe we will discover that the genes for right and left are identical.

Let us begin with experimental studies of the paw preferences of inbred laboratory mice. The term *inbred strain* has a precise meaning. A strain may be regarded as inbred if it was derived by single-pair brother-by-sister matings for at least 20 consecutive generations, or by parent-by-offspring matings for the same length of time where each mating is made to the younger parent (Staats, 1972). After about 20 generations of inbreeding, approximately 99% of the genetic loci are considered to be in a homozygous condition. A number of inbred strains have been inbred beyond 150 generations. Because differing genetic alleles become fixed in each inbreeding process, and because there is no way to predict in advance just which alleles will become fixed, each inbred strain harbors a unique set of hereditary differences distinguishing it from every other inbred strain. Because members of an inbred strain are virtually identical genetically, any variability observed in the characteristics of inbred mice is usually considered to have nongenetic or environmental causes. Readers unfamiliar with the advantages of using highly inbred laboratory animals in research may wish to consult Green (1975) for general information and Collins (1972) for useful applications in neurobiological research.

Mice exhibit handedness. If food is withheld for 24 hr and a mouse is then placed into a test apparatus in which food grains are available through a feeding tube, it will begin to reach with one or the other paw to retrieve food. These reaches can be counted conveniently. The test apparatus I use consists of five in-line cubicles 3.8 cm wide, 5.5 cm deep, and 11.5 cm high (inside dimensions). A 9-mm feeding tube is attached to the front wall of each cubicle 5.75 cm from the floor. The feeding tube is filled with sweetened rolled wheat (Maypo). Fifty reaches for food are routinely counted for every mouse, and the number of right paw entries (RPEs) is used as one index of laterality. For example, if a mouse scores 48 RPEs, it has reached only twice with its left paw and it would be considered dextral. If a mouse scores 2 RPEs, 48 left-handed reaches were observed, and the mouse would be considered sinistral. Another way to treat paw preference scores is to assign R to a mouse that scores more than 25 RPEs, and L to one that scores fewer than 25 RPEs. R or L classifications would ordinarily not be assigned to a mouse that scored exactly 25 RPEs.

To date, several thousand tests of paw preference have been performed, using mice of the highly inbred C57BL/6J strain. This strain has been carefully and continuously inbred for beyond 120 generations. Several general findings from these data are noteworthy. Mice appear to be either strongly right-handed or strongly left-handed. Very few mice could be considered ambilateral. The paw preference scores of individual mice are remarkably consistent from test to test. The correlations of laterality classifications for these mice are also high (Collins, 1968). The paw preference scores of mice tested in the standard apparatus have been found to be positively correlated with paw preferences measured in a different test apparatus, which demanded differing response topographies (Collins, 1970). Thus, the paw preferences of mice are reliable, consistent within tasks, and consistent across differing tasks (cf. Warren, this volume).

Approximately one-half of the C57BL/6J mice tested were classified as dextral, and one-half, sinistral. Similar proportions were observed in tests of eight other inbred strains or genetically uniform $F_1$ hybrids (Collins, 1968). It appears then that differing genetic alleles are not required to explain the near maximum variation of right- and left-handedness in C57BL/6J mice. Furthermore, phenotypic selection studies were performed *within* C57BL/6J mice. The proportions of dextral and sinistral progeny from matings between two right-handed parents, two left-handed parents, or mixed parental matings did not change through three generations of intensive selective breeding (Collins, 1969). This indicates that it is unlikely that right- and left-handedness in these mice is being maintained by a residue of nonfixed genetic variation that escaped the rigors of continuous inbreeding. It also indicates that the laterality of these mice is not likely to have been inherited culturally through mechanisms of social learning.

The results described were obtained when mice were tested in an unbiased or U-world, a test apparatus in which the feeding tube was located equidistantly from the right and left sides of the cubicle. We will shortly consider in detail research in which mice were tested in biased worlds. I define a right- or R-world as one in which the feeding tube is located flush against the right wall as faced by the mouse, and a left- or L-world as one in which the feeding tube is located flush with the left wall. The apparatus used for both worlds is identical; it only needs to be inverted. The relationships between the expressed handedness of mice tested in unbiased and biased worlds will, I believe, aid in understanding genetic effects upon lateralization itself. They will also lead us toward an admissible genetic model for the inheritance of sense of asymmetry. Data analyses to be presented are an extension of those reported in Collins (1975).

Figure 1 (upper graph) illustrates the paw preference scores of

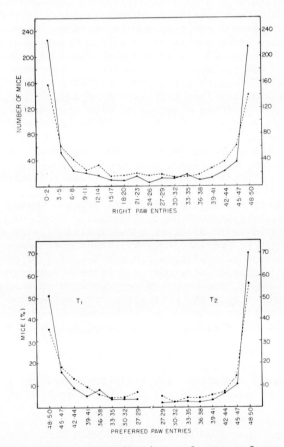

Fig. 1. *Upper graph: Distributions of paw preference scores expressed as right paw entries (RPEs) for 709 C57BL/6J mice tested in an unbiased or U-world. Test 1 is the dashed line and Test 2 is the solid line. From Collins (1975) with permission of the publisher. Lower graph: Preferred paw entries (PPEs) for male mice (dashed line) and female mice (solid line) on Test 1 and Test 2 in the U-world.*

709 C57BL/6J mice aged 8 to 12 weeks that were tested for paw preference in an unbiased or U-world. One week after initial testing, mice were retested under the same conditions. The abscissa has been divided into 17 class intervals of three RPEs. First note the general appearance of the two frequency distributions. They are markedly U-shaped. Most mice were either strongly right-handed or strongly left-handed. Only a few expressed ambilaterality. On Test 1, 41.8% of mice scored in the region of 0-2 and 48-50 RPEs and in Test 2, 62.2% were in this region. The strength of expressed laterality had increased on the second testing. Ignoring mice that scored exactly 25 RPEs, we find that 368 of 702 or 52.42% of mice in Test 1 and 370 of 707 or 52.33% of mice in Test 2 could be classified as sinistral. There were no significant differences between the sexes in the proportions of dextral and sinistral mice. For 341 female mice tested in the U-world, the product moment correlation of Test 1 and Test 2 scores was $r = .912$ ($t = 40.96$, $df = 339$), and for 368 male mice, this correlation was $r = .904$ ($t = 40.43$, $df = 366$). In both cases the correlation was highly significant ($p < .0001$).

Let us now consider differences in lateralization between the sexes in U-world performance. The lower graph in Figure 1 presents the paw preference scores of the same female and male mice as in Test 1 and Test 2 expressed as preferred paw entries (PPEs). The PPE score depicts the strength of laterality without regard to the direction of the asymmetry. For example, RPE scores of 5 (indicating a left-handed mouse) and of 45 (indicating a right-handed mouse) both become a PPE score of 45.

For both Test 1 and Test 2, female mice exhibited stronger unimanual lateralization than did male mice. The difference in the degree of expressed lateralization between the sexes is dramatic. In Test 1, 169 of 334 or 50.60% of females and 128 of 359 or 35.65% of males occupied PPE intervals 48-50 ($\chi^2 = 15.78$, $p = 7.1 \times 10^{-5}$). In Test 2, these proportions were 237 of 340 or 69.71% and 204 of 364 or 56.04% respectively ($\chi^2 = 14.02$, $p = 1.8 \times 10^{-4}$).

Female C57BL/6J mice were more strongly lateralized in an unbiased world than were male mice. This is a basic finding. I offer no explanation why this is the case. We will simply consider this sex difference to be a genetic difference, albeit of sex-chromosomal rather than autosomal origin, and we will follow the effects of this sex difference in further experiments.

Let us consider now the paw preference scores of other C57BL/6J mice that were tested for paw preference in biased worlds. An additional 435 mice aged 6 to 8 weeks were assigned randomly to biased worlds (217 to the R-world and 218 to the L-world).

Figure 2 (upper graph) illustrates the paw preference scores of 435 C57BL/6J mice tested in biased worlds expressed as biased world paw entries (BWPEs). The distributions of RPE scores for L- and R-world mice may be found in Collins (1975). BWPE scores were derived by a mirror-image superposition of the L-world

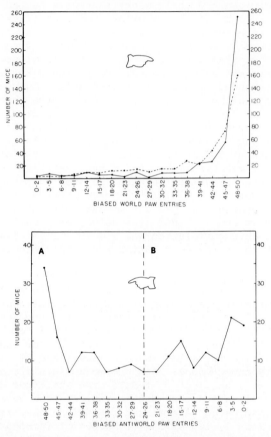

*Fig. 2. Upper graph: Distributions of paw preference scores, expressed as the number of entries consistent with the world bias (biased world paw entries, BWPEs) for 435 C57BL/6J mice. Test 1 is shown as a dashed line, and Test 2, a solid line. Lower graph: Distribution of biased antiworld paw entires (BAWPEs) is shown for 215 mice retested in a world that was a mirror image of their original biased world. Group A consists of mice that exhibited paw preference scores in the direction consistent with the antiworld bias, and Group B, those with scores in the direction opposite to the antiworld bias. From Collins (1975) with permission of the publisher.*

distribution onto the R-world distribution. For example, RPE scores of 10 in an L-world and of 40 in an R-world are both equivalent to a BWPE score of 40. The biased worlds exerted a pronounced effect upon the expressed paw preferences of mice. Note that the distributions are now rather J-shaped. Most mice exhibited BWPE scores consistent in direction with the world bias. However, between 8.7 and 14.7% of mice produced paw preferences opposite to the world bias. In the L-world, 27 of 218 mice in Test 1 and 19 mice in Test 2 scored in the region of 26-50 RPEs. In the R-world, 32 of 217 mice in Test 1, and 23 mice in Test 2 scored in the region of 0-24 RPEs. The strength of laterality was increased on the second testing. The average BWPE score on Test 1 was $40.147 \pm .567$ and on Test 2, it was $43.012 \pm .567$.

Before examining possible sex differences in the paw preferences of mice in biased worlds, we must address the issue of whether the tests measured an already existing lateral specialization or whether the paw preferences themselves were acquired during the actual testing. Does the handedness of mice arise de novo during initial testing?

To answer this question, I assigned the first 320 mice randomly to R-, L-, or U-worlds for a third paw-preference test. If the first and second biased world tests are designated R-R and L-L, then we will now be concerned with the scores of mice tested in worlds of the opposite bias or antiworlds, test sequences R-R-L and L-L-R. The remaining 115 mice from a replicated experiment were assigned to antiworlds.

Figure 2 (lower graph) presents the biased antiworld paw entries (BAWPEs) for 215 mice tested in a world that was the mirror image of the world in which they were originally tested. The figure is partitioned at the BAWPE score of 25. Group A mice are those that produced BAWPE scores consistent with the antiworld bias (BAWPE 26-50), and Group B mice are those with scores opposite to the antiworld bias (BAWPE 0-24). By identifying mice that gravitated toward the antiworld bias and those that resisted it, we can partition the original Test 1 and Test 2 biased world scores into A and B parts. If mice acquire their paw preferences during initial testing, the A and B partitions should not differ. If mice entering the original biased worlds comprised one group possessing a native laterality consistent with the bias and another group with a native laterality opposite to the bias, then we should expect the paw preference scores for Group A to be significantly less than those for Group B.

The results of this partitioning across sexes is but briefly described here. Additional information may be found in Collins (1975). The average BWPE score of 108 mice in Group A for Test 1 was $34.24 \pm 1.28$, and for 106 mice in Group B, $45.75 \pm .58$ ($t = -8.131$). For Test 2 the mean for Group A was $37.56 \pm 1.39$, and for Group B, $48.69 \pm .24$ ($t = -7.813$). The probabilities that the mean differences in the predicted direction arose by chance are infinitesimal. Group A mice appear to consist of right-handed mice tested in left-handed worlds and left-handed mice tested in right-handed worlds. On the basis of their BWPE performance, Group A mice can be described as being ambilateral. Group B mice appear to consist of right-handed mice tested in right-handed worlds and left-handed mice tested in left-handed worlds. Their performance expressed strong lateralization in a direction consistent with their biased worlds.

These findings are inconsistent with the view that mice learn their handedness in the paw preference tests. The analyses are consistent with the view that mice arrive for paw preference testing with an already established sense of lateral specialization (cf. Glick, Jerussi, & Zimmerberg; Stamm, Rosen, & Gadotti, this volume).

Now let us examine differences between the sexes in Group A and Group B mice. Figure 3 (upper graph) presents Test 1 replotted in cumulative percent for 107 female and 107 male mice.

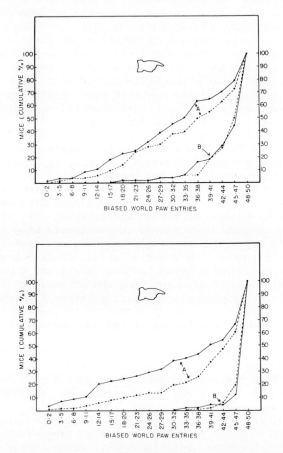

Fig. 3. Upper graph: Biased world paw entries for Test 1 originally plotted in upper graph in Figure 2 are replotted in cumulative percent for Group A and Group B mice. Male mice are shown as a dashed line, and female mice as a solid line. Lower graph: Similar information for Test 2.

Given that female mice were more strongly lateralized than males in the U-world, and that Group A mice were mainly native right-handers tested in a left-world and native left-handers tested in a right-world, we should expect Group A females to resist the influence of an uncongenial environmental bias better than males. Therefore we should predict that the BWPE scores of Group A females ought to be less than those of Group A males. The mean BWPE score of Group A females was $32.93 \pm 1.832$ ($n = 57$), and for males, $35.71 \pm 1.776$ ($n = 51$). This 2.78 BWPE difference in Test 1 is consistent in direction with that predicted, but it is not statistically significant ($t = -1.083$, $p = .141$). Figure 3 (lower graph) presents a similar partition of Test 2 scores. The mean BWPE score for Group A females was $34.77 \pm 2.121$, and for males, $40.67 \pm 1.666$. This 5.90 BWPE difference in average performance is consistent in direction with that predicted and it is statistically significant ($t = -2.149$, $p = .017$).

Consider now the case of Group B mice. Given that female mice were more strongly lateralized than males in the U-world, and that Group B mice were mainly native right-handers tested in a right-world and native left-handers tested in a left-world, we would expect Group B females to be more strongly lateralized than Group B males. Therefore we expect that the BWPE scores of females should be larger than those of males. However, because both males and females will produce BWPE scores near the ceiling of the paw preference range, any sex difference will be minimized, masked, and more difficult to detect. For this reason, we should employ a stricter criterion than that affordable by treating the data in BWPE class intervals of three paw reaches. Consider instead the proportions of male and female mice of Group B exhibiting the strongest lateralization possible in biased worlds, that is, a BWPE score of 50. For Test 1, 17 of 50 or 34% of female mice and 17 of 56 or 30.4% of male mice had a BWPE score of 50. This slight difference of proportions in the predicted direction is not statistically significant. For Test 2, 34 of 50 or 68.0% of female mice and 26 of 56 or 46.4% of male mice exhibited the maximum BWPE score. This difference of proportions is in the predicted direction and statistically significant ($\chi^2 = 5.00$, $p = .025$).

Now we may return to consider the overall pattern of sex differences in the paw preferences of mice tested in biased worlds. We know that female mice possessing a native lateral sense opposite to an environmental bias resist the pressure of this bias better than male mice. We also know that female mice possessing a native lateral sense consistent with an environmental bias will be slightly more strongly lateralized in biased worlds than male mice. Therefore we should predict male mice to be more strongly lateralized in biased worlds than female mice, and this difference between the sexes to be much smaller than the differences observed in the U-world.

Figure 4 (upper graph) presents the Test 1 performance of 215 female and 220 male mice in BWPE scores. The mean BWPE score

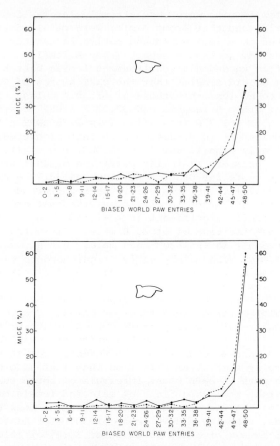

*Fig. 4.* Upper graph: *Distributions of biased world paw entries for 435 C57BL/6J mice tested in biased worlds according to sex for Test 1. Male mice are shown as a dashed line, and females as a solid line.* Lower graph: *Distributions by sex for Test 2 scores.*

for males was 40.99 + .744 and for females 39.28 + .855. Although males were 1.71. BWPEs more strongly lateralized than females in Test 1, this difference does not exceed a conventional level of statistical significance ($t$ = 1.509, $p$ = .066). The lower graph in Figure 4 presents similar information for Test 2. Greater numbers of male mice occupied the extreme intervals of 39–50 BWPEs. The mean BWPE score for males was 44.64 + .657 and for females it was 41.34 + .916. The increase in expressed laterality of 3.30 BWPEs for male mice is again consistent in direction with that expected. The difference is statistically significant ($t$ = 2.934, $p$ = .0018).

The experimental findings I have presented have some

important implications. Let us review. Genetic differences
giving rise to sex differences are associated with variation in
the strength of expressed laterality. Female mice harbor a
genetic complement associated with stronger expressed laterality.
Male mice harbor a genetic complement associated with weaker expressed laterality. The sense of laterality itself appears to
be established in individual mice prior to the initial paw-
preference testing. Consider now the genetic effects on degree
of lateralization in mice placed into worlds biased for and
against their native lateralities. For simplicity, consider the
biased world to be an R-world.

Native left-handed female mice placed into an R-world tend
to be more left-handed and native right-handed females tend to
be more right-handed. The genetic complement in female mice
associated with increases in the degree of expressed lateralization is associated with increasing right-handedness as well as
increasing left-handedness. Native left-handed male mice placed
into an R-world tend to be less left-handed and native right-
handed males tend to be less right-handed. The genetic complement in male mice associated with decreases in the degree of
expressed lateralization is associated with decreasing left-
handedness as well as decreasing right-handedness. The genes
increasing right-handedness appear to be the same genes increasing left-handedness. The genes decreasing right-handedness
appear to be the same genes decreasing left-handedness. Even
more simply, the genes for right and left appear to be identical.
Although genetic alternatives themselves appear to be inherently
indifferent to the senses of asymmetry, we have seen that genetic differences responsible for variation in the degree of
lateralization may take on the appearance of an inheritance of
left-right forms when organisms exist in biased worlds.

Thus far we have examined the effects of a genetics of lateralization on the expressed senses of a single asymmetry. Let
us briefly consider a mental experiment in which two asymmetries
are considered jointly. Suppose we are interested in the possible physiological interdependence between the two asymmetries,
and that individuals studied exist in a biased environment that
favors the expression of one of the two senses of each asymmetry.
It makes no difference whether the same or opposite senses are
favored. We consider that the initial senses of the asymmetries
arise randomly, and that there exists genetic variation affecting the strength of lateralization common to both asymmetries.
We now expect that the proportions of dextral and sinistral
forms of both asymmetries will be altered by the genes affecting
lateralization. Let $R_1$ and $L_1$ refer to the senses of the first
asymmetry, and $R_2$ and $L_2$, of the second asymmetry. For a subpopulation of individuals possessing one type of genetic complement affecting lateralization, let the numbers of individuals
observed in classes $R_1$ - $R_2$, $R_1$ - $L_2$, $L_1$ - $R_2$, and $L_1$ - $L_2$ be
360, 90, 40, and 10, respectively. The correlation between the
senses of the two asymmetries is zero ($\chi^2$ = 0.0). For the other

subpopulation, individuals possessing the alternative genetic complement affecting lateralization, let the observed frequencies be 150, 150, 100, and 100, respectively. Although there are differences in the marginal frequencies for the forms of the asymmetries, there is again no association between the senses of the two asymmetries ($\chi^2 = 0.0$). But now let the populations be mixed. The frequencies in the four phenotypic classes now become 510, 240, 140, and 110 ($\chi^2 = 11.87$, $p < .001$). If a fourfold point correlation were calculated, its value would be $\phi = .109 \pm .032$.

A researcher having just examined this population of 1000 individuals would probably be pleased at finding this highly significant correlation. For example, the first asymmetry might reflect lateral dominance of an important cerebral process, and the second asymmetry might be a respected measure of handedness. Our hypothetical researcher might be tempted to search the neuroanatomical literature for reasons why the first asymmetry may influence the second. If he later discovered that the second asymmetry tends to run in families, he might be inclined to devise a sophisticated two-locus four-allele genetic model for the inheritance of the senses of both asymmetries. And much later he might even be tempted to speculate on the occasions during evolution that gave rise to the newly mutated right and left genetic alleles (see Levy, this volume).

I believe that this mental experiment serves a useful purpose. First, it shows that associations between the directions of two asymmetries may emerge quite naturally as a consequence of genetic effects upon lateralization itself, and not upon primary lateral sense. Second, I believe it sounds a note of gentle caution that should be heeded by investigators who report modest correlations between the senses of asymmetries. The correlations will be indeed real, but they just might arise from heterogeneity of subpopulations.


DISCUSSION

On a prior occasion I have likened the bond existing between genetics and the senses of asymmetry to a Gordian knot, more neatly cut than untied (Collins, 1970). The experimental evidence presented herein prompts me to recast this early view. I now tend to regard the bond as an aerial image of a Gordian knot that just might be capable of being untied so long as attention is focused not on it, but elsewhere. The modern debate over the manner of inheritance of the direction of asymmetry has centered on whether left and right are properties of alternative nuclear genes. Not only am I unaware of any evidence supporting the existence of right and left genes in animal and human populations, but I believe that the very formulation of the issue in terms of the possible sense-properties of DNA has misdirected our attention and clouded the issue (see Levy; Morgan, this volume; Corballis and Morgan, 1976).

The research reported here and in Collins (1975) has led me to conclude that genetic variation plays two important roles in the maintenance of the senses of asymmetries. I have proposed that each individual's initial asymmetric sense arises according to a seemingly random process, an "asymmetry lottery," the outcomes of which are responsible for initial sense direction. Transmissible genetic variation could well maintain this asymmetry lottery and thereby engender the senses of asymmetry. The probabilities of the initial sense outcomes, it is stressed, need not be equal. Genetic variation may also give rise to differences in the degree to which lateralization is achieved. For the case in which organisms develop in or exist in an environment that differentially favors the expression of one sense of asymmetry, these genetic differences may lead to variation in the proportions of expressed asymmetric forms.

It has been observed in the majority of studies that adult human males show a greater average degree of lateralization than do adult human females in tests of verbal, visuospatial, and overall lateralization. A review of this literature has been provided by Harshman and Remington (1976; see also Gur & Gur, this volume). In interpreting this finding in light of the research reported herein, we may raise the question of whether the greater lateralization of human males implies that males indeed possess inherently greater cerebral specialization or whether males possess a weaker, more diffuse, cerebral organization that leads to a greater lability to adapt to persistent environmental biases.

## ACKNOWLEDGMENTS

Supported in part by NSF Grant BMS 75-15966 and by institutional funds of the Jackson Laboratory. The Jackson Laboratory is fully accredited by the American Association for Accreditation of Laboratory Animal Care.

## REFERENCES

Collins, R. L. On the inheritance of handedness: I. Laterality in inbred mice. *Journal of Heredity*, 1968, *59*, 9-12.
Collins, R. L. On the inheritance of handedness: II. Selection for sinistrality in mice. *Journal of Heredity*, 1969, *60*, 117-119.
Collins, R. L. The sound of one paw clapping: An inquiry into the origin of left-handedness. In G. Lindzey & D. Thiessen (Eds.), *Contributions to behavior-genetic analysis: The mouse as a prototype*. New York: Appleton, 1970. Pp. 115-136.
Collins, R. L. Audiogenic seizures. In D. Purpura, J. Penry,

ROBERT L. COLLINS

D. Tower, D. Woodbury, & R. Walter (Eds.), *Experimental models of epilepsy--A manual for the laboratory worker.* New York: Raven Press, 1972. Pp. 347-372.

Collins, R. L. When left-handed mice live in right-handed worlds. *Science*, 1975, *187*, 181-184.

Corballis, M. C., and Morgan, M. J. On the biological basis of human laterality. Submitted for publication, 1976.

Green, E. L. *Biology of the laboratory mouse.* (2nd ed.) New York: Dover Publications, 1975.

Harshman, R. A. & Remington, R. Sex, language and the brain: A review of adult sex differences in lateralization. Part I. *Brain and Language.* Submitted for publication, 1976.

Staats, J. Standardized nomenclature for inbred strains of mice: Fifth listing. *Cancer Research*, 1972, *32*, 1609-1646.

150

# 10.

# Handedness and Cerebral Dominance in Monkeys

The Pennsylvania State University

Jung clearly articulated the classical neurological view on handedness and cerebral dominance in animals when he said,

Up to this point, nothing has been found in these animal experiments that would bear on cerebral dominance. I believe this shows clearly the limitations of animal experiments. It is evident that real hemispheric dominance does not occur in any of these infrahuman species. We have no evidence whatsoever for cerebral dominance in monkeys, not to mention the carnivores. . . . In my opinion, preference for one side of the body, in animals, is very different from handedness. Many experiments show this. Cole and Glees (1951) have shown that hand preference in monkeys is rather evenly distributed, in contrast to the preponderant preference for the right hand in man. Besides, preference for a particular hand, right or left, is much less pronounced in the monkey. Similarly, J. M. Warren (1958) has shown that paw preferences in cats, and hand preferences in monkeys, are rather plastic: the 'favoring' of one upper extremity over the other increases as a function of prolonged testing and is much more easily reversed than in man.

Thus, I think that we must distinguish between the preference for one hand in animals, and the dominance of one side of the brain in man. As I said, no evidence whatsoever has been presented that cerebral dominance really occurs in monkeys [Jung, 1962, pp. 268-269].

---

*Supported by NIMH Grant MH-04726.

Some years ago we (Warren, Abplanalp, & Watten, 1967) argued that the experiments Jung cited were inadequate to support his negative conclusion, and we presented evidence that lateral preferences in monkeys and cats are relatively strong, moderately stable over time, and rather resistant to change by training. The conclusion was that one cannot categorically deny the possibility of handedness in these species.

After further analyses of that 1967 data and examination of the results of other recent studies of laterality in monkeys, we are seriously considering the possibility that Jung was more nearly correct than we were. The rest of this paper is an exposition of the grounds for doubt and skepticism regarding the presence of handedness and cerebral dominance in monkeys.

METHOD

Subjects

Fourteen young rhesus monkeys were studied. The animals were about 2 years old on arrival, and eight were about 4 years old when subjected to unilateral frontal ablations (Warren, Cornwell, & Warren, 1969), between the second and third series of handedness tests.

The monkeys were tested on learning problems (Beck, Warren, & Sterner, 1966; Coutant & Warren, 1966; Warren, 1966; Warren & Ebel, 1967) that required manipulatory responses during the interval between the first and second series.

Apparatus

The handedness tests were carried out in the Wisconsin General Test Apparatus (WGTA), illustrated in Harlow (1949, Figure 1).

Handedness Tests

Lateral preferences were observed on 10 manipulation tests designed to elicit a variety of manual responses and postural adjustments. The manipulanda and incentive were presented in positions corresponding to the locations of the left, right, and center food wells of a standard WGTA test tray containing three food wells. The placement of the incentive was varied over trials in a balanced irregular sequence to control for position biases (see Glick, Jerussi, & Zimmerberg; Stamm, Rosen & Gadotti, this volume), and the food was never placed so far toward one side of the test tray as to force the monkey to use one hand because of gross physical constraints. In five (unimanual) tests visible food was presented well within the monkeys' reach and the animals responded with one hand or the other. The remaining five (potentially bimanual) tests required the subjects to perform an instrumental response to gain access to the food incentive; they had either to displace an object covering concealed food or to draw food within reach by manipulating a chain or rod. Since the two motor acts needed to secure the reinforcement in these tests were successive rather than simultaneous, both could be carried out with the same hand, and most monkeys did make both responses in a given sequence with the same hand.

## UNIMANUAL TESTS

### Reach

A WGTA test tray with no food wells was divided into three equivalent sectors. A raisin, peanut, or small piece of other high-preference food was placed in the center of the right, left, or central areas on the tray. The monkey had only to pick up the food from the surface of the test tray.

### Trough

A single piece of food was placed at the end of one of three wooden troughs, 10 cm long with a 1.5-cm opening. The troughs were intended to force the monkey to slide the piece of food the length of the trough rather than pick it up directly, but the subjects were often able to pick up the food with one finger. We decided not to change the trough, however, since both the sliding and one-finger-reach responses differed from those made on the other tests.

### Wire

A fruit-flavored cereal ring (Froot Loops) was presented on horizontal wires, 10 cm long and 10 cm above the surface of the test tray. The test was intended to force the monkeys to slide the cereal rings the length of the wire, with the direction of movement required varying from trial to tiral since the wires on the right and left required lateral movements (to the right and left, respectively), and the wire in the central position, which was oriented toward the cage, demanded movement in a plane normal, rather than parallel, to the cage. Frequently the monkeys simply broke the dry cereal off the wire rather than sliding the ring in the anticipated direction. Again, it was decided not to alter the character of the test since the responses made on this task differed from those made on the other tests.

### Horizontal Bottle

The incentive was placed about halfway into one of the three test tubes (4.8 cm in diameter and 18 cm long) lying on the test tray. The monkey had to insert its hand and wrist into the tube to secure the reward.

## Vertical Bottle

The monkeys were obliged to reach into one of three vertically oriented clear-plastic containers (7.7 cm high and 5.1 cm in diameter) to obtain a raisin or peanut.

*BIMANUAL TESTS*

## Block, Extension, and Card

A raisin or peanut was placed under a single object in one of the three food wells of the test tray. The subject was required to push the object aside to uncover the food. Three sorts of objects were used; each required somewhat different patterns of hand movements. The manipulandum used in the block test was a small rectangular tin (7.7 x 6.4 x 2.6 cm) and in the card test, a 7.7 x 7.7 cm square of sheet metal about 2 mm thick. In both these tests, the subject was free to displace the object in any way it chose. This was not so with the extension test, in which the objects were wooden boocks (7.7 x 10.2 x 5.1 cm) that slid on metal rails. The rails prevented any lateral movement of the blocks and forced the animal to push the block directly back toward the rear of the test tray to uncover the food.

## Chain

A raisin was impaled on a 1.3-cm-long pin at the end of one of three 30-cm lengths of light chain that were clipped to eyelets on a 43.5 x 61.4 cm tray. In order to obtain the raisin the monkey had to draw the chain in closer to the restraining cage.

## Handle Box

The incentive was placed in a wooden box, 12.8 cm square and 7.7 cm deep, with a handle 1.3 cm in diameter and 12.8 cm long. The box was presented far enough (approximately 23 cm) from the cage to make it impossible for the monkey to reach the food directly. The subject had, instead, to grasp the handle and drag the 300-g box toward the cage before it could take the food.

In all the bimanual tests it was possible for a monkey to use one hand to handle the manipulandum and the other to take the food. For this reason, both the hand used in manipulation (M) and the hand used in securing the incentive (I) were recorded on these tests.

*HANDEDNESS TESTING PROCEDURE*

The initial series of handedness tests was designed to adapt the subjects to the WGTA as well as to yield data on lateral preferences. It consisted of the following stages:

1. *Pretest Adaptation*. The subjects were tested 25 trials per day for 20 days on the reach test only.

2. *Unimanual Tests*. The monkeys were tested 25 trials per day for 8 days on each of the five unimanual tests, over a period of 40 days. Each test was given once in successive blocks of 5 days, and the order of presentation was varied from block to block to prevent confounding tests and cumulative practice effects. Preference scores in this series were based upon a total of 200 responses per test (8 days x 25 trials).

3. *Bimanual Tests*. The subjects were tested for 25 trials on each bimanual test on 8 days over the next 40 days of testing. The five tests were again given once in successive 5-day periods and the order of presentation varied between blocks. A total of 200 trials was given on every test.

The entire series of handedness tests was repeated twice 2 years after the initial tests (Series 1), just prior to and immediately after the unilateral lesions were made. The procedures followed in the preoperative Series 2 and postoperative Series 3 were identical with those of Series 1 with two exceptions. There was no extensive pretest adaptation on the simple reach task, and each test was presented for 100 rather than 200 trials.


RESULTS

If the monkeys' performance is evaluated in terms of composite scores, the percentage of total right or left responses, averaged over all 15 response measures in a single series of tests, one can make a fairly strong case for handedness in this species. This is shown in Figures 1 and 2.

The stability of individual monkeys' preferences may be judged from Figure 1, scatter plots of the scores on successive series

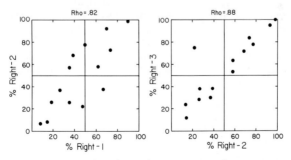

*Fig. 1. Scatter plots showing the mean preference scores of 14 monkeys on all 15 handedness measures in Series 1 and 2 (left panel) and Series 2 and 3 (right panel).*

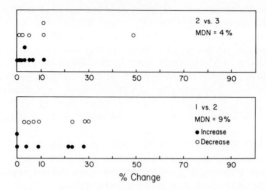

*Fig. 2. Percentage of change in individual monkeys' overall preference scores between successive series of handedness tests.*

of tests. The ordinates and abscissas are given as 0 to 100% right responses; extremely low and extremely high scores represent decided left- and right-handedness, respectively. One's immediate response to the visual display and the magnitude of the rank order correlations is that there is a high positive relation between scores of successive administrations of the test battery.

The distributions of the changes in total preference scores for individual monkeys between Series 1 and 2, and between Series 2 and 3, are shown in Figure 2. The greatest change was 50%. No monkey shifted from a 100%-right to a 100%-left preference, nor from an 80%-right to an 80%-left preference. The average monkey showed less than 10% change between series.

The findings just presented are impressive, and it is easy to see how they could be construed as supporting the idea that monkeys have handedness just as people do. We began to have misgivings when we started to examine the pattern of interrelations between tasks, and found that curious but compelling pattern shown in Figure 3. The population of 15 measures of hand preference divides itself into three distinct subgroups (see Table 1). One set, H, consists of tasks that are *highly* correlated with one another throughout the experiment. The tasks in sets L and C̆ were not correlated among themselves nor with any other tasks in Series 1. The tests in set L tended to remain that way. But the tasks in set C became more consistently correlated with one another and also with the tasks in set H in series 2 and 3.

These relationships are shown in a somewhat more conventional if less dramatic, way in Figure 4, where the correlations *within* sets are plotted on the left, and the correlations *between* sets on the right. The average correlation involving tests in the L set is initially low and stays low. Intercorrelations among tests in the H set start high and stay high. Correlations involving tests in the C group are low at the beginning, but the

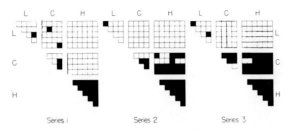

Fig. 3. *The patterns of correlations between handedness-test scores at three stages in training the same group of 14 monkeys. Black and white cells in the matrices represent statistically significant and nonsignificant rank order correlations, respectively. Letters L, C, and H identify sets of tasks with typically low, changing, and high intercorrelations.*

TABLE 1

*Tests Comprising the Three Sets*

| *Set L* | *Set H* |
|---|---|
| Wire | Block (M) |
| Horizontal bottle | Block (I) |
| Chain (M) | Extension (M) |
| Chain (I) | Extension (I) |
| Handle box (M) | Card (M) |
| | Card (I) |
| *Set C* | |
| Handle Box (I) | |
| Vertical bottle | |
| Trough | |
| Reach | |

correlations among C tests and between C and H tests increase considerably in Series 2 and 3.

The further we looked, the more evidence we found of substantial differences among the handedness tests. The median percentage of preference responses elicited by the tasks in the three sets is compared in Figure 5, which shows that sets H, C, and L are quite differentially effective in producing strong preferences.

Figure 6 also deals with preferences; it shows the percentage of tests on which monkeys manifested statistically significant

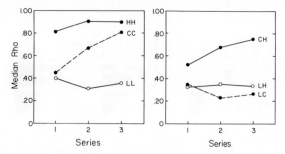

Fig. 4. *Median rank order correlations between scores within (left panel) and between (right panel) the subgroups of tests characterized as having low (L), changing (C), or high (H) intertest correlations.*

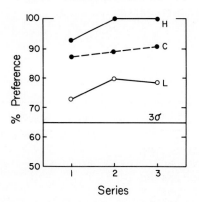

Fig. 5. *Median percentage of responses with the preferred hand on the sets of tests with low (L), changing (C), and high (H) intertest consistency.*

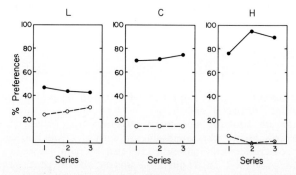

Fig. 6. *Percentage of tests in sets L, C, and H that elicited preference scores significantly different from chance in individual monkeys. Filled and open cirlces indicate preferences consistent and inconsistent with the monkeys' overall preferences.*

preferences that were consistent or inconsistent with their overall preference. It is apparent that tasks in set L evoked few significant preferences, and that many of these were inconsistent. Tests in set H, in contrast, produced many significant preferences, and almost all were consistent with the animals' preferences over all tests.

The median percentage of change in hand preference between Series 1 and 2, and Series 2 and 3 is displayed in Figure 7. The average change in performance on the tasks in set H is markedly less than for the tests in sets L and C.

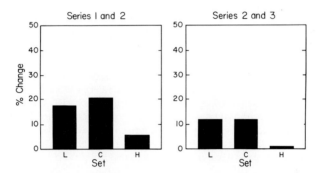

*Fig. 7. Median percentage of change in the monkeys' preference scores on the tests of sets L, C, and H between successive replications of the handedness test battery.*

Figure 8 presents the median reliability correlations for the tasks in sets L, C, and H. A very modest relationship between scores on the tests of set C on Series 1 and 2 is evident. More important, in spite of the low correlations among the tasks of set L and between tasks in set L and sets C and H, the L tests individually yield tolerably consistent manual preference scores on successive tests. The results obtained in successive

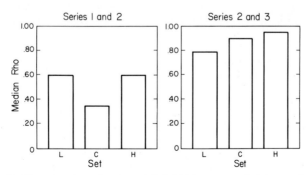

*Fig. 8. Median test-retest reliability correlations for the tests in sets L, C, and H.*

replications of the set L tests are in almost as good agreement
as sets H and C. Thus, one cannot dismiss the fact that they
correlate poorly with one another and with the tests in sets C
and H as due to intrinsic noisiness and low reliability.

There is only one conclusion possible from the findings just
reviewed. Hand preferences in rhesus monkeys are quite specific.
The six response measures that comprise set H can easily be considered as very minor variants of a single task. Card-M requires displacement of a thin object, extension-M, displacement
of a thick object in a single direction, and block-M, displacement of a moderately thick object, free style. The movements
required to obtain the incentive in these tasks (card-I, exten-
sion-I, and block-I) are even more patently isomorphic with one
another. Given this degree of similarity in the structure of
the tasks, we could be surprised only if they did not correlate
with one another.

The tasks in set L require quite different movement patterns,
to pick Froot Loops from a wire above the test tray (wire test),
to draw in and remove food from a flexible chain (chain M and I),
to drag a heavy container some distance to the cage (handle box-
M), or to place an arm into a horizontal test tube (horizontal
bottle). After the fact, it seems obvious that these different
tasks which require idiosyncratic movement patterns ought not to
be correlated with one another or the tasks in set H.

The motor requirements for coping with the tests in set C
seem more like those of set H than set L; the monkeys certainly
acted as if this were the case.

The consistency and the stability of the total preference
scores, averaged over all handedness tests (Figures 1 and 2),
now seem due largely to the quality of the monkeys' performance
that is selectively elicited by the object-displacement tasks of
set H. These, of course, were the tasks on which the animals
were most practiced between series of handedness tests.

Thus far the results obtained in the pretest have not been
considered. They consisted of 500 trials on the reach test,
which was the monkeys' first experience in the WGTA and preceded Series 1. In the left panel of Figure 9 the rank order
correlations between scores on the pretest and subsequent scores
on the reach tests and on the total of all tests excluding the
reach test, are plotted for the three series. It is readily
apparent that performance on the pretest is not a very good pre-
dictor of later performance on handedness tests. Only one of
six correlations, the one between pretest and the reach test on
Series 1, is statistically significant, and two of the remaining
five correlations are negative. The panel on the right in
Figure 9 shows that the reach test is neither a stronge nor a
bizarre task; performance on reach is well correlated with performance on all other tasks on Series 1, 2, and 3. This indicates that the reach test fairly accurately reflects the monkeys'
predominant tendency to prefer the right of left hand at a
given moment, but that early preferences on the reach task, even

if based on 500 trials, provide no valid basis for judgments concerning the animals' later lateral preferences.

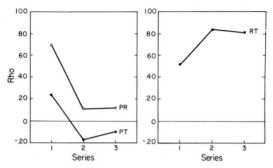

*Fig. 9. Left: Correlations between scores on the pretest with reach and on reach in subsequent series (PR), and between pretest scores and the total preference score on all measures except reach in Series 1 through 3 (PT). Right: Correlations between preference on the reach test and preference on all measures except the reach test (RT) at three stages of training.*

DISCUSSION

The results of these experiments can be regarded as grounds for doubting that hand preferences in monkeys imply any major organismic asymmetry. Fortunately, the findings of the present study need not stand entirely on their own. Three additional experiments provide more information on the questions of whether hand preferences in inexperienced monkeys are largely task-specific, relatively poor predictors of later performance and strongly affected by experience on manipulation tasks. Warren (1958), and Warren and Nonneman (1976) tested rhesus monkeys on three of the tasks used in the present experiment and observed the animals on the same tests after intervals of 3 months (Warren, 1958), 8 months (Warren & Nonneman, 1976) or 24 months (this experiment).

The rank order correlations between pairs of tests on the first and second series in each experiment are presented in Table 2. The intercorrelations in the first replications are generally modest, but vary greatly between experiments. In contrast, the correlations on the second repetitions of the tests with now more experienced subjects are fairly high in all three experiments, suggesting a similar response to extended practice and experience.

Reliability correlations for the tests used in these experiments are given in Table 3. The values indicate low to moderately high agreement between performance on the first and second series in each experiment, but slow marked variability between studies and tasks.

TABLE 2

*Intertest Correlations in Three Experiments*

| Tests | Warren, 1958 Series | | This study Series | | Warren & Nonneman, 1976 Series | |
|---|---|---|---|---|---|---|
| | 1 | 2 | 1 | 2 | 1 | 2 |
| Reach & block (I) | .01 | .69 | .36 | .90 | .64 | .92 |
| Reach & card (I) | .29 | .91 | .39 | .82 | .62 | .94 |
| Block (I) & card (I) | .54 | .79 | .94 | .91 | .90 | .98 |

TABLE 3

*Reliability Correlations in Three Experiments*

| Test | Warren, 1958 | This study | Warren & Nonneman |
|---|---|---|---|
| Reach | .16 | .38 | .62 |
| Block (I) | .89 | .57 | .62 |
| Card (I) | .24 | .84 | .73 |
| | | | |
| Interest interval (months) | 3 | 24 | 8 |

Brookshire and Warren's (1962) experiment permits a more extensive comparison of different groups of inexperienced monkeys' performance on handedness tests. They observed 19 experimentally naive monkeys on seven of the measures used in the current experiment, and retested their subjects on five tasks after an interval of 2 weeks. The results of the two studies are compared in Figure 10, which shows, on the left, the agreement between the 21 correlations among seven tasks, and, on the right, the agreement between the reliability correlations obtained in the two experiments. Neither chart reveals a high level of agreement between the two sets of observations.

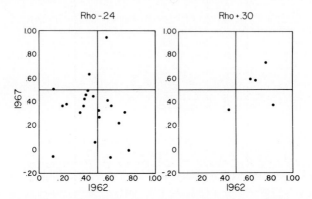

Fig. 10. *Repeatability of the results of handedness tests with experimentally naive monkeys. The panel on the left shows the agreement between the values of 21 intercorrelations between scores on the same seven tests obtained by Brookshire and Warren (1962) and Warren et al. (1967). The panel on the right shows the correspondence in the test-retest reliability correlations for five tests that were repeated in the same two experiments.*

The comparisons between four similar experiments yield a picture of extreme variability in the magnitude of intertask and reliability correlations for naive subjects. Yet they all agree in suggesting that early performance on handedness tests is largely task-specific and not highly predictive of later performance on the same task; they also agree in showing that prolonged experience has a marked effect on many measures of hand preference in monkeys.

The total pattern of results obtained from monkeys tested on multiple manipulation tasks over an appreciable period of time is most compatible with the following model of apparent handedness in monkeys. The initial performance of inexperienced monkeys is somewhat unstable, inconsistent, and largely task-specific. Measures of the strength, consistency, and value of initial preference scores for predicting future handedness test performance, vary markedly between experiments, probably because of differences in adaptation and pretraining procedures, the number of particular types of handedness tests used, and other experimental conditions.

As monkeys become experienced in performing particular manipulations (during the learning and perception experiments that almost always intervene between bouts of handedness testing), they develop skills and strong hand preferences for dealing with limited classes of manipulanda. The animals may later generalize the motor skills and hand preferences to tasks requiring somewhat similar manual and postural responses. But some tests lay well beyond the range of potential generalization and require a separate set of motor skills. Performance on such tests remains independent of, or uncorrelated with, the tests that can be managed with the skills acquired in displacing objects or cards, during other kinds of experiments.

This is the most parsimonious view of handedness and its development in monkeys. But it must be admitted that the behavioral data are not completely unequivocal. An ingenious advocate of genetically determined cerebral dominance and handedness in macaques might be able to create a clever Ptolemaic explanation to account in a fairly plausible manner for the data summarized here. (See also Collins; Morgan; Levy, this volume.)

There are, however, no comparable opportunities for alternate interpretations of the relevant neurobehavioral experiments. Warren, Cornwell, and Warren (1969) observed that monkeys with unilateral lesions in the frontal granular cortex were significantly impaired on delayed response, but subjects with lesions contralateral to the preferred hand made no more errors than animals with ablations ipsilateral to their preferred hand. Warren and Nonneman (1976) found that rhesus monkeys with unilateral lesions in the posterior temporal cortex were significantly inferior to controls in pattern discrimination learning, but there was no difference between monkeys with lesions in the hemispheres that appeared to be dominant and nondominant, on the basis of handedness scores (cf. Hamilton, this volume). Ettlinger and Gautrin (1971) report a similar result for monkeys with unilateral ablations of ventral temporal cortex. The unilateral preparations were inferior to controls, but the magnitude of the deficit in visual discrimination learning in the operated subjects was not affected by their suffering damage to the hemisphere ipsi- or contralateral to the preferred hand.

The failure of these attempts to demonstrate cerebral dominance in problem solving indicates that right- and left-handed monkeys are not left- and right-brained. Other investigators are free to make their own interpretations, but the chances that the rhesus monkey will become a useful animal model for cerebral dominance phenomena are so small that further efforts in research on this subject do not appear promising (cf. Dewson; Hamilton; Rubens; Stamm *et al.*, this volume).

SUMMARY

Fourteen inexperienced rhesus monkeys (*Macaca mulatta*) were observed on a battery of 10 handedness tests on three separate occasions. During the 24 months that intervened between the first and second series of tests, the subjects participated in several learning experiments that required movements like the manipulations required for some of the handedness tests.
The chief results of the experiment were as follows:

1. The correlations between the total number of right-hand responses by individual monkeys on all tests within successive series were high and positive (> .80). The median percentage of change in overall preferences was less than 10% between replications.
2. The intercorrelations between tests showed, however, that they could be divided into three distinct groups. Performances on tests in set L (low) were not significantly correlated with performance on any other tests. Scores on the tests in set H (high) were highly and significantly correlated with one another at all stages of the experiment; the tasks in this set were very similar or identical to the manipulations required in the intervening learning experiments. The tests in set C (changing) were initially statistically independent of one another and of the tests in sets L and H. On Series 2 and 3, however, scores on the tests in set C were consistently correlated with one another and with the tests included in H.
3. The tasks in set H elicited much stronger and more consistent preferences than those in set L. Set C was intermediate in this respect.

The data suggest that macaques, when first brought to the laboratory, have typically weak, somewhat inconsistent and task-specific hand preferences that do not correlate with later preferences on the same test with a high degree of accuracy. If the monkeys are given, as the present subjects were, much practice in manipulation in the test situation, they develop considerable skill and strong and consistent manual preferences in performing the highly practiced responses. The learned skills and preferences may be transferred to tasks that are sufficiently similar to permit response generalization to occur, as from set H to set C. Response generalization fails, of course, if the familiar and highly practiced tasks and the special tests require distinctly different motor responses; this may be the reason why tests in set L remain poorly correlated among themselves and with the tests in sets H and C.
This is the best guess as to the causes for the grouping of the tests in this sample. It can hardly be an accident that all the H tests require the monkey to push one kind of object or another aside to uncover a hidden piece of food, and this is the skill that the animals practiced almost every day between

handedness test series.

The findings of three other experiments that entailed repeated testing on handedness tasks strongly support the results of this experiment. In all three cases, the first hand-preference scores on different tests were in low-to-modest agreement with each other and were rather fallible predictors of retest performance on the same tasks. In all three studies, experience was observed to have a powerful effect on hand preferences. With increasing experience in the test situation, both intertest and reliability correlations increased, and the monkeys showed stronger average preferences on most tests.

However, the absolute values of the interest and reliability correlations obtained in the early phases of different experiments are almost ludicrously variable and inconsistent. This chaotic variation probably reflects the influence of differences in several contextual variables on a trait that is labile and apparently highly sensitive to environmental conditions--the handedness of naive monkeys.

It now seems far more likely that handedness in *M. mulatta* is primarily the result of experience, and not the expression of any organismic asymmetry. (See also Collins; Levy, this volume.)

The view that hand preferences in monkeys do not reflect any functional asymmetry between the cerebral hemispheres is supported by experiments showing that lesions in the association cortex ipsi- and contralateral to the preferred hand produce equivalent defects in cognitive tasks in rhesus monkeys. (See also Dewson; Hamilton, this volume.)


POSTSCRIPT

In the group discussion of the material presented in this chapter, conference participants raised several questions about handedness in nonhuman primates. Three questions are of sufficient interest and importance to consider here:

*1. Do manipulation tasks that require complementary asymmetrical use of both hands evoke stronger and more consistent hand preferences than unimanual tasks?* Beck and Barton (1972) have made a comprehensive study of the relation between manipulation task complexity and handedness in monkeys. They observed 10 stump-tail macaques on 7 unimanual and 10 bimanual tests that yielded 31 handedness scores, 14 for preliminary manipulation (M) and 17 for incentive-taking (I) responses. The bimanual tasks required from one to three manipulations to gain access to the food reward and demanded simultaneous or sequential use of both hands. Simultaneous coordination was necessary to hold open a spring-loaded drawer while extracting a raisin from it, and to hold a counterweighted food box in a position where food could be removed from it. Sequential tests did not force the monkeys to use both hands at the same time and are typified by tasks that

obliged the subject to undo a series of catches to open a box
containing food. The macaques had to be taught how to do several
of the more complicated tasks by shaping procedures; no handedness scores were recorded until the subjects acquired a substantial level of skill on these tasks.

Beck and Barton's findings on the strength of the preferences
elicited by one- and two-hand tests are summarized in Table 4.

TABLE 4

*Monkeys' Hand Preferences on Five Types of Motor Responses*[a]

| Tests | % of Monkeys with Significant Preferences | Mean % Preference |
|---|---|---|
| Unimanual (I) | 37 | 21 |
| Bimanual | | |
| Sequential | | |
|   M | 82 | 39 |
|   I | 75 | 32 |
| Simultaneous | | |
|   M | 90 | 40 |
|   I | 85 | 37 |

[a]Based on Beck and Barton (1972).

This table shows the percentage of monkeys with significant hand
preferences and average percentage of preference on the manipulation (M) and incentive (I) elements of the unimanual, and
simultaneous and sequential bimanual tests. Bimanual tasks elicited more significant and stronger preferences than unimanual
tests. The differences in performance between the simultaneous
and sequential tasks are not impressive.

Intertest correlations do not, however, reveal a comparable
disparity between unimanual and bimanual tests with respect to
the consistency of hand preferences. Ten of the 21 correlations
(48%) between unimanual tests were statistically significant,
but only 20 of 136 correlations (15%) between bimanual tests
were significant.

The data indicate that bimanual tasks involving more or less
elaborately coordinated activities of both hands produced preferences that are stronger but less consistent than those obtained
in unimanual tests. This pattern immediately suggests that the
preferences observed on two-hand tasks are highly specific. Two
bits of evidence compatible with this interpretation are found in
Beck and Barton's paper. More than half the significant correla-

tions between measures of bimanual performance were between performance scores on a single type of motor response, hasp-manipulation, included in several of the sequential bimanual tests. This indicates a high degree of specificity, with the monkeys displaying a consistent preference for one hand predominantly on variants of a single act.

The most likely way that bimanual tests could yield high preference scores and low intertest consistency would be for the monkeys to have a rather large number of significant preferences that did not agree with their overall preference. Beck and Barton show the following percentages for preferences on the manipulation components of their bimanual tasks: consistent with overall preference, 56%; inconsistent with overall preference, 31%; no preference, 13%. Comparison of these values with those presented in Figure 6 indicates that fairly complicated bimanual tasks do in fact elicit an unusually large number of significant but discordant preferences.

Beck and Barton's experiment thus affords little or no support for the notion that monkeys tested on elaborate motor sequences will display consistent hand preferences like those seen in humans (Annett, 1972). On the other hand, their finding that preferences on bimanual tasks are strong but largely uncorrelated with one another lends strong support to the argument that hand preferences in monkeys are probably much more strongly determined by experiential and environmental variables than by organismic factors.

2. *What is the relation between handedness and other functional asymmetries in monkeys?* Monkeys, like humans, exhibit lateral differences in several behavioral and physiological responses other than handedness. Both humans and monkeys have eye and foot preferences, but eye and foot preferences are not highly correlated with one another, nor with hand preferences in either macaques or humans (Cole, 1957; Hecaen & de Ajuriaguerra, 1964; Kruper, Boyle, & Patton, 1966). The potential usefulness of such measures for investigating cerebral dominance in nonhuman primates is questionable.

The approach of Stamm *et al.* (this volume), however, appears to hold much more promise. They succeeded in demonstrating cerebral dominance in monkeys when they showed that unilateral disruptive electrical stimulation only impaired delayed response performance when applied to the frontal cortex which showed the greater steady potential shift during the delay period. They also describe a marked preference for visual orientation in one direction, toward the side contralateral to the hemisphere showing the larger macropotentials (cf. Anderson; Glick *et al.*, Heilman and Watson, this volume).

Stamm *et al.* believe the dominance they find in monkeys is acquired, and unrelated to innate processes or hand preferences, because the hemisphere contralateral to the initially trained hand becomes dominant, independent of hand preference. It may be well

to reserve judgment on this point until the phenomenon has been
studied more extensively.  One would like answers to these questions:  What is the relation between visual orientation preference and larger macropotentials on the side contralateral to the
trained hand?  (See Anderson, this volume.)  Which asymmetry can
be detected first?  What is the time course of differentiation
between the activity of the hemispheres ipsi- and contralateral
to the trained hand?  (See Donchin, Kutas, & McCarthy, this
volume.)  Is more training required to produce differential activity if the trained hand is the monkey's nonpreferred rather than
its preferred hand?  (See Glick *et al.*, this volume.)  The last
question is meant to suggest that there may be a preexperimental
bias that can be overcome by training, but only with more training than in cases where the subject's initial bias does not coincide with the training regime (cf. Collins, this volume).

No matter what the outcome of developmental studies of the
dominance effect described by Stamm *et al.* may be, there is an
important problem concerning its usefulness as a potential model
for cerebral dominance in humans.  How specific or general is the
dominance induced in monkeys?  If, for example, the frontal cortex on one hemisphere is trained to become dominant for delayed
response in a primate chair, will it also be dominant for delayed response in the WGTA and for other delayed responselike
tasks, such as delayed alternation, in the primate chair?

It is difficult to restrain one's impulse to speculate about
additional profitable ways to follow up the provocative findings
of Stamm *et al.*  Perhaps it is now best simply to concur en-
thusiastically in their view that this may indeed be a profitable
area for further research.

3. *Is handedness more highly developed in the great apes than
in monkeys?*  The data regarding manual preferences in apes are
meager and contradictory.

## Chimpanzees

Chimpanzees have been described as ambidextrous (Gijzen, 1972;
Grzimek, 1949) and as having pronounced preferences that are inconsistent for different activities (Yerkes, 1943) or consistent
for different sorts of manipulations (Wrangham, personal communication).  Finch (1941) and Wrangham agree that the frequency of
right- and left-handed chimpanzees is approximately equal, as is
true of monkeys but not of people.

## Gorillas

The skulls of mountain gorillas (*Gorilla gorilla beringei*) are
often asymmetrical, the left side being more than 2% longer than
the right in about half the specimens examined by Groves and
Humphrey (1973).  The significance of this observation for cerebral dominance research is obscure.  Schaller (1963) reported

that all eight male mountain gorillas he observed began chest beating displays with the right hand more often than with the left, but he was quite unable to discern any preferential use of one hand rather than the other in the gorillas' feeding behavior. Of five mountain gorillas tested in the Antwerp zoo, two were left-handed and three ambidextrous in taking food and eating; all three lowland gorillas (*Gorilla gorilla gorilla*) were ambidextrous (Gijzen, 1972).

## Orangutans

Both Grzimek (1949) and Gijzen (1972) report that orangutans are ambidextrous.

The literature cannot possibly sustain any claim that handedness is more highly developed in pongids than in simians. It must be pointed out, however, that the published studies on great apes are generally quite inferior to the investigations with monkeys. Too few apes have been tested; the number of trials have been inadequate and the number of tasks insufficient. Neither has there been proper concern for retests to evaluate the stability of preferences. The only safe conclusion is that the question of handedness in apes should be carefully reexamined using the techniques developed for research monkeys. (See also Rubens, this volume.)

REFERENCES

Annett, M. The distribution of manual asymmetry. *British Journal of Psychology*, 1972, *63*, 343-358.

Beck, C. H. M., & Barton, R. L. Deviation and laterality of hand preference in monkeys. *Cortex*, 1972, *8*, 339-363.

Beck, C. H. M., Warren, J. M., & Sterner, R. Overtraining and reversal learning by cats and rhesus monkeys. *Journal of Comparative and Physiological Psychology*, 1966, *62*, 332-335.

Brookshire, K. H., & Warren, J. M. The generality and consistency of handedness in monkeys. *Animal Behaviour*, 1962, *10*, 222-227.

Cole, J. Laterality in the use of hand, foot and eye in monkeys. *Journal of Comparative and Physiological Psychology*, 1957, *50*, 296-299.

Cole, J., & Glees, P. Handedness in monkeys. *Experientia*, 1951, *8*, 224-225.

Coutant, L. W., & Warren, J. M. Reversal and nonreversal shifts by cats and rhesus monkeys. *Journal of Comparative and Physiological Psychology*, 1966, *61*, 484-487.

Ettlinger, G., & Gautrin, D. Visual discrimination performance in the monkey: The effect of unilateral removals of temporal cortex. *Cortex*, 1971, *7*, 317-331.

Finch, G. Chimpanzee handedness. *Science*, 1941, *94*, 117-118

Gijzen, A. Bonnes manières á table chez les anthropoïdes en

captivité. *Zoo* (Antwerp), 1972,  , No. 1.

Groves, C. P., & Humphrey, N. K. Asymmetry in gorilla skulls: Evidence of lateralized brain function? *Nature*, 1973, *244*, 53-54.

Grzimek, B. Rechts und Linkshandigkeit bei Pferden, Papageien und Affen. *Zeitschrift für Tierpsychologie*, 1949, *6*, 406-432.

Harlow, H. F. The formation of learning sets. *Psychological Reivew*, 1949, *66*, 51-76.

Hecaen, H., & de Ajuriaguerra, J. *Left-handedness*. New York: Grune & Stratton, 1964.

Jung, R. Summary of the conference. In V. B. Mountcastle (Ed.), *Interhemispheric relations and cerebral dominance*. Baltimore: Johns Hopkins Press, 1962.

Kruper, D. C., Boyle, B. E., & Patton, R. A. Eye and hand preference in rhesus monkeys (*Macaca mulatta*). *Psychonomic Science*, 1966, *5*, 277-278.

Schaller, G. B., *The mountain gorilla*. Chicago: Univ. of Chicago Press, 1963.

Warren, J. M. The development of paw preferences in cats and monkeys. *Journal of Genetic Psychology*, 1958, *93*, 229-236.

Warren, J. M. Reversal learning and the formation of learning sets by cats and rhesus monkeys. *Journal of Comparative and Physiological Psychology*, 1966, *61*, 421-428.

Warren, J. M., Abplanalp, J. M., & Warren, H. B. The development of handedness in cats and rhesus monkeys. In H. Stevenson, E. H. Hess, & H. Rheingold (Eds.), *Early behavior*. New York: Wiley, 1967.

Warren, J. M., Cornwell, P. R., & Warren, H. B. Unilateral frontal lesions and learning by rhesus monkeys. *Journal of Comparative and Physiological Psychology*, 1969, *69*, 498-505.

Warren, J. M., & Ebel, H. C. Generalization of responses to intermediate size by cats and monkeys. *Psychonomic Science*, 1967, *9*, 5-6.

Warren, J. M., & Nonneman, A. J. The search for cerebral dominance in rhesus monkeys. In *Origins and evolution of language and speech*. *Annals of the New York Academy of Sciences*, 1976, in press.

Yerkes, R. M. *Chimpanzees*. New Haven, Connecticut: Yale Univ. Press, 1943.

# 11.
# Embryology and Inheritance of Asymmetry

*MICHAEL MORGAN*

University of Cambridge

Although the term *inherited* is often used by nonbiologists synonymously with *genetically inherited*, there are ways other than the Mendelian by which organisms can transmit information to their offspring. We inherit not only genes but also a cell with a highly complex spatial structure, the oocyte; there is evidence that the spatial information carried in this cell is vital in determining the form of the developing embryo. The argument in this chapter will be that the inheritance of asymmetries is very probably oocytic, and that brain asymmetries, instead of being considered in isolation, should be viewed as a special case of a much more fundamental asymmetry in the body plan of vertebrates. I will present evidence that there is a general factor operative in vertebrates, as well as in their ancestors, favoring more rapid development of the left side of the embryo. That is the constructive part of the argument. The destructive part will be evidence that genes themselves may well be *left-right agnosic*: able to produce asymmetries, but unable to code for the direction of those asymmetries (Dahlberg, 1943; see also Collins; Levy, this volume).

## OOCYTIC ASYMMETRY

The problem of the coding of left-right differences is conveniently discussed in terms of Wolpert's (1969) concept of *positional information*. Wolpert argues that each cell must have, in addition to strictly genetic information, some information that

tells it where it is situated in relation to key reference
points.  A much-discussed example is that of the vertebrate limb
(MacCabe, Saunders, & Pickett, 1973; Stark & Searls, 1973;
Wolpert, 1969; Zwilling, 1961).  In models of limb development it
has proved unnecessary to provide the limb with left-right positional information.  Once the anteroposterior and dorsoventral
axes have been specified, it is entirely determinate that a limb
bud on the left side of the animal shall develop as a mirror
image of the limb on the right.  But matters are quite otherwise
when the structures on the two sides of the body are not mirror
images.  What is the positional information that makes presumptive heart tissue on the left side develop in a way that has no
counterpart on the right?  The evidence of experimental embryology is that this information inheres in the spatial structure
of the embryo at a very early stage.

Spemann and Falkenberg (1919) tied a child's hair around a
developing newt embryo in the plane corresponding to the midsaggital (left-right) plane of the adult.  This constriction prevented normal development and produced Siamese twins joined by
their medial surfaces.  Thus two almost-separate individuals developed from the sides of the embryo that would normally have
grown into the left and right halves of a single individual.  The
result was that the twin developing from the presumptive left
side of the embryo usually had normal *situs* of the heart and
other internal organs, but the right-side twin was often disturbed in its development.  Sometimes it had normal *situs*, sometimes it was neither one thing nor the other, and sometimes it
showed mirror imaging (*situs inversus viscerum et cordis*) like
the executed criminal referred to by Molière.  Spemann was also
successful in inducing *situs inversus* by removing a piece of the
medullary place and reimplanting it after a $180^0$ rotation.

From these experiments, Spemann concluded that left-right differences must exist in the embryo at a very early stage, probably
before the oocyte is even fertilized.  As Spemann and Falkenberg
(1919) put it:

> By whatever meridian the sperm enters the egg, the
> cytoplasm must always be different on the left and right
> sides of entry.  If it were otherwise, given the well-
> known undifferentiation of the spermatazoon, it would be
> impossible to provide an explanation of the different de-
> velopment of the left and right sides following fertili-
> zation.  This implies that the cytoplasm of the egg
> possesses a bilaterally asymmetrical structure around
> the ovular axis, to which one can attribute the overt
> bilaterally asymmetrical development [p. 398].

This statement goes beyond the facts, but more recent research
has confirmed Spemann's speculation that lateral asymmetry is
established before the genetic material of the embryo has had an
opportunity to determine the direction.  A clear case is the

spiral cleavage of worms and molluscs (Nemertea, Annelida, and Mollusca). In these animals there is an asymmetry visible as early as the second cell division of the embryo. Instead of occurring at right angles, successive cleavages occur obliquely, with a regular alternation between clockwise and counterclockwise rotation. The cleavage pattern is determined in at least one case (*Limnaea peragra*) not by the embryo's own genotype but by the mother's (Sturtevant, 1923); therefore the asymmetry of the future embryo seems to be laid down during oogenesis. Raven (1967) has suggested that blueprint positional information is transmitted to the egg cortex by way of the follicle, which surrounds the developing oocyte with an asymmetric circle of follicle cells. A possible sign of the blueprint is the asymmetric arrangement of six subcortical accumulations (SCAs) around the equator of the oocyte. However, it has not yet been possible to demonstrate a correlation between the follicular arrangement and the SCA pattern (Ubbels, Bezem, & Raven, 1969). See also Raven (1974) and the important experiments of Guerrier (1970).

The asymmetries in cleavage pattern arise before the organism's own genes become active. Evidence for this will be found in Davidson (1968) and Gurdon (1969). According to Gurdon, "from the end of oogenesis until the midblastula stage (some 10 divisions after fertilization) nuclear RNA synthesis is very largely if not entirely deficient." Actinomycin, which prevents RNA synthesis, does not affect the morphological development until the stage of tissue differentiation. Spiral cleavage of the snail *Ilyanassa* is unaffected by actinomycin (Davidson, 1968, p. 29). Since this cleavage is chiral and species-specific in direction, we can conclude that here is a clear case in which the determination of asymmetry is oocytic. Rather than genes being the determiners of the asymmetry, there is in fact evidence that the expression of the genetic material itself can be affected by the preexisting asymmetry; thus Donohoo and Kafatos (1973) have reported differences in the proteins synthesized by cell lines originating from the first two blastomeres of *Ilyanassa*.

It is clear, then, that the just-fertilized ovum is not an undifferentiated bowl of broth in which the genes multiply like so many viruses. There is a complex structure laid down beforehand. We turn now to the question of how prototype asymmetries can be translated into the complex morphological asymmetries of the adult. A possible mechanism is a different growth rate between the two sides of the body. If this sort of mechanism exists, we can expect to find correlations between asymmetries of different organs of the body. Evidence for this will now be assessed in relation to the heart and brain of vertebrates.

EMBRYOLOGY OF THE HEART

There are many asymmetries in the fully developed chordate

heart. The first sign of asymmetry in development is this: The tube that will give rise to the heart is given a bend by more rapid development on the left side (Lepori, 1969). Thus the very early heart looks like a letter *C*, with the ventricle and developing aortic arches at the top, and the future atrium at the bottom. The process of curvature becomes more complex so that the ventricle is bent into a complete loop lying to the left of the atrium and posterior to it. In birds and mammals the ventricle becomes divided; it is the left half that takes on the task of pumping oxygenated blood to the body; the right chamber pumps blood to the lungs. There are extensive asymmetries in the development of the aortic arches. In mammals the right fourth arch breaks down and it is the left that persists as the aorta; in birds, however, it is the left arch that breaks down. There are also asymmetries in the venous system: In the heart of cyclostomes, for example, only one ductus Cuvieri is preserved, on the right in lampreys and the left in Myxinoids (Robb, 1965).

Obviously, the statement "the heart lies on the left" is a gross oversimplification. In sharks the heart is outwardly almost symmetrical; in the frog it does not noticably deviate from the midline. However, since the C-asymmetry appears so early in development, it is suggestive of being a fundamental feature. Further evidence exists for more advanced development on the left side. In Urodeles left rudiments develop pulsations but right ones do not; in Amblyostoma left rudiments more frequently develop into functional hearts (see Copenhaver, 1955, for a re view). In birds, the heart developed from a left rudiment is larger than that from the right in 96% of cases (Lepori, 1969). Rawles and Willier (1934) report the results of attempting to grow pieces of bird blastoderm on chorioallantoic membrane: "Of the lateral pieces, grafts were obtained from the left side more frequently, and showed better growth." This applied not only to heart, but to thyroid, liver, ear, eye, and "brain parts." Could the factor determining asymmetry of the heart be part of a more general asymmetry extending even to the nervous system? What we want here is evidence for correlation between *situs* of the brain and other internal organs. For this purpose, we now turn to studies of the asymmetries in the habenular ganglion. The following is in part a paraphrase of Braitenberg and Kemali (1970) and of Morgan, O'Donnell, and Oliver (1973).

ASYMMETRY IN THE HABENULAR GANGLION

The habenular nuclei in the brains of vertebrates are found in the dorsal anterior diencephalon, under the epiphysis, on either side of the third ventricle. It has been known since 1899 that there is a striking asymmetry in the habenulae of frogs. The left habenula is longer than the right one and consists of two nuclei, the lateral and the medial; the habenula on the right consists of a single nucleus only (Figure 1). In

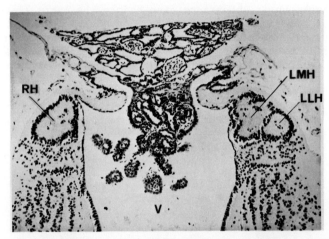

*Fig. 1. From a Nissl preparation, frontal section, of the habenula region of an adult frog (Rana temporaria). In this, as in all subsequent figures, the specimen is being viewed from the front (anteriorly) so that the left side of the animal appears on the right side of the figure. The left habenula consists of two distinct nuclei: the left medial habenual (LMH) and the left lateral habenula (LLH). The right habenula (RH) consists of a single nucleus. The nuclei border on the III ventricle (V).*

newts the asymmetry is not quite so obvious, but the left nucleus has a thin lateral extension that is missing on the right; in the eel (*Anguilla*) the left nucleus is partially divided by a vertical septum protruding into the central core from the shell (Braitenberg & Kemali, 1970). Previous reports of asymmetry are also reviewed by Braitenberg & Kemali. The asymmetry does not always favor the left-hand side; a larger right nucleus has been reported in the fish *Cyclothone acclinidens* and in the slime eel *Myxine glutinosa*. In the lamprey (*Petromyzon*) the right habenulopenduncular tract is predominant.

It is possible that the habenular asymmetry is connected to a more general asymmetry in the roof of the diencephalon. One view on the dorsal evaginations of the roof holds that there were originally two lateral eyes and that these rotated during evolution to occupy a medial position, forming respectively the pineal (epiphysis cerebri) and parapineal (parietal) organs. In different vertebrates one or the other of these two organs comes to predominate, except that in some instances (e.g., *Rana temporaria*) the rudiments of the two organs fuse. This whole matter of pineal and parapineal asymmetry is somewhat complicated and controversial (Holmgren, 1965; Oksche, 1965; Sivak,

1974).

An investigation of the development of the habenula (Morgan
*et al.*, 1973) has shown that there are several asymmetries, some
of which make their appearance even before the extra (lateral)
nucleus is visible on the left side. An unexplained fact, one
suggestive of chemical communication, is that there is an incom-
pleteness in part of the medial wall of the left habenula, so
that it is separated from the third ventricle by only a single
layer of epithelial cells (Figure 2). Another asymmetry consists

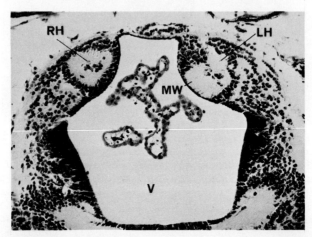

*Fig. 2. Anterior region of the habenula in a frog tadpole with
developed hindlimbs, but no forelimbs. There is only a single
nucleus on the left, but it differs from the one on the right by
having a thinner medial wall (MW). From a Nissl preparation,
frontal section.*

in the presence of a tongue or partial septum of cells invading
the lumen of the left lateral nucleus (Figure 3). Also, as
Braitenberg and Kemali (1970) noted, there are more free cells
lying in the lumen of the right nucleus than in the lumen of
the left.

The asymmetry in the frog may be contrasted with the case of
*Xenopus laevis*, in which the habenula is multilobulate and shows
no obvious morphological asymmetry (Figure 4).

Von Woellwarth (1950) has investigated *situs* of the habenula
in newts with both naturally occurring and experimentally induced
*situs inversus viscerum et cordis*. His finding is that there is
a perfect correlation: When the internal organs are mirror
images, so is the habenula. "Although the (habenular) nuclei are
far removed from the surgical intervention and other asymmetric
organs, and separated from them by undisturbed organs, they were
inverted along with the other asymmetric organs, and behave like

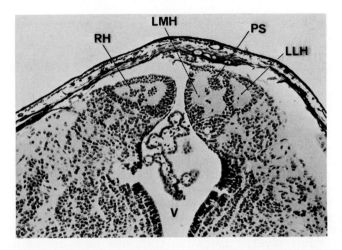

Fig. 3. From a Nissl preparation, frontal section, of the habenula region in a frog (Rana temporaria) several weeks after metamorphosis. A second nucleus has made its appearance on the left-hand side. The right habenula (RH) still consists of a single nucleus. A partial septum (PS) of cells is seen on the dorsal wall of the left medial habenula nucleus (LMH).

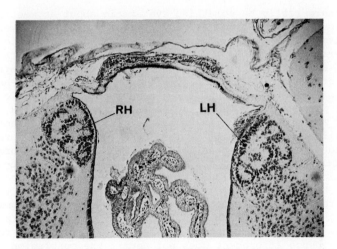

Fig. 4. From a Nissl preparation, frontal section, of the habenula region in an adult zenopus laevis (South African toad). The habenula structure is more complex than that of the frog, and there is no obvious asymmetry. Abbreviations: LH, left habenula; RH, right habenula.

the liver and the heart; this was so in all investigations and in all developmental stages [p. 255]." Was this because of some direct effect of the heart upon the habenula by the blood supply? Carmon and Gambos (1970) have shown that there is an asymmetrical blood flow through the ophthalmic arteries in man; conceivably some such asymmetry could determine unequal development of the two halves of the brain. This possibility, as far as the habenula is concerned, was decisively eliminated by von Woellwarth (1969) in an experiment showing that habenular asymmetry developed in the absence of a heart. Isolates from the head region of neurulae of *Triturus alpestris*, consisting of cephalic ectoderm and mesoderm and sometimes also endoderm, could, under favorable conditions, develop brains with habenular nuclei. These showed the normal asymmetry in spite of the absence of the blood supply and of other organs. The conclusion of von Woellwarth is that habenular asymmetries and those of other asymmetrical organs develop under the influence of a common cause, which he terms the *allgemeinen asymmetriebestimmenden Faktor des Keimes* ("the general asymmetry-determining factor of the embryo"). This supports the claim by Rawles and Willier (1934) that there is a general factor determining more rapid and complete development on the left side.

## OTHER ASYMMETRIES FAVORING THE LEFT SIDE

Can there really be something systematic about asymmetries of bodily form? It would not be too surprising, given the very fundamental and systematic asymmetry of the underlying biochemical material (Monod, 1969). A clear causal chain links the asymmetry of amino acids to the asymmetry of secondary and tertiary protein structure. For example, the energy of the right-handed $\alpha$-helix of poly-L-alanine is a few tenths of a kilocalorie per mole per residue lower than that of the left-handed helix, implying that as soon as they get to any length, the right-handed chains will be more stable. Poly-$\beta$-benzyl-L-aspartate forms left-handed helices, whereas poly-$\gamma$-benzyl-L-glutamate forms right-handed helices. This result also agrees with least-energy calculations (Scheraga, 1969). So, as soon as the sequence of building blocks in a large molecule has been determined, the higher order spatial structure follows, including the asymmetry (Liquori, 1969). The next step in the chain might well take one up to the level of macroscopic asymmetry (cf. Levy, this volume).

The evidence at present does not permit the conclusion that all consistent macroscopic asymmetries in vertebrates favor the left side. Nevertheless, there are extremely interesting indications that such a principle may have wide validity. Examples are as follows:

1. The starfish and other echinoderms, because of the

chordate features of their larvae, are often considered to have some distant relationship to the ancestors of the vertebrates. It may therefore be noteworthy that they show a very fundamental asymmetry favoring the left. The hydrocoel (body cavity) appears originally as pouches on the left and right of the gut, but the right pouch regresses, so that the whole adult hydrocoel arises from the left (Child, 1941; Horstadius, 1973).

2. The asymmetries of heart and habenula have already been discussed; see also the observations of Rawles and Willier (1934) on asymmetries in the rate of development of left and right (cf. Taylor, 1969).

3. In constricted newt embryos there are more cases of *situs inversus* in the "right" twin than in the "left" twin, according to Spemann and Falkenberg (1919). Spemann accounted for this by postulating a gradient favoring more rapid development of the left side of the embryo. It was further assumed that in the region of the cut or constriction there was a lack of material (*Materialmangel*) that retarded development of the medial surfaces of both twins. In the left twin the normal developmental gradient and the *Materialmangel* would reinforce one another, leading to normal *situs;* in the right twin they would be in competition, and would lead to less determinate results. A major piece of evidence in favor of this theory was the observation that univitteline twins were less well developed on their (medial) joined surfaces.

4. In the human brain there is anatomical asymmetry favoring the left over the right temporal cortex (Geschwind & Levitsky, 1968; Rubens, this volume). The difference is present at birth, with possible sex differences (Witelson & Pallie, 1973).

5. Song in canaries is dependent on the left-hypoglossal nerve (Nottebohm, this volume). Lesions on the left in the adult prevent singing but those on the right do not.

6. In the mountain gorilla the left side of the skull is larger than the right (Groves & Humphrey, 1973), as it is in man (Halperin, 1931). Other asymmetries in the axial skeleton are reviewed by Latimer and Lowrance (1965) and by Halperin (1931). In man the bones of the upper half tend to be more developed on the *right*, but this is plausibly a result of right-handedness, which depends of course on *left*-hemisphere control. In the lower skeleton, where handedness would be expected to exert a smaller influence, and particularly in the femur, it is the left side that shows superior development.

7. In chickens the transverse process of the cervical vertebrae is longer on the left than on the right (Kawahara, 1974).

8. In birds the right ovary is smaller than the left. If the left ovary is removed, the right one increases in size, suggesting that the left ovary normally exerts an inhibitory effect (Young, 1950; cf. Mittwoch and Kirk, 1975; see also the work of Wilson, Przibram, Zeleny, Abeloos in Goss, 1969).

It needs only a few counterexamples to spoil this general
picture. Therefore, the larger *right* ovary in certain elasmo-
branchs (Romer, 1962) and the presence of the heart on the right
in the colonial protochordate *Botryllus schlosseri* (Sabbadin,
Zaniolo, & Majone, 1975) must be taken seriously. Functional
superiority of the right hemisphere for certain tasks in man (see
Milner, 1971 for a review) is also problematic, but since there
is no anatomical basis established for the latter asymmetry, it
can be argued (Corballis & Morgan, 1976) that it is secondary to
a developmental gradient favoring language development in the
left hemisphere. Other asymmetries, such as the migration of the
eye and the crossing of the optic nerves in flatfish, go in different directions in different species, and thus cannot be interpreted on the basis of a model claiming absolute cross-species
dominance of the left side (Parker, 1903; Hubbs & Hubbs, 1944).
The evidence, however, is sufficient to put the celebrated left-
hemisphere speech dominance into a wider biological context.
This asymmetry may be part of a much wider one, starting with the
spatial asymmetry of the oocyte, and possibly stretching down to
the microstructural and molecular level.

I turn now to the destructive part of this chapter: the argument that there is no known case in which the direction of an
asymmetry is determined in an individual by its own genetic
material. If this is true it seriously questions the usefulness
of applying complex Mendelian models to the inheritance of human
laterality.


SOME NON-MENDELIAN DETERMINANTS OF ASYMMETRY

The evidence that the spiral asymmetries of worms and molluscs
are not under control of the individual's genes has been discussed in the preceding sections. Two additional clear examples
of nongenetic determination of asymmetry may be given: (1) Duckweeds retain consistent configuration of their variety of "handedness" during vegatative propagation, but there is a random mixture of dextrals and sinistrals in the first sexual generation,
regardless of the parents' configuration (Kasinov, 1969). (2) In
*Botryllus schlosseri*, the asymmetry of an individual zooid is
that of the colony in which it grows, not the asymmetry of the
colony from which it is removed as a palleal bud (Sabbadin
*et al.*, 1975).

Dahlberg (1943) pointed out that a gene could determine an
asymmetry without determining the *direction* of that asymmetry, in
that it might promote unequal distribution of cytoplasmic material without deciding the orientation of the distribution in a
specified relation to particular morphological axes. In other
words, just because an asymmetry occurs for genetic reasons, it
does not follow that the *positional information* is provided by the
gene. The positional information may be provided by the oocytic

inheritance, or it may be absent entirely, in which case the direction of the asymmetry will be random.

Consider the inheritance of the asymmetric spotting pattern in the beetle *Bruchus quadrimaculatus*, for example (Stern, 1955, p. 163). The normal females possess two black spots bilaterally located on each wing case but in a recessive mutant strain the females have two red spots on one side and two black on the other; individuals with red spots on the right occur with the same frequency as those with red on the left, irrespective of the condition of their ancestors. Thus the gene programs an asymmetry, but its direction is a matter of chance, presumably because the distribution of cytoplasmic factors underlying the unequal expression of the gene is randomly determined.

In other cases, the cytoplasmic asymmetry through which the gene is expressed may be a consistent one, and there will be an illusion that the gene provides positional information. In *Drosophila melanogaster* there is a mutant form that has a chiral penis, with a counterclockwise rotation, to a varying degree. This apparent asymmetry is actually the partial *absence* of a still greater asymmetry seen in the normal male. In the normal nonmutant male the external genitalia are rotated clockwise through 360° during development, as may be seen from the spiral counterclockwise looping of the sperm duct around the intestine. In the mutant the rotation is only partially accomplished (Bridges, cited by Stern, 1955). This shows just how careful one must be before concluding that a gene embodies positional information for left and right.

When a gene gives rise to a developmental anomaly its expression on two sides of the body may be unequal because of a preexisting asymmetry. This, as we saw, is the case with the wing markings in *Bruchus*; it may also be involved in unilateral anomalies in man. Walker (1950) described discordant unilateral anomalies in a pair of monozygotic twins; one twin had a retinoblastoma in the left eye, the other had a normal left eye and cleft palate. The elder of two sisters described by Cotterman and Falls (1949) had a left-sided deformity of ear, nose, and mouth; the sister had a right-sided pectoralis defect. It is clear that if these abnormalities have any genetic base at all, the expression of the gene on the two sides depends upon some further factor. In other instances the nongenetic determining factors may have some systematic relationship to preexisting asymmetry. For example, when harelip and cleft palate occur unilaterally in man, they are more frequently expressed on the left-hand side; conversely, hemifacial microsomia is more common on the right (Schnall & Smith, 1974). The direction of the asymmetry appears to be species-specific, in that cleft lip is overwhelmingly *right*-sided in the rat (further instances of species-specific asymmetries are described by Schnall and Smith). These facts argue that genes can have *variable penetrance* on the two sides of the body (Stern, 1955), just as they can have very different effects in different invididuals (e.g., Bingle, Dillon and Hurwitz, 1975).


SITUS INVERSUS

Consider next *situs inversus*. This condition is extremely rare. In newts, a series of investigations reviewed by von Woellwarth (1950) gives the frequency as varying between .67 and 2.1%. The condition is equally rare in frogs, although Schwind (1934) described a batch of *Rana sylvatica* eggs in which there were 27 Siamese twins, many members of which had *situs inversus*. In man, Gunther found a frequency of .104% in 150,000 cases (cited by von Woellwarth). Torgersen (1950), in a mass x-ray study of Norwegians, found 200 cases among 1,800,000 individuals above 15 years of age, and an additional 70 cases in hospitals. Certain inbred strains of mice and fish have been described having a much higher than usual frequency (see Campbell, 1963). There is also evidence for a familial concordance in man, although, as we shall presently see, the facts do not support any particular genetic model.

*Situs inversus* does not always involve all the asymmetric organs. In dextrocardia (see Oram, 1971) the apex of the heart is displaced to the right instead of to the left. This may occur either with mirror-imaging of the left and right chambers (mirror-image dextrocardia) or without (complete dextrocardia). Mirror-image dextrocardia may occur with reversal of the other internal organs (*situs inversus totalis*) or it may occur by itself (isolated dextrocardia). A very suggestive fact is that *situs inversus totalis* is considerably more common than isolated dextrocardia (Oram, 1971, p. 571). This is reminiscent of von Woellwarth's correlation between heart and habenula, and it speaks against the existence of an isolated genetic factor determining *situs* of the heart. Furthermore, Campbell (1963) found no cardiac malformations in 14 families, in each of which one member had isolated dextrocardia. This seems more compatible with an environmental-traumatic interpretation than with a genetic model. However, Campbell's data contrast somewhat with Soltani and Li's (1974) description of a kindred with four males affected by dextrocardia. Possibly some kinds of dextrocardia are more familial than others. In any event, the data of Soltani and Li, interesting though they are, are too sparse to justify what they call the "obvious interpretation . . . that an X-linked gene is segregating and is the basis of the serious cardiac defects in the 4 affected males [p. 57]." The data would be just as compatible with intrauterine traumatism or disease, for which evidence is reviewed by Lichtman (1931).

An interesting condition with an apparently high degree of familial association is that of asymmetric septal hypertrophy (ASH) as found in idiopathic hypertrophic subaortic stenosis.

The septum between the ventricles enlarges, more so on the left than on the right, thereby sometimes blocking outflow from the left ventricle and causing heart failure. Clark, Henry, and Epstein (1973) examined the families of 26 patients and found ASH in 48% of parents, 55% of sibs, and 30% of children. The lower incidence in children is very puzzling from a genetic point of view, but may be a result of difficulties in diagnosis of the young. The familial association was confirmed by Bingle, Dillon, and Hurwitz (1975), who point out, however, that the degree of expression of the trait is very variable. This may be a genuine case of a genetic factor affecting an asymmetry. But as I have pointed out several times, this does not mean that the gene encodes the asymmetry, or provides positional information. The part of the heart affected by ASH is highly asymmetrical in normal circumstances; the gene is merely interacting with this asymmetry.

Let us now return to *situs inversus totalis*. The familial data are clearly inconsistent with a strict Mendelian interpretation. To start with, the condition has been described discordantly in monozygotic (MZ) twins, and despite the objections of Nagylaki and Levy (1973) to overenthusiastic interpretation of MZ data, this point is bound to carry some weight. Torgersen (1950) observes that in the case history literature, *situs inversus* has been observed in 12 pairs of probable MZ twins, six times concordantly and six times discordantly. In the pair described by Cockayne, one twin showed complete transposition of the viscera and was right-handed, the other twin was normal except for left-handedness. The data for sibs are also difficult to interpret genetically, as Torgersen (1950) notes: "The number of sibs is known in 229 unselected families, the ratio of affected (*situs inversus*) sibs to normal sibs being 11 : 1, index cases being, of course, excluded. In 221 families, the index case was found to be the only individual affected. Three sibs were affected in 3 sibships, 2 in 5 sibships; in all 36 normal sibs were present in these 8 sibships. These data do not agree with the supposition of a single recessive gene. In fact, they can hardly be considered as proof of an influence of the genes at all, environmental factors not being excluded [p. 365]."

Spemann and Falkenberg's method of producing *situs inversus* by dividing the embryo suggests that one of the ways in which it could result naturally is by twin-formation, with the two twins originating from the left and right halves of the embryo. However, the work of Lepori (1969) on the development of birds, which mammals resemble in development more than they do the amphibia, suggests that MZ twin formation is not a way to produce *situs inversus*. In line with this, Torgersen (1950) exploded the myth that there is an association between *situs inversus* and MZ twinning in man: In his sample, neither twinning nor left-handedness was observed with greater frequencies than those expected on the basis of chance association. He concludes that the "mirror-image mechanism, as revealed in experimentally produced amphibian twins, is of relatively little importance in human polyembryony [p. 369]."

The factors causing *situs inversus* are thus unknown; they are not straightforwardly genetic, because of the MZ twin data, and they are not a result of polyembryony per se. The simplest view seems to be that they are associated with disturbances in oogenesis, leading to an abnormally structured oocyte. This would explain why the parents of individuals with *situs inversus*, according to Torgersen (1950, p. 365) frequently show other anomalies, such as bronchiectasis, nasal polyps, and heart defects, and why there is a higher incidence of inbreeding. These defects, possibly genetic, may be part of a syndrome of which abnormal oogenesis is a further expression. Note that this does *not* implicate the genes responsible for the anomalies in programming the direction of an asymmetry in the oocyte; they may merely alter it in a random way. The fact that parents of children with *situs inversus* are quite capable of producing normal children as well argues against a determinate form of maternal inheritance such as that found in *Limnaea*.

## HAIR-WHORL DIRECTIONALITY

It is sometimes claimed that the direction of hair whorling is genetically determined--e.g., by Rife (1933), who said that a single-factor Mendelian determination of hair-whorling had been demonstrated by Bernstein (1925) in a moderately inaccessible paper. Reference to the paper itself, instead of to Rife's over-enthusiastic interpretation, might shake the confidence of those who have since quoted Bernstein's speculations as if they were solid fact. The paper begins in the following vein: "Die Bedeutung mendelnder Merkmale für die menschliche Rassenforschung besteht darin dass as durch die statistische Auszählung derselben möglich erscheint, die Rassengemische, welche wir allenthalben antreffen, in ihre ursprünglichen Bestandteile zu zerlegen." Loosely translated, this means that genetics is a useful way of sorting out the results of miscegenation--for purposes Bernstein does not state. Previous investigations, Berstein continues, have shown that there is a "Bass-Soprano" Mendelian factor that characterizes the dolicocephalic, fair, blue-eyed Nordic race. Now along comes hair-whorling to delineate this race still further. Apparently, clockwise whorling is dominant over counter-clockwise; this is shown by a study of a group of 41 families that includes two families in which both parents are clockwise. In one of these there were three counterclockwise offspring. The geographical facts show that the dominant gene is characteristic of the Nordic race along with the Bass-Soprano feature. (The same issue of the journal contains two papers by Albert Einstein on the behavior of ideal gases.)

In the cases of asymmetry reviewed so far, there is not one that on close examination supports the hypothesis that the genes of an individual can encode the *direction* of its own asymmetry. A genetic factor may be expressed unequally on the two sides because of a preexisting asymmetry (harelip, cleft palate), it may reduce an existing asymmetry (rotated penis in *Drosophila*), it may introduce an asymmetry that is inconsistent in direction (*Bruchus*), it may affect oogenesis and determine the asymmetry in the following generation (*Limnaea*), or it may be entirely imaginary (hair-whorling), but there seems to be no simple case in which a Mendelian factor determines the direction of asymmetry in its carrier. This leads us to question the idea that human handedness is genetically determined.

## HANDEDNESS

That human left-handedness is *familial* is beyond dispute (Zangwill, 1960). To take just one fact illustrating this, Rife (1940) observed a high frequency of left-handedness among relatives of twins showing interpair differences in handedness, in contrast to a low frequency of left-handed relatives of twins where both were right-handed. But is the condition genetic? Simple models that have tried to make left-handedness a single recessive gene always founder on the fact that two left-handers do not invariably produce left-handed offspring; in fact they produce right-handers slightly more frequently than left-handers. Invariably, then, genetic models have had to resort to additional determinants of handedness to supplement the hypothetical genetic determinant. One possibility is that the gene has a "variable penetrance," so that it is manifested in under half the individuals who are homozygous for the gene. The variable penetrance is presumably due to other factors, genetic or nongenetic, which determine whether or not the gene in question will produce left- or right-handedness. The trouble is that once these factors have been postulated, the gene itself becomes superrogatory. *A Mendelian factor is one that can be shown to segregate in the offspring by known Mendelian rules:* If it is anything else it is merely an unwanted sacrificial offering to the altar of exact science. There is no distribution of offspring that cannot be made to conform to a Mendelian model by a judicious mixture of imaginary gene frequencies, and degree of variable expression. Therefore such models are academic exercises until such time as the mechanisms of genetic determination and the mechanisms of variable penetrance can be specified or at least guessed at. The present disputes about the genetics of handedness remind one of nothing so much as the internecine disputes among "learning theorists," with the gene taking the role of the S-R bond as a talismanic substitute for physiological reality. It is no use collecting more and more breeding data and subjecting it to more and more elaborate statistical analyses: There is no substitute for opening the system up. And I have tried to argue here that what little we know about the determination of asymmetries in general speaks against a specifically Mendelian mode of inheritance. Why should handedness be such a special case?

One particular model for the inheritance of handedness is worth considering in some detail, because it may be half-right. Annett (1972) has proposed that there may be a gene for right-handedness but not for left-handedness. The theory is that in the absence of the right-handedness gene, laterality is determined by purely random considerations, as seems to be the case in mice (Collins, this volume). Right-handers in the population are a mixture of those having the right-handed gene, and those lacking it but pushed in the direction of right-handedness by random variation. No left-handers (L) have the gene; neither therefore do the offspring of L x L pairings. Annett (1972) succinctly summarizes the model as follows: "The suggestion that a genetic factor may be involved in the shift towards dextrality but not in the origin of the basic bell-shaped distribution which underlies all [sic] lateral asymmetry has the paradoxical implication that right-handedness may be inherited while left-handedness is not. Left-handedness can be thought of as the result of accidental factors which endow the left limb with greater skill, together with a weak dose of the factors which induce most humans towards dextrality. Right-handedness can be thought of as a result of accidental factors giving greater skill to the right limb or to a combination of relative bilateral symmetry and the presence of a factor inducing laterality [p. 355]."

The model can more or less account for the familial data, as would be expected from the fact that it posits two variables, the bell-shaped curve and the frequency of the putative gene in the population. The slight bias toward dextrals in the offspring of L x L marriages is explained by the intrusion of a third variable, having a cultural basis.

The hypothesis of a right-handed gene is certainly not refuted by Annett's data. To say that there is a "factor" that induces right-handedness in the majority of people is undoubtedly correct. But the data do not show that it is a *genetic* factor; it is much more likely that it is a nongenetic factor, as in the case of the heart. The assumption that a gene could determine the direction of human handedness conflicts with the accumulated evidence to date indicating that no such genes exist. Conversely, to deny, as Annett does, a genetic contribution to left-handedness seems strange when examples are known of genes that can work against the background of a preexisting asymmetry (cleft palate, *situs inversus*, rotated penis).

One possible resolution of the problem is that Annett is right in spirit, but has the details backwards. It may very well be that there is a genetic contribution to one kind of handedness but not to the other. The other known cases of genetic asymmetries fit such a picture. But if one had to choose on the basis of existing data, surely it would be more rational to conjecture that it is the majority condition that is nongenetically and oocytically determined (like heart and habenula), whereas the *departure* from the normal condition could in part have a genetic cause, which interferes with normal development. There might, indeed, be a whole constellation of genes that interfere with normal development of laterality, such as those that according to Torgersen contribute to *situs inversus*. These genes could act either during oogenesis or during early development; the importance of oogenesis (as in snails) is indicated by the lower incidence of right-handers in L x R crosses when it is the mother who is the left-hander (Annett, 1972, Table 3).

It must be obvious from considerations of logical symmetry that this hypothesis could do no worse than Annett's in describing the data. This just shows the limitations of arguing from family trees. A decision between alternative models has to be made on the basis of the plausibility of their claims about the mechanics of inheritance in the light of general evidence. My conclusion is that there is not likely to be a genetic determination of the direction of human handedness, because genes do not appear to act in this way, and because in other cases of asymmetry nongenetic factors have been convincingly demonstrated. There is evidence, however, that genetic factors may interact with a previously established asymmetry, and it is in that direction we should look for an explanation of left-handedness.

I finish with the conventional remark that the ultimate nature of the asymmetry determining *situs* of the heart, cerebrum, and habenula, be it microstructural, macroscopic, or macromolecular, is absolutely unknown (cf. Chapple; Glick, Jerussi, & Zimmerberg; Rubens, this volume). Like most people who have thought about the topic, I hope that it will turn out to be molecular, and related to the fundamental asymmetry in our body chemistry (and from thence, perhaps, to failures of parity conservation in the subatomic domain). It was almost exactly 100 years before the time of writing that the tetrahedral structure of the carbon atom was discovered by van't Hoff and Le Bell; the next few years would be a very good time to take the next logical step in explaining our asymmetric bodies.

## ACKNOWLEDGMENTS

I should like to dedicate this work to Professor O. L. Zangwill, who first stimulated my interest in the problems of cerebral asymmetry, and who made many useful comments on earlier drafts of this chapter. Robert Collins, Michael Corballis, Marcel Kinsbourne, and Lyn Beezley drew my attention to much useful material. Carl von Woellwarth introduced me to the classical embryological literature. Responsibility for the more obviously speculative parts of this chapter rests with me. The histological specimens were painstakingly prepared by Mr. Jarvis, of the Institute of Animal Physiology, Babraham, Cambridgeshire.

REFERENCES

Annett, M. The distribution of manual asymmetry. *British Journal of Psychology*, 1972, *63*, 343-358.

Bernstein, F. Beiträge zur mendelistischen Anthropologie. II. Quantatative Rassenanalyse auf Grund von statistischen Beobachtungen über den Drehsinn des Kopfhaarwirbels. *Sitzungsberichte der preussische Akademie der Wissenschaft (Phys-Math Klasse)*, 1925, pp. 71-82.

Bingle, G. J., Dillon, J., & Hurwitz, R. Asymmetric septal hypertrophy in a large Amish kindred. *Clinical Genetics*, 1975, *7*, 255-261.

Braitenberg, V., & Kemali, M. Exceptions to bilateral symmetry in the epithalamus of lower vertebrates. *Journal of Comparative Neurology*, 1970, *138*, 137-146.

Campbell, M. The mode of inheritance in isolated laevocardia and dextrocardia and situs inversus. *British Heart Journal*, 1963, *25*, 803-813.

Carmon, A., & Gambos, M. A physiological vascular correlate of hand preference: possible implications with respect to hemispheric cerebral dominance. *Neuropsychologia*, 1970, *8*, 119-128.

Child, C. M. *Patterns and problems of development*. Chicago: Univ. of Chicago Press, 1941.

Clark, C. E., Henry, W. L., & Epstein, S. E. Familial prevelance and genetic transmission of idiopathic hypertrophic sub-aortic stenosis. *New England Journal of Medicine*, 1973, *289*, 709-714.

Copenhaver, W. M. Heart, blood vessels, blood, and endodermal derivatives. In B. H. Willier, P. A. Weiss, & V. Hamburger (Eds.), *Analysis of development*. New York: Hafner, 1955. Pp. 440-461.

Corballis, M. C. & Morgan, M. J. On the biological basis of human laterality. Submitted for publication, 1976.

Cotterman, C. W., & Falls, H. F. Unilateral developmental anomalies in sisters. *American Journal of Human Genetics*, 1949, *1*, 203-213.

Dahlberg, G. Genotypic asymmetries. *Proceedings of the Royal Society of Edinburgh (B)*, 1943, *62*, 20-31.

Davidson, E. H. *Gene activity in early development*. New York: Academic Press, 1968.

Donohoo, P., & Kafatos, F. C. Differences in the proteins synthesised by the progeny of the first two blastomeres of Ilyanassa, a "Mosaic" embryo. *Developmental Biology*, 1973, *32*, 224-229.

Geschwind, N., & Levitsky. W. Human brain: Left-right asymmetries in temporal speech region. *Science*, 1968, *161*, 186-187.

Goss, R.J., *Principles of Regeneration*. New York: Academic Press, 1969.

Groves, C. P., & Humphrey, N. K. Asymmetry in gorilla skills: Evidence of lateralised brain function? *Nature (London)*, 1973, *244*, 53-54.

Guerrier, P. Les charactères de la segmentation et la détermination de la polarité dorsoventrale dans le développement de quelques Spiralia. I. Les formes à premier clivage égal. *Journal of Embryology and Experimental Morphology*, 1970 *23*, 611-637.

Gurdon, J. B. The importance of egg cytoplasm for the control of RNA and DNA synthesis in early amphibian development. In E. W. Hanly (Ed.), *Problems in biology: RNA in development*. Salt Lake City: Univ. of Utah Press, 1969. Pp. 217-229.

Halperin, G. Normal asymmetry and unilateral hypertrophy. *Archives of Internal Medicine*, 1931, *48*, 676-682.

Harrison, R. G. Relations of symmetry in the developing embryo. *Transactions of the Connecticut Academy of Arts and Sciences*, 1945, *36*, 227-230.

Holmgren, U. On the ontogeny of the pineal and parapineal organs in teleost fishes. In J. A. Kappers & J. P. Schade (Eds.), *Structure and function of the epiphysis cerebri*. Amsterdam: Elsevier, 1965. Pp. 172-182.

Horstadius, S. *Experimental embryology of echinoderms*. Chapter 8. Oxford: Clarendon, 1973.

Hubbs, C. L., & Hubbs, L. C. Bilateral asymmetry and bilateral variation in fishes. *Papers of the Michigan Academy of Sciences*, 1944, *30*, 229-311.

Kappers, J. A. Survey of the innervation of the epiphysis cerebri and the accessory pineal organs of vertebrates. In J. A. Kappers & J. P. Schade (Eds.), *Structure and function of the epiphysis cerebri*. Amsterdam: Elsevier, 1965.

Kasinov, V. B. Inheritance of left- and right-handedness in duckweeds and other organisms. *Genetika*, 1969, *5*, 22-29.

Kawahara, R. Bilateral asymmetry in the transverse processes of the cervical vertebrae of chickens. *Japanese Journal of Genetics*, 1974, *49*, 1-9.

Kraft, A. von. Situs inversus beim Alpenmolch (*Triturus alpestris*) nach UV-Bestahlung von Gastrula-Keimen. *Wilhelm Roux' Archiv*, 1968, *161*, 351-374.

Latimer, H. B., & Lowrance, E. W. Bilateral asymmetry in weight and length of human bones. *Anatomical Record*, 1965, *152*, 217-224.

Lichtman, S. S. Isolated congenital dextrocardia. *Archives of Internal Medicine*, 1931, *48*, 683-717.

Lepori, N. G. Sur la genèse des structures asymmétriques chez l'embryon des oiseauz. *Monitore Zoologico Italiano*, 1969,

*3*, 33-53.

Liquori, A. M.   Stereochemical code of amino acid residues in polypeptides and proteins.   In A. Engstrom & B. Strandberg (Eds.),   *Symmetry and function of biological systems at the macromolecular level*.   Stockholm:   Almquist and Wiksell, 1969.   Pp. 101-121.

MacCabe, J. A., Saunders, J. W., & Pickett, M.   The control of antero-posterior and dorso-ventral axes in embryonic chick limbs constructed of dissociated and reaggregated limb-bud mesoderm.   *Developmental Biology*, 1973, *31*, 323-335.

Milner, B.   Interhemispheric differences in the localization of psychological processes in man.   *British Medical Bulletin*, 1971, *27*, 272-277.

Mittwoch, U., & Kirk, D.   Superior growth of the right gonad in human foetuses.   *Nature (London)*, 1975, *275*, 791-792.

Monod, J.   On symmetry and function in biological organisms.   In A. Engstrom & B. Strandberg (Eds.),   *Symmetry and function of biological systems at the macromolecular level*.   Stockholm: Almquist and Wiksell, 1969.   Pp. 15-27.

Morgan, M. J., O'Donnell, J., & Oliver, R. F.   Development of left-right asymmetry in the Habenular nuclei of Rana temporaria.   *Journal of Comparative Neurology*, 1973, *149*, 203-214.

Nagylaki, T., & Levy, J.   "The sound of one paw clapping" isn't sound.   *Behavior Genetics*, 1973, *3*, 279-292.

Oksche, A.   Survey of the development and comparative morphology of the pineal organ.   In J. A. Kappers & J. P. Schade (Eds.),   *Structure and function of the epiphysis cerebri*.   Amsterdam:   Elsevier, 1965.

Oram, S.   *Clinical heart disease*.   London:   Heinemann, 1971.   Pp. 568-575.

Parker, G. H.   The optic chiasma in teleosts and its bearing on the asymmetry of the Heterosomata (Flatfishes).   *Bulletin of the Museum of Comparative Zoology at Harvard College*, 1903, *40*, 221-242.

Raven, C. P.   The distribution of special cytoplasmic differentiation of the egg during early cleavage of *Limnaea stagnalis*.   *Developmental Biology*, 1967, *16*, 407-437.

Raven, C. P.   Further observations on the distribution of cytoplasmic substances among the cleavage cells of *Limnaea stagnalis*.   *Journal of Embryology and Experimental Morphology*, 1974, *131*, 37-59.

Rawles, M., & Willier, B. H.   A study in the localisation of organ-forming areas in the chick blastoderm of the head process stage.   *Anatomical Record*, 1934, *58*, supplement 34.

Rife, D. C.   Genetic studies of monozygotic twins.   III.   Mirror imaging.   *Journal of Heredity*, 1933, *24*, 443-446.

Rife, D. C.   Handedness with special reference to twins.   *Genetics*, 1940, *25*, 178-186.

Robb, J. A.   *Basic comparative cardiology*.   New York:   Grune and

Stratton, 1965.

Romer, A. S. *The vertebrate body*. London: W. B. Saunders, 1962. Pp. 392-393.

Sabbadin, A., Zaniolo, G., & Majone, F. Determination of polarity and bilateral asymmetry in palleal and vascular buds of the Ascidian *Botryllus schlosseri*. *Developmental Biology*, 1975, *46*, 79-87.

Scheraga, H. A. Calculation of conformation of polypeptides from amino acid sequences. In A. Engstrom & B. Strandberg (Eds.), *Symmetry and function of biological systems at the macromolecular level*. Stockholm: Almquist and Wiksell, 1969. Pp. 43-78.

Schnall, B. S., & Smith, D. W. Nonrandom laterality of malformation in paired structures. *Pediatrics*, 1974, *85*, 509-511.

Schwind, J. L. Symmetry in spontaneous twinning in *Rana sylvatica*. *Anatomical Record*, 1934, *58*, supplement 37.

Sivak, J. G. Historical note: The vertebrate median eye. *Vision Research*, 1974, *14*, 137-140.

Soltani, H. C., & Li, M. D. Hereditary dextrocardia associated with other congenital heart defect: Report of a pedigree. *Clinical Genetics*, 1974, *5*, 51-58.

Spemann, H., & Falkenberg, H. Uber asymmetrische Entwicklung und Situs inversus bei Zwillingen und Doppelbildungen. *Wilhelm Roux' Archiv*, 1919, *45*, 371-422.

Stark, R. J., & Searls, R. L. A description of chick wing bud development and a model of limb morphogenesis. *Developmental Biology*, 1973, *33*, 138-153.

Stern, C. Gene Action. In B. H. Willer, P. A. Weiss, & V. Hamburger (Eds.), *Analysis of development*. New York: Hafner, 1955. Pp. 151-169.

Sturtevant, A. H. Inheritance of direction of coiling in *Limnaea*. *Science (New York)*, 1923, *58*, 269.

Taylor, D. C. Differential rates of cerebral maturation between sexes and between hemispheres. *Lancet*, 1969, *2*, 140-142.

Torgersen, J. Situs inversus, asymmetry and twinning. *American Journal of Human Genetics*, 1950, *2*, 361-370.

Ubbels, G. A., Bezem, J. J., & Raven, C. P. Analysis of follicle cell patterns in dextral and sinistral *Limnaea paragra*. *Journal of Embryology and Experimental Morphology*, 1969, *21*, 445-466.

Walker, N. F. Discordant MZ twins with retinoblastoma and cleft palate. *American Journal of Human Genetics*, 1950, *2*, 375-384.

Witelson, S. F., & Pallie, W. Left hemisphere specialization for language in the newborn: Neuroanatomical evidence for asymmetry. *Brain*, 1973, *96*, 641-646.

Woellwarth, C. von. Experimentelle Untersuchungen uber den Situs Inversus der Eingeweide und der Habenula des Zwischenhirns bei Amphibien. *Wilhelm Roux' Archiv*. 1950, *144*, 178-256.

Woellwarth, C. von. Die Ausbildung der Asymmetrie der Nuclei habenulae des Zwischenhirns bei Amphibien in Unabhangigkeit vom Blutkreislauf. *Wilhelm Roux' Archiv*, 1969, *162*, 306-308.

Wolpert, L. Positional information and the spatial pattern of cellular differentiation. *Journal of Theoretical Biology*, 1969, *25*, 1-47.

Young, J. Z. *The life of vertebrates*. Oxford: Clarendon Press, 1950. Pp. 452-453.

Zangwill. O. L. *Cerebral dominance and its relation to psychological function*. Edinburgh: Oliver and Boyd, 1960.

Zwilling, E. Limb morphogenesis. *Advances in Morphogenesis*, 1961, *1*, 301-330.

# 12.
# The Origins of Lateral Asymmetry

*JERRE LEVY*

University of Pennsylvania

During the first half of the twentieth century there were essentially two opposing positions regarding the origins of human manual asymmetry. Some investigators proposed that the direction of hand dominance was solely a consequence of sociocultural conditioning; others attributed part of the variation in handedness to genetic variation and part to sociocultural factors. The environmental school attempted to demonstrate that the degree of pressure exerted on children to be right-handed was related to the proportion of dextrality in the population, and the genetic school sought to prove that there were various asymmetric traits present in the neonate that were predictive of handedness. The evidence currently available can leave little doubt that both prenatal and postnatal factors affect the direction of manual dominance (see Levy, 1976a, for a review).

Recently, the question has arisen as to whether any prenatally influenced asymmetries, in man or other animals, are based on genetic factors at all (Corballis & Morgan, 1976; Collins; Morgan Morgan, this volume). Both Morgan and Collins state that there is no instance of genetic determination of the direction of any asymmetry in any animal whatsoever. Morgan believes that all asymmetries may be attributed to maternal cytoplasmic effects operative during oogenesis, and Collins believes that asymmetries are due to an interaction between a genetic determination of the *degree* of asymmetry and a laterally biased environment.

The question as to whether the direction of any lateral asymmetry can have a genetic basis, thus, reduces to the question of whether or not any asymmetries present at birth can be attributed to information encoded in nuclear DNA.


NONGENETIC FACTORS INFLUENCING ASYMMETRIES

There are a number of factors that can influence the direction
of a lateral asymmetry. That sociocultural factors affect writing
hand cannot be doubted. The frequency of left-handed writing in
the United States was only 2.1% in 1932, and had risen to over
11% by 1972 (see Levy, 1974). In a recent study by Annett in
England (1973), over 11% of propositi wrote with the left hand;
only 3.5% of their parents did. The change of frequency of left-
handed writing from 1932 to the present fits a model in which
there has been a constant reduction in the proportion of factors
(parents and teachers?) that serve to repress native handedness,
and in which the asymptotic frequency of sinistrality in the
absence of cultural pressure is approximately 12% (see Levy,
1976a).

The percentage of sinistrality is also affected by perinatal
brain damage. In brain-damaged, epileptic, and mentally retarded populations its rate is unusually high (see Nagylaki &
Levy, 1973, for review).

In monozygotic twins, ectodermal *situs inversus* is not infre-
quent, being observed in dermatoglyphic patterns, direction of
hair growth, facial features, and handedness itself (Newman,
1917, 1928; Rife, 1933). Newman attributes these mirror-imaging
effects to splitting of the zygotic tissue at a time when ectodermal cells have begun to differentiate, and considerably prior
to endodermal differentiation. Based on his work with the nine-
banded armadillo, an animal that regularly undergoes monozygotic
quadrupling, Newman reached the conclusion that there was a
greater probability of observing mirror-imaging effects in any
ectodermally derived tissue the later in development that zygotic
separation occurred. It is very likely that zygotic splitting,
in mammals, depending on the developmental stage at which it
occurs, can induce mirror-imaging. There is no reason to expect,
however, that various manifestations of mirror-imaging would be
correlated, since whether a particular feature will display inversion would depend on the particular region of the zygote in
which separation occurred and on the degree of differentiation
in various portions of the ectoderm.

*Situs inversus totalis* is extremely rate (1/10,000 in Norway;
Torgersen, 1950), and the rarity is probably due to late splitting of the zygote in cases of monozygotic twinning, after endodermal differentiation has begun. The endoderm does not differentiate from ectoderm until the gastrula stage, and does not differentiate from mesoderm until the midgastrula stage. There can
be little doubt that such late splitting of the zygote would
almost always be fatal to both resultant embryos, and it is
highly improbable that even if one embryo survived (possibly

because it received an unequal share of zygotic tissue), the other would do so as well. One would therefore expect to see, if late zygotic splitting is indeed the explanation for *situs inversus totalis*, almost no cases of twins in which one or both display visceral inversion. One would expect also to observe a relatively high frequency of anatomical abnormalities in people with *situs inversus totalis*, as a consequence of zygotic splitting in the gastrula stage. Torgersen's investigation of *situs inversus totalis* (1950) is consistent with these expectations, and his results do not, as Morgan suggests, imply that *situs inversus totalis* is independent of monozygotic twinning and a consequence of abnormal oogenesis.

It should be mentioned that monozygotic twinning, unlike dizygotic twinning, is without a genetic basis (Bulmer, 1970; Guttmacher, 1937), so one expects neither a correlation between the rate of *situs inversus* and twinning rate across various breeding populations, nor an increase in the twinning rate in families of people with *situs inversus*. It is conceivable, however, that there is a genetic predisposition that tends to induce zygotic splitting, not at the normal pre- or early-blastula stage when most twins are produced, but rather at the gastrula stage. Monozygotic twinning rate would not be increased in such families since, as pointed out, such splitting would usually be fatal, if not to both, then at least to one embryo. Even if both embryos survived, they would constitute such a tiny fraction of all monozygotic twin births that no familial trend could be discerned. One might see, however, a higher rate of rare abnormalities in families of people with *situs inversus totalis*, reflecting survival of one embryo derived from zygotic splitting of the gastrula. Again, such abnormalities would not imply maternally caused oogenic abnormality unless the familial pattern were seen only in the maternal line. There is no evidence for such maternally restricted inheritance, and there is positive evidence to show occasional paternal inheritance (Pernkopf, 1937; Torgersen, 1946, 1949).

As Spemann and Falkenberg (1919), among others, have shown, constriction of an amphibian embryo down the midsaggital plane can induce both monozygotic twinning and *situs inversus*, an obviously nongenetic effect. The observation of these researchers that *situs inversus* typically occurred in the twin produced from the right side of the animal suggests that the left half of the embryo was developmentally advanced over the right side and, perhaps, served as an inducer for dextral organization.

The mechanisms by which monozygotic twinning produces mirror reversal are unknown. However, one might imagine that if, for example, the left half of an embryo is more differentiated than the right, the tissue lying just to the left of the midsaggital plane is the inducer for dextral differentiation, and that induction proceeds from the midline toward the right. At the beginning of right-side differentiation, the most medial cells to the right of midline would be most dextral-determined, and the

lateral cells on the right would be least determined. If the
embryo is now constricted down the midsaggital plane, thus removing the inducer region on the left, the cells of the right-
half embryo which formerly lay in a medial position, are fated
to differentiate as the right half of the animal, albeit this
region now lies on the new embryo's left side. A new midsaggital
coordinate is established, and the cells lying to the left of
this induce differentiation on the right. However, the new left
half of the animal contains dextral-determined cells, so the
right half of the embryo is induced to differentiate as a left
side. Under this model induction proceeds from the more to the
less differentiated tissue.

One sees in the phenomenon of *situs inversus* the interplay between the cellular environment and genetic expression in the control of morphogenesis. If the cellular environment is changed,
by whatever means, cellular differentiation also changes, presumably because those portions of the genome that are transcribed in any given cell differ depending on the cell's environment. *Situs inversus* reflects not a genomic change, but a
change in genomic expression.

Collins' elegant experiments on paw preference in mice (this
volume) also demonstrate an environmental influence on a
lateralized trait. The proportions of dextral or sinistral mice
are directly related to whether the mice are raised in an unbiased or laterally biased world, even in mice who are genetically identical. Collins' finding that at the beginning of the experiment homozygous mice already display a left or right paw
preference of varying degrees of strength suggests that unimanual
preference was partially established during the first 6 or 8
weeks of life through accidental contingencies of reinforcement
in the environment, strengthened through positive feedback. If
a mouse happened to use, say, his right paw for some task and
achieved his aim, he would be more likely to use that paw for
subsequent activities, thus having paw preference strengthened.
Such random environmental factors would be expected to lead to
varying degrees of unimanual preference in any given population
of mice. Collins also found that female mice were more strongly
lateralized than males at the beginning of the experiment and
were more resistant to change from being placed in a biased world.
One would guess that the maturational rate of female mice was
faster than that of males, and hence that in the preexperimental
period they learned a unimanual preference more rapidly, with the
resulting habit stronger and more resistant to extinction.

One may thus see that there are a variety of asymmetric
traits whose directions can be influenced, or even determined
entirely, by nongenetic factors such as cultural pressures,
brain damage, monozygotic twinning, and instrumental conditioning. In addition, however, there are asymmetric traits whose
directions are entirely determined by information encoded in the
genes, and many more in which directional variance appears to be
partially genetic.

CONTROL MECHANISMS IN MORPHOGENESIS

Morgan seeks to establish on theoretical grounds that it is, in principle, imposiible for the direction of lateral asymmetry to be encoded in the DNA. The main thrust of his argument is that in order for a left-right asymmetry to develop, the embryo must have information with respect to critical reference points at an early stage of development--information that cannot inhere, Morgan says, in the structure of DNA itself. In the first place, the establishment of an anterior-posterior gradient also necessitates access to information regarding critical reference points at an early stage of development, as, in fact, does the morphogenesis of any part of the animal. In deuterostomes, the transplantation of a piece of embryonic tissue into a new cellular environment can, depending on the stage of transplantation, induce a morphogenesis in the transplant that is radically different from what would have been observed had the embryo been allowed to develop normally. Critical reference points are a necessity and determinant for all morphogenetic development, not just for the differentiation of left from right.

A particularly elegant example of this in the case of anterior-posterior differentiation is seen in the work of Hibbard (1965). In the normal amphibian embryo a pair of very large cells, the Mauthner neurons, develop in the medulla. Their axons grow posteriorly along the whole length of the animal. Hibbard implanted an extra medulla in salamander embryos, just anterior to the normal medulla. The implant was reversed in rostrocaudal orientation so that if the anterior-posterior gradient within the extra medulla determines the direction of Mauthner axon growth, the axons from the supernumerary Mauthner cells should grow in a rostral instead of a caudal direction. In fact, the axons initially began to grow anteriorly, but then they made a complete $180^{\circ}$ turn and continued their growth toward the spinal cord. The rostrocaudal gradient of the animal apparently overrode that of the extra medulla and/or induced a gradient change in the medulla itself. The consequence was that an environmental event (rostrocaudal reversal of a medulla) induced the Mauthner axons to grow in a direction opposite to that, relative to the medullary gradient, which would have occurred in the absence of the event.

It is clear that the genetic control over anterior-posterior differentiation is mediated through an anterior-posterior gradient whose chemical properties control morphogenesis as dictated by the animal's genome. That it is genetic information itself that determines how cells will respond morphogenetically to the chemical environment is demonstrated in the bithorax mutants of *Drosophila melanogaster* (Lewis & Craymer, 1971).

A clear distinction must be kept in mind between the *mechanisms* by which genetic information is expressed in embryogenesis and the *source* of information guiding the development of some structure. No molecular or developmental biologist doubts

199

that morphogenesis involves the constant interplay between the cytoplasmic environment of a nucleus and information transcribed from chromosomal DNA.  Although all cells of a multicellular organism are genetically identical, only the smallest portion of DNA is actually transcribed in any differentiated cell, the vast portion being repressed.  The repressors are themselves gene products, and may very well be under control of negative and positive feedback systems.  That the cellular environment is both controlled by and controls which portions of DNA are repressed is obvious from hundreds of embryological transplantation experiments, but such control does *not* imply cytoplasmic *inheritance*.


MOLECULAR POLARITIES

   The proteins manufactured by cells are of a single isomeric form, polarizing light either to the left or to the right.  No known protein occurs in living organisms in both the levo and dextro varieties, though some proteins are levorotatory and others are dextrorotatory.  It is quite irrelevant that the amino acids of which they are composed are all levorotatory. Were organisms based on dextro amino acids, proteins could nevertheless be produced whose tertiary structures would be very similar to naturally occurring proteins, although the primary structures would have to differ.  It is not only conceivable, but probable, that the proteins manufactured in cells composing right and left differentiated organs also differ.  It is also probable that left-right differentiation itself proceeds under control of the interplay between (1) selective differential repression of DNA in cells on the left and right of the animal's midline and (2) the differentiating cellular environments.
   The polarity of the tertiary structures (as well as the secondary structures) of proteins is a function of the sequence of amino acids.  The particular sequences found in living organisms are determined by the codon-sequence along *one* strand of the DNA helix, moving from the 3' end toward the 5' end within any given region of the helix.  Transcription of messenger RNA always proceeds in the 3'-5' direction of DNA, and only on one strand in that region, producing a messenger RNA of opposite polarity.  During translation, the ribosome moves from the 5' end of messenger RNA toward the 3' end, constructing a growing polypeptide chain in which amino acids are attached in the same order that their DNA codons were originally transcribed.  The determination of which of the two DNA strands is to be transcribed results, at least in the case of the *N* and *tof* genes of the lambda phage, from the spatial relations among structural genes, operator genes, and a repressor gene (Maniatis & Ptashne, 1976).
   There are two operators, one for each of the two structural genes, which are separated by a repressor.  In consequence,

transcription of the structural genes must proceed in a direction away from the medially placed repressor, and since transcription must occur in the 3'-5' direction of DNA, and since the
two strands of the helix are oppositely polarized, the *N* gene is
transcribed from one strand of DNA, and the *tof* gene from the
other.

Thus, although there are four different mRNA's that could be
transcribed from any given region of DNA if both strands could
be copied and if transcription could proceed in either the 3'-5'
of 5'-3' direction, in fact, only one of the four possibilities
is actually realized. Ultimately, the particular asymmetry of
the tertiary structure of a protein derives from those factors
determining *which* strand of DNA is to be copied, the direction in
which it must be copied, and the sequence of codons along the
copied strand. The biological activity of a protein is a function of its tertiary, or even higher-order, structure. It is
not difficult to imagine that asymmetric proteins can, during
the course of morphogenesis, result in morphological asymmetry.

Morgan's suggestion that the left sides of animals are more
developed than the right may be correct, but his proposal that
this is due to the levoisometry of amino acids cannot be valid
for the theoretical reasons outlined, and is refuted, in any
case, by the occurrence of any single instance of asymmetric
dextral development, of which there are hundreds of examples.

Given that the possibility exists for the genes to encode the
direction of an asymmetry, one may ask whether any such cases
are known. Morgan cites the best known case, but interprets it
as evidence opposing the genetic hypothesis.


ASYMMETRIES WHOSE DIRECTIONS ARE DETERMINED BY GENES

The coiling direction of the snail *Limnaea peragra* is determined by a single diallelic locus, dextral coiling being dominant (Srb, Owen, & Edgar, 1965). However, in this protostomic
animal, in which development is determined by the four-cell
stage, this gene acts, not on the developmental course of the
animal possessing it, but rather on its zygote. In protostomes,
cell division, rather than being radial as in deuterostomes such
as the Chordata, is spiral, and the direction of the cleavage
pattern is determined by the gene products of the mother. The
mother's phenotype is totally irrelevant. If she is heterozy-
gotic for coiling direction, her progeny will always display
dextral coiling. If these progeny, however, have received recessive alleles from both mother and father, the next generation
will all display sinistral coiling. The alleles derived from
the grandparental generation, equally in the maternal and paternal lines of the mother, segregate according to Mendelian laws
in producing the coiling phenotype of the second-generation offspring. Clearly, information determining coiling direction is

encoded in the DNA and it is irrelevant to the genetic question that this information is expressed phenotypically in the germ cells, rather than in the somatic cells, of an animal possessing it.

In protostomic phyla, it is not only chirality that is trans-generationally genetically controlled, but also anterior-posterior differentiation. If the four cells resulting from two cleavages are separated in such animals, each cell will develop into only one quadrant of the animal; yet morphological develop-ment is independent of embryonic genomic activity at this stage of development.*

It is obvious that in protostomes a great deal of DNA is irreversibly repressed by the four-cell stage and subsequent development is fated.

That morphogenesis in protostomes necessarily depends on maternally conferred genetic products at the earliest stages of development is of relevance in understanding the mechanisms of differentiation, but it says nothing with respect to whether the source of information guiding differentiation is coded in DNA. As Srb *et al.* (1965, p. 345) say, "All of the systems detected on the basis of extrachormosomal transmission interact with chromosomal genes or their products. In many instances, these systems seem to be concerned with the expression and integration of gene action or with determining whether a gene is active in a particular cell. They are systems, therefore, that appear to be

---

*The following points warrant emphasis. Although in sea urchins, urochordates, and amphibia, actinomycin treatment has no effects on morphogenesis until the blastula, gastrula, or even early larval stage, this does not imply that RNA synthesis does not occur in the preblastula stages of these embryos. It is known, in fact, that DNA-like RNA (messenger RNA) is synthesized by the embryonic genome from the earliest cleavage stages. Fur-ther, early morphogenesis in sea urchins, though unaffected by actinomycin, does *not* appear to be independent of embryonic genome activity. Gontcharoff and Mazia (1967) found that treat-ment of sea urchin embryos in the eight-cell stage with bromo-deoxyuridine, a thymine analogue that is incorporated into DNA, resulted in unequally sized blastomeres, lack of animal-vegetal differentiation (which sets the anterior-posterior axis), and failure of correct development of blastular form. Since other experiments demonstrate that bromodeoxyuridine must be incorpor-ated into DNA to produce these effects, it follows that early genomic activity is important for early morphogenesis.

A final consideration is that in mammals and birds the embry-onic genome synthesizes both messenger and ribosomal RNA by the two-cell stage and possibly even before cleavage. In these higher vertebrates, actinomycin treatment blocks development by the four-cell stage, showing that the course of morphogenesis is under control of embryonic activity from the time the fertilized egg first cleaves (see Davison, 1968, for review).

concerned with cellular differentiation." In other words, the maternal effect on phenogenesis acts *through* control of chromosomal activity, in precisely the same way that the organism's own differentiating cells act to control further differentiation. It should be obvious that extrachromosomal transmission in animals is, as Srb *et al.* suggest (p. 345) "only concerned in the expression of specific potentialities transmitted through the *chromosomes* /italics mine/."

In the cases of so-called cytoplasmic inheritance in animals, the information in genes determines the phenotype, if not in the organism itself, then in its progeny. *When* the genes will produce their effects depends on the time course of development, and it hardly matters that in protostomes some of the genes act by the second cell division of the organism's zygote, rather than on its own early zygotic development. It is important to keep in mind Jinks' (1964, p. 134) statement that "wherever an adequate investigation has been carried out, it has been found that the action, stability, and reproduction of extrachromosomal determinants are under chromosomal gene control. . . ." The cytoplasmic characteristics of the ovum are necessarily determined by the mother's genome, and after fertilization the differentiation of the zygote depends on what gene products are present in the cells. These gene products derive both from the mother, and, after nuclear RNA synthesis in the zygote begins, from the zygote itself. The genetic potentialities of any differentiated cell are, by definition, much broader than the genetic realization. Cytoplasmic constituents, from the mother or the zygote's own gene products, serve selectively to repress or activate only portions of the DNA, thereby determining the future course of morphogenesis.

One cannot establish that some structure develops in the absence of genetic information simply because the cytoplasm is critical for phenogenesis. Cytoplasm is *always* critical for phenogenesis and its biochemistry and structure are determined by genes. On the one hand is the question as to whether nuclear DNA codes the information to determine some trait, and on the other is the question of the control mechanisms by which this information gains morphologic expression, a developmental issue.

It would appear, however, that transgenerationally mediated chromosomal inheritance is insufficient evidence to convince all researchers either of the theoretical possibility that the direction of lateral asymmetries can be encoded in nuclear DNA or of its actual realization. It would seem that the only evidence acceptable as proof of the proposition here offered is an instance of the genetic determination of the direction of an asymmetry by an animal's own genes. The ever-useful fruit fly, *D. melanogaster*, provides the clearest possible example.

In the wild-type fly the abdomen of the animal is perfectly straight and untwisted. There are two loci, however, one on chromosome IV, the abdomen rotatum (*ar*) locus, and one on chromosome I, the twisted locus ($tw$), which can produce rotation of the entire abdomen if mutant alleles are present. At the $ar$ locus, there are four mutant alleles that have so far been discovered, $ar$, $ar^2$, $ar^{57d}$, and $ar^{57g}$. The $ar$ allele causes clockwise rotation (as viewed from the rear of the animal). The $ar^2$ allele produces clockwise pupal rotation, which reverses as the fly matures to produce counterclockwise rotation in the adult. Both the $ar^{57d}$ and $ar^{57g}$ mutants are counterclockwise rotated.

There are two mutant alleles at the twisted locus, $tw$ and $tw^2$, both of which produce clockwise rotation, $tw$ by about $30^0$ and $tw^2$ by $30-60^0$. The various mutants are described in Lindsley and Grell (1967) and the normal morphology in Demerec (1950).

It should be noted that these mutants represent a case very different from that of penile chirality, discussed by Morgan. As Morgan says, in the wild-type fly the ejaculatory ducts are rotated a full $360^0$, so that the anterior duct begins from a ventromedial position, extends to the left, bends right and then courses over the dorsal surface of the rectum to connect with the ejaculatory bulb on the right. The posterior ejaculatory duct then leaves the bulb, extending leftward and ventrally, to exit in a medial position, just ventral to the anus. The spiraling of the ejaculatory ducts around the rectum results from a $360^0$ rotation of the terminal abdominal segments during development. In the mutant, the direction of the spiral is unchanged, but a full rotation has not occurred.

In contrast to this internal rotation seen in the normal male fly, the external morphology of the abdomen displays no sign of rotation. In the *abdomen rotatum* mutants, one allele, $ar$, produces clockwise rotation in the adult and three alleles, $ar^2$, $ar^{57d}$, and $ar^{57g}$, produce counterclockwise rotation in the adult. At the twisted locus, both mutant alleles cause clockwise rotation. The rotations are not merely changes in the *degree* of rotation as a function of what mutant allele is present, but changes in the *direction* of rotation. It might be mentioned also that if the $ar$ mutation is present, the direction of rotation it produces can be reversed in the male fly if a second mutation, the minute deficiency $/Df(4)M/$, is also present on chromosome IV. If both these mutations are present, the abdomen of males will have a counterclockwise rotation.

Though it is possible to construct complex models that might account for species-invariant directional asymmetries in the absence of genetic information, at least in the cases of the snail and the fly, genetic determination of the direction of asymmetries has been empirically demonstrated. Morgan's claim (this volume) that "there seems to be no simple case in which a Mendelian factor determines the direction of asymmetry in its carrier" cannot be maintained. By his own definition, the direction of abdominal rotation in *D. melanogaster* is under control of Mendelian factors, and by the definition of most geneticists, the same holds for coiling direction in the snail.

HUMAN ASYMMETRIES WHOSE DIRECTIONS ARE LIKELY TO BE INFLUENCED
BY GENETIC FACTORS

In addition to the proven cases of genetic determination for
rotational direction of the abdomen in the fruit fly and for
coiling direction in the snail, there is a substantial body of
evidence supporting the view that some of the variance in the
direction of a number of asymmetries in people is also genetic.

As shown earlier in this chapter, under Nongenetic Factors
Influencing Asymmetries, handedness itself is highly susceptible
to cultural influence, especially if it is defined by writing
hand. In the absence of cross-fostering studies, no set of
familial correlations for handedness itself can be taken as
proof or disproof of the action of genetic factors. Particularly when the parental and filial populations display widely differing handedness distributions, it becomes impossible to assess
either the degree or nature of possible genetic influences (see
Levy, 1976b). Any attempt to determine prenatal maternal influences on handedness is doomed when it is known that handedness
can be strongly postnatally affected. A brief review of the
literature on this issue makes clear that maternal influences may
or may not appear in any given study, and that if they do, they
can be at least as easily attributed to postnatal sociocultural
effects as to postulated oogenic effects. Annett (1973) found
more sinistral progeny born to R♂ x L♀ than to L♂ x R♀ matings.
Merrell (1957 found the reverse, whereas Rife (1940) found no
significant difference in the frequency of sinistral offspring
born to the two types of matings.

If any progress is to be made in determining whether asymmetric traits in people have a genetic basis, attention should
be directed toward those traits that are present in the neonate,
which are unlikely to be much affected by learning and cultural
factors, or toward the relationships between these and culturally affected traits.

There are a variety of asymmetries present in the newborn
infant, including dermatoglyphic patterns (Rife, 1943, 1955),
direction of tonic neck reflex (Gesell & Amatruda, 1945; Gesell &
Ames, 1947; Turkewitz, this volume), and direction of cerebral
asymmetry (Entus & Corballis, 1976; LeMay, 1976; Witelson &
Pallie, 1973; Gardiner & Walter, Rubens, this volume), all of
which are correlated with handedness. The correlation of handedness with these asymmetries is important for two reasons. First,
it illustrates that whatever prenatal factors determine neonatal
asymmetries also, to some extent, affect handedness. Second,
since handedness is such an easily measured phenotype, it has
been used in a large number of studies as an index of other
asymmetries, and familial relations have been assessed.

Luria (1970) found that the presence or absence of sinistral
family members was predictive of the probability of recovery
from aphasia following left-hemisphere lesions, in both left-

and right-handers. Hines ans Satz (1971) found in dextrals, and
Zurif and Bryden (1969) in sinistrals, that a history of familial
sinistrality reduced the magnitude of sensory half-field differences in tachistoscopic or dichotic tests. Hécaen and Sauguet
(1971) observed that aphasia occurred with lesions to either
hemisphere in sinistrals from left-handed families, but only
after left-hemisphere lesions in those from dextral families.
None of these investigators reported that the familial effect was
only manifested through the maternal line. For asymmetries such
as direction of brain lateralization, which is present at birth
and unlikely to be affected by sociological factors, paternal
influence can only be mediated by the genes.

Further, in a recent study by Levy and Reid (1976), direction
of brain lateralization, as measured by two tachistoscopic tests,
one for verbal and one for spatial specialization, could be
almost perfectly predicted by writing hand and hand position in
writing. Dextrals with a normal writing position and sinistrals
with a hooked or inverted posture (hand held above the line of
writing, pen pointing toward bottom of the page) had verbally
specialized left hemispheres and spatially specialized right
hemispheres. Sinistrals with a normal writing position and a
dextral with an inverted position manifested the reverse. Out of
73 subjects, 71 showed this pattern when the average of the two
tests was taken as the index of cerebral lateralization. The
two exceptions were both sinistral females with inverted
postures. Such a correlation cannot be attributed to peculiar
frequency distributions for handedness, hand position, and cerebral dominance in postulated, but unidentified, subpopulations
in the sample (see Collins, this volume). It is hard to doubt
that the relationship is causal.

There are other human asymmetries that, although never investigated in the neonate, are unlikely to reflect cultural
influence. Eye dominance is a trait of which most people are
unaware, and, in fact, in the Asher Test (1961), subjects are
usually unable to recognize with which eye they have sighted.
Merrell (1957) found not only that breeding ratios for eye dominance deviate significantly from random expectations, but also
that there is no evidence for a maternal effect. In R♂ x L♀
matings, 44.8% of the progeny were left-eye dominant; in L♂ x R♀
matings, 43.4% of the progeny were left-eye dominant, a totally
nonsignificant difference. Merrell also found a strong and significant correlation of eye dominance with handedness, though by
incorrectly assuming three degrees of freedom instead of one in
testing his frequency distributions, he reached the opposite
conclusion.

Finally, Sutton (1967) investigated the relation between nasal
asymmetry and handedness in 772 Australians of European ancestry
and in 257 Polynesians. Though postnatal factors, such as nose
fractures, may affect nasal asymmetry, it is very unlikely that
postnatal environmental events could produce a covariance be-

tween the anatomy of the nose and handedness. The correlation between the two traits was .37 in Australians and .35 in Polynesians, each significant at $p < .001$, the correlations not differing from each other. The near-identity of the correlations in two entirely different breeding populations makes it extremely improbable that they are spurious artifacts of odd subpopulation distributions. It would be of some interest to investigate the inheritance pattern for nasal asymmetry. If it is found to have a positive correlation with the maternal line, but a zero correlation with the paternal line, even through two generations, genetic factors would be ruled out. If positive correlations were seen with both parents, and if the paternal correlation were too large to be attributed to any assortative mating that may exist, one would be led to conclude that the direction of nasal asymmetry was encoded in genes.

There can be no doubt that many human asymmetries whose directions are variable across the population are either entirely determined or strongly affected by prenatal factors. These factors must be such that the produce familial correlations, that they produce correlations between different asymmetric traits that are of the same magnitude in entirely different breeding populations, and in one case (the brain-hand-hand position relationship), a correlation approaching unity. Where is the source of information producing these effects? If it is in cytoplasm, then since cytoplasmic structure is itself a consequence of information in DNA, the ultimate informational source is the genome. Morgan (this volume) says, "A decision between alternative models has to be made on the plausibility of their claims about the mechanics of inheritance, in the light of general evidence." In this we concur.

BIBLIOGRAPHY

Annett, M. Handedness in families. *Annals of Human Genetics*, *Lond.*, 1973, *37*, 93-105.
Asher, H. *Experiments in seeing.* New York: Basic Books, 1961.
Bulmer, M. G. *The biology of twinning in man.* Oxford: Clarendon Press, 1970.
Corballis, M. C., & Morgan, M. J. On the biological basis of human laterality. Submitted for publication, 1976.
Davidson, E. H. *Gene activity in early development.* New York: Academic Press, 1968.
Demerec, M. *Biology of drosophila.* New York: Wiley, 1950.
Entus, A. K., & Corballis, M. C. Hemispheric asymmetry in processing of speech and nonspeech sounds by infants. Submitted, 1976.
Gesell, A., & Amatruda, C. S. *The embryology of behavior.* New York: Harper, 1945.
Gesell, A., & Ames, L. B. The development of handedness.

*Journal of Genetic Psychology*, 1947, *70*, 155-175.

Gontcharoff, M., & Mazia, D. Developmental consequences of introduction of bromouracil into the DNA of sea urchin embryos during early division stages. *Experimental Cell Research*, 1967, *46*, 315-327.

Guttmacher, A. F. An analysis of 521 cases of twin pregnancy: I. Differences in single and double ovum twinning. *American Journal of Obstetrics and Gynecology*, 1937, *34*, 76-84.

Hécaen, H., & Sauguet, J. Cerebral dominance in left-handed subjects. *Cortex*, 1971, *7*, 19-48.

Hibbard, E. Orientation and directed growth of Mauthner's cell axons from duplicated vestibular nerve roots. *Experimental Neurology*, 1965, *13*, 289-301.

Hines, D., & Satz, P. Superiority of right visual half-fields in right-handers for recall of digits presented at varying rates. *Neuropsychologia*, 1971, *9*, 21-25.

Jinks, J. L. *Extrachromosomal inheritance*. Englewood Cliffs, New Jersey: Prentice-Hall, 1964.

LeMay, M. Cerebral asymmetries in nonhuman primate, Neanderthal and modern man. In *Origins and evolution of language and speech*. *Annals of the New York Academy of Sciences*, 1976, in press.

Levy, J. Psychogiological implications of bilateral asymmetry. In S. Dimond, & J. G. Beaumont (Eds.), *Hemisphere function in the human brain*. London: Paul Elek, Ltd., 1974.

Levy, J. A review of evidence for a genetic component in handedness. *Behavior Genetics*, 1976, in press. (a)

Levy, J. A reply to Hudson regarding the Levy-Nagylaki model for the genetics of handedness. *Neuropsychologia*, 1976, in press. (b)

Levy, J., & Reid, M. Variations in writing posture of the hand and cerebral organization. Submitted, 1976.

Lewis, E. B., & Craymer, L. *Drosophila Information Service*, 1971, *47*, 133-134.

Lindsley, D. L., & Grell, E. H. *Genetic variations of drosophila melanogaster*. Carnegie Institute of Washington, publication no. 627, 1967.

Luria, A. R. *Traumatic aphasia*. Paris: Mouton, 1970.

Maniatis, T., & Ptashne, M. A DNA operator-repressor system. *Scientific American*, 1976, *234*, 64-76.

Merrell, D. J. Dominance of hand and eye. *Human Biology*, 1957, *29*, 314-328.

Nagylaki, T., & Levy, J. The sound of one paw clapping is not sound. *Behavior Genetics*, 1973, *3*, 279-292.

Newman, H. *The biology of twins*. Chicago: Univ. of Chicago Press, 1917.

Newman, H. Asymmetry reversal or mirror imaging in identical twins. *Biological Bulletin*, 1928, *55*, 298-315.

Pernkopf, E. Asymmetrie, Inversion, und Vererbung. *Zeitschrift fur menschliche Vererbungs-und Konstitutionslehre,* 1937, *20,* 606-656.

Rife, D. C.  Genetic studies of monozygotic twins.  I, II, III. *Journal of Heredity,* 1933, *24,* 339-345, 407-414, 443-446.

Rife, D. C.  Handedness with special reference to twins. *Genetics,* 1940, *25,* 178-186.

Rife, D. C.  Genetic interrelationships of dermatoglyphics and functional handedness.  *Genetics,* 1943, *28,* 41-48.

Rife, D. C.  Hand prints and handedness. *American Journal of Human Genetics,* 1955, *7,* 170-179.

Spemann, H., & Falkenberg, H.  Uber asymmetrische Entwicklung und Situs inversus bei Zwillingen und Doppelbildungen. *Wilhelm Roux' Archiv,* 1919, *45,* 371-422.

Srb, A., Owen, R., & Edgar, R.  *General genetics.* (2nd ed.) San Francisco: W. H. Freeman, 1965.

Sutton, P. R.  Handedness and facial asymmetry:  Lateral position of the nose in two racial groups.  *Nature,* 1967, *198,* 909.

Torgersen, J.  Familial transposition of viscera.  *Acta Medica Scandinavica,* 1946, *126,* 319-322.

Torgersen, J.  Genic factors in visceral asymmetry and in the development and pathologic changes of the lungs, heart, and abdominal organs.  *Archives of Pathology,* 1949, *47,* 566-593.

Torgersen, J.  Situs inversus, asymmetry, and twinning. *American Journal of Human Genetics,* 1950, *2,* 361-370.

Witelson, S. F., & Pallie, W.  Left hemisphere specialization for language in the newborn:  Neuroanatomical evidence of asymmetry.  *Brain,* 1973, *96,* 641-647.

Zurif, E. B., & Bryden, M. P.  Familial handedness and left-right difference in auditory and visual perception. *Neuropsychologia,* 1969, *7,* 179-187.

# Part IV

# TURNING TENDENCIES

# 13.

# Behavioral and Neuropharmacological Correlates of Nigrostriatal Asymmetry in Rats

*S. D. GLICK, T. P. JERUSSI AND B. ZIMMERBERG*

City University of New York
Mount Sinai School of Medicine

In research, the brain of the rat is treated as a bilaterally symmetrical organ. In behavioral as well as neuroanatomical and neurochemical studies, unilateral brain lesions are typically placed on either the left or the right side of the brain at random, on an implicit assumption that the two sides are identical. We have been led to question this assumption by the serendipitous observation of amphetamine-induced unidirectional circling behavior in normal rats, a phenomenon previously noted only in unilaterally lesioned rats. We have subsequently been able to demonstrate that, in at least one bilateral stuucture in the rat brain, there is a marked left-right asymmetry of function. This chapter will review our research on the behavioral significance of this asymmetry as well as the mechanisms responsible for it.

ROTATION AND LESIONS OF THE NIGROSTRIATAL SYSTEM

Following a unilateral lesion in any part of the nigrostriatal system (i.e., in either the substantia nigra, nigrostriatal bundle, or corpus striatum), rats will rotate or turn in circles toward the side of the lesion (*ipsiversive rotation*). The cause of such circling is presumed to be an imbalance in nigrostriatal function on the two sides of the brain. If the lesions are

*Supported by NIMH Grant MH 25644 and NIMH Research Scientist Development Award DA70082 to S.D.G.

subtotal, which they usually are, animals will gradually recover from the spontaneous tendency to rotate. However, the administration of amphetamine will potentiate spontaneous rotation during postsurgical recovery and reelicit ipsiversive rotation in fully recovered animals (Ungerstedt, 1971a; Christie & Crow, 1971). Amphetamine, which releases dopamine from nigrostriatal nerve endings, apparently enhances the imbalance between the two nigrostriatal systems by acting predominantly on the intact side.

In contrast, apomorphine, a drug that directly stimulates dopamine receptors, has very different circling effects depending upon the location of the lesion within the nigrostriatal system. That is, following a unilateral lesion of the corpus striatum, apomorphine, like amphetamine, will potentiate or induce ipsiversive circling behavior (e.g., Anden, 1970; Jerussi & Glick, 1975). This would be expected on the grounds that apomorphine should predominantly activate receptors in the intact striatum. Following a unilateral lesion of either the substantia nigra or the nigrostriatal bundle, the circling effects of apomorphine will vary with the duration of the time interval after the lesion (Ungerstedt, 1971b). Immediately after such a lesion, apomorphine produces very little effect. With increasing time after surgery, however, apomorphine increasingly induces contraversive turning behavior (toward the side opposite the lesion).

This result has been attributed to the development of denervation supersensitivity. The nigral lesion denervates dopamine receptors in the striatum, which then become progressively supersensitive as a function of time following the denervation. As supersensitivity occurs, therefore, apomorphine has a greater effect on the denervated striatum than on the intact striatum such that the imbalance produced by the lesion (i.e., intact side more active than denervated side) is reversed by the drug (i.e., denervated side more active than intact side). Since amphetamine's action depends upon intact presynaptic terminals containing dopamine, its ipsiversive circling effect varies very little with time after surgery. Haloperidol, a drug that blocks dopamine receptors, antagonizes these effects of both amphetamine and apomorphine.

Further studies concerned with this lesion-rotation paradigm have established that rotation is specific* to the nigrostriatal system (Crow, 1971), that rats consistently rotate in the direction contralateral to the more active nigrostriatal system (Arbuthnott & Crow, 1971; Zimmerberg & Glick, 1974) and that similar results occur in mice (Von Voigtlander & Moore, 1973; Thornburg & Moore, 1975). Although there is general agreement that an

---

*A recent report (Yehuda & Wurtmàn, 1975) that amphetamine induces ipsiversive rotation in rats with unilateral lesions of the tuberculum olfactorium has not been confirmed in this laboratory. We (Fleisher & Glick, 1975) have found no change from the preoperative level of rotation following such lesions.

asymmetry in striatal dopaminergic function is of primary importance for rotation, there is also evidence, although controversial, for modulation of rotation by noradrenergic (Marsden & Guldberg, 1973), cholinergic (Anden & Bedard, 1971; Costall, Naylor, & Olley, 1972; Muller & Seeman, 1974) and serotonergic (Costall & Naylor, 1974; Neill, Grant, & Grossman, 1972) mechanisms.

Interpretation of rotation data may sometimes be confounded by two methodological problems:

1. Some investigators measure rotation in automated testing devices whereas other investigators measure rotation by visual observations only. In view of the fact that the latter method can often produce unrepresentative and erroneous results, particularly when test sessions are of short duration (e.g., Costall & Naylor, 1975), we have designed and used an automated rotometer that distinguishes complete 360° rotations from incomplete oscillatory turns (Greenstein & Glick, 1975).

2. As will be discussed, it has been established that normal rats will also rotate following the administration of the same drugs (though usually in higher doses) that elicit rotation in lesioned rats. The magnitude of rotation following a unilateral nigrostriatal lesion has been found to depend upon whether the lesion is on the side ipsilateral or contralateral to the preoperative direction of rotation. If the preoperative direction and magnitude of rotation are not considered (as they frequently are not), erroneous conclusions may be reached with regard to the kind or magnitude of effect produced by a lesion (cf. Watson & Heilman, this volume). For example, the lesion may actually have no effect whatsoever even though it appears to have an effect inasmuch as the animal rotates postoperatively as much as it would have rotated preoperatively; or the results may be enormously variable, because of inconsistent placements of the lesion with respect to preoperative direction of rotation. These problems may also be of considerable importance in efforts to understand certain contradictory effects that have been reported following lesions outside the nigrostriatal system (e.g., Marsden & Guldberg, 1973 vs. Costall & Naylor, 1974 for the median raphe; also see footnote on p. XXX).

AMPHETAMINE-INDUCED ROTATION IN NORMAL RATS

In all our rotation studies, rats are placed individually in a rotometer for 15 min before administration of a test drug. Left and right rotations (360° turns) are then separately recorded on a printout counter at 5-min intervals for the 15 min before and 60 min after injection. Rotations to the left and to the right during the pre- and postinjection periods are separately totaled. The net positive rotations (i.e., rotations in the dominant

direction minus rotations in the opposite direction) are calculated.

Figure 1A shows a dose-response curve generated after the

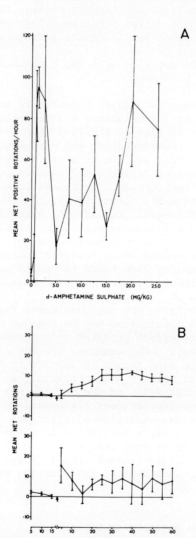

Fig. 1.  (A) Dose-response relationship for d-amphetamine-induced
rotation (mean net rotations + SE).  Rats were placed in the rotometer for 15 min prior to injection (i.p.) of d-amphetamine; rotations were then recorded for 60 min; N = 6 rats per dose.
(B) Time course of rotation (mean net rotations + SE) preceding
and following injection (arrow) of 1.25 mg/kg (upper figure) and
20.0 mg/kg (lower figure) of d-amphetamine (from Jerussi & Glick,
1976).

administration of d-amphetamine sulfate to naive rats. At all doses except .625 and 5.0 mg/kg, rotations are significantly greater ($p$ <.01 - .001) for d-amphetamine-treated rats as compared to saline-injected controls. There appears to be a biphasic dose-response relationship with peak rotations occurring at 1.25 and 20.0 mg/kg. Figure 1B shows the time-course of d-amphetamine-induced rotation. The 1.25 mg/kg dose has its peak effect between 25 and 45 min, whereas the 20.0 mg/kg dose induces the greatest rotation within the first 5 min after injection. The 20.0 mg/kg dose produces more variability from animal to animal and more frequent rotation to the opposite direction. The rotation elicited by low doses (1-2 mg/kg) appears to be qualitatively different from the rotation elicited at high doses (15-25 mg/kg). At low doses, rats rear on their hind limbs and rotate by moving their front paws around the inner surface of the spherical rotometer. However, at high doses, rats rotate in tight circles very similar to the d-amphetamine-induced rotation occurring with lower doses in rats with unilateral nigrostriatal lesions (Anden, 1970; Ungerstedt, 1971a; Ungerstedt & Arbuthnott, 1970).

The spherical nature of the apparatus seems to be an important factor in eliciting rotation. Perhaps other investigators have failed to report rotation in intact rats with low doses of amphetamine because rotation was observed either on a flat surface or in a hemispherical rotometer. On a flat surface, low doses of d-amphetamine initially appear only to cause rats to become hyperactive. However, careful observation reveals that there are slight postural and locomotor asymmetries that are masked by the hyperactivity and difficult to quantify. In a spherical rotometer, this hyperactivity is channeled into rotational behavior; it is probable that the enclosed apparatus also eliminates distracting environmental influences and induces the animal to move in an upright position. In contrast, with high doses of d-amphetamine, rotation may be observed in any testing condition.


MECHANISMS UNDERLYING ROTATION

As already discussed, amphetamine-induced rotation in rats with unilateral lesions of the nigrostriatal system appears to be due to the greater release of dopamine from the intact striatum. Amphetamine-induced rotation in normal rats could be explained by the same mechanism. Amphetamine would release more dopamine from one striatum than the other if it were the case that one striatum intrinsically contained more dopamine, or its content of the monoamine were more labile in response to the releasing action of the drug. The biphasic dose-response relationship could

be accounted for by the proposition that under normal physiological conditions there occurs an unequal release of dopamine.
Small doses of *d*-amphetamine would augment the normal unequal release of dopamine from either the left or right striatum. As the
dose of *d*-amphetamine is increased, the left-right postsynaptic
difference in the content of dopamine would increase and rotation
would be observed. With further increases in dose, the side that
initially contained the greater amount of the more labile pool of
dopamine would be close to depletion and the postsynaptic dopamine
content would be nearly equal in the two striata. Thus at these
doses of *d*-amphetamine (5-15 mg/kg), rotation would be expected
to be at a minimum. High doses of *d*-amphetamine cause massive
dopamine depletion (Brodie, Cho, & Gessa, 1970; Leonard &
Shallice, 1971) in both striata (Glick, Jerussi, Waters, & Green,
1974). However, the striatum that had initially released the
larger amount of dopamine would be depleted to a greater extent
than the contralateral side, where the postsynaptic dopamine content would now be relatively higher. Again, postsynaptic differences would be large, but now the animal would be expected to
rotate in the direction contralateral to that elicited by low
doses of *d*-amphetamine. Thus at high doses of the drug, the selective release from one striatum would lead to eventual depletion of dopamine on that side and the release of more transmitter
from the contralateral side. If this were the case, then rats
would not rotate in the same direction with low and high doses of
*d*-amphetamine.

When rats are tested twice, 1 week between tests, with 1.0
mg/kg of *d*-amphetamine, the direction of rotation remains unchanged for each rat and the magnitude of rotation is signifi
cantly correlated (Table 1). In contrast, rats (*n* = 9) do not
necessarily rotate in the same direction when they are tested a
week apart with 1.0 and 20.0 mg/kg, respectively. During the
first few minutes of the test session with the high dose, rats
rotate in the same direction as with the low dose. However,
during the last 30 min of the test session with the high dose,
rats rotate predominantly in the opposite direction.

Drug interaction studies support the premise that *d*-ampheta
mine-induced rotation in normal rats is mediated via dopamine.
Both α-methyl-*p*-tyrosine, an inhibitor of tyrosine hydroxylase,
and haloperidol, a dopamine-blocking agent, antagonize *d*-
amphetamine-induced rotation (Tables 2 and 3). The fact that
diethyldithiocarbamate, an inhibitor of dopamine-β-hydroxylase,
does not inhibit rotation induced by *d*-amphetamine (Table 4) indicates that dopamine rather than norepinephrine is primarily
involved.

All the foregoing rotation data suggest that normal rats have
an intrinsic asymmetry between left and right nigrostriatal systems that is accentuated by *d*-amphetamine. Such an asymmetry
has recently been demonstrated more directly (Glick *et al.*, 1974).
The dopamine contents of normal left and right striata have been

TABLE 1

*CONSISTENCY OF D-AMPHETAMINE-INDUCED ROTATION*

| Rat no. | Net rotations per hour for 1/0 mg/kg, i.p.[a, b] | |
| --- | --- | --- |
| | Day 1 | Day 8 |
| 1 | + 113 | + 136 |
| 2 | - 113 | -  80 |
| 3 | -  67 | - 133 |
| 4 | -  53 | -  50 |
| 5 | + 147 | +  66 |
| 6 | +  15 | +  18 |
| 7 | +  12 | +  36 |
| 8 | + 225 | +  86 |
| 9 | -  75 | -  46 |
| 10 | + 149 | + 216 |
| 11 | +  85 | + 128 |
| 12 | -  48 | - 105 |
| 13 | -  76 | - 134 |
| 14 | +  44 | +  11 |
| 15 | - 158 | - 164 |
| $\overline{X}$ | 92.0 | 93.9 |

[a]For Day 1 vs. Day 8, the magnitude of net rotation is significantly correlated ($r$ = .51, $p$ <.05, linear regression analysis) and the means are not significantly different ($p$ >.1, paired $t$ tests).

[b]+, net rotations to the left; -, net rotations to the right.

TABLE 2

*d-Amphetamine-AMPT (α-methyl-p-tyrosine) dose-response interactions*

| Dose (mg/kg, i.p.)[a] | Net rotations per hour (mean ± SE) | |
| | d-Amphetamine | d-Amphetamine-AMPT[b] |
| --- | --- | --- |
| 0.1 | 3.8 ± 1.7 | 1.8 ± 0.9 |
| 1.0* | 85.0 ± 19.9 | 10.7 ± 3.5 |
| 2.5** | 88.7 ± 31.9 | 12.0 ± 4.9 |
| 5.0 | 17.2 ± 9.0 | 20.3 ± 5.9 |
| 15.0 | 27.2 ± 7.1 | 52.3 ± 16.0 |
| 25.0 | 74.7 ± 22.5 | 51.7 ± 18.8 |

[a] $n$ = 6 rats per dose.

[b] For the d-amphetamine-AMPT interaction, rats were pretreated with AMPT (150.0 mg/kg) 135 min prior to the injection of d-amphetamine. Although AMPT did not significantly antagonize high doses of d-amphetamine, in terms of rotations for the whole hour, AMPT did prevent the rapid onset of rotation following high doses such that the time course resembled that of lower doses.

*, **Significant difference between treatments at $p < .005$ and .05, respectively ($t$ tests).

TABLE 3

d-*Amphetamine-haloperidol dose-response interactions*

| Dose (mg/kg, i.p.)[a] | Net rotations per hour (mean ± SE) | |
| | d-Amphetamine | d-Amphetamine-haloperidol[b] |
| --- | --- | --- |
| 0.0 | 3.8 ± 1.7 | 0.8 ± 0.5 |
| 1.0* | 85.0 ± 19.9 | 0.8 ± 0.3 |
| 2.5** | 88.7 ± 31.9 | 0.8 ± 0.3 |
| 5.0 | 17.2 ± 9.0 | 3.7 ± 1.1 |
| 15.0 | 27.2 ± 7.1 | 34.2 ± 11.3 |
| 25.0 | 74.7 ± 22.5 | 57.2 ± 11.4 |

[a] $n$ = 6 rats per dose.

[b] For the d-amphetamine-haloperidol interaction, rats were pretreated with haloperidol (1.0 mg/kg) 60 min prior to the injection of d-amphetamine. Although haloperidol did not significantly antagonize high doses of d-amphetamine, it did, like AMPT, prevent the rapid onset of rotation.

*,**Significant difference between treatments at $p < .005$ and .05, respectively ($t$ tests).

TABLE 4

d-

*Amphetamine-DDC (Diethyldithiocarbamate) dose-response inter-actions*

| Dose (mg/kg, i.p.)[a] | Net rotations per hour (mean $\pm$ SE) | |
| --- | --- | --- |
| | *d*-Amphetamine | *d*-Amphetamine-DDC[b] |
| 0.0 | 3.8 $\pm$ 1.7 | 13.0 $\pm$ 4.5 |
| 1.0 | 85.0 $\pm$ 19.9 | 156.0 $\pm$ 68.4 |
| 2.5 | 88.7 $\pm$ 31.9 | 61.7 $\pm$ 24.1 |
| 5.0 | 17.2 $\pm$ 9.0 | 33.3 $\pm$ 11.8 |
| 15.0* | 27.2 $\pm$ 7.1 | 121.0 $\pm$ 26.3 |
| 25.0 | 74.7 $\pm$ 22.5 | 87.0 $\pm$ 21.6 |

[a] $n$ = 6 rats per dose.

[b] For the *d*-amphetamine-DDC interaction, rats were pretreated with DDC (200.0 mg/kg) 45 min prior to the injection of *d*-amphetamine.

*Significant difference between treatments at $p$ <.05 (*t* test).

found to differ significantly by 10-15%. Following the administration of *d*-amphetamine (20 mg/kg), the dopamine contents of left and right striata differ by approximately 25%. Moreover, in response to *d*-amphetamine, rats rotate in the direction contralateral to the side containing the higher level of dopamine (Table 5). There is no such intrinsic asymmetry or rotation-effect associated with acetylcholine levels in the striatum or forebrain, nor with forebrain norepinephrine levels. The enhanced striatal dopamine asymmetry after *d*-amphetamine cannot be attributed to an asymmetrical distribution of the drug, which we have found (Jerussi & Glick, 1976) to be equally distributed in both striata as well as in both forebrains (Table 6).

ROTATION WITHOUT DRUGS

In view of the finding of a striatal dopamine asymmetry in normal rats, it might be expected that rats would rotate without any drug. As indicated by the zero dose in Figure 1A, almost no rotation occurs in the hour following a saline injection. Not shown, however, are the data for the 15-min preinjection period. These data were initially ignored because, in the design of a paradigm for testing rotation, it seemed reasonable to allow

TABLE 5

*Unilateral dopamine (DA), acetylcholine (Ach) and norepinephrine (NE) levels[a,b] ($\mu g/g$) in brains of rats treated with d-amphetamine sulfate (amphet.)[c]*

| | Group | Left | Right | High | Low |
|---|---|---|---|---|---|
| Striatal DA | Saline | 7.04 ± 1.29 | 6.83 ± 1.14 | 7.39 ± 1.06 | 6.48 ± 1.08 |
| | Amphet. | 4.75* ± 0.68 | 4.99* ± 0.88 | 5.43* ± 0.43 | 4.31* ± 0.30 |
| Striatal Ach | Saline | 4.01 ± 0.69 | 3.89 ± 0.74 | 4.06 ± 0.68 | 3.84 ± 0.73 |
| | Amphet. | 4.61* ± 1.47 | 4.51* ± 1.35 | 4.74* ± 1.40 | 4.37* ± 1.40 |
| Tel-dienceph. NE | Saline | .327 ± .048 | .344 ± .056 | .347 ± .055 | .324 ± .050 |
| | Amphet. | .194* ± .039 | .199* ± .039 | .201* ± .036 | .192* ± .031 |
| Tel-dienceph. Ach | Saline | 2.06 ± 0.25 | 2.06 ± 0.15 | 2.12 ± 0.18 | 2.00 ± 0.21 |
| | Amphet. | 2.13 ± 0.39 | 2.10 ± 0.03 | 2.18 ± 0.40 | 2.05 ± 0.28 |

Continued on next page

222

TABLE 5

Unilateral dopamine (DA), acetylcholine (Ach) and norepinephrine (NE) levels[a,b] ($\mu g/g$) in brains of rats treated with d-amphetamine sulfate (amphet.)[c]

| | Group | Ratio H/L | Ipsi | Contra | Ratio C/I |
|---|---|---|---|---|---|
| Striatal DA | Saline | 1.14 ± 0.10 | 6.67 ± 1.15 | 7.20 ± 1.17 | 1.08 ± 0.09 |
| | Amphet. | 1.26**± 0.16 | 4.33*± 0.32 | 5.41*± 0.46 | 1.25**± 0.16 |
| Striatal Ach | Saline | 1.06 ± 0.04 | 3.93 ± 0.71 | 3.97 ± 0.75 | 1.01 ± 0.07 |
| | Amphet. | 1.09 ± 0.11 | 4.46*± 1.52 | 4.66*± 1.41 | 1.05 ± 0.09 |
| Tel-dienceph. NE | Saline | 1.07 ± 0.06 | .328 ± .052 | .343 ± .051 | 1.05 ± 0.07 |
| | Amphet. | 1.05 ± 0.03 | .196*± .030 | .197*± .041 | 1.01 ± 0.06 |
| Tel-dienceph. Ach | Saline | 1.06 ± 0.06 | 2.06 ± 0.16 | 2.06 ± 0.12 | 1.00 ± 0.08 |
| | Amphet. | 1.06 ± 0.05 | 2.14 ± 0.39 | 2.09 ± 0.35 | 0.98 ± 0.05 |

[a]Values are mean ± SD.

[b]DA, Ach, and NE levels were computed in three ways: left side vs. right side, side containing highest level vs. side containing lowest level, and side ipsilateral to the direction of rotation vs. side contralateral to the direction of rotation. In addition, the high side/low side (H/L) and contralateral/ipsilateral (C/I) ratios were also computed.

[c]Dose, 20 mg/kg (i.p.).

[d]$n$ = 12 rats in each group; rats were killed 30 min after injection.
*Levels significantly different from saline control ($t$ tests, $p < .05-.01$).
**Ratios significantly different from saline control ($t$ tests, $p < .02$).

TABLE 6

*Unilateral levels of* d-amphetamine *(mean $\pm$ SD)*[a]

| d-Amphetamine sulfate (mg/kg, i.p.) | | d-Amphetamine ($\mu$g/g) | |
|---|---|---|---|
| | | Tel-diencephalon | Striatum |
| 2.0 | L | 2.25 $\pm$ 0.91 | 2.26 $\pm$ 0.96 |
| | R | 2.02 $\pm$ 0.90 | 2.24 $\pm$ 0.94 |
| | C | 2.11 $\pm$ 0.98 | 2.28 $\pm$ 0.96 |
| | I | 2.16 $\pm$ 0.84 | 2.23 $\pm$ 0.92 |
| 5.0 | L | 8.59 $\pm$ 3.48 | 9.77 $\pm$ 3.99 |
| | R | 8.47 $\pm$ 2.90 | 9.01 $\pm$ 2.59 |
| | C | 8.63 $\pm$ 3.38 | 9.79 $\pm$ 3.48 |
| | I | 8.42 $\pm$ 3.02 | 8.99 $\pm$ 3.24 |
| 10.0 | L | 15.52 $\pm$ 3.26 | 13.84 $\pm$ 1.78 |
| | R | 14.52 $\pm$ 1.45 | 14.79 $\pm$ 2.20 |
| | C | 15.25 $\pm$ 2.57 | 15.10 $\pm$ 2.14 |
| | I | 14.79 $\pm$ 2.56 | 13.53 $\pm$ 1.59 |
| 20.0 | L | 37.74 $\pm$ 3.58 | 32.62 $\pm$ 3.19 |
| | R | 35.82 $\pm$ 2.34 | 31.86 $\pm$ 2.77 |
| | C | 37.39 $\pm$ 3.20 | 32.04 $\pm$ 2.74 |
| | I | 36.17 $\pm$ 3.06 | 32.44 $\pm$ 3.26 |

[a]L, left; R, right; C, contralateral; I, ipsilateral. Each group had 7-14 rats; rats were killed 30 min after injection. There were no significant ($p$ >.1) differences between sides.

some time for the rat to habituate to the apparatus.

More recently, we (Fleisher, Glick, & Jerussi, unpublished results) have analyzed such preinjection data from approximately 100 rats subsequently tested with *d*-amphetamine (1.0 mg/kg). When first placed in the rotometer, rats are typically very active, making rotations in both directions; this activity decreases over time such that, after 10 min, there is very little activity. Net positive rotations for the entire 15-min period may be as high as 10 with a mean of about 4. This analysis reveals that 70% of all rats tested have net positive rotations in the preinjection period that are in the same direction as their rotations following the injection of *d*-amphetamine. This association is significant in a chi-square test at $p$ <.001.

It appears, then, that environmental influences, e.g., novelty, that increase activity or arousal, will result in a behavioral manifestation of the striatal dopamine asymmetry; alternatively, perhaps the arousal-enhancing variable potentiates the dopamine asymmetry to the extent that it is behaviorally evident. Consistent with this idea is our finding (Jerussi & Glick, unpublished results) that rats stressed with either air puffs or electrical tail shocks while in the rotometer rotate in the same direction as when subsequently tested with $d$-amphetamine (1.0 mg/kg).

EFFECTS OF OTHER DRUGS: PRESYNAPTIC AND POSTSYNAPTIC ASYMMETRIES

Besides $d$-amphetamine, we have tested several other drugs for their efficacy in eliciting rotation. Among those tested, apomorphine, L-dopa +MK-486 (a peripheral decarboxylase inhibitor), and scopolamine induce rotation whereas pentobarbital, pilocarpine, and haloperidol (except at a very low dose, .125 mg/kg) do not. The rotation elicited by scopolamine (Figure 2) appears to be the result of disinhibiting a cholinergic mechanism that normally modulates the dopaminergic mechanism primarily involved in rotation. Thus peak rotation is much less with scopolamine than with $d$-amphetamine, rats rotate in the same direction with $d$-amphetamine and scopolamine, and scopolamine potentiates $d$-amphetamine-induced rotation. Moreover, pilocarpine partially antagonizes $d$-amphetamine-induced rotation. The rotation elicited by a low dose of haloperidol may be attributable to greater blockade of the intrinsically more active nigrostriatal pathway; with increasing dose, both pathways are blocked and catalepsy ensues. Rotation elicited by L-dopa is hardly surprising inasmuch as it should be more readily converted to dopamine in the more active nigrostriatal pathway.

Rotation elicited by apomorphine (Figure 3), however, is more intriguing inasmuch as apomorphine directly activates postsynaptic dopamine receptors; its effects should not be dependent upon and cannot be attributed to an asymmetry in striatal dopamine content. Indeed, α-methyl-$p$-tyrosine does not antagonize apomorphine (Jerussi & Glick, 1975). Rather, the apomorphine data suggest that there is an intrinsic postsynaptic asymmetry, as well as a presynaptic asymmetry, in the nigrostriatal system. Either there are more receptors in one striatum as compared to the other, or receptors in one striatum are more sensitive than those in the other. With small doses of apomorphine, differential stimulation of the receptors in the two striata would occur and reach a maximum as the dose was increased. At 10 mg/kg, rotation plateaus and it would appear that all receptors are then saturated. As with $d$-amphetamine, rotation induced by apomorphine is remarkably consistent from week to seek (Table 7).

Rats tested with apomorphine 1 week and $d$-amphetamine the following week do not necessarily rotate in the same direction with each drug. Much evidence (Dominic & Moore, 1969; Gianutsos,

225

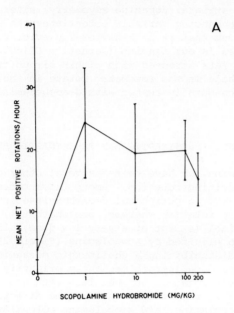

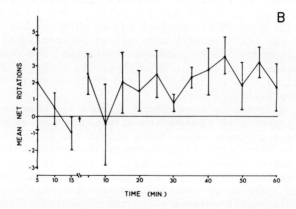

*Fig. 2.* (A) *Dose-response relationship for scopolamine-induced rotation (mean net rotations per hour ± SE); n = 6 rats per dose. (B) Time course of rotation (mean net rotations ± SE) preceding and following injection (arrow) of scopolamine, 1.0 mg/kg (from Jerussi & Glick, 1976).*

Drawbaugh, Hynes, & Lal, 1974; Tarsy & Boldessarini, 1974; Ungerstedt, 1971b) has indicated that procedures that reduce the concentration of a transmitter at postsynaptic sites in the central nervous system (e.g., surgical denervation, inhibition of transmitter synthesis, pharmacological receptor blockade)

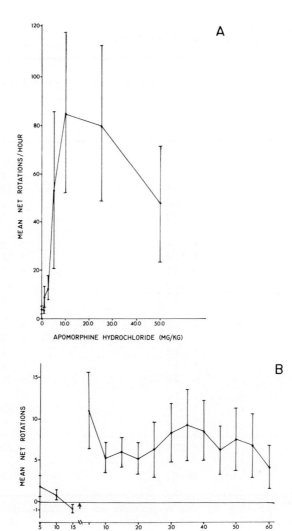

*Fig. 3.* (A) *Dose-response relationship for apomorphine-induced rotation (mean net rotations $\pm$ SE); n = 6 rats per dose. (B) Time course of rotation (mean net rotations $\pm$ SE) preceding and following injection (arrow) of apomorphine, 10.0 mg/kg (from Jerussi & Glick, 1976).*

increase the sensitivity of the receptors to that transmitter (i.e., a postsynaptic "supersensitivity" develops). Conversely, an excess of transmitter at postsynaptic sites appears to result

TABLE 7

*Consistency of apomorphine-induced rotation*

| Rat no. | Net rotations per hour for 10.0 mg/kg, i.p.[a,b] | |
| --- | --- | --- |
| | Day 1 | Day 8 |
| 1 | + 226 | + 276 |
| 2 | − 49 | − 29 |
| 3 | − 26 | − 126 |
| 4 | − 62 | − 60 |
| 5 | − 70 | − 49 |
| 6 | + 42 | + 62 |
| 7 | + 123 | + 126 |
| 8 | − 71 | − 56 |
| 9 | − 200 | − 215 |
| 10 | − 12 | − 33 |
| 11 | + 12 | + 24 |
| 12 | + 40 | + 99 |
| 13 | + 24 | + 33 |
| 14 | + 83 | + 23 |
| 15 | − 24 | − 10 |
| 16 | − 171 | − 169 |
| 17 | + 39 | + 83 |
| 18 | + 111 | + 83 |
| 19 | − 124 | − 226 |
| $\overline{X}$ | 79.4 | 93.8 |

[a]For Day 1 vs. Day 8, the magnitude of net rotation is significantly correlated ($r$ = .84, $p$ <.001, linear regression analysis) and the means are not significantly different ($p$ >.1, paired $t$ test).

[b]+, net rotations to the left; −, net rotations to the right.

in decreased receptor sensitivity (Overstreet, Vasquez, & Russel, 1974). Perhaps variations in postsynaptic receptor sensitivity are normally related, in a reciprocal way, to variations in presynaptic input. Thus a transmitter released from more active terminals would activate less sensitive receptors. From this regulatory and homeostatic model, one would then predict that if receptors are more sensitive in the left striatum, nigrostriatal terminals would be more active in the right striatum. Since the direction of rotation induced by $d$-amphetamine is presumably the result of both pre- and postsynaptic asymmetries, one might surmise that in rats that rotate to the same side with $d$-amphetamine and apomorphine the dominant asymmetry is postsynaptic. In animals where the direction of rotation is different for each drug, the dominant asymmetry would be presynaptic.

## INTERACTION OF CAUDATE LESIONS WITH ROTATIONAL ASYMMETRY

As mentioned earlier, drug-induced rotation after a unilateral nigrostriatal lesion should be influenced by the preoperative direction of rotation. We have tested this prediction using apomorphine and lesions of the caudate nucleus (Jerussi & Glick, 1975). Rats were initially tested with a 10 mg/kg dose of apomorphine hydrochloride. Ten rats then received unilateral lesions of the caudate nucleus contralateral to the preoperative direction of rotation; 10 other rats received ipsilateral lesions. Postoperatively, rats were again tested with apomorphine. Although both groups of rats rotated toward the side of the lesion, the mean number of rotations was approximately twice as great in the group with ipsilateral lesion (Table 8). Recently, we

TABLE 8

*Net rotations (Mean $\pm$ SE) per hour elicited by apomorphine[a] before and after unilateral lesions of the caudate nucleus either ipsilateral or contralateral to the preoperative direction of rotation*

|  | Preoperative | Postoperative[b] |
|---|---|---|
| Ipsilateral ($n = 10$) | 55.7 $\pm$ 14.8 | 242.7 $\pm$ 56.1 |
| Contralateral ($n = 10$) | 59.2 $\pm$ 19.5 | 123.3 $\pm$ 39.9 |

[a]Dose, 10.0 mg/kg.

[b]Difference between ipsilateral and contralateral groups significant at $p < .05$ (paired $t$ test); there was no significant difference preoperatively ($p > .1$).

(Fleisher & Glick, unpublished results) have obtained similar results using $d$-amphetamine (1.0 mg/kg) instead of apomorphine. Thus it may no longer be assumed that a unilateral lesion in one hemisphere of the rat will produce effects identical to those of a lesion in the other hemisphere (cf. Watson & Heilman, this volume).

Lastly, with respect to rotation, some species generalizations should be noted. We have tested *d*-amphetamine and apomorphine in mice and gerbils and found that both species readily rotate in response to both drugs (Jerussi & Glick, unpublished results). Apomorphine-induced rotation has also been described in dogs (Nymark, 1972). Thus, rotation may be a fairly general phenomenon (cf. Anderson; Gur & Gur; Stamm, Rosen, & Gadotti, this volume).

STRIATAL ASYMMETRY AND SPATIAL BEHAVIOR

Several experiments have been conducted to determine the more general functional significance of the nigrostriatal asymmetry revealed by the rotation studies. In particular, we have postulated that the asymmetry may be related to spatial behavior. This hypothesis was originally based on earlier findings concerned with the effects of *d*-amphetamine on side preferences in two-lever bar-pressing studies (Glick, 1973; Glick & Jerussi, 1974). In such studies, rats have been allowed to use either of two levers (left or right) while bar-pressing on a FI 15 (fixed interval 15 sec) schedule for water. We have found that baseline rates are directly related to the strength of side preferences: Higher rates are significantly correlated with greater preferences.

Videotape observations of paw use during bar-pressing have also revealed interesting relationships between paw use and the effects of *d*-amphetamine on lever-side preference (cf. Collins; Nelsen, Phillips, & Goldstein; Stamm *et al.*, this volume). If baseline lever and paw preferences are to the same side (as in approximately 75% of rats), then *d*-amphetamine enhances side preferences; if baseline lever and paw preferences are to opposite sides (e.g., pressing right lever with left paw), then *d*-amphetamine diminishes side preferences (Figure 4).

This relationship cannot be explained on a rate-dependent basis. That is, since high rates of responding are more sensitive than low rates to being depressed by *d*-amphetamine (Clark & Steele, 1966; Kelleher & Morse, 1968; Glick & Muller, 1971), it might have been expected that *d*-amphetamine would decrease side preferences overall (i.e., the lever sustaining the higher rate being affected to a greater degree than the lever with the lower rate). However, rats with very similar baseline rates and lever preferences may sustain opposite drug-induced effects on the strength of their side preference. The relationship between paw and lever-side preferences appears to be the only obvious difference between such rats (see Figure 4).

The initial suggestion that side preferences are related to nigrostriatal asymmetry was the result of testing rats for *d*-amphetamine-induced rotation at the completion of bar-pressing studies. Of 18 rats tested, we have found that 16 rotate in the

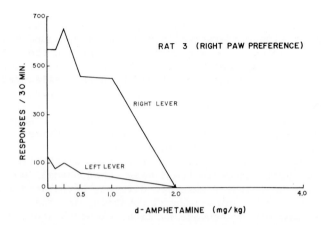

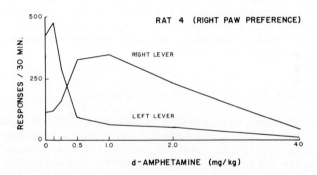

Fig. 4. *Dose-response* d-amphetamine *data for two rats bar-pressing on a FI 15 sec schedule for water reinforcement; rates on preferred and nonpreferred levers are shown separately. Note that although baseline rates of the two rats are similar, the relative proportion of responses made on the nonpreferred lever decreases in rat 3 and increases in rat 4 with increasing drug dosage. Baseline paw and lever preferences were to the same side for rat 3 but to opposite sides for rat 4 (from Glick & Jerussi, 1974).*

same direction as their normal baseline lever-side preference.

In order to examine such correlations more closely we have developed a simpler paradigm for the reliable determination of spatial preferences in rats. Rats are placed individually in the long arm of a T maze with scrambled foot shock administered through a grid floor. When a rat enters either the left or right arm of the T maze the shock is terminated and the rat is removed from the maze. Testing consists of 10 consecutive trials, with 5-15 sec between trials. Out of the 10 trials most rats (92%)

have a side preference that is stable from day to day and from week to week.

When the brains of rats were assayed following the determination of their side preferences in the T maze we found the concentration of dopamine to be significantly higher in the striatum contralateral to the preferred side than in the ipsilateral striatum. No such differences were found between ipsilateral and contralateral forebrain norepinephrine levels (Table 9). Other results have indicated that the small asymmetry in striatal dopamine is not due to any learning or stress-related change induced by the testing procedure but is most probably inherent in normal rats (Zimmerberg, Glick, & Jerussi, 1974).

In further studies, we have observed that *d*-amphetamine increases side preferences in the T maze, that normal (nondrug) side preferences in the T maze are directly correlated with the direction of *d*-amphetamine-induced rotation, and that small unilateral lesions of the caudate nucleus, although inducing spontaneous ipsiversive rotation for only a couple of hours after surgery, induce persistent (i.e., for many days or weeks) ipsilateral side preferences in the T maze. All of these results suggest, therefore, that rotation is an exaggerated or stereotyped form of spatial behavior and that spatial tendencies derive from a nigrostriatal asymmetry.

## CAUDATE STIMULATION AND SPATIAL PREFERENCES

We have employed electrical stimulation of the caudate nucleus in two studies. Unilateral stimulation elicits stimulus-bound contraversive turning or rotation resembling that induced by drugs. In one experiment, we attempted to determine the relationship between rotation and other behaviors (e.g., rearing, sniffing, gnawing) characteristic of the stereotypy also induced by the drugs that induce rotation. We found that bilateral caudate stimulation elicits such stereotypy if both nuclei are stimulated simultaneously at unilateral rotation threshold (i.e., the current that elicits contraversive rotation when each caudate nucleus is stimulated alone). Bilateral stimulation below rotation threshold produces no effect, but stimulation at currents above the threshold exacerbates the stereotypy. When rats are stimulated with one electrode at rotation threshold and the other below, rotation occurs in the direction contralateral to the threshold stimulation. Similarly, with one electrode above threshold and the second at threshold, rotation is contralateral to the suprathreshold stimulation. Stereotypy therefore appears to be the net effect of bilateral activation of the same system that subserves rotation (Zimmerberg & Glick, 1974).

In another experiment, the effect of unilateral caudate stimulation on spatial preferences was studied. We administered unilateral caudate stimulation at currents 10-20% below rotation

TABLE 9

*Unilateral dopamine (DA) and norepinephrine (NE) levels[a] (µg/g)*

| Group[b] | Left | Right | High | Low |
|---|---|---|---|---|
| | | Striatal DA (mean ± SD)[b] | | |
| 1. Pref. (2 min) | 7.26 ± 1.11 | 7.56 ± 1.16 | 7.87 ± 1.07 | 6.95 ± 1.06 |
| 2. Pref. (10 days) | 7.51 ± 1.20 | 7.13 ± 1.18 | 7.74 ± 1.10 | 6.90 ± 1.05 |
| 3. Shock | 7.29 ± 1.19 | 7.33 ± 1.24 | 7.82 ± 1.11 | 6.80 ± 1.09 |
| 4. Control | 7.97 ± 1.28 | 7.58 ± 1.21 | 8.25 ± 1.15 | 7.30 ± 1.07 |
| | | Forebrain NE (mean SD)[c] | | |
| 1. Pref. (2 min) | .411 ± .051 | .421 ± .056 | .428 ± .064 | .404 ± .058 |
| 2. Pref. (10 days) | .417 ± .061 | .428 ± .058 | .433 ± .055 | .412 ± .059 |
| 3. Shock | .404 ± .048 | .416 ± .057 | .420 ± .072 | .400 ± .051 |
| 4. Control | .405 ± .052 | .423 ± .061 | .426 ± .062 | .401 ± .058 |

Continued on next page

TABLE 9

*Unilateral dopamine (DA) and norepinephrine (NE) levels* [a] *(μg/g)*

| Group [b] | Pref. | Nonpref. | Ratio (H/L) |
|---|---|---|---|
| | | Striatal DA (mean $\pm$ SD) [b] | |
| 1. Pref. (2 min) | 7.00 $\pm$ 1.08 | 7.82 $\pm$ 1.07 | 1.13 $\pm$ 0.09 |
| 2. Pref. (10 days) | 6.94 $\pm$ 1.06 | 7.70 $\pm$ 1.11 | 1.12 $\pm$ 0.06 |
| 3. Shock | | | 1.15 $\pm$ 0.08 |
| 4. Control | | | 1.13 $\pm$ 0.09 |
| | | Forebrain NE (mean SD) [c] | |
| 1. Pref. (2 min) | .420 $\pm$ .050 | .412 $\pm$ .059 | 1.06 $\pm$ .05 |
| 2. Pref. (10 days) | .414 $\pm$ .060 | .431 $\pm$ .054 | 1.05 $\pm$ .05 |
| 3. Shock | | | 1.05 $\pm$ .04 |
| 4. Control | | | 1.06 $\pm$ .06 |

[a] DA and NE levels were computed in three ways: left side vs. right side, side containing highest level vs. side containing lowest level, and side ipsilateral to a preference (Pref.) vs. side contralateral to a preference (nonpref.). The high side/low side ratio (H/L) was also computed.

[b] Group 1 and Group 2 were tested for preference then killed 2 min and 10 days, respectively, after test; Group 3 received foot shock but no preference test; Group 4 received neither shock nor test.

[c] There were no significant differences (analysis of variance and $t$ tests, $p > .1$) among the four groups in left, right, high, or low DA levels or in H/L ratios. Within each group, there was a significant difference (paired $t$ tests) between high and low sides ($p < .01$) but not between left and right sides ($p > .05$). In both groups tested for preferences, the difference between the preferred and nonpreferred sides was significant (paired $t$ tests, $p < .02$ and .05 for the 2-min and 10-days groups, respectively). For each group, DA H/L ratios were significantly greater (paired $t$ tests, $p < .05$ in each case) than NE H/L ratios.

[d] There were no significant preferences (analysis of variance and $t$ tests, $p > .11$) among the four groups in left, right, high, or low NE levels or in H/L ratios. Within each group, there was no significant difference (paired $t$ tests, $p > .1$) between left and right sides, between high and low sides, or between preferred and nonpreferred sides in the groups tested for preferences.

NIGROSTRIATAL ASYMMETRY IN RATS

threshold to rats bar- pressing (continuous reinforcement for
water) in a two-lever operant chamber. Stimulation of the caudate nucleus ipsilateral to a rat's side preference induces the
rat to switch levers for the duration of the stimulation; upon
termination of the stimulation, rats immediately return to the
original lever (Figure 5). Stimulation of the caudate nucleus
contralateral to a rat's side preference has no effect on bar
pressing (Zimmerberg & Glick, 1975). In both cases (ipsilateral
or contralateral), the stimulation is such that independent observers (unaware of the experimental design) watching a closed-
circuit TV monitor cannot tell whether or not a rat is being
stimulated. Thus, electrical stimulation of the caudate nucleus
accurately mimics some of the effects of drugs thought to act in
the caudate nucleus and further implicates a striatal asymmetry
in spatial behavior.

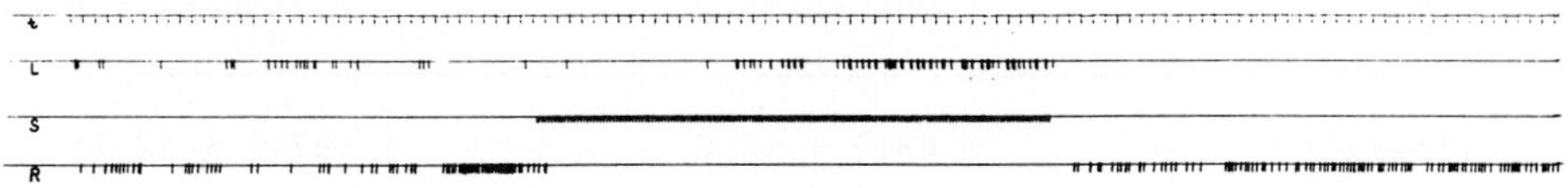

*Fig. 5. Representative event recording showing the effect of
unilateral caudate stimulation on bar- pressing; stimulation was
administered to the caudate nucleus ipsilateral to the initial
(prestimulation) side preference. Abbreviations: t, time with
15 sec between markers; L, left lever; S, stimulation; R, right
lever. (From Zimmerberg & Glick, 1975.)*

REGULATION OF STRIATAL ASYMMETRY: COMMISSURAL CONNECTIONS

The finding of a normal striatal dopamine asymmetry suggested
that there might be interhemispheric mechanisms to regulate or
modulate the asymmetry. Recently, both functional and anatomical
interrelationships between the two striata have been demonstrated.
Unilateral lesions of the caudate nucleus in cats have been reported to inhibit unit firing in the contralateral caudate
nucleus (Levine, Hull, Buchwald, & Villablance, 1974). More important, an intercaudate pathway coursing through the ventral
corpus callosum has been described in rats (Mensah & Deadwyler,
1974). It seemed reasonable to speculate that this commissural
system between the two caudate nuclei was responsible for maintaining a specific degree of asymmetry in striatal function. On
this hypothesis, striatal asymmetry of function ought either to
increase or decrease following commissural damage.

As a preliminary test of this hypothesis, we conducted an experiment to examine the effects of callosal section on *d*-
amphetamine-induced rotation and on striatal dopamine and acetylcholine levels. After callosal section, we found that *d*-
amphetamine elicits approximately twice as much rotation as that

235

occurring before the section. The callosal section has no effect
on mean total levels of either dopamine or acetylcholine in the
striatum but it does potentiate the striatal dopamine asymmetry
as well as inducing a striatal acetylcholine asymmetry (Tables 10
and 11). These results suggest that a callosal pathway may
normally function to synchronize the activity of the two striata

TABLE 10

*Potentiation of striatal asymmetry by callosal section: Rotation
induced by* d-Amphetamine *(1.0 mg/kg, i.p.)*

| Group | Net rotations per hour (mean SE) | |
| | Preoperative | Postoperative |
| --- | --- | --- |
| Callosal | 48.2 + 14.6 | 97.7 + 12.2* |
| Sham-operated | 46.8 + 14.5 | 49.0 + 15.1 |

*Significantly different from preoperative value at $p < .01$,
paired $t$ test.

(Glick, Crane, Jerussi, Fleisher, & Green, 1975). The finding of
a striatal acetylcholine asymmetry after callosal section further
suggests that this synchronizing function of commissural connections operates at different setpoints for different neurochemical
systems within the same structure, and possibly for different
structures as well. Perhaps, in the normal state, the activity of
some structures is bilaterally synchronized to a much greater extent than the activity of other structures; after section of interhemispheric commissures, inherent asymmetries may be revealed.
(See also Sechzer, Golstein, Geiger, & Mervis, this volume.)

SPATIAL TENDENCIES AND NONSPATIAL BEHAVIOR

A few years ago, well before any of the previously mentioned
studies were begun, one of us (Glick) participated in a study
concerned with analyzing response strategies of rhesus monkeys
performing a nonspatial delayed color-matching-to-sample test.
Although the test was specifically designed to minimize the operation of side preferences, monkeys were found, nevertheless, to
utilize significant spatial tendencies (cf. Stamm, *et al.*, this
volume). The strength of spatial tendencies was found to be an
important error factor accounting for differences among monkeys
in overall accuracy: Monkeys having stronger side preferences

TABLE 11

*Potentiation of striatal asymmetry by callosal section: Unilateral striatal dopamine (DA) and acetylcholine (Ach) levels (µg/g)[a,b]*

| | Group | Left | Right | High | Low | Ratio (H/L) |
|---|---|---|---|---|---|---|
| Striatal DA | Callosal | 6.87 ± .51 | 6.57 ± .49 | *7.67 ± .44 | 5.77 ± .43 | **1.33 ± .07 |
| | Sham-operated | 6.73 ± .39 | 6.56 ± .53 | *7.11 ± .46 | 6.18 ± .38 | 1.15 ± .04 |
| Striatal | Callosal | 5.13 ± .47 | 4.70 ± .41 | *5.35 ± .40 | 4.48 ± .41 | **1.19 ± .05 |
| | Sham-operated | 4.82 ± .32 | 4.65 ± .23 | 4.94 ± .34 | 4.53 ± .25 | 1.08 ± .04 |

[a] Values are mean ± SE.

[b] Dopamine (DA) and acetylcholine (Ach) were computed in two ways: left side vs. right side, and side containing higher level vs. side containing lower level. In addition, the high side/low side (H/L) ratio was also computed.

*High side significantly different from low side (t tests, $p < .05-.01$).

**Callosal-sectioned significantly different from sham-operated (t test, $p < .05$).

performed worse than monkeys with weaker side preferences. More-over, *d*-amphetamine lowered accuracy to the extent that it also increased side preferences (Glick, Levin & Jarvik, 1970).

At the time that this study was completed, there was very little idea that the results had any significance beyond the im-mediate goal of understanding how monkeys can undermine experi-menters' attempts to design a test resistant to irrelevant re-sponse biases. However, if species generalizations can be made, to the extent that side preferences in monkeys are related, as in rats, to an inherent asymmetry in striatal function, the associa-tion between matching-to-sample accuracy and side preference would suggest that the asymmetry may have a much broader influ-ence on behavior. In this context, it should be noted, as men-tioned earlier, that rates of bar- pressing on the FI 15 schedule were positively correlated with the strength of rats' side pre-ferences. Recently, we have conducted several studies concerned with examining other possible associations of side preference with behaviors not obviously spatial in nature.

SIDE PREFERENCE AND TIMING PERFORMANCE

Bar- pressing has been studied on both FR 30 (fixed ratio 30) and DRL 16 (differential reinforcement of low rate  16 sec) schedules for water in the two-lever situation. On the FR 30 schedule, as on the FI 15 schedule, rats' baseline rates of responding are directly related to the strength of side prefer-ences; higher rates are positively correlated with greater pre-ferences (Glick & Jerussi, 1974). On the DRL 16 schedule, how-ever, baseline rates are inversely correlated with the strength of side preferences (Glick, *et al.*, 1975). The different corre-lations among schedules may be attributable to different schedule-dependent determinants of reinforcement frequency. That is, on an FR schedule and, to a lesser extent, on an FI schedule, more reinforcements are received when rates of responding are higher. However, on a DRL schedule, less reinforcements are gen-erally received when rates of responding are higher (i.e., when timing performance is poor). Thus, on all three schedules, greater side preferences are associated with response rates that yield more reinforcements. Side preferences per se may there-fore have some adaptive significance related to a way, perhaps, in which the organism can most effectively cope with or strate-gically explore its environment.

The effects of *d*-amphetamine on DRL timing performance (i.e., percentage of correct or rewarded responses) are particularly in-teresting with respect to side preferences. First, as on the FI 15 schedule, the effects of *d*-amphetamine on side preferences on the DRL 16 schedule are closely linked to the relationship be-tween side and paw preferences. If baseline lever and paw pre-ferences are to the same side, then *d*-amphetamine enhances side

preferences; if baseline lever and paw preferences are to opposite sides, then d-amphetamine diminishes side preferences; if
both paws are used equally for lever pressing, then d-amphetamine
has no effect on side preferences (Figure 6).

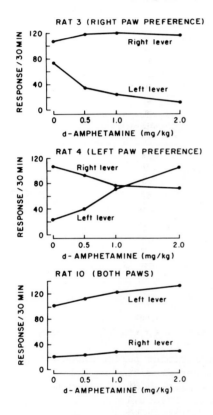

Fig. 6. Dose-response d-
amphetamine data for three rats
bar- pressing on a DRL 16 sec
schedule for water reinforcement; rates on preferred and
nonpreferred levers are shown
separately. Note that although
baseline rates of the three
rats are similar, the relative
proportion of responses made on
the nonpreferred lever decreases in rat 3, increases in
rat 4, and remains unchanged in
rat 10 with increasing drug
dosage. Baseline paw and lever
preferences were to the same
side for rat 3 but to opposite
sides for rat 4; rat 10 always
used both paws simultaneously
to respond (from Glick, Cox,
and Greenstein, 1975).

The effect of d-amphetamine on timing performance is related
to its effect on side preferences. In rats with paw preferences,
d-amphetamine decreases side preferences when it impairs timing
performance and increases side preferences when it facilitates or
has no effect on timing performance (Figure 7). We have conducted similar studies using a modified DRL 16 test in which an
external cue (a light situated above the water dipper) signals
the availability of reward (Glick et al., 1975). In this paradigm the rat does not have to rely on its timing ability to obtain rewards. (The test may be regarded as a successive visual
discrimination.) In this test, there is no relationship between
baseline rates of responding and the strength of side preferences, nor is there a relationship between the effects of d-
amphetamine on cue discrimination and side preferences. d-
Amphetamine affects side preferences as it does in the nonsignaled DRL test, but it does not affect cue discrimination

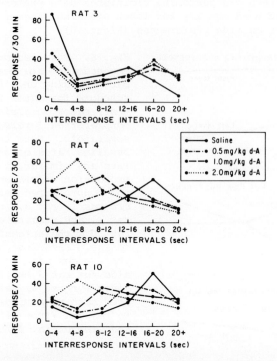

Fig. 7. *IRT distributions of DRL rats 3, 4, and 10 following saline or* d-amphetamine. *The timing performance of rat 3 was improved by* d-amphetamine *whereas the timing performances of rats 4 and 10 were impaired by* d-amphetamine; *the majority of rats behave like rats 4 and 10 (from Glick, Cox, & Greenstein, 1975).*

Figure 8).

The specificity of the relationship between side preferences and timing performance suggests that side preferences may be related to mechanisms involved in the control of behavior by internal stimuli. Some support for this notion has been obtained while observing (via a closed-circuit TV monitor) rats performing the DRL test. During nondrug sessions, most rats appear to conduct characteristic stereotyped patterns of motor behavior between successive lever-presses; such patterns have also been reported by others (Morrison & Stephenson, cf. Stamm *et al.*, this volume). For example, two rats have been observed to gnaw on a bar of the grid floor for the duration of the interresponse intervals. Upon receiving a reward, each of these rats quickly positions itself 1-2 in. in front of its preferred lever and gnaws at the floor. Upon cessation of gnawing, the rat immediately presses the lever and goes to the water dipper to receive

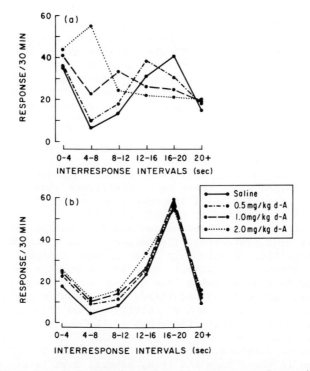

Fig. 8. *Mean IRT distributions for 12 rats tested on either the nonsignaled DRL test (a).or the signaled DRL test (b). Note that d-amphetamine affects timing performance but not discrimination of a visual cue (i.e., signaled DRL), even though its effects on side preferences (as in Figure 6) in the two tests are similar (from Glick, Cox, & Greenstein, 1975).*

the reward. If a reward is not forthcoming (i.e., responding has been premature), the rat usually returns to the lever and then the dipper again, before resuming gnawing behavior. For both rats, rewards are normally received only after a period of gnawing.

When *d*-amphetamine is administered, however, this interresponse sequence is dramatically disrupted--periods of gnawing are of much shorter duration and interspersed with periods of locomotor hyperactivity. This disruption results in many more premature responses and hence poorer timing performance. Patterns of interresponse behaviors have also been observed for other rats (*n* = 10), although the place at which such occurs varies. Some rats continually sniff and gnaw at the dipper recess whereas others gnaw at the floor to the immediate left or right of the dipper. Generally, *d*-amphetamine disrupts these patterns and induces premature responding.

On the basis of these observations, it might be speculated that motor feedback functions as a counting mechanism in normal timing behavior and that *d*-amphetamine affects timing behavior as a consequence of its motor effects. To the extent that these interresponse motor patterns are associated with side preferences, it would appear that such preferences facilitate the stereotyped programming of such patterns; that is, such patterns are most useful when they are linked to a stable side preference, which in turn is most stable when linked to a stable paw preference (cf. Collins; Warren, this volume).

Aside from investigating bar- pressing, we have looked for associations of side preference with locomotor activity as well as with learning of both active and passive avoidance behavior. For both rats and mice, there is a significant inverse correlation between activity level (recorded in a photocell apparatus) and strength of side preference (determined in the T maze): Animals with stronger side preferences are less active than animals with weaker side preferences (Zimmerberg & Glick, unpublished results). A similar relationship holds between *d*-amphetamine-induced rotation and activity: More active animals rotate less in response to *d*-amphetamine than do less active animals (Glick & Greenstein, unpublished results). These results suggest that normal variations in locomotor activity may be related or attributable to individual differences in the degree of striatal asymmetry.

In other experiments, rats and mice have been tested for side preferences in the T maze and then, several days later, trained to perform either a discriminated active avoidance response in a shuttle box or a passive avoidance response in a step-through apparatus (Jarvik & Kopp, 1967). We have found a significant inverse correlation between side preference and learning of the active avoidance response and a significant positive correlation between side preference and learning of the passive avoidance response (Zimmerberg & Glick, unpublished results). In other words, animals with greater striatal asymmetry are less active, learn passive avoidance responses better, and learn active avoidance responses slower than animals with lesser striatal asymmetry.

The only exception to this generalization appears to occur in the case of those animals (less than 10%) that display no evidence of striatal asymmetry (i.e., those animals having no preference for either side in the T maze). Although such animals are the most active and the poorest passive avoidance learners, they are also the poorest active avoidance learners. Their presence suggests that a moderate degree of striatal asymmetry may be optimal for maximal overall learning ability.

STABILITY OF SIDE PREFERENCES

We have recently determined that inherent side preferences are particularly important in the learning of spatial tasks (Zimmerberg & Glick, unpublished results). As discussed earlier, we have found that the striatal dopamine asymmetry is correlated with spontaneous side preferences of rats tested in the T maze (Zimmerberg et al., 1974). It appears, at present, that the direction of the dopamine asymmetry is intrinsic and is related *only* to spontaneous side preferences. That is, we have assayed left and right striata of rats trained in the T maze to reverse their initial side preferences. The direction of the dopamine asymmetry in each rat is related to the initial spontaneous preference but not to the learned preference (i.e., dopamine is higher in the side contralateral to the initial preference, as reported earlier for untrained rats).

However, although the direction of the striatal dopamine asymmetry is unrelated to a learned side preference, the intrinsic asymmetry appears to continue modulating or interacting with the effects of learning. After training rats to reverse their initial side preferences in the T maze (reversal training is accomplished by shocking rats if they choose their initially preferred side; a criterion of 5/6 correct choices is used), we have retested rats for spontaneous side preferences (i.e., when allowed to choose either side) once a week for 2 months. Although all rats exhibit learned preferences for the first 2-3 weeks, thereafter rats begin to revert to their initial preferences such that, eventually, most rats exhibit their initial preferences (cf. Collins; Stamm et al.; Warren, this volume). The greater the strength of the initial preference before training, the more trials it takes for rats to reach the reversal criterion and the less time it takes for rats to revert to their initial preferences. These results indicate that, although side preferences can be modified as a result of learning, such learning is superimposed upon an intrinsic and persistent bias. It would appear that mechanisms other than the striatal dopamine asymmetry are primarily responsible for learning per se, although the asymmetry, if it is the basis for the intrinsic bias, will influence learning depending upon the importance of spatial cues and tendencies in particular situations.

SOME IMPLICATIONS

It is undoubtedly premature to attempt extensive generalization of our findings to other species and phenomena. We would, however, like to offer a few speculative thoughts that may have some bearing on some human clinical disorders. Obviously, our work is potentially most relevant to the concept of cerebral dominance. Although we have identified one neuronal system that functions asymmetrically, it is by no means clear whether this particular system is in fact the substrate for cerebral dominance in man or whether other neuronal systems are also asymmetrically organized and together result in a dominant hemisphere (cf. Ruben, this volume). It has been reported that patients with unilateral parkinsonism exhibit differential deficits in tests of motor ability and spatial orientation depending upon whether the disease affects their dominant or nondominant hemispheres (Bowen, Hoehn, & Yahr, 1972a, b). This suggests that at least the motor component of cerebral dominance in man may be related to nigrostriatal function.

Our observations relating the striatal asymmetry to many aspects of behavior, together with the well-known actions of *d*-amphetamine on dopamine metabolism in the nigrostriatal system (e.g., Snyder & Meyerhoff, 1973), may be helpful in understanding the etiology and current treatment of Minimal Brain Dysfunction (MBD), a disorder in children characterized by hyperactivity and learning difficulties. MBD is frequently associated with poor cerebral dominance. Learning and motor disabilities as well as electrophysiological abnormalities may be manifested asymmetrically (Conners, 1973; Reitan & Boll, 1973). It has been hypothesized that a fundamental problem in MBD may be related to the failure of normal cerebral dominance to develop (Gazzaniga, 1973). Amphetamines and related drugs are particularly useful in treating MBD, especially when neurological evidence of minimal but real brain damage is demonstrable (Millichap, 1973; Satterfield, Lesser, Saul, & Cantwell, 1973). We may speculate, therefore, that amphetamine's therapeutic effects in MBD are attributable to enhancement of nigrostriatal asymmetry and/or of cerebral dominance generally (cf. Sechzer *et al.*, this volume; Shaywitz, Yager, & Klopper, 1976). The small percentage of animals having minimal or no striatal asymmetry, noted earlier, may be a possible model for MBD (cf. Sechzer *et al.*, this volume). Such animals are hyperactive and appear to have overall impairments in learning ability. They are also hypersensitive to *d*-amphetamine-induced depression of locomotor activity, a finding consistent both with the rate-dependent principle of behavioral pharmacology and with the empirical sedative effect of amphetamine in MBD (Glick & Milloy, 1973). One might predict that amphetamine would facilitate learning of such animals, and of children with MBD, by increasing nigrostriatal asymmetry, i.e., by inducing a more optimal degree of asymmetry. It might be expected, in fact, that excessive doses of amphetamine would impair learning; and this is certainly the case, at least in many animal studies (e.g., Glick, 1971; Rensch & Rahmann, 1960). Of course, a great deal of further research will be required to substantiate these ideas.

SUMMARY

Recent work has revealed a possible neuroanatomical and neurochemical basis for side preferences.  Such a basis was initially
suggested by the accidental finding that d-amphetamine induces
circling behavior or rotation in normal rats.  Because rotation
had previously been reported only in rats with unilateral lesions
of the nigrostriatal system, it was postulated that rotation in
normal rats reflects an intrinsic nigrostriatal asymmetry.  Subsequently, it was found that normal rats have a 10-15% asymmetry
in dopamine content of the two striata.  Following a large dose
(20 mg/kg) of d-amphetamine, the asymmetry increases to 25-30%
and rats rotate toward the side with the lower level of dopamine.
The direction in which rats rotate following d-amphetamine is
correlated with their normal side preferences in a two-lever
operant task and in a T maze.  Striatal dopamine levels of normal
rats tested in the T maze are lower in the striatum ipsilateral
to a side preference than in the striatum contralateral to a side
preference.  Electrical stimulation of the striatum will induce
contralateral side preferences and, at higher currents, contraversive rotation.  Unilateral lesions of the striatum will induce
ipsiversive tendencies but will have quantitatively different
effects depending upon whether the lesion is in the more or less
active side.  These and other results indicate that the striatal
asymmetry is intrinsic and is not the result of learned preferences.  A normal degree of striatal asymmetry appears to be regulated or maintained by an intercaudate callosal pathway.
Further studies have attempted to understand the functional
importance of side preferences per se.  On three different operant schedules involving bar pressing for water, greater side preferences of rats have been associated with response rates that
yield more reinforcements.  Animals with greater side preferences
are also less active, learn passive avoidance responses better,
and learn active avoidance responses slower than animals with
lesser side preferences.  Animals (less than 10%) having no side
preferences are the most active and the poorest overall learners
of all tasks studied.  A moderate degree of striatal asymmetry
may be optimal for maximal overall learning ability and side preferences may have some adaptive significance in terms of how the
organism can most effectively cope with or strategically explore
its environment.

REFERENCES

Anden, N. E.  Effects of amphetamine and some other drugs in cen-
    tral catecholamine mechanisms.  In E. Costa & S. Garattini
    (Eds.) *Amphetamines and related compounds*.  New York:  Raven
    Press, 1970.  Pp. 447-462.
Anden, N. E., & Bedard, P.  Influences of cholinergic mechanisms

of the function and turnover of brain dopamine. *Journal of Pharmacy and Pharmacology*, 1971, *23*, 460-462.

Arbuthnott, G. W., & Crow, T. J. Relation of contraversive turning to unilateral release of dopamine from the nigro-striatal pathway in rats. *Experimental Neurology*, 1971, *30*, 484-491.

Bowen, F. P., Hoehn, M. N., & Yahr, M. D. Parkinsonism: Alterations in spatial orientation as determined by a route-walking test. *Neuropsychologia*, 1972, *10*, 355-351.(a)

Bowen, F. P., Hoehn, M. N., & Yahr, M. D. Cerebral dominance in relation to tracking and tapping performance in patients with Parkinsonism. *Neurology*, 1972, *22*, 32-39.(b)

Brodie, B. B., Cho, A. K., & Gessa, G. L. Possible role of p-hydroxynorephedrine in the depletion of norepinephrine, induced by d-amphetamine and in tolerance to this drug. In E. Costa & A. Garattini (Eds.), *Amphetamine and related compounds*. New York: Raven Press, 1970.

Christie, J. E., & Crow, T. J. Turning behavior as an index of the action of amphetamine and ephedrines on central dopamine-containing neurons. *British Journal of Pharmacology*, 1971, *43*, 658-667.

Clark, F. C., & Steele, B. J. Effects of d-amphetamine on performance under a multiple schedule in the rat. *Psychopharmacologia*, 1966, *9*, 157-169.

Conners, K. C. Psychological Assessment of children with minimal brain dysfunction. *Annals of the New York Academy of Science*, 1973, *205*, 283-302.

Costall, B., & Naylor, R. J. Stereotyped and circling behaviour induced by dopaminergic agonists after lesions of the midbrain raphe nuclei. *European Journal of Pharmacology*, 1974, *23*, 206-222.

Costall, B., & Naylor, R. J. A comparison of circling models for the detection of anti-Parkinson activity. *Psychopharmacologia*, 1975, *41*, 57-64.

Costall, B., Naylor, R. J., & Olley, J. E. Catalepsy and circling behavior after intracerebral injections of neuroleptic, cholinergic and anticholinergic agents into the caudate-putamen, globus pallidus and substantia nigra of rat brain. *Neuropharmacology*, 1972, *11*, 645-663.

Crow, T. J. The relationship between lesion site, dopamine neurons, and turning behavior in the rat. *Experimental Neurology*, 1971, *32*, 247-255.

Dominic, J. A., & Moore, K. E. Supersensitivity to the central stimulant actions of adrenergic drugs following discontinuation of a choonic diet of a-methyl-tyrosine. *Psychopharmacologia*, 1969, *15*, 96-101.

Fleisher, L. N., & Glick, S. D. A telencephalic lesion site for D-amphetamine-induced contralateral rotation in rats. *Brain Research*, 1975, *96*, 413-417.

Gazzaniga, M. S. Brain theory and minimal brain dysfunction. *Annals of the New York Academy of Sciences*, 1973, *205*, 89-92.

Gianutsos, G., Drawbaugh, R. B., Hynes, M. D., & Lal, H. Behavioral evidence for dopaminergic supersensitivity after chronic haloperidol. *Life Sciences*, 1974, *14*, 887-898.

Glick, S. D. Facilitation or impairment of learning by d-amphetamine as a function of stimuli. *Psychopharmacologia*, 1971, *21*, 353-360.

Glick, S. D. Enhancement of spatial preferences by (+)-amphetamine. *Neuropharmacology*, 1973, *12*, 43-47.

Glick, S. D., Cox, R. S., & Greenstein, S. Relationship of rats' spatial preferences to effects of d-amphetamine on timing behavior. *European Journal of Pharmacology*, 1975, *33*, 173-182.

Glick, S. D., Crane, A. M., Jerussi, T. P., Fleisher, L. N., & Green, J. P. Functional and neurochemical correlates of potentiation of striatal asymmetry by callosal section. *Nature*, 1975, *254*, 616-617.

Glick, S. D., & Jerussi, T. P. Spatial and paw preferences in rats: their relationship to rate-dependent effects of d-amphetamine. *Journal of Pharmacology and Experimental Therapeutics*, 1974, *188*, 714-725.

Glick, S. D., Jerussi, T. P., Waters, D. H., & Green, J. P. Amphetamine-induced changes in striatal dopamine and acetylcholine levels and relationship to rotation (circling behavior) in rats. *Biochemical Pharmacology*, 1974, *23*, 3223-3225.

Glick, S. D., Levin, B., & Jarvik, M. E. Role of monkeys spatial preferences in performance of a nonspatial task. *Journal of Comparative and Physiological Psychology*, 1970, *73*, 56-61.

Glick, S. D., & Milloy, S. Rate-Dependent effects of d-amphetamine on locomotor activity in mice: possible relationship to paradoxical amphetamine sedation in minimal brain dysfunction. *European Journal of Pharmacology*, 1973, *24*, 266-268.

Glick, S. D., & Miller, R. U. Paradoxical effects of low doses of d-amphetamine in rats. *Psychopharmacologia*, 1971, *22*, 396-402.

Greenstein, S., & Glick, S. D. Improved automated apparatus for recording rotation (circling behavior) in rats or mice. *Pharmacology, Biochemistry and Behavior*, 1975, *3*, 507-510.

Jarvik, M. E., & Kopp, R. An improved one-trial passive avoidance learning situation. *Psychological Reports*, 1967, *21*, 221-224.

Jerussi, T. P., & Glick, S. D. Amphetamine-induced rotation in rats without lesions. *Neuropharmacology*, 1974, *13*, 283-286.

Jerussi, T. P., & Glick, S. D. Apomorphine-induced rotation in normal rats and interaction with unilateral caudate lesions. *Psychopharmacologia*, 1975, *40*, 329-334.

Jerussi, T. P., & Glick, S. D. Drug-induced rotation in rats without lesions: Behavioral and neurochemical indices of a normal asymmetry in nigro-striatal function.

*Psychopharmacology*, 1976, *47*, 249-260.

Kelleher, R. T., & Morse, W. H.   Determination of the specificity of behavioral effects of drugs. *Ergebnisse der Physiologie, Biologischen Chemie und Experimentallen Pharmakelogie*, 1968, *60*, 1-56.

Leonard, B. E., & Shallice, S. A.   Some neurochemical effects of amphetamine, methylamphetamine and p=bromomethylamphetamine in the rat. *British Journal of Pharmacology*, 1971, *41*, 198-212.

Levine, M. S., Hull, C. D., Buchwald, N. A., & Villablanca, J. The spontaneous firing patterns of forebrain neurons:  II. Effects of unilateral caudate nuclear ablation. *Brain Research*, 1974, *78*, 411-424.

Marsden, C. A., & Guldberg, H. C.   The role of monoamines in rotation induced or potentiated by amphetamine after nigral, raphe and mesencephalic reticular lesions in the rat brain. *Neuropharmacology*, 1973, *12*, 195-224.

Mensah, P., & Deadwyler, S.   The caudate nucleus of the rat:   Cell types and the demonstration of a commissural system. *Journal of Anatomy*, 1974, *117*, 281-293.

Millichap, g. L.   Drugs in management of minimal brain dysfunction.   *Annals of the New York Academy of Sciences*, 1973, *205*, 321-334.

Morrison, C. F., & Stephenson, J. A.   Effect of stimulants on observed behavior of rats on six operant schedules. *Neuropharmacology*, 1973, *12*, 297-310.

Muller, P., & Seeman, P.   Neuroleptics:  A relation between cataleptic and anti-turning actions, and role of the cholinergic system. *Journal of Pharmacy and Pharmacology*, 1973, *26*, 981-984.

Neill, D. B., Grant, L. D., & Grossman, S. P.   Selective potentiation of locomotor effects of amphetamine by midbrain raphe lesions. *Physiology and Behavior*, 1972, *9*, 655-657.

Nymark, M.   Apomorphine provoked stereotypy in the dog. *Psychopharmacologia*, 1972, *26*, 261-268.

Overstreet, D. H., Vasquez, B. J., & Russel, R. W.   Reduced behavioral effects of intrahippocampally administered carbachol in rats with low cholinesterase activity. *Neuropharmacology*, 1974, *13*, 911-917.

Reitan, R. M., Boll, T. J.   Neuropsychological correlates of minimal brain dysfunction. *Annals of the New York Academy of Sciences*, 1973, *205*, 65-88.

Rensch, B., & Rahmann, H.   EinfluB des Previtins auf das Gedachtnis von Gold-Hamstern. *Pfluegers Archiv fuer die Gesamie Physiologie*, 1960, *271*, 693-704.

Satterfield, J. H., Lesser, L. L., Saul, R. E., & Cantwell, D. P. EEG aspects in the diagnosis and treatment of minimal brain dysfunction. *Annals of the New York Academy of Sciences*, 1973, *205*, 274-282.

Shaywitz, D. A., Yager, R. D., & Klopper, J. H.   Selective brain dopamine depletion in developing rats: An experimental model of minimal brain dysfunction. *Science*, 1976, *191*, 305-307.

Snyder, S., & Meyerhoff, J. L. How amphetamine acts in minimal brain dysfunction. *Annals of the New York Academy of Sciences*, 1973, *205*, 310-320.

Tarsy, D., & Baldessarini, R. J. Behavioral supersensitivity to apomorphine following chronic treatment with drugs which interfere with the synaptic functions of catecholamines. *Neuropharmacology*, 1974, *13*, 923-940.

Thornburg, J. E., & Moore, K. E. Supersensitivity to dopamine agonist following unilateral, 6-hydroxydopamine-induced striatal lesions in mice. *Journal of Pharmacology and Experimental Therapeutics*, 1975, *192*, 42-49.

Ungerstedt, U. Striatal dopamine release after amphetamine or nerve degeneration revealed by rotational behavior. *Physiologica Scandinavica*, 1971, *367*, 49-68.

Ungerstedt, U. Postsynaptic supersensitivity after 6-hydroxydopamine induced degeneration of the nigro-striatal dopamine system. *Acta Physiologica Scandinavica*, 1971, *367*, 69-93.

Ungerstedt, U., & Arbuthnott, G. W. Quantitative recording of rotational behavior in rats after 6-hydroxydopamine lesions of the nigro-striatal dopamine system. *Brain Research*, 1970, *24*, 485-493.

Von Voightlander, P. F., & Moore, K. E. Turning behavior of mice with unilateral 6-hydroxydopamine lesions in the striatum, effects of apomorphine l-dopa, amantadine, amphetamine and other psychomotor stimulants. *Neuropharmacology*, 1973, *12*, 451-462.

Yehuda, S., & Wurtman, R. J. Dopaminergic neurons in the nigrostriatal and mesolimbic pathways: Mediation of specific effects of d-amphetamine. *European Journal of Pharmacology*, 1975, *30*, 154-158.

Zimmerberg, B., & Glick, S. D. Rotation and stereotypy during electrical stimulation of the caudate nucleus. *Research Communications in Chemical Pathology and Pharmacology*, 1974, *8*, 195-196.

Zimmerberg, B., & Glick, S. D. Changes in side preference during unilateral electrical stimulation of the caudate nucleus in rats. *Brain Research*, 1975, *86*, 335-338.

Zimmerberg, B., Glick, S. D., & Jerussi, T. P. Neurochemical correlate of a spatial preference in rats. *Science*, 1974, *185*, 623-625.

# 14.
# The Development of Lateral Differences in the Human Infant

*GERALD TURKEWITZ*

Hunter College

As indicated in other papers in this volume (Collins; Gardiner & Walter; Levy; Morgan; Rubens), there has been a recent growth of concern for identifying developmentally early lateral differences in the structure or function of the nervous system. Although such identification is of obvious importance for understanding the development of lateral differentiation, there has been a tendency to use data concerning early lateralization to support oversimplifications concerning the nature of the development of lateralization. As has previously been claimed with regard to a variety of species-typical behaviors, it has been suggested that the early appearance of certain types of lateralized structure and function is indicative of a maturational unfolding of what are essentially genetic processes. Such interpretation may divert attention from the study of subtle though important developmental changes and may hinder the further exploration of developmental problems that still exist.

Recent data have indicated that the human infant is asymmetric in its response to auditory (Hammer & Turkewitz, 1975; Turkewitz, Birch, Moreau, Levy, & Cornwell, 1966a), tactile (Hammer & Turkewitz, 1974; Siqueland, 1964; Turkewitz, Gordon, & Birch, 1965), and visual (Wickelgren, 1967) stimulation and that such asymmetries are present at 24 hr of age. When the corner of an infant's mouth is touched with an artist's paintbrush, the infant turns its head in the direction of the contact. Although such an ipsiversive response is the most characteristic response to stimulation of either side, the response occurs more reliably when the stimulus is applied to the infant's right side than when it is applied to its left side (Turkewitz *et al*., 1965). In a somewhat similar fashion, infants will make ipsiversive tongue movements more reliably to somesthetic stimulation of the right margin of the tongue than of the left margin (Weiffenbach, 1972). When presented with visual targets, infants spend more time looking at the target on the right than at a comparable target on the left (Wickelgren, 1967). Finally, infants will turn their eyes in the direction of laterally presented complex auditory stimuli (Turkewitz, Birch, & Cooper, 1972a, 1972b; Turkewitz *et al*., 1966a; Turkewitz, Moreau, Birch, & Davis, 1971; Wertheimer, 1961). Although such ipsiversive eye turns are elicited by stimuli presented at either the left or the right ear, the threshold for this response to stimulation at the left is higher than for stimulation at the right (Turkewitz *et al*., 1966a). The fact that all these asymmetries are present at or shortly after birth is potentially important for an understanding of the development of lateral differences and hemispheric differentiation, but it is largely irrelevant to the question of whether lateralization of function is innate or acquired.

The early appearance of lateralization does not rule out the possibility that it is dependent on intrauterine or very early postnatal experiential factors. More than 50 years ago, Kuo (1924) in his classical discussion of the origin of behavior patterns pointed out that equating behavior present at birth with behavior that is unaffected by individual experience is highly questionable. Indeed, it has become a truism in psychology that birth does not represent the point of origin for behavioral development. Since both Schneirla (1956, 1957, 1959, 1965) and Lehrman (1953, 1956) have discussed this point extensively, it will not be discussed here. However, it should be noted that the postulation of effects of prenatal experience should not be viewed as the substitution of an explanation in terms of learning for one in terms of genetics. As Schneirla (1957) has pointed out, there are many effects of experience that are not mediated by any learning process.

In an attempt to understand the sources for order underlying some of the ontogenetically early lateral differences, a phenomenon was noted that had previously been described by Gesell (Gesell & Ames, 1947). If one goes into a nursery for healthy, full-term newborn infants and is attuned to the phenomenon, two things will be noted. First, the posture of the infant is asymmetrical; the infant lies with its head turned out of the midline. Second, this asymmetry is highly uniform; almost all the infants lie with their heads turned to the right. A series of observations (Turkewitz & Birch, 1971) of the head positions of 100 healthy infants (ranging in age from several minutes to slightly over 100 hr) revealed that when infants are in the supine position they lie with their heads turned to the right of the body midline 88% of the time, and to the left of the midline only 9% of the time. Although there was some variation in the

amount of time individual infants spent with their heads turned
to the right (a *head-right* posture), most of the infants were
observed to be in this posture well over 90% of the time.  No
infant was observed to spend more time with his head to the left
than to the right of the midline.

It was our belief that the maintenance of such a stable position preference would affect sensitivity to stimulus input and
that such effects might account, at least in part, for the kinds
of lateral differences in the infant's responsiveness to the
laterally presented stimuli we have thus far discussed.  For
example, when the supine infant lies with its head turned to the
right, its right ear is occluded, resulting in a lower level of
ambient auditory input at the right than at the left ear.
Adaptation to different levels of input at the two sides could
then result in the input to the side adapted to the lower level
of stimulation being effectively louder than an identical input
at the other side.  Such a mechanism has been found to operate
with adults.  When sounds of equal loudness are simultaneously
presented to the left and right ears, the sound source will usually be localized in the midline.  If, however, one ear is pre-
adapted to a higher level of stimulation by being primed with a
continuous sound at that ear, following which the subject is
simultaneously and equally stimulated at the two ears, the sound
source is identified as being displaced in the direction of the
ear adapted to the lower level of input (Carterette, Friedman,
Linder, & Pierce, 1965).

To determine whether a comparable mechanism might be operating
in the newborn, two groups of infants were examined.  Prior to
testing for auditory responsiveness, infants in one group were
allowed to maintain their characteristic head-right posture with
its concomitant occlusion of the right ear.  Infants in the other
group had their heads maintained in a midline position for 15
min.  Subsequent presentations of lateralized auditory stimuli
resulted in lateral differences in ipsiversive eye-turning responses by subjects allowed to maintain their asymmetrical head
positions prior to testing but no such differences in subjects
who had their heads maintained in a midline position (Turkewitz,
Moreau, & Birch, 1966b).

To determine whether asymmetries of input consequent upon
maintenance of a head-right posture might be basic to lateral
differences in responsiveness to stimulus modalities other than
audition, the effect of prior head position on the head-turning
response to somesthetic stimulation of the perioral region
(around the mouth) was studied.  As was found in the case of
audition, forced maintenance of the head in a midline position
resulted in the elimination of the lateral difference characteristic of infants tested following a period in which there is no
interference with the head position (Turkewitz, Moreau, Birch, &
Crystal, 1967).  Those infants permitted to maintain their head-
right posture prior to testing made more ipsiversive head-turning

responses to somesthetic stimulation of the perioral region on the right than on the left side. Infants whose heads were maintained in a midline position for 15 min before identical testing showed no such lateral difference in response. The finding that infants whose heads were experimentally held to the right of the midline also exhibit greater responsiveness to stimulation of the right than of the left indicates that it is not head holding per se that eliminates the lateral difference in response.

When the infant lies with its head turned to the right there is differential tonus of the neck muscles on the two sides. In addition, there is differential stimulation to the two sides of the infant's face. In a study that separated the occurrence of these two concomitants of an asymmetrical head posture, it was found that both were capable of affecting lateral differences in the infants' responsiveness (Turkewitz, Moreau, Davis, & Birch, 1969). Four groups of infants were involved in this study. Asymmetry of both muscle tonus and of somesthetic input was reduced in one group by having the infant's head held in the midline. Asymmetry of tonus without an associated asymmetry of somesthetic input was produced in a second group by holding the infant's head to the right without allowing the cheek to make contact with the substrate. Asymmetry of input without accompanying asymmetry of tonus was produced by maintaining the head in the midline and intermittently stroking the infant's cheek. The third group of infants was stroked on the right cheek and the final group on the left cheek. In each case the prestimulation period lasted 15 min. Following these treatments the infants were tested for lateral differences in their head-turning response to somesthetic stimulation of the perioral region. Those infants exposed to a lateral difference in tonus or prestimulated on the right cheek were more responsive to stimulation of the right than of the left. Those who had reduced asymmetries of both tonus and somesthetic input exhibited no lateral difference in response.

The picture was complicated somewhat by the finding that identical prestimulation of the left and right cheeks did not have equal and opposite effects. Whereas prestimulation of the right cheek resulted in greater responsiveness to stimulation of the right than of the left, prestimulation of the left cheek resulted in the absence of a lateral difference in responsiveness to subsequently applied somesthetic stimulation.

This failure to obtain equivalent effects from stimulation at the two sides means that the effects of prior somesthetic stimulation on lateral differentiation cannot be understood in terms of a simple and direct effect of immediately preceding stimulation on an organism that is otherwise laterally undifferentiated. Rather, it suggests that the effect of asymmetry of somesthetic input interacts with at least one other form of asymmetry to determine the nature of lateral differences in responsiveness. Although the nature of this asymmetry is unknown (cf. Rubens, this volume), it is likely that the effects of prior stimulation of the right side summate with it to produce greater responsiveness to stimulation of the right than of the left. Prior stimulation of the left, however, produces an effect that is not great enough to overcome the preexisting right-side advantage; it merely serves to neutralize this advantage, resulting in equivalent degrees of responsiveness to stimulation of the two sides.

These findings, substantiating the importance of the infant's asymmetrical head position for determining lateral differences in its responsiveness to various forms of stimulation, should also call attention to the complexities that exist in determining lateral differences even during the first days of life. Further evidence of these complexities is provided by examination of age-related changes in the infant's assumption of the head-right posture. The evidence presented thus far suggests that the infant's head-right posture serves as the keystone in the development of various lateral differences in responsiveness to stimulation. Despite the critical role the infant's posture plays there is evidence suggesting that the relationship between posture and responsiveness may be reciprocal rather than unidirectional.

Recent evidence (Turkewitz & Creighton, 1974) suggests that the lateral differences in responsiveness that accompany and follow maintenance of a head-right posture may serve to increase the likelihood of the infant's assuming such a posture. Infants between 12 and 72 hr of age usually show a head-right posture even after lateral differences in responsiveness have been eliminated by holding their heads in a midline position for 15 min. That is, when the infant's head is released following such a procedure, approximately 75% of infants make their initial turn toward the right. Furthermore, when the side first making contact with the mattress is noted, it is found that almost 90% of such contacts are made with the right side of the face. These findings suggest that in these infants the assumption of a head-right posture is independent of lateral differences in responsiveness. However, when very young infants, those under 12 hr of age, are examined, it is found that the assumption of a head-right posture may not be independent of lateral differences in responsiveness. Thus, even in these very young infants, if the lateral differences in responsiveness are not interfered with and the infant's head is released from a momentarily maintained midline position, most of the infants turn their heads toward the right. If, however, lateral differences are reduced or eliminated in these very young infants by maintenance of their heads in a midline position for 15 min, the tendency to assume a head-right posture is eliminated. The infants are as likely to turn left as right following such a procedure.

Although alternative explanations of various features of these data are possible, the data do suggest a complex set of developmental relationships between the assumption and maintenance of an asymmetrical head position and lateral differences in response to various aspects of stimulation. The picture that emerges is one in which an initially systematic but relatively impermanent asymmetric head-position bias gives rise to lateral differences in response to auditory and somesthetic stimulation and possibly to lateral differences in response to stimuli in other modalities as well. These lateral differences in response, by making it more likely that the infant will turn to the right than to the left, may serve to strengthen the initially modifiable position bias so that its maintenance comes to be independent of the lateral differences in responsiveness that nurtured it. In a similar manner, it is possible that, with subsequent development, lateral differences in responsiveness can come to be independent of the asymmetrical head position upon which they were initially based (cf. Anderson; Berlin; Gur & Gur; Springer, this volume).

It should be apparent that the basis for the infant's initial head-right bias has not yet been identified. The following fairly reasonable hypothesis has been eliminated but others remain to be tested or developed: Since most babies are born in a left occipital anterior position (i.e., a position in which the head is turned to the right), it seemed possible that passage through the birth canal might be involved in the establishment of the right turning bias. In order to examine this possibility, Turkewitz and Creighton (unpublished), examined the head position of a group of infants who, because they were born via cesarean section, had not passed through the birth canal in the usual manner. It was found that such infants did not differ from normally born infants with regard to the assumption of a head-right posture following release from a midline position. It is still possible, however, that the position bias is related to the infant's position in utero. Gottlieb and Kuo (1965) have suggested an association between the position of the duckling in the egg and subsequent lateral differences in its response to tactile stimulation. (See also Chapple; Morgan, this volume.)

Whatever the basis for the head position bias turns out to be, it is unlikely that the solution of the problem will be aided by simplistic formulations in terms of innate or acquired, or even--in a more modern guise--between prewired and learned. The data thus far are sufficient to indicate that ontogenetically early lateral differences in responsiveness are the outcome of complexly interrelated factors in the developmental history of the infant. It appears unlikely that further investigation will result in any marked simplification of the picture thus far obtained. In fact, it appears more reasonable to believe that further investigation will reveal other factors relating to the early manifestation of lateral differences. When one attempts to relate these early lateral differences to later aspects of lateral differentiation, it would be wise to be prepared to find complex and not necessarily self-apparent relationships between early development and later functioning.

LATERAL DIFFERENCES IN THE HUMAN INFANT

SUMMARY

The 2-day-old human infant is asymmetrical in its response to auditory and somesthetic stimuli.
These lateral differences can be eliminated by holding the infant's head in a midline position prior to testing. It seems likely therefore that these asymmetries are in part dependent on the infant's prior maintenance of a head-right posture. This posture probably affects lateral differences in responsiveness because it results in both differential input to the two sides and differential muscle tonus. This hypothesis is supported by the finding that lateral differences in either prestimulation or tonus result in lateral differences in response to somesthetic stimulation.
Although much evidence suggests that the infant's asymmetrical posture is basic to the early appearance of lateral differences in its response to stimulation, there is also evidence that suggests a possible reciprocal relationship between posture and responsiveness. Although infants over 12 hr of age assume a head-right posture following the elimination of lateral differences in responsiveness, infants below this age do not.
The data support the view that lateral differences present during early stages of development are the result of a complex set of interrelationships among a variety of factors.

REFERENCES

Carterette, E. C., Friedman, M. P., Lindner, W., & Pierce, J. Lateralization of sounds at the unstimulated ear opposite a noise-adapted ear. *Science*, 1965, *147*, 63-65.
Gesell, A., & Ames, L. B. The development of handedness. *Journal of Genetic Psychology*, 1947, *70*, 155-175.
Gottlieb, G., & Kuo, Z. Y. Development of behavior in the duck embryo. *Journal of Comparative and Physiological Psychology*, 1965, *59*, 183-188.
Hammer, M., & Turkewitz, G. A sensory basis for the lateral difference in the newborn infant's response to somesthetic stimulation. *Journal of Experimental Child Psychology*, 1974, *18*, 304-312.
Hammer, M., & Turkewitz, G. Relationship between effective intensity of auditory stimulation and directional eye turns in the human newborn. *Animal Behaviour*, 1975, *23*, 287-290.
Kuo, Z. Y. A psychology without heredity. *Psychological Review*, 1924, *31*, 427-448.
Lehrman, D. S. A critique of Lorenz' "objectivistic" theory of animal behavior. *Quarterly Review of Biology*, 1953, *28*, 337-363.
Lehrman, D. S. On the organization of maternal behavior and the problem of instinct. In P. P. Grasse (Ed.), *L'instinct dans*

*le comportement des animaux et de l'homme*. Paris: Masson, 1956.

Schneirla, T. C. Interrelationships of the "innate" and the "acquired" in instinctive behavior. In P. P. Grasse (Ed.), *L'instinct dans le comportement des animaux et de l'homme*. Paris: Masson, 1956.

Schneirla, T. C. The concept of development in comparative psychology. In D. B. Harris (Ed.), *The concept of development*. Minneapolis: Univ. of Minnesota Press, 1957.

Schneirla, T. C. An evolutionary and developmental theory of biphasic processes underlying approach and withdrawal. In M. R. Jones (Ed.), *Current theory and research on motivation*. Vol. 7. Lincoln: Univ. of Nebraska Press, 1959.

Schneirla, T. C. Aspects of stimulation and organization in approach/withdrawal processes underlying vertebrate behavioral development. In D. S. Lehrman, R. A. Hinde, & E. Shaw (Eds.), *Advances in the study of behavior*. Vol. 1. New York: Academic Press, 1965.

Siqueland, E. Operant conditioning of head turning in four-month infants. *Psychonomic Science*, 1964, *1*, 223-224.

Turkewitz, G., & Birch, G. H. Neurobehavioral organization of the human newborn. In J. Hellmuth (Ed.), *Exceptional infant, 2: Studies in abnormalities*. New York: Brunner/Mazel, 1971.

Turkewitz, G., Birch, H.G., & Cooper, K. K. Responsiveness to simple and complex auditory stimuli in the human newborn. *Developmental Psychobiology*, 1972, *5*, 7-19.(a)

Turkewitz, G., Birch, H. G., & Cooper, K. K. Patterns of response to different auditory stimuli in the human newborn. *Developmental Medicine and Child Neurology*, 1972, *14*, 487-491.(b)

Turkewitz, G., Birch, H. G., Moreau, T., Levy, L., & Cornwell, A. C. Effect of intensity of auditory stimulation on directional eye movements in the human neonate. *Animal Behaviour*, 1966, *14*, 93-101.(a)

Turkewitz, G., & Creighton, S. Changes in lateral differentiation of head posture in the human neonate. *Developmental Psychobiology*, 1974, *8*, 85-89.

Turkewitz, G., Gordon, E. W., & Birch, H. G. Head turning in the human neonate: Spontaneous patterns. *Journal of Genetic Psychology*, 1965, *107*, 143-158.

Turkewitz, G., Moreau, T., & Birch, H. G. Head position and receptor organization in the human neonate. *Journal of Experimental Psychology*, 1966, *4*, 169-177.(b)

Turkewitz, G., Moreau, T., Birch, H. G., & Crystal, D. Relationship between prior head position and lateral differences in responsiveness to somesthetic stimulation in the human neonate. *Journal of Experimental Child Psychology*, 1967, *5*, 548-561.

Turkewitz, G., Moreau, T., Birch, H. G., & Davis, L. Relation-

LATERAL DIFFERENCES IN THE HUMAN INFANT

ships among responses in the human newborn: The non-association and non-equivalence among different indicators of responsiveness. *Psychophysiology*, 1971, 7, 233-247.

Turkewitz, G., Moreau, T., Davis, L., & Birch, H.G. Factors affecting lateral differentiation in the human newborn. *Journal of Experimental Child Psychology*, 1969, *8*, 483-493.

Weiffenbach, J. M. Discrete elicited motions of the newborn's tongue. In J. F. Bosma (Ed.), *Third symposium on oral sensation and perception*. Springfield, Illinois: C. C. Thomas, 1972.

Wickelgren, L. W. Convergence in the human newborn. *Journal of Experimental Child Psychology*, 1967, *5*, 74-85.

# 15.
# Correlates of Conjugate Lateral Eye Movements in Man

*RAQUEL GUR AND RUBEN GUR*

University of Pennsylvania

Localization of function within the brain is generally studied by integrating clinical findings obtained from brain-injured patients with more closely controllable laboratory investigations on animals. Human clinical data are frequently difficult to interpret, however. There is usually little information concerning performance prior to injury; moreover, the precise extent of injury is often difficult to determine. As a consequence, conclusions tend to be *post hoc*. Mapping of higher cognitive functions of the human brain through inference from animal experimentation, on the other hand, is limited by various apparent discontinuities between man and nonhuman species, particularly with regard to hemispheric asymmetries of function (Levy, 1969; cf. Dewson; Doty & Overman; Hamilton; Stamm, Rosen, & Gadotti; Warren, this volume). It is these peculiarly human lateralized cognitive functions and their performance and personality correlates that are the objects of study in the research described in this chapter.

Both the discovery of functional differences between the two cerebral hemispheres of the human brain and the first major steps toward identifying the specific functions subserved by each hemisphere have been accomplished primarily through the study of patients with unilateral brain damage (see Hécaen, 1969 or McFie, 1969 for a summary of the effects of left-hemisphere lesions, and Bogen, 1969, for a review of the reported effects of lesions to the right hemisphere). A major advance in the study of lateral differentiation of function in the human brain came with the

investigation of patients in whom the hemispheres had been surgically separated by midline section of the neocortical commissures
(Gazzaniga, Bogen, & Sperry, 1962; Sperry & Gazzaniga, 1967).
Here, for the first time, interhemispheric comparisons could be
made in the same individual, permitting more direct conclusions to
be drawn concerning the nature of the functional asymmetries.

In spite of the richness of information that can be obtained
from studying split-brain patients, the small number of such
patients available for study is a drawback. Furthermore, the results obtained are open to the criticism that some of the effects
are probably influenced by preoperative conditions, since all
these patients were epileptics prior to the operation. Finally,
the way the two hemispheres *interact* in the normal person cannot
be studied with patients in whom either one hemisphere is damaged
or the callosal connections between hemispheres are severed.

It is partly for these reasons that a number of techniques
have been developed to study functional brain asymmetry in normal,
intact subjects. These techniques make use of lateralized input
and output modes, capitalizing on partially separate pathways in
the intact nervous system. They include procedures such as dichotic presentation of auditory stimuli (Kimura, 1967; Knox &
Kimura, 1970; see Berlin; Springer, this volume), tachistoscopic
presentation of visual stimuli to the left and right visual half-
fields (Kimura, 1966; Rizzolatti, Umilta, & Berlucchi, 1971; see
Springer, this volume), tactile stimulation of the two hands
(Benton, 1972; Carmon, 1971; Ingram, 1973), and monitoring the
direction of conjugate lateral eye movements during various types
of mental activity (Gur, Gur, & Harris, 1975; Kinsbourne, 1972;
Kocel, Galin, Ornstein, & Merrin, 1972; see Anderson, this volume). Other methods to investigate activity in the two hemispheres of intact subjects have included recording scalp EEG activity over the two hemispheres during the performance of various
tasks thought to engage the hemispheres differentially (Galin &
Ornstein, 1972; McKee, Humphrey, & McAdam, 1973; Morgan,
MacDonald & Hilgard, 1974; see Gardiner & Walter, this volume),
bilateral recording of evoked potentials (Bigum, 1969; Morrell &
Salamy, 1971; see Donchin, Kutas, & McCarthy; Thatcher, this volume), and, recently, monitoring of manual gestures (Kimura,
1973a, 1973b).

A number of global dichotomies have been suggested to describe
the overall differences between the two hemispheres. The early
verbal (left) versus spatial (right) dichotomy was amplified by
others such as analytic-synthetic (Levy, 1969), propositional-
appositional (Bogen, 1969), logical and rational versus holistic
and intuitive (Ornstein, 1972), and serial-parallel (Cohen, 1973).
These dichotomies are not mutually exclusive, nor do they necessarily reflect any basic disagreement over fact or theory.
Rather, they seem to convey differences in emphasis and perspective.

Along with the discovery of functional differences between the hemispheres, evidence has started to accumulate suggesting that there are individual differences in the tendency to use modes of information processing and problem solving characteristic of one hemisphere or the other. Thus, Bogen (1969) observed individual differences in what he called *hemisphericity*, Ornstein (1972) discussed individual differences in logical versus intuitive cognitive styles, and Bakan (1969) offered the typology of right-hemisphere and left-hemisphere people.

If individuals do indeed differ in a tendency to rely on one or the other hemispheric mode of information processing, one might expect this to be reflected in differences on psychological variables, ranging from cognitive to conative in nature. The investigation of these correlates may shed light on the nature of hemispheric differences as well as interhemispheric interactions in various tasks and situations. The purpose of this chapter is to report a series of studies aimed at validating a measure of asymmetric hemispheric activation and examining individual differences with respect to this variable and some of its correlates. The optimal measure would reflect the hemispheric information-processing mode employed by an individual and would enable quantitative comparisons between individuals. The measure chosen for these purposes was *direction of conjugate lateral eye movement* (see also Anderson; Turkewitz, this volume).

## VALIDATION OF CONJUGATE LATERAL EYE MOVEMENTS AS AN INDEX OF HEMISPHERIC ACTIVATION

It has been observed since 1890 (Mott & Shafer, 1890; Penfield & Roberts, 1959) that electrical stimulation of a number of sites in one cerebral hemisphere can produce a deviation of the eyes toward the opposite side. The biological basis for this association between asymmetric hemispheric activation and orientation toward the contralateral field was discussed by Trevarthen (1972). He suggested that bilaterally symmetric animals have had to evolve a system of sensorimotor integration that would generate an orientation reflex toward a source of stimulation. In vertebrates in which each sensory half-field is projected to the contralateral hemisphere (see Gross & Mishkin, this volume), this implies the evolution of a system that produces contralateral orientation in the presence of asymmetric hemispheric activity. Concerning other species, it is not yet clear whether, apart from (1) asymmetric sensory input, (2) asymmetric motor output, or (3) direct electrical stimulation, anything *else* may involve asymmetric cerebral activity (cf. Stamm *et al.*, this volume). However, it is known that in man this can also be caused by laterally specialized processing. Trevarthen claims that, irrespective of the factors responsible for asymmetric activity, an orientation reflex (or its covert homologue, an attentional bias) toward the side of space contralateral to the more active side has a tendency to accompany the activity (see Glick, Jerussi, & Zimmerberg; Heilman & Watson, this volume). Conjugate lateral eye movements are a component of this contralateral orienting response.

A series of recent experiments has investigated the conditions under which conjugate lateral eye movements occur in human subjects. Teitelbaum (1954) was the first to report the observation that when a subject is faced by a questioner he usually breaks eye contact following the presentation of a question and moves his eyes either to the right or to the left. This phenomenon was later investigated more thoroughly by Day (1964), who found that the direction in which the eyes move is fairly consistent for a given individual. Duke (1968) offered further experimental support for these observations and suggested a new typology, *left-movers* and *right-movers*. A series of investigations by Day (1964, 1967a, b, 1968) revealed various differences between right-movers and left-movers. These differences were "most clearly related to differences in the experience of anxiety, language styles, cognitive styles and thus to personality variables [Day, 1967b, p. 51]."

Bakan and Shotland (1969) found that right-movers performed better than left-movers on specific tasks that require visual attention. Left-movers, on the other hand, reported clearer visual images (Bakan, 1969) and were more fluent verbally than were right-movers. In addition, left-movers were likely to display more resting EEG alpha activity. They also more frequently majored in the humanities and social sciences in college and performed better on the verbal than on the mathematical section of the Scholastic Aptitude Test (SAT). Right-movers tended to display less alpha activity, preferred majors in science, and had relatively higher mathematical SAT scores (Bakan, 1969, 1971; Bakan & Svorad, 1969).

Bakan (1971) attempted to account for the differences between left-movers and right-movers by interpreting eye movement directionality as an indication of relative "predominance" of one of the two cerebral hemispheres. According to Bakan (1971), lateral eye movement indicates easier triggering of activity in the hemisphere contralateral to the direction of eye movement irrespective of the content of the problem put to the subject (see Anderson, this volume).

At first glance these findings appear inconsistent with the results of studies by Kinsbourne (1972) and Kocel *et al.* (1972). These investigators recorded eye and head movements of undergraduate sbujects as the subjects responded to questions asked by an experimenter seated behind them. The recordings were made by a hidden videotape camera. It was found that direction of movement was related to problem type: Subjects showed a significant tendency to move their eyes to the right for verbal problems, and either upward or to the left for spatial problems.

Is the direction of conjugate lateral eye movement an enduring personality trait, as suggested by Bakan (1971), or does it depend on the types of problems presented to the subject, as suggested by Kinsbourne (1972)? We conjectured that differences in procedure might account for the apparent inconsistency in these results. The most obvious difference between the procedures is that in Kinsbourne's (1972) study the experimenter was seated behind the subject and the eye movements were recorded by a hidden videotape camera. Kinsbourne (1971) had suggested that the face-to-face findings may be attributable to errors caused by the experimenter's own subconscious lateral gaze behavior, as well as from lack of control of the appearance of the background. However, in at least some of the face-to-face studies (Baken & Shotland, 1969; Gur & Reyher, 1973), both factors were carefully controlled. Furthermore, it is unlikely that these results were artifacts since various personality and behavioral differences were found to be significantly associated with an individual's characteristic eye-movement directionality in those studies in which a consistent directional bias was observed.

The difference between the two lines of results may indeed be linked with aspects of the experimental situation, but, contrary to the implication in Kinsbourne's criticism, perhaps in a systematic and meaningful way. We conjectured that the face-to-face situation, being obviously interpersonal, may be more threatening and anxiety provoking. Under such conditions an anxious subject may tend to fall back on certain characteristic modes of response. That is, when questioned, he may tend to "rely" on the hemisphere that is more compatible with his characteristic cognitive style, even though it might be the "wrong" hemisphere for a particular kind of problem. When the testing situation is impersonal (the experimenter is behind the subject), less anxiety would be elicited, permitting optimal hemispheric information-processing in accordance with the type of problem.

We tested this hypothesis by directly comparing both procedures on the same subjects. The subjects were 32 right-handed and 17 left-handed undergraduate males. Handedness was determined by a 20-item questionnaire (Humphrey, 1951). Following Kinsbourne (1972), three types of questions were used: verbal (explanation of proverbs), numerical (solution of arithmetic problems), and spatial (visualization and identification of spatial relationships of familiar places and visual arrangements). There were 20 pairs of parallel questions for each type, constituting a pool of 120 questions. From this pool, two test forms of 60 questions each were constructed, each form with 20 verbal, 20 spatial, and 20 numerical questions. Within each form, the 60 questions were randomly ordered, with the constraint that within each triad of questions, each problem type appeared once. Examples of proverbs to be explained by the subject follow: "Rome was not built in a day," "All that glitters is not gold," and "A bird in the hand is worth two in the bush." Examples of numerical questions are "69 times 14 equals (?)" "1935 minus 829 equals (?)" and "Square 75 minus 62." Examples of spatial questions are "Imagine the map of the United States. Where is Chicago relative to Minneapolis?"

"Visualize sitting in front of a typewriter. Where is the letter
R relative to B?" and "Visualize your library card. Where is
your student number relative to your name?"

Subjects were tested individually in a 2.5 x 2 m portable experimental room placed within a laboratory. The walls of the
room were 2 m high and were completely covered with cloth to provide a perfectly homogeneous surrounding.

The two experimental sessions, separated by 1 week, were presented in a counterbalanced order. Each of the two 60-item forms
was presented in one session. The order of presentation of the
forms was counterbalanced across subjects.

## Experimenter behind the subject

The subject was seated at a small table 1.2 m from the wall,
with the experimenter seated about .8 m behind him. The subject
was told to concentrate on answering a series of questions, to
remain seated, and not to look behind him. The experimenter then
read the questions and recorded the subject's answers. Each trial
was concluded either when the subject answered or after 30 sec.
Eye movements were recorded by a hidden television camera and
scored from a monitor by two independent judges seated in a
separate room of the laboratory.

## Experimenter facing the subject

The subject sat in the same position as in the prior condition
but now the experimenter sat directly opposite him at a distance
of .8 m. The instructions were the same as when the experimenter
was behind the subjects. The experimenter read the questions and
recorded both the answers and eye-movement directionality.

The experimenters were two 20-year-old undergraduate women unaware of the experimental predictions. Each subject was tested
by the same experimenter for his two sessions. Each session
lasted approximately 30 min.

The results for right-handed subjects were clear-cut. As can
be seen in Figure 1, when the experimenter was behind the subjects, the subjects moved their eyes predominantly to the right
for the verbal questions (indicating left-hemisphere activation),
and primarily to the left for spatial questions (indicating
right-hemisphere activation).

When the experimenter was in front, however, problem type had
no effect on eye-movement directionality (see Figure 2). Rather,
the lateral eye-movement distribution for the same subjects
appeared bimodal under this condition, suggesting that regardless
of problem type one group of subjects tended to move their eyes
predominantly to the right, whereas another group of subjects
moved their eyes predominantly to the left.

Left-handers showed the tendency to move their eyes characteristically in one direction when the experimenter faced them, but

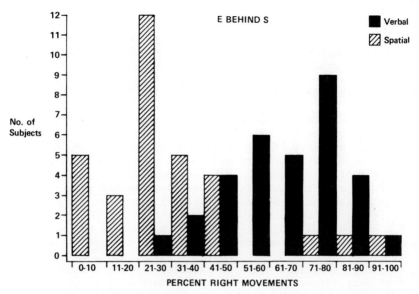

Fig. 1.  *Number of right-handed subjects within each range of proportions of eye movements to the right, for verbal and spatial problems, when the Experimenter (E) was behind the subject (S). From Gur, Gur, & Harris, 1975.*

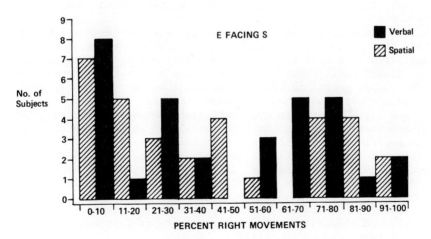

Fig. 2.  *Number of right-handed subjects within each range of proportions of eye movements to the right, for verbal and spatial problems, when the experimenter (E) was facing the subject (S). From Gur, Gur, & Harris, 1975.*

they did not move their eyes according to the type of problem when the experimenter was behind them. Some moved their eyes in the same direction for both verbal and spatial questions, others showed a pattern of eye movements that was the reverse of that shown by right-handers (i.e., left for verbal and right for spatial problems), and still others seemed to move their eyes haphazardly. This finding supports the notion that left-handers, as a group, are not as lateralized in terms of hemisphere function as are right-handers (Hécaen & Ajuriaguerra, 1964).

In light of these findings and other data pertaining to the functional asymmetry of the brain, the question arises as to whether directionally "appropriate" eye movements would be correlated with superior performance on a task. Specifically, since a movement of the eyes to the left presumably indicates relatively greater activation of the right cerebral hemisphere, a movement to the left in response to a spatial question ought to be associated with a more accurate answer than would a movement to the right. Conversely, rightward movement, in response to a verbal question, ought to be associated with greater accuracy than leftware movement. These relations would be expected for right-handers. For left-handers, directional predictions would be less clear-cut.

To assess these relationships, we compared the accuracy of each subject's performance on those verbal and spatial questions to which the direction of eye movements was appropriate with his accuracy on those questions to which the direction was inappropriate. We included only those subjects who made at least two movements in each direction within a set of 20 questions. Each response was scored for completeness and correctness.

For right-handers, with the experimenter behind them, performance on verbal questions was better with right movements than left movements to a marginally significant degree ($t = 1.68$, $df = 22$, $.05 < p < .06$, one-tailed). On spatial questions, performance was slightly better with left movements, but the difference was not significant. With the experimenter in front, performance on the spatial questions was significantly better ($t = 2.67$, $df = 18$, $p < .01$, one-tailed) when eye movements were to the left.

For left-handers, in contrast, right movements were associated with better performance on both verbal and spatial questions when the experimenter was in front, but this difference was significant only for the spatial questions ($t = 2.62$, $df = 15$, $p < .02$, two-tailed). These results, like the main findings, support the view that left-handers are not as lateralized for hemispheric functioning as are right-handers.

Finally, none of the differences among the numerical questions approached significance for either right- or left-handers, in either testing condition (all $t$'s $< 1.0$).

We concluded from the results obtained in both experimental paradigms that gaze direction in response to questions is determined both by problem type and by the individual's characteristic tendency to "use" a certain hemisphere. The influence of the first factor seems to be maximized when the experimenter is seated behind the subject, whereas the influence of the second factor is maximized when the experimenter faces the subject.

Having taken a step toward validating the measure of conjugate lateral eye-movement directionality in the face-to-face situation as indicative of individual differences in *hemisphere activation bias*, we have proceeded to explore behavioral correlates of these differences.

## CONJUGATE LATERAL EYE MOVEMENTS AND HYPNOTIC SUSCEPTIBILITY

Hypnotic susceptibility, as measured by standardized scales, appears to be a relatively stable and enduring personality trait (Hilgard, 1965; R. C. Gur, 1974).

Hyponsis has been described as a regressive mode of relating interpersonally (Gill & Brenman, 1959), requiring an "imaginative involvement" on the part of the subject (J. R. Hilgard, 1970), and an ability to concentrate on an object without thinking discursively or analytically (Van Nuys, 1973). These characteristics are reminiscent of some current views of right-hemisphere functioning (Ornstein, 1972). One might accordingly expect hypnotizability (in right-handed subjects) to be related to a bias toward right-hemisphere activation.

This prediction was supported by Bakan's (1969) finding that right-movers tend to be less hypnotizable than left-movers. He asked subjects five questions and found a significant negative correlation of -.44 between number of eye movements to the right in response to questioning and hypnotic susceptibility as measured by the Stanford Hypnotic Susceptibility Scale, Form C (SHSS:C; Weitzenhoffer & Hilgard, 1962). Morgan, McDonald, & MacDonald (1971) have replicated this finding, again obtaining a significant, albeit lower (-.22) negative correlation between the number of eye movements to the right and hypnotic susceptibility. There is also some evidence that right- and left-movers differ in terms of the kind of hypnotic induction technique to which they are most responsive (Gur & Reyher, 1973).

If hypnotic susceptibility is somehow related to interhemisphere differences, one might expect sex and handedness to be variables moderating this relationship, since there is evidence that males differ from females, and right-handers from left-handers, in the degree to which their hemispheres are functionally lateralized. Left-handers (Benton, 1962; Hécaen & Ajuriaguerra, 1964) and females (Harshman & Remmington, 1976; McGlone & Davidson, 1973; cf. Collins, this volume) appear to be less lateralized, with their language functions represented relatively more bilaterally; in particular, the normally nonverbal right hemisphere is more like the left in its linguistic capabilities. In addition, both these groups demonstrate difficulties in performing spatial tasks when compared to male right-handers (Harris,

1975; Knox & Kimura, 1970; Lansdell, 1961, 1962; Levy, 1969; Miller, 1971; Nebes, 1971). This is thought to be a consequence of bilateral language preempting some of the specialization of the right hemisphere.

Some evidence suggesting that handedness may be related to hypnotizability was provided by Bakan (1970), who found that left-handers tended to score at the extremes, either high or low, on a hypnotic susceptibility scale, rather than the middle. Left-handers, however, also vary much more than do right handers in terms of strength and consistency of hand use and eyedness (Humphrey, 1951). One might accordingly expect that degree of lateralization and concordance of hand-eye preference would serve as another moderator variable among left-handers in the relation between hypnotizability and eye-movement directionality in this group.

Sex was not taken into account in Bakan's (1969, 1970) studies, and only right-handed males were used in Gur and Reyher's (1973) study. Our purpose was to explore the relation between eye-movement directionality and hypnotic susceptibility and the possible moderating effect of sex, handedness and eyedness (as an additional indicator of lateralization).

Sixty right-handers (30 male, 30 female) were randomly selected from a total sample of 270 undergraduate volunteers. From this total sample, 30 left-handers (19 males and 11 females) were also selected. Initially, handedness was defined on the basis of the response to the question "Are you right-handed, left-handed, or ambidextrous?" Subsequently, the subjects chosen were administered Part A of Humphrey's (1951) questionnaire, which assesses hand usage for a variety of tasks. Eye-movement directionality and eye dominance were measured as described in Gur and Gur (1974).

Hypnotic susceptibility was measured both by a group scale (the Harvard Group Scale of Hypnotic Susceptibility; Shor & Orne, 1962) and by a more advanced scale administered individually (the Stanford Hypnotic Susceptibility Scale, Form C; Weitzenhoffer & Hilgard, 1962). The experimenters were seven male and four female undergraduate honors students unfamiliar with the experimental hypotheses.

The main findings were as follows:

1. For the total sample, eye movements to the left and hypnotic susceptibility were moderately related ($n = 90$, $r = -.21$, $p < .05$).

2. When handedness was introduced as a moderating variable, the results showed that this relationship existed for right-handed subjects only.

3. When sex was introduced as a moderating variable, the results showed the relationship to be present only for males.

4. When the combined moderating effect of both sex and handedness were considered, the results still showed that the sole

significant association, that between hypnotizability and leftward eye movements, was only exhibited by right-handed males. There appeared to be a trend toward the reverse association (hypnotizability with rightward eye movements) in left-handed females (see Figure 3).

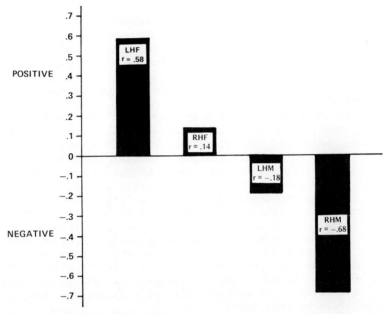

*Fig. 3. Magnitude and direction of correlations between number of eye movements to the right and hypnotic susceptibility for right-handed males (RHM), left-handed males (LHM), right-handed females (RHF), and left-handed females. From Gur & Gur, 1974.*

5. When eye dominance was introduced as a moderating variable for left-handed males and right-handed females (the two groups showing no association between eye-movement bias and hypnotizability), the results showed that for left-handed, *left-eyed* males, hypnotizability is associated with rightward eye movements ($r$ = .52) whereas for left-handed *right-eyed* males hypnotic susceptibility is associated with leftward eye movement ($r$ = −.41; $z$ = 1.75; $p$ <.05). For the right-handed females, the correlations were not significantly different although there was again a trend toward a reverse association with the correlation between leftward eye movements and hypnotic susceptibility positive for the left-eyed ($r$ = .35) and negative for the right-eyed ($r$ = −.20; $z$ = 1.37; not significant).

The results support the idea that the ability to become

271

hypnotized is related to a hemisphere bias as measured by eye-movement directionality, but the relation is complex, depending on other variables such as degree and direction of functional lateralization, as well as peripheral eye and hand laterality.

## CONJUGATE LATERAL EYE MOVEMENTS AND PERSONALITY

If, indeed, left- and right-movers differ in a tendency to rely on one or the other hemisphere, one would also expect them to show corresponding differences in their characteristic modes of coping with problems and conflicts. Left-movers would be expected to be more holistic and nonverbal, whereas right-movers should be more analytic and should use more verbal elaborations in their coping or defense mechanisms.

Using an inventory developed by Gleser and Ihilevich (1969; Gleser & Sacks, 1973) to measure individual differences in modes of defense, we tested the hypothesis that left-movers differ from right-movers in their characteristic defense clusters. It was predicted that left-movers would score higher on a defense cluster that internalized conflict in a holistic and preverbal fashion, whereas right-movers would score higher on defense clusters that externalized conflict and involved verbal elaborations.

The Defense Mechanism Inventory (DMI) was administered to a group of 28 right-handed males, whose eye-movement directionality had been previously determined using the battery of 60 questions developed by Gur, Gur, and Harris (1975). The DMI classifies people according to the kinds of defense they tend to use most frequently. Five major defenses (Gleser & Ihilevich, 1969, p. 52) are identified by this test:

1. Turning Against Others (TAO), characterized as dealing with conflict: "through attacking a real or presumed external frustrating object."
2. Projection (PRO), characterized as expressing aggression toward an external object "through first attributing to it, without unequivocal evidence, negative intent, or characteristics."
3. Principalization (PRN), characterized as dealing with conflicts "through invoking a general principle that 'splits off' affect from content and represses the former."
4. Turning Against Self (TAS), characterized as "directing aggressive behavior toward S [subject] himself."
5. Reversal (REV), characterized as defenses such as repression, denial, negation, and reaction formation, which "deal with conflict by responding in a positive or neutral fashion to a frustrating object."

The results (see Figure 4) indicate that the three groups differed on three of the five defense mechanisms. Scheffé's (1959) method for multiple comparisons was used to determine which

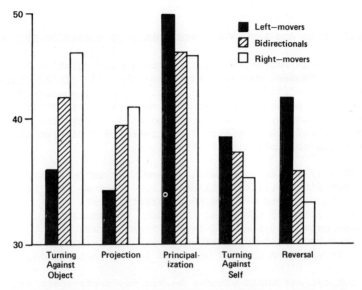

*Fig. 4. Comparisons among left-movers, right-movers, and bidirectional subjects on the Defense Mechanism Inventory.*

differences among the group means contributed significantly to the between-group variance. On TAO, right-movers scored significantly higher than left-movers, but not significantly higher than bidirectionals, whose mean score fell between the two. On the PRO, both right-movers and bidirectionals scored significantly higher than left-movers and were not significantly different from each other. On REV, left-movers scored significantly higher than right-movers, but not significantly higher than bidirectionals.

These results have been replicated in a recent investigation by Packer (1975), with the exception that bidirectional subjects did not exhibit any consistent pattern, whereas in the previous study they had consistently scored between the other two groups.

The finding that left-movers differed from right-movers on the REV defense cluster led us to expect the groups to differ also in terms of amount of reported psychosomatic symptomatology, since both in laboratory (Perkins & Reyher, 1971; Reyher, 1961; Sommerschield & Reyher, 1973) and field studies (Reyher & Basch, 1970), degree of repression has been found to be related to psychosomatic complaints (e.g., headaches, ulcer). Left-movers were therefore expected to report a larger amount of psychosomatic symptomatology.

A physical health questionnaire, administered to the same 28 subjects, showed this to be the case. Left-movers reported an average of 9.5 psychosomatic symptoms (SD = 4.99), right-movers reported an average of 5.5 symptoms (SD = 2.88), whereas bidirectional subjects reported 5.4 symptoms (SD = 3.02) on the

273

$[F\ (2,25)\ =\ 3.59;\ p\ <\ .05]$.

## HEMISPHERE BIAS AND LEFT-RIGHT PREFERENCE IN CLASSROOM SEATING

Gur, Gur, and Marshalek (1975) examined the relation between lateral eye-movement directionality and the side of the classroom on which individuals prefer to sit. Ninety undergraduates who had participated in the hypnotic susceptibility study described previously were contacted by mail. They were asked to fill out a brief questionnaire that presented a diagram of a classroom and the following instructions:

> This is a diagram of a classroom. It is an inside room with artificial illumination. Assume that it is possible to see and hear perfectly well from all points of the room. The door is exactly at the back center of the room. Please check the seat you would typically occupy. Think about the seat you have usually occupied in the last period.

The subject was asked whether he had any preferences for "soft" topics, such as art, and for "hard" topics, such as mathematics or physics. If he had, he was asked to mark his preference by inserting $S$ for "soft" and $H$ for "hard." Seventy-four subjects responded (41 males and 33 females) and were included in the study.

Following Bakan (1971) and Gur (1975), subjects had been classified as left-movers if 70% or more of their eye movements were to the left, right-movers if 70% of more of their eye movements were to the right, and bidirectional otherwise. Of the 74 subjects who responded, 21 had been classified as left-movers, 23 as right-movers, and 30 as bidirectionals.

As seen in Figure 5, left-movers preferred to sit on the right side of the classroom more often than right-movers, and, conversely, right-movers preferred to sit on the left side of the classroom more often than left-movers.

Furthermore, of the 28 subjects who indicated preferential seating location for hard (mathematics, physics) compared to the soft (art, music) topics, 22 indicated they preferred to sit more to the left for the former compared to the latter. There were no differences between right- and left-movers on this question, but of the 6 who indicated a reversed pattern of preference, 5 were left-handed.

These results suggest that left-right preferences in classroom seating may be influenced by a hemisphere activation bias factor as measured by conjugate lateral eye movements.

In a recent investigation, Gur, Sackeim, and Gur (1976) have replicated and extended these findings. If the relationships between hemisphere bias (as measured by lateral eye movements) and

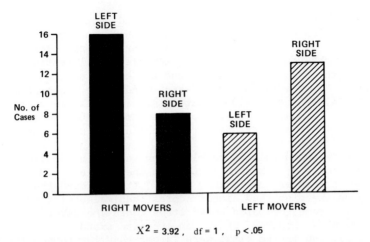

$X^2 = 3.92$, df = 1, p < .05

*Fig. 5. Seating preference of left-movers and right-movers. From R. E. Gur, R. C. Gur, & Marshalek, 1975.*

*personality variables* (as measured by questionnaire), on the one hand, and *lateral seating preference*, on the other hand, were robust and reliable ones, then one would expect both these correlates of hemisphere bias also to be correlated with one another. Accordingly, a new study was undertaken to examine their relation jointly. Gur and Gur (1975) had investigated a restricted range of symptomatology (psychosomatic complaints) using male subjects only. For the present study, the range of symptomatology was expanded and subjects of both sexes were included so as to allow for possible sex differences. Finally, a validation of self-reported seating preference was obtained by comparing this measure with actual seating location.

The subjects were 228 introductory psychology students (116 male, 112 female). As each student entered the classroom, he was handed a battery of questionnaires. These included a handedness and laterality questionnaire, which included the items used by Gur, Gur, and Marshalek (1975) to assess classroom seating preference, and the Manifest Symptom Questionnaire (MSQ). The MSQ (Gur & Sackeim, 1975) consists of a set of 124 items, which elicit self-reports on the symptoms listed under diagnostic categories in the *Diagnostic and Statistical Manual of Mental Disorders (DSM-II)* (APA, 1968). The questionnaire employs a seven-point Likert-type scale to measure the intensity or frequency of symptomatic behavior. Scores on this questionnaire are determined for each of 65 disorders and 11 superordinate categories.

The classroom was a large auditorium with no windows, structurally symmetrical, divided into four sections. Subjects could hear equally well from all points in the classroom and illumination was homogeneous. When the subjects were given general instructions for filling out the inventories, they were also requested to mark down their seat, row, and section.

The relation between *expressed* and *actual* seating preference was examined by dividing subjects into three groups--left, middle, and right--on both measures. (On the actual seating measure this was achieved by considering the two center sections together as "middle.") The two measures were found to be associated ($\chi^2 = 13.94$, $df = 4$, $p < .01$), but, since it is likely that response bias from *actual* seating at the time influenced *expressed* preference in this study, no strong conclusions can be drawn from this association alone.

MSQ scores were related to classroom seating by considering the mean scores of subjects sitting on the left and right extreme sections on each of the 124 MSQ items. It was found that males sitting on the right had higher scores than males sitting on the left on 71 items, compared to 48 items where the reverse was the case. Females, however, showed an opposite trend. Means for females sitting on the right were larger than for those sitting on the left for only 28 items, as contrasted with 93 items where the reverse was the case. This pattern is highly significant ($\chi^2 = 33.02$, $df = 1$, $p < .001$).

These results indicate that left-side seating preference is associated with higher MSQ scores in males, whereas the opposite is true for females. They also show that there is considerable variability in this regard. Although we noted some systematic trends in terms of the kinds of items that departed from the male and female pattern, these will not be discussed here. How the sex differences found in this study might relate to sex differences in lateralization (Harris, 1975; Harshman & Remmington, 1976) and to what extent they are genetically or culturally determined can at this stage only be a matter of conjecture, and will likewise be deferred for future work.


SUMMARY

In this chapter we have summarized a number of studies investigating the effects of a hypothesized hemisphere activation factor on a number of variables. We started by validating conjugate lateral eye movements as an index of individual differences in hemisphere activation bias and then examined tasks and measures that one would expect to correlate with this index. So far we have found some evidence suggesting that hemisphere bias is correlated with certain personality traits, task performances, and classroom lateral seating preferences. The pattern of the relations among these variables appears to be different for males and females.

It must be pointed out that, although a rather suggestive network of correlations has been demonstrated by these studies, and although hemisphere activation bias appears to be a plausible candidate for one of the primary factors underlying these correlations, we can hardly claim that the *causal* basis of these findings has been accounted for, or even clearly understood. This must wait on further research.

## ACKNOWLEDGMENTS

The writing of this chapter and the research reported in it were partly supported by USPHS Biomedical Sciences Support Grant 07083 (Donald N. Langenberg, Program Director). We thank the editors of this volume, as well as Jonquil M. Drinkwater, Jerre Levy, and Harold A. Sackeim, for their comments.

## REFERENCES

American Psychiatric Association. *Diagnostic and statistical manual of mental disorder* (2nd ed.), (DSM-II). Washington, D.C.: Author, 1968.

Bakan, P. Hypnotizability, laterality of eye movement and functional brain asymmetry. *Perceptual and Motor Skills*, 1969, *28*, 927-932.

Bakan, P. Handedness and hypnotizability. *The International Journal of Clinical and Experimental Hypnosis*, 1970, *18*, 99-104.

Bakan, P. The eyes have it. *Psychology today*, 1971, *4*, 64-69.

Bakan, P., & Shotland, J. Lateral eye movement, reading speed, and visual attention. *Psychonomic Science*, 1969, *16*, 93-94.

Bakan, P., & Svorad, D. Resting EEG alpha and asymmetry of reflective lateral eye movements. *Nature*, 1969, *223*, 975-976.

Benton, A. L. Clinical symptomatology in right and left hemisphere lesions. In Mountcastle, V. B. (Ed.), *Interhemispheric relations and cerebral dominance*. Baltimore: Johns Hopkins Press, 1962. Pp. 253-261.

Benton, A. L. The "minor" hemisphere. *Journal of the History of Medicine and Allied Sciences*, 1972, *27*, 5-14.

Bigum, H. Visual and somatosensory evoked responses from mongoloid and normal children. Unpublished doctoral dissertation, Univ. of Utah, 1969.

Bogen, J. E. The other side of the brain II: An appositional mind. *Bulletin of the Los Angeles Neurological Societies*, 1969, *34*, 135-162.

Carmon, A. Disturbances of tactile sensitivity in patients with unilateral cerebral lesions. *Cortex*, 1971, *7*, 83-97.

Cohen, G. Hemispheric differences in serial versus parallel processing. *Journal of Experimental Psychology*, 1973, *97*, 349-356.

Day, M. E. An eye-movement phenomenon relating to attention, thought and anxiety. *Perceptual and Motor Skills*, 1964, *19*, 443-446.

Day, M. E. An eye-movement indicator of type and level of anxiety. Some clinical observations. *Journal of Clinical Psychology*, 1967, *23*, 433-441.(a)

Day, M. E. An eye-movement indicator of individual differences in the psychological organization of attentional processes and anxiety. *Journal of Psychology*, 1967, *66*, 51-62.(b)

Day, M. E. Attention, anxiety and psychotherapy. *Psychotherapy Theory, Research and Practice*, 1968, *5*, 146-149.

Duke, J. Lateral eye-movement behavior. *Journal of General Psychology*, 1968, *78*, 189-195.

Galin, D., & Ornstein, R. Lateral specialization of cognitive mode: An EEG study. *Psychophysiology*, 1972, *9*, 412-418.

Gazzaniga, M. S., Bogen, J. E., & Sperry, R. W. Some functional effects of sectioning the cerebral commissures in man. *Proceedings of the National Academy of Sciences*, 1962, *48*, 1965.

Gill, M. M., & Brenman, M. *Hypnosis and related states*. New York: International Universities Press, 1959.

Gleser, G. C., & Ihilevich, D. An objective instrument for measuring defense mechanisms. *Journal of Consulting and Clinical Psychology*, 1969, *33*, 51-60.

Gleser, G. C., & Sacks, M. Ego defenses and reaction to stress: A validation study of the defense mechanisms inventory. *Journal of Consulting and Clinical Psychology*, 1973, *40*, 181-187.

Gur, R. C. An attention-controlled operant procedure for enhancing hypnotic susceptibility. *Journal of Abnormal Psychology*, 1974, *83*, 644-650.

Gur, R. C., & Gur, R. E. Handedness, sex and eyedness as moderating variables in the relation between hypnotic susceptibility and functional brain asymmetry. *Journal of Abnormal Psychology*, 1974, *83*, 635-643.

Gur, R. C., & Sackeim, H. S. The manifest symptom questionnaire. Unpublished manuscript, Univ. of Pennsylvania, 1975.

Gur, R. C., Sackeim, H. A., & Gur, R. E. Classroom seating and psychopathology: Some initial data. *Journal of Abnormal Psychology*, 1976, *85*, 122-124.

Gur, R. E. Conjugate lateral eye movements as an index of hemispheric activation. *Journal of Personality and Social Psychology*, 1975, *31*, 751-757.

Gur, R. E., & Gur, R. C. Defense mechanisms, psychosomatic symptomatology, and conjugate lateral eye movements. *Journal of Consulting and Clinical Psychology*, 1975, *43*, 416-420.

Gur, R. E., Gur, R. C., & Harris, L. J. Cerebral activation, as measured by subjects' lateral eye movements, is influenced by experimenter location. *Neuropsychologia*, 1975, *13*, 35-44.

Gur, R. E., Gur, R. C., & Marshalek, B. Classroom seating and functional brain asymmetry. *Journal of Educational Psychology*, 1975, *67*, 151-153.

Gur, R. E., & Reyher, J.   The relationship between style of hypnotic induction and direction of lateral eye movement. *Journal of Abnormal Psychology*, 1973, *82*, 499-505.

Harris, L. J.   Sex differences in spatial ability, possible environmental, genetic and neurological factors.   In M. Kinsbourne (Ed.), *Hemispheric asymmetry of function*.   New York:  Cambridge Univ. Press, 1975.

Harshman, R. A., & Remmington, R.   Sex, language and the brain. Part I:  A review of the literature on adult sex differences in lateralization.   Submitted for publication, 1976.

Hécaen, H.   Aphasic, apraxic and agnostic syndromes in right and left hemisphere lesions.   In P. J. Vinken, & G. W. Bruyn (Eds.), *Handbook of Clinical Neurology*.   Vol. IV. Amsterdam:  North-Holland Publishing Co., 1969.

Hécaen, H., & Ajuriaguerra, J. de.   *Left-handedness*.   New York: Grune & Stratton, 1964.

Hilgard, E. R.   *Hypnotic susceptibility*.   New York:  Harcourt, 1965.

Hilgard, J. R.   *Personality and hypnosis:  A study of imaginative involvement*.   Chicago:  Univ. of Chicago Press, 1970.

Humphrey, M. E.   Consistency of hand usage:  A preliminary inquiry.   *British Journal of Educational Psychology*, 1951, *21*, 214-225.

Ingram, D.   Motor asymmetries in young children.   *Research Bulletin #269*, Univ. of Western Ontario, London, Canada, 1973.

Kimura, D.   Dual functional asymmetry of the brain in visual perception.   *Neuropsychologia*, 1966, *4*, 275-285.

Kimura, D.   Functional asymmetry of the brain in dichotic listening.   *Cortex*, 1967, *3*, 163-178.

Kimura, D.   Manual activity during speaking - I.   Right-handers. *Neuropsychologia*, 1973, *11*, 45-50.(a)

Kimura, D.   Manual activity during speaking - II.   Left-handers. *Neuropsychologia*, 1973, *11*, 51-55.(b)

Kinsbourne, M.   The control of attention by interaction between the cerebral hemispheres.   Paper presented to the Fourth International Symposium on Attention and Performance, 1971, Boulder.

Kinsbourne, M.   Eye and head turning indicates cerebral lateralization.   *Science*, 1972, *176*, 539-541.

Knox, C., & Kimura, D.   Cerebral processing of nonverbal sounds in boys and girls.   *Neuropsychologia*, 1970, *8*, 227-238.

Kocel, K., Galin, D., Ornstein, R., & Merrin, E.   Lateral eye movement and cognitive mode.   *Psychonomic Science*, 1972, *27*, 223-224.

Lansdell, M.   The effect of neurosurgery on a test of proverbs. *American Psychologist*, 1961, *16*, 448.

Lansdell, M.   A sex difference in effect of temporal lobe neurosurgery on design preference.   *Nature*, 1962, *194*, 852-854.

Levy, J.   Possible basis for the evolution of lateral specialization of the human brain.   *Nature*, 1969, *224*, 614-615.

McFie, J. The diagnostic significance of disorders of higher nervous activity. In P. J. Vinken, & G. W. Bruyn (Eds.), *Handbook of clinical neurology*. Vol. IV. Amsterdam: North-Holland Publishing Co., 1969.

McGlone, J., & Davidson, W. The relation between cerebral speech laterality and spatial ability with special reference to sex and hand preference. *Neuropsychologia*, 1973, *11*, 105-113.

McKee, G., Humphrey, B., & McAdam, D. W. Scaled lateralization of alpha activity during linguistic and musical tasks. *Psychophysiology*, 1973, *4*, 441-443.

Miller, E. Handedness and the pattern of human ability. *British Journal of Psychology*, 1971, *62*, 111-112.

Morgan, A. H., MacDonald, H., & Hilgard, E. R. EEG alpha: Lateral asymmetry related to task, and hypnotizability. *Psychophysiology*, 1974, *11*, 275-282.

Morgan, A. H., McDonald, P. J., & MacDonald, H. Differences in bilateral alpha activity as a function of experimental task with a note on lateral eye movements and hypnotizability. *Neuropsychologia*, 1971, *9*, 459-469.

Morrell, L. K., & Salamy, J. G. Hemispheric asymmetry of electrocortical responses to speech stimuli. *Science*, 1971, *174*, 164-166.

Mott, F. W., & Shafer, E. On associated eye movements produced by cortical faradization of the monkey's brain. *Brain*, 1890, *13*, 165-173.

Nebes, R. Handedness and the perception of part-whole relationship. *Cortex*, 1971, *7*, 350-356.

Ornstein, R. E. *The psychology of consciousness*. San Francisco: W. H. Freeman, 1972.

Packer, I. Some cognitive and affective characteristics associated with lateral eye movements. Unpublished manuscript. Univ. of Pennsylvania, 1975.

Penfield, W., & Roberts, L. *Speech and brain mechanisms*. Princeton, New Jersey: Princeton Univ. Press, 1959.

Perkins, K. A., & Reyher, J. Repression, psychopathology and drive representation: An experimental hypnotic investigation of impulse inhibition. *American Journal of Clinical Hypnosis*, 1971, *18*, 249-258.

Reyher, J. Posthypnotic stimulation of hypnotically induced conflict in relation to psychosomatic reactions and psychopathology. *Psychosomatic Medicine,* 1961, *23*, 384-391.

Reyher, J., & Basch, J. A. Degree of repression and frequency of psychosomatic symptoms. *Perceptual and Motor Skills*, 1970, *30*, 559-562.

Rizzolatti, G., Umilta, D., & Berlucchi, G. Opposite superiorities of the right and left cerebral hemispheres in discriminative reaction time to physiognomical and alphabetical material. *Brain*, 1971, *94*, 431-442.

Scheffé, H. *The analysis of variance*. New York: Wiley, 1959.

Shor, R. E., & Orne, E. C. *Harvard group scale of hypnotic sus-*

*ceptibility*. Palo Alto, California: Consulting Psychologists Press, 1962.

Sommerschield, H., & Reyher, J. Posthypnotic conflict, repression and psychopathology. *Journal of Abnormal Psychology*, 1973, *82*, 278-290.

Sperry, R. W., & Gazzaniga, M. S. Language following surgical disconnection of the hemispheres. In C. H. Milikan, & F. L. Darley (Eds.), *Brain mechanisms underlying speech and language*. New York: Grune & Stratton, 1967.

Teitelbaum, H. A. Spontaneous rhythmic ocular movement. Their possible relationship to mental activity. *Neurology*, 1954, 350-354.

Trevarthen, C. Brain bisymmetry and the role of the corpus callosum in behavior and conscious experience. In J. Cernacek, & F. Podivinsky (Eds.), *Cerebral interhemispheric relations*. Bratislava: Publishing House of the Slovak Academy of Sciences, 1972.

Van Nuys, D. Meditation, attention, and hypnotic susceptibility: A correlational study. *International Journal of Clinical and Experimental Hypnosis*, 1973, *21*, 59-69.

Weitzenhoffer, A. M., & Hilgard, E. R. *Stanford Hypnosis Susceptibility Scale, Form C*. Palo Alto, California: Consulting Psychologists, 1962.

# Part V

# ASYMMETRIES IN ATTENTION AND PERCEPTION

# Part V

# ASYMMETRIES IN ATTENTION AND PERCEPTION

# 16.
# The Neglect Syndrome—A Unilateral Defect of the Orienting Response

*KENNETH M. HEILMAN AND ROBERT T. WATSON*

University of Florida College of Medicine

## THE ORIENTING RESPONSE

Pavlov (1927) wrote that when a novel stimulus is presented to animals or man "they immediately orient their receptor organs in accordance with the perceptible quality in the agent bringing about the change, making interpretation of it. The biological significance of this reflex is obvious. If the animal were not provided with such a reflex its life would hang at any moment by a thread. . . ." Sokolov (1963) noted that "the orienting reflex is the first response of the body to any type of stimulus. . . The orienting reflex involves muscular activity resulting in specific movements of eyes, lids, ears, head, or trunk. . . ." Associated with the orienting reflex is also a general increase in muscle tone. In addition to overt movement, there are autonomic reactions (i.e., changes in pupil size, respiratory rate, vascular size, heart rate, and cutaneogalvanic response) as well as electrophysiologic alterations (e.g., in the electroencephalogram).

Although novel stimuli may induce an orienting reflex, meaningful stimuli (i.e., those with signal significance), even though not novel, also induce this reflex. However, this orienting reflex differs from the classic type in that it may be stronger and habituate more slowly (Lynn, 1966). The function of the orienting reflex is to prepare the organism to deal with novel or signal stimuli more efficiently (Lynn, 1966). Sensory organs become more sensitive, and sensorimotor responses become more rapid (Lansing, Schwartz, & Lindsley, 1969).

The purpose of this chapter is to examine neglect syndromes in terms of the orienting response and some of the neurological systems underlying it.

## THE SYNDROME OF UNILATERAL NEGLECT

The present research began with an investigation of the conditions involving loss of the orienting reflex. Occasionally in clinical practice one sees a patient with a unilateral brain lesion, who, in the apparent absence of sensory deficit, exhibits a behavioral response pattern suggestive of an "asymmetrical orienting reflex." Because there is some controversy about the pathophysiology of this syndrome, it has been called by a variety of names, such as *unilateral neglect, unilateral inattention, extinction to simultaneous stimulation, hemispatial agnosia,* and *amorphosynthesis.* Although this behavioral syndrome can be caused by a variety of diseases, the behavioral picture of these patients is similar in most instances. The following is a prototypic case.

The patient was a right-handed, middle-aged teacher who had previously enjoyed excellent health. Although the patient denied having any difficulties, his family noted the sudden onset of left-sided weakness and brought him to the hospital. He was alert and oriented to time, place, and person; he had a good digit span and did not appear to have any anterograde or retrograde amnesia. His fund of information was excellent. The patient was not aphasic, agraphic, or apraxic. He did not have finger agnosia, right-left confusion, or acalculia. When asked to read, he read only those words found on the right side of the page. When words like *toothpick* and *baseball* were presented to him, he read *pick* and *ball.* He was able to recognize faces. However, when he dressed, he did not attempt to put on the left side of his clothing. He shaved only the right side of his face. When asked to draw a daisy, he drew petals only on the right side. When asked to bisect a horizontal line he would quarter it (three quarters on the left and one quarter on the right). When asked to cross out lines on a page, he would cross out only those lines on the right side of the page. When eating, he would eat food only from the right side of the plate.

Cranial nerve examination of the patient showed that he had mild head and eye deviation to the right. He appeared not to be able to see anything in the left visual field, and when a sound was made on his left, he did not orient to the sound. Motor examination revealed what appeared to be almost flaccid left extremities. Occasionally the patient could be observed sitting on his left hand. When asked to move his left extremeties, he denied that they belonged to him. When his left arm was carried to his normal visual field and he was asked to move this arm, he could not move it, denied it was his arm, and insisted it was the examiner's arm. His deep tendon reflexes were hypoactive on the left side, and he demonstrated a left extensor plantar response. When somesthetic sensation was tested, the patient did not respond to any stimuli to his left side, but he appeared to respond normally to stimuli on his right.

After several days the patient improved somewhat. Head and eye deviations were no longer present. Now when a sound was made or someone spoke to him from his left, he would orient to the right. When touched on his left and asked to indicate the side of stimulation, he would indicate to the examiner that he had been touched on his right. He continued to respond to right-side stimulation normally. He did not appear to show a hyperreactive orienting reflex to right-sided stimulation (cf. Glick, Jerussi, & Zimmerberg, this volume) but this possibility is still being investigated in other patients.

After several weeks the patient showed further improvement. He now seemed to realize that something was wrong with his left side. He admitted he owned his left arm but felt compelled to name it as if it were a prosthesis (e.g., "it" or "this thing"). When asked to move his left arm, he was capable of movements of good strength, but in general was reluctant to move this extremity (akinesia). When he was asked to sustain any bilateral posture, his left extremity would be the first to fall, but he even had difficulty sustaining posture on the normal side (i.e., motor impersistence). When his visual fields were tested, he was able to detect unilateral stimulation in either field. Bilateral simultaneous stimulation, however, induced a response to stimuli in the right visual field only. If fingers were snapped beside his left ear, he was able to recognize that the sound came from the left; however, when fingers were simultaneously snapped on both sides, the patient responded only to the sound coming from the right. The patient was also able to recognize stimuli applied to the left side of his body, but if both sides were simultaneously stimulated, he recognized only the stimuli applied to his right.

Functional recovery predictably occurs in stages. Initially, the patient fails to respond to stimuli contralateral to the side of the lesion, or the subject orients and responds to stimuli applied to the contralateral side as if he were stimulated on the side ipsilateral to the lesion. Subsequently, the subject may orient and respond appropriately to unilateral stimulation on the side contralateral to the lesion, but with bilateral simultaneous stimulation he responds only to the stimulus presented to the side ipsilateral to the lesion. This has been termed *extinction to simultaneous stimulation* (Bender, 1952). Although some patients go through all the stages, a patient may start off at any stage, depending on the severity of the lesion.

Patients with the neglect syndrome just described may also display a unilateral memory defect (Heilman, Watson, & Shulman, 1974), disturbed comprehension of affective aspect of speech (Heilman, Scholes, & Watson, 1975), motor impersistence (Joynt, Benton, & Fogel, 1962), and anosognosia (Critchley, 1966); however, the present discussion will be limited to defects in the orienting reflex.

EARLIER THEORIES OF NEGLECT

Many theories have been proposed to explain these deficits, but most attempt to explain only part of the picture (e.g., extinction), rather than the full clinical manifestation of the neglect syndrome. This problem may have arisen because some investigators are unaware that neglect, allesthesia, and extinction represent a clinical spectrum determined by such factors as severity, location, and duration of the pathological process. In this chapter the term *neglect* will be used, to emphasize the unity of the phenomenon.

There are several theories of neglect that propose that it is caused by defective sensation. Battersby, Bender, and Pollack (1956) felt that neglect in humans resulted from decreased sensory input superimposed on a background of decreased mental function. Sprague, Chambers, and Stellar (1961) made unilateral lateral mesencephalic lesions in cats, which produced unilateral neglect involving smell and vision: "The lateral regions of the mesencephalon containing the specific, highly localized long and direct sensory pathways have been thought by many to be restricted to the function of bearing specific information to the reticular formation and forebrain structures. Because one animal with reticular formation damage was asymptomatic and another with more medial damage was hypokinetic but without sensory defects, Sprague and co-workers concluded that neglect was due to loss of of patterned sensory input to the forebrain, particularly to the neocortex, rather than to reduced ascending reticular activity.

More recently Eidelberg and Schwartz (1971) proposed a hypothesis similar to that of Sprague *et al*. They postulated that neglect was caused by decreased sensory input and is a passive phenomenon due to quantitatively asymmetrical input to the two hemispheres. Eidelberg and Schwartz based this conclusion on the finding that they could produce neglect from neospinothalamic lesions but not from medial lemniscal lesions. They thought that the neospinothalamic tract carried more tactile information to the hemisphere than did the medial lemniscus. However, since they recognized that neglect could also be brought about by primary and secondary sensory cortical lesions, they postulated that neglect was also caused by relative reductions of functional mass in areas concerned with somatic sensation.

Denny-Brown and associates (Denny-Brown & Banker, 1954; Denny-

Brown, Meyer, & Horenstein, 1952) thought that the parietal lobes were important for synthesizing multiple sensory data and were concerned with spatial summation of sensation (morphosynthesis). Neglect induced by parietal lobe dysfunction was therefore felt to be caused by amorphosynthesis.

Other investigators have felt that neglect has an attentional basis. Critchley (1949) was a strong proponent of this viewpoint. However, due to the vagueness of the underlying construct of "attention," hypotheses of this sort have not been further developed.

AREAS WHERE LESIONS PRODUCE UNILATERAL NEGLECT

To help determine why patients with unilateral neglect do not orient to stimuli presented to the side contralateral to the lesion, we felt it important to examine systematically the specific areas in which a lesion has been found to produce neglect Denny-Brown et al. (1952). Denny-Brown and Banker (1954), and others have reported cases of unilateral neglect in patients with unilateral parietal lobe lesions. Heilman and Valenstein (1972a) studied 17 patients with unilateral neglect. Ten patients had positive brain scans, and in nine of these the lesion was in the region of the inferior parietal lobule. More recently we have studied 23 patients with unilateral neglect (Watson & Heilman, in preparation), 20 left-sided, and 3 right. Nineteen of these patients had a verified lesion site, and in 14 the site involved the inferior parietal lobule (Figure 1). According to this study the most common site of lesions inducing unilateral neglect involves the inferior parietal lobule of the right hemisphere.

According to the work of Pandya and Kuypers (1969) on cortico-cortical connections in monkeys, the primary sensory areas (i.e., visual, auditory, and somesthetic) project to their association areas, which in turn project to the inferior parietal lobule and the caudal portion of the superior temporal gyrus.

To ascertain whether the region of the inferior parietal lobule and the caudal portion of the superior temporal gyrus in monkeys was homologous to the inferior parietal lobule in man as far as the neglect syndrome was concerned, this area was unilaterally ablated by subpial suction in monkeys (Heilman, Pandya, Karol, & Geschwind, 1971). Visual fields and visually guided behavior were tested under conditions of distraction, response to threat, and reaching for food on a tray. Auditory fields and acoustically guided behavior were tested by having animals turn to the side on which a sound was being made. Somesthetic sensation and somesthetically guided behavior were tested by blindfolding the monkeys and testing touch distraction and pain avoidance. Bilateral simultaneous stimulation was used to test visual, auditory, and somesthetic fields. After surgery the animals exhibited extinction to simultaneous visual and somesthe-

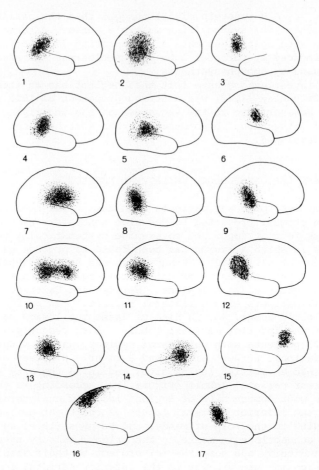

*Fig. 1. Diagrammatic representation of the 17 patients who had abnormal brain scans (from a group of 19 patients who had discrete anatomical lesions).*

tic stimulation and a decreased blink to threat on the side contralateral to the lesion. Occasionally, although hungry, the animals would fail to pick up apples from the side contralateral to the lesion. To unilateral auditory stimuli the animals would show an allesthetic response (turning toward the side ipsilateral to the lesion when stimuli were presented on the side contralateral to the lesion). It appears that these animals displayed a mild form of some of the deficits seen in man after parietal lobe lesions. Three control animals with lesions in different portions of the temporal lobe did not demonstrate this neglect phenomenon. Schwartz and Eidelberg (1968) have also made parietal lesions in monkeys and produced somesthetic neglect and recently

Mountcastle, Lynch, Georgopoulos, Sakata, & Acuna (1975) have demonstrated that cells in area VII perform a "command" function, directing visual attention toward contralateral space.

Initially we postulated that since the inferior parietal lobule is a secondary association area and since the destruction of this area produces neglect, neglect is caused because one-half of the brain is unable to synthesize sensory input. These observations appeared to support Denny-Brown and Banker's (1954) hypothesis of amorphosynthesis.

Pandya and Kuypers (1969) have shown that the sensory association areas also project to the dorsolateral frontal lobe in the region of the arcuate gyrus and that the inferior parietal lobule also projects to this region. Several investigators (Kennard & Ectors, 1938; Welch & Stuteville, 1958) have also demonstrated that lesions in this region can produce unilateral neglect in the monkey. Neglect from dorsolateral frontal lesions in man has also been described (Heilman & Valenstein, 1972b). The observation that neglect can result from lesions in a frontal tertiary association area further supports a hypothesis of amorphosynthesis. Also described, however, were three patients with unilateral neglect from unilateral cingulate gyrus lesions (Heilman & Valenstein, 1972b), an area that receives projections from the arcuate gyrus (Pandya & Kuypers, 1969).

To confirm these observations and to ascertain that the causative lesion can indeed be in the cingulate gyrus, we (Watson, Heilman, Cauthen, & King, 1973) trained four monkeys (*Macaca speciosa*) to open a left door to left-leg stimulation, the right door to right-leg stimulation, and the left door when both legs were simultaneously stimulated. The anterior portion of the right cingulate cortex was ablated in all four monkeys. Two subjects received simultaneous right supplementary motor area and cingulate lesions. One monkey had the motor lesion prior to cingulectomy, and another monkey had it afterward. Following surgery the cingulectomized animals showed either no response or an allesthetic response to left-leg stimulation, and opened the right door to bilateral simultaneous stimulation rather than making the trained left-door response. The supplementary motor cortex ablations did not alter performance on the tactile task. Neglect is thus produced by lesions in both the arcuate gyrus and cingulate cortex.

Because it was possible to produce neglect with lesions entirely outside the sensory and sensory-association areas, we felt that the mechanism of neglect could not be completely explained by a sensory hypothesis. In addition, because the cingulate gyrus is limbic rather than association cortex, the synthetic or perceptual hypothesis, although perhaps a first-order explanation, did not seem to provide the requisite unifying concept. In search of the latter, we turned our attention to the arousal system.

## THE CORTICO-LIMBIC-RETICULAR ACTIVATING LOOP

The cingulate gyrus has extensive connections with the mesencephalic components of the diffuse ascending and descending reticular system (Nauta, 1964). There is also a connection between
the frontal eye fields (arcuate gyrus) and the mesencephalic reticular system (Astruc, 1971). Stimulation studies corroborate
the existence of functional connections between these cortical
areas and the reticular system (French, Hernandez, & Livingston,
1955; Segundo, Naguet, & Buser, 1955). Since neglect is manifested as a defect of the orienting reflex and since the extensive, reciprocal cortico-reticular connections include prominent-
ly the areas known to produce neglect we proposed that unilateral neglect consists of a unilateral defect of arousal (alerting)
produced by a lesion that disrupts a cortico-limbic-reticular
pathway (Heilman & Valenstein, 1972b; Watson *et al.*, 1973). (See
Figure 2.)

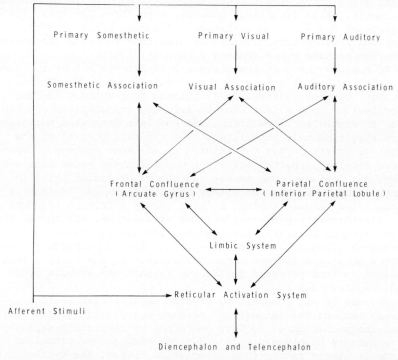

*Fig. 2. Cortico-limbic-reticular loop, important in the induc-
tion of neglect.*

To test this hypothesis, we made discrete unilateral mesencephalic reticular formation lesions in four macaques (Watson,

Heilman, Miller, & King, 1974). Three monkeys received control lesions and two of these three subsequently received experimental lesions. Two additional animals received experimental lesions. (There were seven lesions in five subjects--four experimental lesions, three control lesions.) On clinical examination experimental subjects showed profound multimodal neglect. On the tactile task described previously, the subjects also demonstrated profound neglect.

Neglect-like behavior following various subcortical lesions in animals had been observed by a number of investigators (Reeves & Hagamen, 1971; Orem, Schlag-Rey, & Schlag, 1973). Unilateral lesions in the superior colliculus of cats also caused unilateral neglect (Sprague & Meikle, 1965). Such animals orient poorly not only to visual stimuli but also to acoustic and tactile stimuli (trimodal neglect).

Unlike lesions of the colliculus, lesions of its brachium, which contains fibers from the optic tract and from the visual cortex, result in transient visual neglect but do not produce trimodal neglect. Perhaps collicular lesions cause trimodal neglect because the superior colliculus in the cat receives somesthetic projections from the spinotectal tract. This, however, would not explain the auditory neglect.

Another possibility is that damage to the tectoreticular pathway decreases reticular driving and thereby produces trimodal neglect. In addition to somesthetic projections, Astruc (1971) has demonstrated that the colliculus receives projections from the arcuate gyrus. Sprague and Meikle (1965) doubt that the superior colliculus is a reflex center controlling eye movement but rather think of it as a "sensory integrative center." Denny-Brown et al. (1952) made large superior collicular lesions in monkeys and found a similar type of neglect. Denny-Brown thought that the tectum may be a "primary driver" of the reticular system. With unilateral collicular lesions the ipsilateral reticular system cannot be driven; therefore, the animal shows a unilateral defect of the orienting response. Since the spinothalamic tract has input into the reticular system, and the medial lemniscus has not (Wall & Dubner, 1972), Eidelberg and Schwartz's spinothalamic lesions could have induced neglect by decreasing reticular driving rather than by the concurrently created differential sensory input.

In rats Marshall, Turner, and Teitelbaum (1971) found that unilateral lesions of the lateral hypothalamus cause marked unilateral neglect. Turner (1973) found that lesions of the medial portion of the amygdala produce a syndrome similar to that seen after lateral hypothalamic lesions. However, the relationship of the amygdala to the hypothalamus in the induction of the orienting reflex is uncertain. In one study Bagshaw and Benzies (1968) found that although amygdalectomized monkeys had a defective vegatative orienting reflex (e.g., galvanic skin response, heart rate, respiratory rate), somatic and EEG indices of orienting were intact; but in a more recent paper (Bagshaw, MacKworth, & Pribram, 1972) amygdalectomized monkeys were found to have an abnormal visual-orienting response. However, all these studies involved bilateral lesions, which, as has been repeatedly shown (Isaacson, 1974), produce placid animals. And although placidity may be produced by a bilateral decrease of the orienting reflex, other mechanisms may also be involved. We have examined nine human patients following unilateral anterior temporal lobectomy that included the amygdala. None of these patients showed evidence of the unilateral neglect syndrome.

Since the stria terminalis is one of the main connections between the hypothalamus and amygdala, Turner (1973) sectioned the stria in rats but was not able to produce neglect. There are, however, ventral amygdalofugal pathways that connect these structures; therefore, the relationship between these structures and the orienting reflex remains unclear. In a recent article Marshall, Richardson, and Teitlebaum (1974) have proposed that the pathway described by Nauta (1964), which goes from the frontal cortex to the lateral hypothalamus, as well as the corticofugal pathway, which passes through the subthalamus and terminates in the reticular formation, may be involved in neglect. This hypothesis appears to coincide with our own.

Let it be noted, however, that systems other than the proposed cortico-limbic-reticular loop are also involved in neglect. Ungerstedt (1973) found that, after the unilateral removal of the nigrostriatal dopamine system by stereotaxic injections of 6-hydroxydopamine hydrobromide, there is an almost complete lack of orienting reflexes to all sensory stimuli on the contralateral side. There is also a motor asymmetry with deviation toward the side of the lesion. The lateral hypothalamus contains ascending fibers of the dopamine system, and perhaps the neglect reported by Marshall et al. (1974) is caused by an interruption of this system. It is quite probable that the monoamine systems, which are mainly ipsilateral systems, are important in the mediation of the orienting reflex. The head and eye deviation, akinesia, and other symptoms of neglect may be caused by a lesion-induced imbalance in the catecholamine system (see Glick et al., this volume).

EEG STUDIES

For the most part, the discussion up to this point has been based on behavioral observations. Since unilateral neglect has been considered as a lateralized defect of arousal (alerting) induced by a cortico-limbic-reticular disconnection, it should be possible to elicit electrophysiologic changes in subjects having neglect. When Lindsley and colleagues (Lindsley, Schreiner, Knowles, & Magoun, 1950; Skinner & Lindsley, 1973)

made bilateral lesions of the midbrain tegmentum, the electroen-
cephalograms (EEGs) of their animals showed large recurring slow
waves.  Initially, ordinary stimuli had no effect on the EEG.
After several days the animals would show some desynchronization
to stimuli, but intensity had to be higher, and the desynchronization was short-lived.  Watson and associates (1974) produced
unilateral neglect by unilateral mesencephalic reticular lesions
in four monkeys and observed high-voltage EEG slowing ipsilateral
to the lesions (as has been reported by other authors, e.g, Berlucchi, 1966; Reeves & Hagaman, 1971).  Control EEGs were normal.
Contralateral neglect, together with ipsilateral EEG slowing
were also produced in five monkeys (*Macaca speciosa*) by frontal
arcuate lesions and in four with cingulate lesions.  Clinical
deficits and EEG signs improved concurrently,

Twenty-two of the 23 human patients with unilateral neglect
exhibited diffuse unilateral hemispheric slowing in the theta
and delta ranges (Heilman, Musella, & Watson, 1973; Watson &
Heilman, in preparation).  Eighteen of these patients also
showed discrete lesions (14 parietal, 3 frontal, 1 thalamic, 1
parietal convexity).  Of 20 aphasic control patients with left-
hemisphere lesions (17 with positive brain scans showing discrete lesions), only 7 had diffuse EEG slowing.

Although the preceding EEG data appear to support the arousal
hypothesis of neglect, the physiological evidence as given does
not rule out the possibility that an asymmetrical sensory input
may be causing these EEG abnormalities.

Another electrophysiological technique that may provide information on the question of asymmetrical sensory input versus
arousal is the cortical evoked potential.  The earliest portions
of evoked potentials are considered to be produced by registra-
tion of sensory information, whereas the late waves are thought
to be decisional or attentional (see Anderson; Donchin, Kutas,
& McCarthy; Thatcher, this volume).

We studied four unanesthetized monkeys (*Macaca speciosa*) by
applying 64 unilateral nonpainful stimuli to the peroneal nerve
and by recording cortical evoked potentials from the hindlimb
area of the sensory cortex (Watson *et al.*, 1976).  After
7 days of preoperative recording, these four animals underwent unilateral frontal arcuate ablations.  Postoperatively, all
four animals demonstrated the unilateral neglect syndrome.  Beginning on the third postoperative day, 7 days of somatosensory
cortical evoked potentials were again obtained.  The amplitude
and latency of each of the five major waves ($P_1$, $N_1$, $P_2$, $N_2$, $P_3$)
was measured.  A two-way analysis of variance for the effects of
*side* (nonlesioned, lesioned) and *condition* (preoperative, postoperative) revealed a significant interaction ($p < .01$) between
the factors, indicating that there is a change from preoperative
to postoperative condition between the lesioned and the nonlesioned side.  Only the latency for $N_2$ and $P_3$ and the amplitude
of $P_3$ were significantly changed.  On the lesioned side, follow-

ing surgery, there was a relative increase (when compared with the nonlesioned side) in the latency of $N_2$ and $P_3$ and the amplitude of $P_3$. The fact that the early potentials were unaltered suggests that in these animals neglect was not produced by decreased sensory input but by the attentional factors involved in the later components.

Most reports suggest that the amplitude of $P_3$ increases with increased attention; however, some studies have reported a decrease in amplitude with increased attention. (See Goff, 1969; also Donchin et al.; Stamm, Rosen, & Gadotti, this volume.) The precise significance of an increased $P_3$ remains to be determined.


INTERHEMISPHERIC EFFECTS

In light of the anatomic, behavioral, and physiological data presented in this chapter, there is little to support the sensory hypotheses. Although Denny-Brown's amorphosynthesis hypothesis may be a first-order explanation, the evidence that neglect can be brought about by lesions outside the parietal lobes, in areas not considered to be sensory association areas, suggests that the amorphosynthesis postulate cannot be the entire explanation of the neglect phenomenon.

Besides the sensory and arousal hypotheses, there are other ways of accounting for neglect. One hypothesis is that of Birch, Belmont, and Karp (1967) who have proposed an inertia-interference model of extinction whereby the damaged hemisphere, because it processes information more slowly, is subject to interference from the normal side. These authors showed that although stimulating the intact side prior to stimulating the abnormal side induced the same degree of extinction as did simultaneous stimulation, extinction could be reduced if the stimulus on the abnormal side came first. Central to their hypothesis is the fact that the abnormal hemisphere processes stimuli more slowly.

Defective arousal may be in part responsible for the delayed responsiveness of the abnormal hemisphere; however, there is an alternative way to account for the extinction. When one side is stimulated, sensory information is transmitted not only to the contralateral hemisphere but also to the ipsilateral hemisphere. Thus, allesthesia need not be caused by a perceptual error of the impaired hemisphere, but perhaps by the normal hemisphere responding as if the stimulus were a signal for it to perform. This hypothesis would imply some type of reciprocal interhemispheric inhibition (e.g., under normal circumstances the hemisphere contralateral to a stimulus may inhibit the ipsilateral hemisphere from performing).

As previously mentioned, during recovery the organism goes from the stage of allesthesia to extinction. At this stage the normal hemisphere can direct an appropriate response to either a contralateral or ipsilateral stimulus. However, when simul-

taneous stimuli are presented, the contralateral stimulus pre-
dominates. If this hypothesis concerning allesthesia and extinction is correct, then corpus callosum lesions ought to extend the neglect stage and eliminate the allesthetic and extinction stage of the syndrome (cf. Glick *et al.*; Sechzer,
Folstein, Geiger, & Mervis, this volume).

The reciprocal inhibition model has been elaborated by
Kinsbourne (1970b) who postulated that neglect may be caused by
lesion-induced imbalance between hemispheric orientational tendencies in favor of the uninjured side. On the basis of this
theory Kinsbourne suggested that neglect be treated with a
callosal lesion.

We also feel that the head and eye deviation seen in neglect
is evoked by an imbalance of orientational tendencies. However,
although Kinsbourne believes the imbalance to be due to relatively increased activity of the nonlesioned side, we think it
is due to decreased activity of the lesioned hemisphere.
Gainotti and Taicci's (1971) observations support our hypothesis.
Patients with left-sided unilateral neglect were presented with
complex visual stimuli. As expected, these patients made more
omissions on their left (neglected) side than they made on their
right side. According to Kinsbourne's hypothesis, their right
side should be normal or even better than normal; however, the
patients with left-sided neglect made more errors on the right
(ipsilateral) side than controls with lesions of the left hemisphere made on their left (ipsilateral) side. Albert (1973)
used a simple line-crossing-out test in aphasics and obtained
similar results concerning left-side injury. Eidelberg and
Schwartz's observations (1971) also failed to confirm
Kinsbourne's hypothesis. These authors were able to induce
neglect in callosally sectioned animals. Finally, if
Kinsbourne's hypothesis were correct, then another lesion in the
opposite hemisphere in regions known to produce neglect should
ameliorate the symptoms of neglect. In humans it is unlikely
that in different hemispheres two arteries going to similar
areas will occlude at the same time. However, there are two
regions of the human brain where both sides may be served by one
arterial feeder, and where unilateral ablation produces neglect.
These regions are the cingulate gyrus and the mesencephalic reticular formation. With bilateral cingulate lesions or bilateral mesencephalic lesions, patients do not respond or orient to
any stimuli from either side. It appears, then, that rather than
ameliorating unilateral neglect symptoms bilateral lesions cause
bilateral neglect or what has been described as the *akinetic
mute state* (Segarra & Angelo, 1970). Since the extinction phenomenon needs at least one normal side, it is not surprising
that these patients do not manifest extinction to simultaneous
stimuli. A similar state has been seen in animals after bilateral destruction of the nigrostriatal dopamine system (Ungerstedt, 1973).

Although we do not think that asymmetrical reciprocal inhibition is causing the neglect syndrome, we do think that the asymmetries of reciprocal inhibition may be producing some of the abnormalities seen in the neglect syndrome, especially allesthesia and related phenomena.

## HEMISPHERIC ASYMMETRIES IN SUSCEPTIBILITY TO NEGLECT

There is disagreement as to whether in man there are hemispheric asymmetries in the production of neglect. Several early reports claimed that neglect is caused predominantly by right-sided lesions (Brain, 1941; Critchley, 1966; McFie, Piercy, & Zangwill, 1950) but Denny-Brown and Banker (1954) reported cases of right-side neglect (amorphosynthesis) from left-parietal lesions. To ascertain whether there were hemispheric asymmetries, Battersby et al. (1956) studied 122 patients with cerebral damage. There were 65 patients with neglect from unilateral lesions; 41 had right-sided lesions, and 24 had left-sided lesions. In the group of 122 subjects there were 10 left-hemisphere-impaired aphasic patients who could not be tested. If these 10 subjects are added to the 24 patients with right-sided neglect, the difference between the groups (i.e., 34 with left-sided lesions and 42 with right-sided lesions) is not significant. Battersby concluded that the occurrence of aphasia after a dominant-hemisphere lesion results in a spuriously high incidence of neglect from nondominant hemispheric lesions.

Albert (1973) had 66 subjects (36 with left-hemisphere lesions and 30 with right-hemisphere lesions) cross out lines distributed over a page. Aphasics were not excluded. In this group, 37% of patients with right-hemisphere lesions and 30% of patients with left-hemisphere lesions failed to cross out lines. Although the frequency of asymmetry was small, when the severity (as determined by the number of errors) was compared, it appeared that right-sided lesions produced a more pronounced defect than did left-sided lesions.

At least four (not incompatible) hypotheses can be proposed to account for the asymmetry. (1) McFie et al. (1950) and Albert (1973) propose that neglect is more marked after right-sided lesions because the right hemisphere is dominant for visuo-spatial organization. (2) Kinsbourne (1970b) has postulated that since patients think in words and verbally communicate with the clinician, this left-hemispheric activation (Bowers & Heilman, 1975; Kinsbourne, 1970a, 1974) would tend to minimize an imbalance between left and right when the left hemisphere is damaged, and to amplify the imbalance when the right is damaged. (3) A third hypothesis could be that the proposed cortico-limbic-reticular loop is more discretely organized in the right hemisphere than it is in the left hemisphere. (4) Finally, perhaps in man there also exist endogenous neurotransmitter asymmetries (like those found in the striatum of the rat by Glick *et al.*, this volume) that may interact differentially with unilateral lesions so as to produce in right-handed man a tendency to orient to the right side of space (cf. Gur & Gur, this volume). Lesions in the right hemisphere would therefore produce a more pronounced asymmetry of the orienting response than lesions in the left.

## SUMMARY

We have proposed that the orienting reflex is mediated by a cortico-limbic-reticular loop and that unilateral dysfunction of this loop produces the clinical syndrome of unilateral neglect. Although we have proposed that a specific cortico-limbic-reticular loop is important in mediating the orienting reflex, it is likely that other parallel systems (such as the neostriatum) are also involved. Finally, the proposed loop will surely have important functional subdivisions (see, e.g., Pribram & Luria, 1973) whose understanding awaits further experimental investigation.

## REFERENCES

Albert, M. C. A simple test of visual neglect. *Neurology*, 1973, *23*, 685-664.

Astruc, J. Corticofugal connections of area 8 (frontal eye field) in *Macaca mulatta*. *Brain Research*, 1971, *33*, 241-256.

Bagshaw, M. H., & Benzies, S. Multiple measures of the orienting reaction and their dissociation after amygdalectomy. *Experimental Neurology*, 1968, *26*, 175-187.

Bagshaw, M. H., Mackworth, N. H., & Pribram, K. H. The effects of resections of the inferotemporal cortex and the amygdala on visual orienting and habituation. *Neuropsychologia*, 1972, *10*, 153-162.

Battersby, W. S., Bender, M. B., & Pollack, M. Unilateral spatial agnosia (inattention) in patients with cerebral lesions. *Brain*, 1956, *79*, 68-93.

Bender, M. B. *Disorders in perception*. Springfield, Illinois: C. C. Thomas, 1952.

Berlucchi, G. Electroencephalographic studies in split brain cats. *Electroencephalography and Clinical Neurophysiology*, 1966, *20*, 348-356.

Birch, H. G., Belmont, I., & Karp, E. Delayed information processing and extinction following cerebral damage. *Brain*, 1967, *90*, 113-130.

Bowers, D., & Heilman, K. M. Material specific hemispheric arousal. *Neuropsychologia*, 1976, *14*, 123-127.

Brain, W. R. Visual disorientation with special reference to lesions of the right cerebral hemisphere. *Brain*, 1941, *64*, 244-272.

Critchley, M. Tactile inattention with reference to parietal lesions. *Brain*, 1949, *72*, 538-561.

Critchley, M. *The parietal lobes*. New York: Harner Publishing, 1966.

Denny-Brown, D., & Banker, B. Q. Amorphosynthesis from left parietal lesions. *Archives of Neurology and Psychiatry*, 1954, *71*, 302-313.

Denny-Brown, D., Meyer, J. S., & Horenstein, S. The significance of perceptual rivalry. *Brain*, 1952, *75*, 434-471.

Eidelberg, E., & Schwartz, A. J. Experimental analysis of the extinction phenomenon in monkeys. *Brain*, 1971, *94*, 91-108.

French, J. D., Hernández-Peón, R., & Livingston, R. Projections from the cortex to cephalic brainstem (reticular formation) in monkeys. *Journal of Neurophysiology*, 1955, *18*, 74-95.

Gainotti, G., & Tiacci, C. The relationships between disorders of visual perception and unilateral spatial neglect. *Neuropsychologia*, 1971, *9*, 451-458.

Goff, W. R. Evoked potential correlates of perceptual organization in man. In C. R. Evans & T. B. Mulholland (Eds.), *Attention and neurophysiology*. New York: Appleton, 1969. Pp. 169-193.

Heilman, K. M., Musella, L., & Watson, R. T. The EEG in neglect. *Neurology*, 1973, *23*, 437.

Heilman, K. M., Pandya, D. N., Karol, E. A., & Geschwind, N. Auditory inattention. *Archives of Neurology*, 1971, *24*, 323-325.

Heilman, K. M., Scholes, R., & Watson, R. T. Auditory affective agnosia: Disturbed comprehension of affective speech. *Journal of Neurology, Neurosurgery, and Psychiatry*, 1975, *38*, 69-72.

Heilman, K. M., & Valenstein, E. Auditory neglect in man. *Archives of Neurology*, 1972, *26*, 32-35.(a)

Heilman, K. M., & Valenstein, E. Frontal lobe neglect in man. *Neurology*, 1972, *22*, 660-664.

Heilman, K. M., Watson, R. T., & Schulman, H. A unilateral memory defect. *Journal of Neurology, Neurosurgery, and Psychiatry*, 1974, *37*, 790-793.

Isaacson, R. *The limbic system*. New York: Plenum Press, 1974.

Joynt, R. J., Benton, A. L., & Fogal, M. L. Behavioral and pathological correlates of motor impersistence. *Neurology*, 1962, *12*, 876-881.

Kennard, M. A., & Ectors, L. Forced circling movements in monkeys following lesions of the frontal lobes. *Journal of Neurophysiology*, 1938, *1*, 45-54.

Kinsbourne, M.   The cerebral basis of lateral asymmetries in attention.  *Acta Psychologia*, 1970, *33*, 193-201.(a)

Kinsbourne, M.   A model for the mechanism of unilateral neglect of space.  *Transactions of the American Neurological Association*, 1970, *95*, 143.(b)

Kinsbourne, M.   Direction of gaze and distribution of cerebral thought processes.  *Neuropsychologia*, 1974, *12*, 279-281.

Lansing, R., Schwartz, E., & Lindsley, D.   Reaction time and EEG activation under alerted and nonalerted conditions.  *Journal of Experimental Psychology*, 1959, *58*, 1-7.

Lindsley, D. B., Schreiner, L. H., Knowles, W. B., & Magoun, H.W.   Behavioral and EEG changes following chronic brainstem lesions in cat.  *Electroencephalography and Clinical Neurophysiology*, 1950, *2*, 483-498.

Lynn, R.   *Attention, arousal, and the orientation reaction*.   Oxford:  Pergamon Press, 1966.

Marshall, J. F., Richardson, J. S., & Teitelbaum, P.   Nigrostriatal bundle damage and the lateral hypothalamic syndrome.  *Journal of Comparative and Physiological Psychology*, 1974, *87*, 808-830.

Marshall, J. F., Turner, B. H., & Teitelbaum, P.   Sensory neglect produced by lateral hypothalamic damage.  *Science*, 1971, *174*, 523-525.

McFie, J., Piercy, F. J., & Zangwill, O. L.   Visual spatial agnosia associated with lesions of the right hemisphere.  *Brain*, 1950, *73*, 167-190.

Mountcastle, V. B., Lynch, J. C., Georgopoulos, A., Sakata, H., & Acuna, C.   Posterior parietal association cortex of the monkey:  Command functions for operations within extrapersonal space.  *Journal of Neurophysiology*, 1975, *38*(4), 871-908.

Nauta, W. J. H.   Some efferent connections of the prefrontal cortex in the monkey.  In J. M. Warren & K. Akert (Eds.), *The frontal granular cortex and behavior*.  New York: McGraw-Hill, 1964.

Orem, J., Schlag-Rey, M., & Schlag, J.   Unilateral visual neglect and thalamic intralaminar lesions in the cat.  *Experimental Neurology*, 1973, *40*, 784-797.

Pandya, D. M., & Kuypers, H. G. J. M.   Cortico-cortical connections in the rhesus monkey.  *Brain Research*, 1969, *13*, 13-36.

Pavlov, I. P.   *Conditioned reflexes*.  New York:  Dover Publication, 1960.  P. 12.

Pribram, K. H., & Luria, A. R.   *Psychophysiology of the frontal lobes*.  New York: Academic Press, 1973.

Reeves, A. G., & Hagamen, W. D.   Behavioral and EEG asymmetry following unilateral lesions of the forebrain and midbrain of cats.  *Electroencephalography and Clinical Neurophysiology*, 1971, *30*, 83-86.

Schwartz, A. S., & Eidelberg, E.   "Extinction" to bilateral simultaneous stimulation in the monkey. *Neurology*, 1968, *18*, 61-68.

Segarra, J. M., & Angelo, J. N. Presentation 1. In A. Benton (Ed.), *Behavioral changes in cerebrovascular disease*. New York: Harper, 1970. Pp. 3-14.

Segundo, J. P., Naguet, R., & Buser, P. Effects of cortical stimulation on electrocortical activity in monkeys. *Journal of Neurophysiology*, 1955, *18*, 236-245.

Sharpless, S. K., & Jasper, H. H. Habituation of the arousal reaction. *Brain*, 1956, *79*, 655-669.

Skinner, J. E., & Lindsley, D. B. The non-specific mediothalamic frontocortical system: Its influence on electrocortical activity and behavior. In K. H. Pribram & A. R. Luria (Eds.), *Psychophysiology of the frontal lobes*. New York: Academic Press, 1973.

Sokolov, Y. N. *Perception and the conditioned reflex*. Oxford: Pergamon Press, 1963. P. 11.

Sprague, J. M., Chambers, W. N., & Stellar, E. Attentive, affective, and adaptive behavior in the cat. *Science*, 1961, *133*, 165-173.

Sprague, J. M., & Meikle, T. H. The role of the superior colliculus in visually guided behavior. *Experimental Neurology*, 1965, *11*, 115-146.

Turner, B. H. Sensorimotor syndrome produced by lesions of the amygdala and lateral hypothalamus. *Journal of Comparative and Physiological Psychology*, 1973, *82*, 37-47.

Ungerstedt, U. Selective lesions of central catecholamine pathways: Application in functional studies. In S. Ehrenpreis & I. Kopin (Eds.), *Neuroscience research*. Vol. 5. *Chemical approaches to brain function*. New York: Academic Press, 1973.

Wall, P. D., & Dubner, R. Somatosensory pathways. *Annual Review of Physiology*, 1972, *34*, 315-336.

Watson, R. T., Dekosky, S. T., Zornetzer, S., & Heilman, K. M. Evoked potential in neglect. Presented before the International Neuropsychological Society, Feb. 1976, Toronto.

Watson, R. T., & Heilman, K. M. The electroencephalogram in neglect (in preparation).

Watson, R. T., Heilman, K. M., Cauthen, J. C., & King, F. A. Neglect after cingulectomy. *Neurology*, 1973, *23*, 1003-1007.

Watson, R. T., Heilman, K. M., Miller, B. D., & King, F. A. Neglect after mesencephalic reticular formation lesions. *Neurology*, 1974, *24*, 294-298.

Welch, K., & Stuteville, P. Experimental production of neglect in monkeys. *Brain*, 1958, *81*, 341-347.

# 17.
# Hemispheric Asymmetry in Auditory Tasks

*CHARLES I. BERLIN*

Louisiana State University Medical Center

Broadbent (1954) first reported that when competing speech messages are presented simultaneously to both ears more messages are processed accurately by the right-ear channel than by the left-ear channel. Kimura (1961) first ascribed this right-ear advantage (REA) to the presumed dominance of the left hemisphere for speech. Using simultaneous digit strings, she confirmed the REA Broadbent originally considered peripheral to his research interests in selective attention. There have been hundreds of papers published since 1954 on the dichotic REA and related phenomena (see for example, Berlin & McNeil, 1976, for review of theories and articles; see also Anderson; Springer, this volume); most of the studies have operated under the assumption that simply giving competing speech messages to both ears will generate a REA, and the size of that REA will be proportional to some linguistic superiority of the left hemisphere.

In this chapter I wish to clarify the following points:

1. Dichotic listening may be a *correlate* of laterality for speech and language functions, but it is by no means an *index* of the magnitude of that laterality. Using dichotic listening to infer the magnitude of left-hemisphere superiority is quite like using noise-level measurements to infer the speed of an automobile; increasing the speed generally increases the noise emanating from an automobile, but unusually high noise readings in no way need reflect the car's true speed.

2. When listening to a list of dichotic pairs, one never

identifies *all* the syllables correctly, although either list
would have been reported with virtually 100% accuracy had it been
given to one ear at a time. This failure of either channel to
approach 100% dichotic transmission implies interference of one
signal by another at some central interference point.

3. There seems to be a time-by-frequency "window" during
which dichotic interference must take place, and this interference need not take place at the temporal lobes. In fact, at
least part of the suppression of the ipsilateral channel by the
contralateral channel may be accomplished at the medial geniculate bodies.

## THE MEANING OF MEASURED ASYMMETRIES

The first issue is this: What do dichotic listening experiments reveal in normal adults? If dichotic listening were first
and above all an *index* of language laterality, the results in
test-retest should be extremely stable. In Figure 1 are group
data from the same subjects for 8 weeks (Porter, Troendle, &
Berlin, 1976). Essentially, the right ear outperformed the left

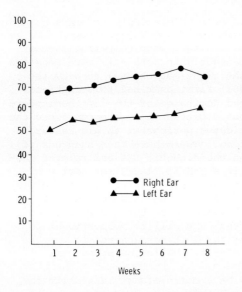

*Fig. 1. Test-retest of
dichotic right-ear advantage
over 8 weeks. Adapted from
Porter et al., 1976.*

in the group although most subjects seemed to get better at the
task as they went along (that is, they progressively reported
more pairs without errors). Figure 2 shows that analysis in terms
of the $[(R - L)/(R + L)]100$ index of asymmetry. The overall picture is in some ways deceptive. For example, some subjects in
the study started weeks 1 and 2 as left-eared subjects and during
weeks 3, 4, and 5 were right-eared subjects; during weeks 6, 7,
and 8 these subjects showed no difference between ears. Needless

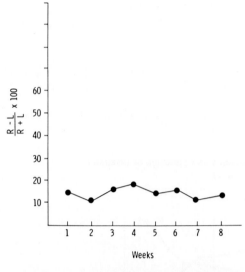

Fig. 2. An index of laterality shown by difference
between right and left ears.
Positive values indicate
right-ear advantages.
Adapted from Porter et al.,
1976.

to say, in any individual normal subject, it is not parsimonious
to assume that the underlying dominant hemisphere for language
shifts so rapidly. Although there are subjects who start out
with large right-ear superiorities and maintain such right-ear
superiorities through retest, they are not to be found universally in populations of so-called normals. As a matter of fact (as
shown later), the most *stable* dichotic listening results over 8
years of testing were seen in patients with circumscribed brain
lesions.

If a dichotic listening task were an immutable index of left-
hemisphere linguistic superiority, it would not be so differentially vulnerable to various acoustic manipulations. In the following sections I will review how adjustments of intensity, frequency, signal-to-noise ratio (S/N), and time of arrival affect
the dichotic REA.


STIMULI

In our work, the stimuli were almost always natural or synthetic consonant-vowel (CV) nonsense syllables (the six English
stops, /pa, ba, ta, da, ka, ga/). (The abbreviation VC, on the
other hand, means vowel-consonant; for example, /ak/.) With the
use of either electromechanical delay lines or computer-control-
ling programs we are able to specify the onsets of the signals
precisely, and can match their amplitudes on the two channels of
a recorded tape. We usually presented the signals to both ears
and asked the subjects to give two CV responses, although we did
not ask the subjects to identify which ear got which signal.

Occasionally there were departures from this general data collection technique; they will be noted where relevant.


INTENSITY

   The first and in some ways most obvious variable to be studied
for its effect on the REA was intensity.  A 10 to 20 dB difference between the ears was necessary (Figure 3) for the left ear
to outperform the right (Berlin, Lowe-Bell, Cullen, Thompson, &
Stafford, 1972a).  Two important points should be made about

**PERCENTAGE CORRECT RESPONSES AS A FUNCTION OF INTENSITY**
**N=11**

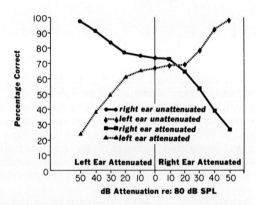

*Fig. 3.  The right-ear advantage as a function of varying inten-
sity in 10-dB steps around 80 dB (SPL = sound pressure level).
From Berlin* et al., *1972a.*

these data:

   1.  As the signal to the right ear was degraded, the performance of the left ear increased and vice versa.
   2.  The entire experiment was run at 80 dB sound pressure
level (SPL).

   The overall SPL at which the task was performed turned out to
be critical, even though the CV syllables were virtually 100%
intelligible if they were given monaurally.  Figure 4 shows that
when the experiment was redone at 50 dB SPL, the asymmetry in
favor of the right ear was reduced to about 5 dB (Cullen, Berlin,
Hughes, Thompson, & Samson, 1975).
   If the REA were related solely to inherent linguistic or
phonological properties of the syllables, the asymmetry should
not be so susceptible to intensity of presentation.

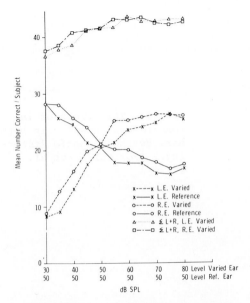

*Fig. 4. The right-ear advantage as a function of varying intensity in 5-dB steps around 50 dB. From Cullen et al., 1975.*

It must be emphasized again that as one channel was degraded, the performance to the other channel increased. One can add the total information out of both channels and find an almost straight-line "constant sum." Departure from this constant sum may reveal something about how speech signals are processed (see later).

Figure 5 shows what happens if the intensity to both channels is reduced simultaneously. A relatively uniform REA is maintained. The apparent convergence of the curves at high intensities was not statistically significant (Cullen *et al.*, 1975).

MANIPULATION OF FREQUENCY

If the usual bandpass of our listening system (roll-off beginning at 4000 Hz) is shifted to 3000 Hz (Figure 6), the REA can be canceled (Cullen *et al.*, 1975). Two things should be noted:

1. The constant superiority of the right over the left ear in comparable conditions.
2. The constant sum generally obtained as the information from one ear is degraded.

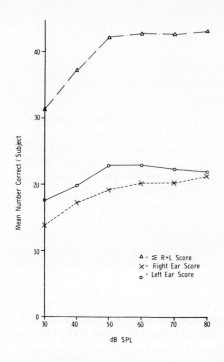

Fig. 5. The effect of intensity manipulation in both ears during dichotic listening. From Cullen et al., 1975.

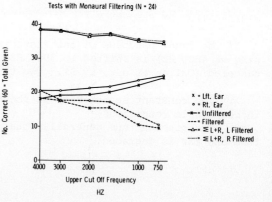

Fig. 6. Dichotic listening results as a function of filtering one ear. From Berlin et al., 1975.

## SIGNAL-TO-NOISE RATIO

Masking one channel has the same effect (Figure 7). That is, as one channel is degraded, the other channel's performance improves, and the constant sum is again observed. An 18 dB signal-to-noise ratio in the left can override the REA (Cullen *et al.*, 1975).

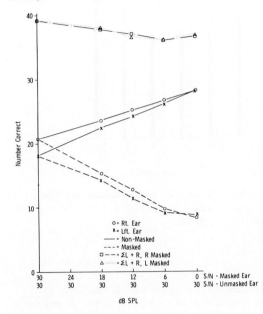

*Fig. 7. Dichotic listening with masking in one ear (S/N = signal-to-noise ratio). From Cullen et al., 1975.*

## TIME

In the time domain, the constant sum effect is absent, apparently indicating a temporal window within which ipsilateral suppression can take place (Figure 8). In presenting these syllables at time separations from 0 to 500 msec, it is observed that in the range of 30 to 60 msec, the *second* signal is the one that is generally better perceived (Berlin, Lowe-Bell, Cullen, Thompson, & Loovis, 1973b). However, when time interval is varied there is no constant sum effect: Better perception of the syllable in the left ear is not accomplished at the expense of the right-ear syllable, but usually in *addition* to right-ear syllable processing, especially beyond 60 msec. Thus the temporal window for ipsilateral suppression does not exceed 60 to 90 msec. It is also clear that the maximum suppression takes place between 0 to 15 msec. As shown later in this chapter, the temporal window suppressing the ipsilateral channel in patients who have undergone temporal lobectomy seems to close around 180 msec.

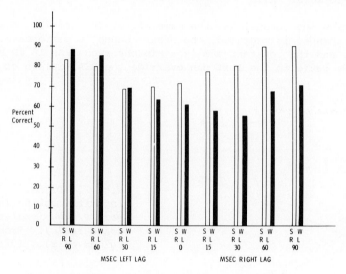

*Fig. 8. The* lag effect: *better dichotic performance in the trailing ear than in the leading ear. S = Strong Ear. W = Weak Ear. Adapted from Berlin et al., 1973b.*

EFFECTS OF AGE

There is some conflict in the literature as to whether language laterality is fixed or develops with age (Porter & Berlin, 1975; cf. Gardiner & Walter; Nottebohm; Rubens; Turkewitz, this volume). If dichotic listening were an *index* of laterality, and if laterality develops with age, one would not obtain results as seen in Figure 9 (Berlin, Hughes, Lowe-Bell, & Berlin, 1973a). Thirty children at each age level were studied (15 males and 15 females). Obviously the laterality index depends on those trials where the syllable is reported correctly only from a single channel. Neither the proportion of such reports nor the predominance of their origin in right-ear syllables varied significantly with age. The score that did develop with age was the number of *double corrects*. Other researchers, using similar tapes, have found that in a geriatric population the right-left ear difference is maintained, but now the double corrects go down again with increasing age (Horning, 1972). In essence, channel capacity, the ability to process signals that overlap temporally and spectrally with one another, seems to be an index of improving brain efficiency, but not necessarily brain laterality. Research with our tapes on dyslexic subjects reveals that they have the same REA as normal children but show a lower double-correct score than the normals (Sobotka, 1974). If this form of dichotic listening is to have any clinical utility, it may come out in the

310

recording and analysis of the double-correct items.

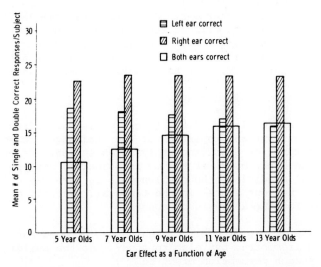

Fig. 9. *Dichotic right-ear advantage in 150 children as a function of age. There were 30 children in each age group (15 males, 15 females). From Berlin et al., 1973a.*

THE CHALLENGES

To clarify the nature of what is meant by a challenge in the dichotic listening paradigm, let me first review some of the logic behind the questions asked:

1. When speech is presented to each ear, in phonetic and acoustic alignment, the right ear generally outperforms the left, *but both ear scores are reduced from their monaural scores of virtually 100%.* If, on the other hand, one musical stimulus is presented to one ear and a different musical stimulus is presented to the other ear, now the *left* ear will outperform the right; *still* both ears fail to get 100% of all the messages presented to them.

2. If speech is presented to one ear, and noise at a level sufficient for *monaural* masking is presented to the other, then (a) the right and left ear perform equally well, and (b) there is almost no interference exerted by the noise on the speech signal.

3. Now, if speech is presented to one ear and music or other nonspeech stimulus to the other, again the right and left ear behave comparably, and there is generally no interference of one signal with another.

This state of affairs, then, leads to the following logic:
We can now designate the CVs in one ear as targets the subject
must identify while various kinds of challenges (to be ignored)
are presented to the other ear.  The functional similarity of
the challenge to speech will be revealed by how much suppression
it generates on the target CV.  Conversely, if the challenge is
*unimportant* to the analysis of speech, there will be no interference with the target CV, just as a masking noise or an irrelevant
sample of music would not interfere with the target CV.  Therefore, it was hypothesized that:

1.  If intelligibility of the target CV is *unimpaired*, then
the acoustical pattern properties of the challenge are essentially unimportant for eliciting analysis as speech.
2.  On the other hand, if the CV is perceived more *poorly* than
in a monaural condition, the challenge is in some way critical to
the auditory nervous system in the temporal, spatial, or intensity domain for the analysis of speech.

In essence, then, dichotic listening can be used not only to
study *brain asymmetry*, but also to study what the building
blocks of speech perception might be.

Figure 10 shows spectral analyses of the challenges used in
various experiments.  These are termed *bleats, CVs, transi-
tionless CV sweeps*, and *CV masks*.  The data plotted in Figure 11
show right- and left-ear performance, respectively, when listening to the CV targets (Berlin, Porter, Lowe-Bell, Berlin,
Thompson, & Hughes, 1973c; Mirabile & Porter, 1975).  The opposite ear always contains one of the challenges and each group of
bars is labeled as a function of what the challenge is in the
*opposite* ear.  As can be seen, CVs and bleats generate suppression of both ears, and also generate REAs when they are used
as challenges.  However, both the size of the REA and the degree
of interference are materially different using the masks, sweeps,

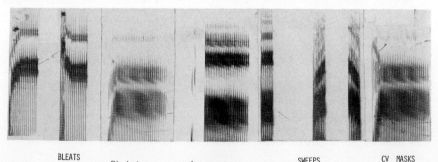

|BLEATS|CV (BA)|P(NO TRANS)+ A|SWEEPS|CV MASKS|

*Fig. 10.  Spectral analyses of challenges used in various ex-
periments.  Adapted from Berlin* et al., *1973c; Mirabile & Porter,
1975; Cullen, 1975.*

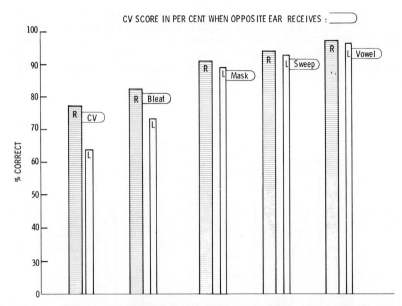

*Fig. 11.* *Right- and left-ear performance when the opposite ear*
*received five of the challenges outlined in the previous figure*
*concurrently with input to other ear. Adapted from the work of*
*Berlin et al., 1973c; Mirabile & Porter, 1975.*

and vowels.  In addition, when an intelligible, voiceless syllable, /pa/, whose transition has been *removed* (Cullen, 1975) is
used, there is *less* interference than with an intact CV, but
there is still a REA.   One major problem in this experimental
design is, of course, that the REA is not seen if one of the
ears is functioning at or near 100%.  Needless to say, however,
some spectral and temporal overlap (as is used in the bleats,
but not in the sweeps, etc.) must be necessary for suppression
to take place.  Some property of the second and third formant
transitions generates a strong contralateral ear suppression.
When this same experiment was performed monotically (putting
both challenge and target in the same ear) the ordering of difficulty for the various challenges as maskers was entirely different.  Thus the dichotic results are not to be explained by masking in its conventional sense.

DICHOTIC INTERFERENCE AFTER CERTAIN BRAIN LESIONS

*INTENSITY*

Temporal lobectomy patients are extremely sensitive to inten-

sity differences between ears (Figures 12, 13, and 14). A syllable in the ear ipsilateral to the lesion is presented at 20 to
30 dB lower than that to the contralateral ear; this is still
enough to overcome the contralateral ear and suppress it considerably. This special susceptibility to intensity differences after
temporal lobectomy probably, in some part, explains why poorly
aligned or poorly controlled dichotic tapes still give large advantages to the ipsilateral ear with these patients (Berlin *et
al.*, 1972a).

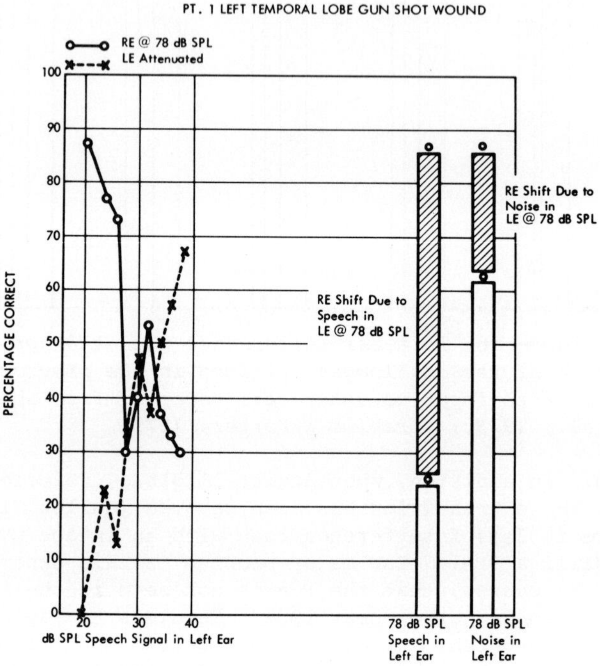

*Fig. 12. Effect of competing intensity on the contralateral ear
of a patient with left temporal lobectomy. Right ear always
received signals at 78 dB SPL. From Berlin et al., 1972a.*

Patients with temporal lobe lesions show no lag effects (Figures 15 and 16). By this I mean that the ear contralateral to
the lesion does not outperform the ipsilateral ear within certain
time separations (Berlin, Lowe-Bell, Jannetta, & Kline, 1972b).
*Note, however, the recovery of the poor ear at or around 180 msec.*
The absence of lag effect (and concomitant release from the
interference with the strong ear) is heightened after hemispherectomy. Performance differs (Figure 17) between normals, patients
with temporal lobectomies, and patients with hemispherectomies
(Berlin, Cullen, Hughes, Berlin, Lowe-Bell, & Thompson, 1975).

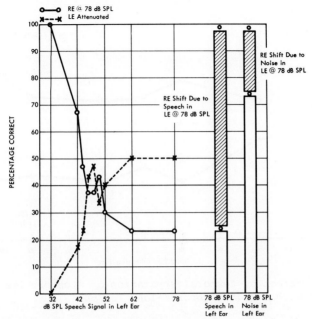

Fig. 13. *Suppression of strong ear by weak ear in another case of left temporal lobectomy. From Berlin* et al., *1973a.*

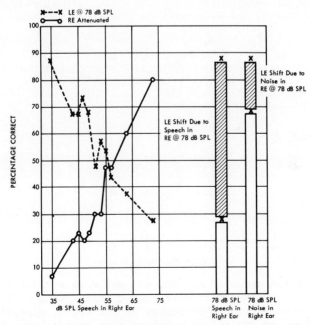

Fig. 14. *Suppression of the contralateral ear in a case of right temporal lobectomy. From Berlin* et al., *1973a.*

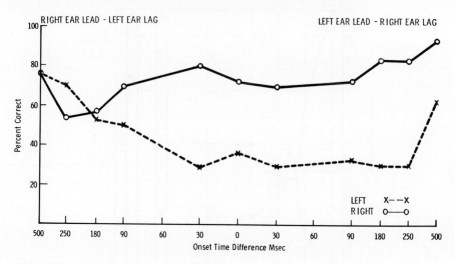

*Fig. 15. Effect of temporal separation on dichotic listening in a patient with a right-temporal-lobe lesion.*

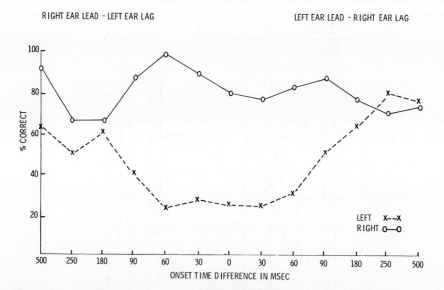

*Fig. 16. Performance of another patient with a right temporal lobectomy on a dichotic time-staggered task. Note in both cases the asymmetrical convergence of the strong versus weak channels between 180 and 500 msec of time separation.*

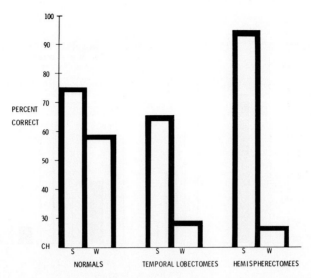

*Fig. 17. A composite of the performances of patients after hemispherectomy or temporal lobectomy and normal subjects on simultaneous message tasks. From Berlin et al., 1975.*

The important thing to notice is that after hemispherectomy the strong ear is performing virtually identically to an ear listening under monaural (no competition) conditions, and certainly better than either ear performs under dichotic conditions in normals. This indicates that one effective level of dichotic interference occurs when partially analyzed information arrives transcallosally from the opposite hemisphere.

When some of the challenges were used with temporal lobectomy or hemispherectomy patients, both groups showed almost complete suppression in the opposite ear and essentially no differentiation between vowels, bleats, and CVs, although noise bursts did have a slight suppressive effect (Figure 18). In patients having brain lesions, the constant sum effect is still seen, with noise, for example, resulting in perfect performance of the contralateral ear after hemispherectomy but with somewhat less efficient performance after temporal lobectomy. What is notable, however, is that the *total percent correct in the brain-injured patients does not approach the total percent correct obtained in normals.*

CASE STUDY OF A PATIENT WITH AN ISOLATED MEDIAL GENICULATE BODY

Figure 19 schematizes the x-ray data localizing the lesion of a patient who is tentatively diagnosed as having a glioma of the brachium of the right inferior colliculus. The interruption of the auditory system on the right side may force ipsilateral and

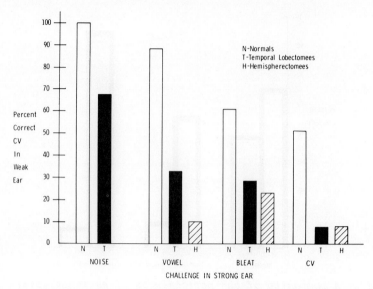

Fig. 18. A composite summary of the effects of challenges on the weak ear of normal, temporal-lobectomized, and hemispherectomized subjects. Adapted from Berlin et al., 1973c.

Glioma, Right Thalamus

CR-26-F

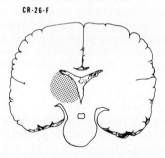

CORONAL SECTION: LEVEL OF POSTERIOR PART OF
THALAMOLENTICULAR PORTION OF INTERNAL CAPSULE

Fig. 19. Frontal view diagram of presumed lesion of the brachium of the inferior colliculus on the right; adapted from x-ray evidence. Courtesy Dr. George Lynn.

contralateral auditory information to pass through the left medial geniculate body.

Figure 20 shows the results on this patient using dichotic

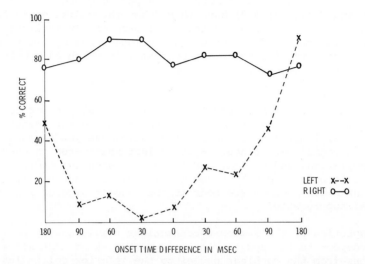

RIGHT EAR LEAD - LEFT EAR LAG        LEFT EAR LEAD - RIGHT EAR LAG

ONSET TIME DIFFERENCE IN MSEC

*Fig. 20. Dichotic-listening results in patient with presumed lesion of the brachium of the right inferior colliculus and presumed isolation of the medial geniculate body on the left. Note that the patient is behaving virtually identically to some-one with a right-temporal-lobe lesion.*

listening. She has almost complete suppression of the left ear and almost but not quite total release from interference of the right ear by the left. Notice a very unusual "catching-up phenomenon" around 90 to 180 msec in which it seems the ipsilateral suppression is diminishing asymmetrically. The suppression of ipsilateral information by contralateral signals becomes ineffi-cient outside the 90-msec range.

If there were no connections between the medial geniculate body and the opposite side, or if the lesion had completely iso-lated the right medial geniculate, *complete* suppression of the left ear might be expected. Since there may be some minor con-nections between the two, it is reasonable to see some interfer-ence in the strong channel in this patient. The original obser-vations suggested that this patient had complete suppression of the left ear and 100% performance in the right ear. However, more careful analysis of the data, especially with respect to forced two-choice responses, reveals that the performance of this patient with isolated medial geniculate body was somewhere between the level of patients with temporal lobectomy and that of total hemispherectomy patients. A similar case has been re-ported by Roeser and Daly (1974). Aside from a possible in-volvement of the commissure of Gudden whose connections are uncertain, no direct commissural connections are known between the pars principalis of the two medial geniculate bodies, and there are no massive connections between the pars magnocellularis. Aitkin and Webster (1972) have shown that the medial geniculate nucleus of the cat has units that will pass either ipsilateral or contralateral information unless impinged upon by two stimuli within a certain time and spectral frame, in which case only contralateral information is passed.

We can conclude from these observations that:

1. It is not exclusively lesions of temporal lobe or corpus callosum that give large and consistent dichotic ear advantages.

2. Only limited ipsilateral information can get through an isolated medial geniculate. What is left unanswered is whether the ipsilateral and contralateral signals reach the medial geniculate body at equal strength. If so, we might conclude that the medial geniculate body is one major source of ipsilateral suppression.

Inspection of the anatomic connections traditionally taught with respect to the auditory nervous system shows that all major stations from the cochlear nuclei to the inferior colliculus are both ipsilaterally and contralaterally related. However, there are specialized regions responding more fully to contralateral than to ipsilateral stimulation. (See, for example, Mountcastle, 1968, p. 1508.) Evidence for a one-way contralateral callosal route for right-hemisphere speech signals is suggested by studies of corpus callosum-sectioned patients in which dichotic-listening results show complete suppression of left-ear and right-hemisphere signals (Milner, Taylor, & Sperry, 1968). It is possible, therefore, that a series of gated pathways for speech-related signals must be postulated between inferior colliculus and temporal lobes, one that operates when spectrally similar signals resembling speech compete within a 90-msec frame. The present case study shows that this competition need not take place at the temporal lobes for ipsilateral suppression to occur. The pathway may furthermore be somewhat asymmetrical. Since there are asymmetries in the left planum temporale (Geschwind & Levitsky, 1968; Witelson & Pallie, 1973), some *asymmetries* might also be expected, either developmental or neonatal, in the projections from the medial geniculate body (and pulvinar) to the temporal-parietal areas. Asymmetries in thalamic function with respect to motor speech have been reported by a number of authors (Guiot, Hertzog, Rondot, & Molina, 1961; Allan, Turner, & Gadea-Ciria, 1966; Bell, 1968; Van Buren & Borke, 1969; Ojemann & Ward, 1971; see also Riklan and Cooper, this volume). The study of functional auditory asymmetries in the *medial geniculate* and other thalamic nuclei might now prove as scientifically profitable as studies of *cortical* asymmetry.

## ACKNOWLEDGMENTS

Support was provided from the National Institutes of Health, USPHS Grants NH 11647-01 and NS 07005, and computer support from the University of New Orleans under NSF Grant GH-131. Critical comments and services were supplied by J. K. Cullen, Jr., Douglas Webster, R. J. Porter, Jr., L. F. Hughes, Sena S. Lowe-Bell, Harriet L. Berlin, Kathy Rich,/and Gae Decker. We thank Drs. Joseph Bogen, Paul Bucy, John Gilroy, George Lynn, and Roger Sperry for access to their patients, and the patients themselves for their cooperation.

## REFERENCES

Aitkin, L. M., & Webster, W. R. Medial geniculate body of the cat: Organization and responses to tonal stimuli of neurons in ventral division. *Journal of Neurophysiology*, 1972, *35*, 365-380.

Allan, C. M., Turner, J. W., & Gadea-Ciria, M. Investigation into speech disturbances following stereotaxic surgery for Parkinsonism. *British Journal of Disorder of Communication*, 1966, *1*, 55-59.

Bell, D. S. Speech functions of the thalamus inferred from the effects of thalamotomy. *Brain*, 1968, *91*, 619-638.

Berlin, C. I., Cullen, J. K., Jr., Hughes, L. F., Berlin, H. L., Lowe-Bell, S. S., & Thompson, C. L. Dichotic processing of speech: Acoustic and phonetic variables (acoustic variables in dichotic listening). *Proceedings of a Symposium on Central Auditory Processing Disorders*, 1975, 36-46.

Berlin, C. I., Hughes, L. F., Lowe-Bell, S. S., & Berlin, H. L. Dichotic right ear advantage in children 5 to 13. *Cortex*, 1973, *9*,(4), 394-402.(a)

Berlin, C. I., Lowe-Bell, S. S., Cullen, J. K., Jr., Thompson, C. L., & Loovis, C. F. Dichotic speech perception: An interpretation of right-ear advantage and temporal offset effects. *Journal of the Acoustical Society of America*, 1973, *53*(3), 699-709.(b)

Berlin, C. I., Lowe-Bell, S. S. Cullen, J. K., Jr., Thompson, C. L., & Stafford, M. R. Is speech "special"? Perhaps the temporal lobectomy patient can tell us. Letter to the Editor. *Journal of the Acoustical Society of America*, 1972, *52*(2), 702-705.(a)

Berlin, C. I., Lowe-Bell, S. S.,Jannetta, P. J., & Kline, D. G. Central auditory deficits after temporal lobectomy. *Archives of Otolaryngology*, 1972, *96*, 4-10.(b)

Berlin, C. I., & McNeil, M. R. Dichotic listening. In Norman J. Lass (Ed.), *Contemporary issues in experimental phonetics*. New York: Academic Press, 1976.

Berlin, C. I., Porter, R. J., Jr., Lowe-Bell, S. S., Berlin, H.L., Thompson, C. L., & Hughes, L. F. Dichotic signs of the recognition of speech elements in normals, temporal lobectomees, and hemispherectomees. *IEEE Transactions on Audio and Electroacoustics*, 1973, AU-21(3), 189-195. (c)

Broadbent, D. E. The role of auditory localization in attenuation and memory span. *Journal of Experimental Psychology*, 1954, *47*, 191-196.

Cullen, J. K., Jr. Tests of a model for speech information flow. Unpublished doctoral dissertation, Louisiana State Univ. Medical Center, Department of Physiology, New Orleans.

Cullen, J. K., Jr., Berlin, C. I., Hughes, L. F., Thompson, C.L., & Samson, D. S. Speech information flow: A model. *Proceedings of a Symposium on Central Auditory Processing Disorders*, 1975, 108-127.

Geschwind, N., & Levitsky, W. Human brain: Left-right asymmetries in temporal speech region. *Science*, 1968, *161*, 186-187.

Guiot, G., Hertzog, E., Rondot, P., & Molina, P. Arrestor acceleration of speech evoked by thalamic stimulation in the course of stereotaxic procedures for Parkinsonism. *Brain*, 1961, *84*, 363-379.

Horning, J. K. The effects of age on dichotic listening. Unpublished master's thesis, San Diego State College, Department of Speech Pathology and Audiology, San Diego, California.

Kimura, D. Cerebral dominance and the perception of verbal stimuli. *Canadian Journal of Psychology*, 1961, *15*, 166-171.

Milner, B., Taylor, L., & Sperry, R. W. Lateralized suppression of dichotically presented digits after commissural section in man. *Science*, 1968, *161*, 184-186.

Mirabile, P., & Porter, R. J., Jr. Dichotic and monotic interactions between speech and nonspeech sounds at different stimulus-onset-asynchronies. *Journal of the Acoustical Society of America*, 1975, *57*(1), S51.

Mountcastle, V. Central neural mechanisms in hearing. In V. Mountcastle (Ed.), *Medical physiology*. Vol. II. St. Louis: C. V. Mosby, 1968.

Ojemann, G. A., & Ward, A. A., Jr. Speech representation in ventrolateral thalamus. *Brain*, 1971, *94*, 669-680.

Porter, R. J., Jr., & Berlin, C. I. On interpreting developmental changes in the dichotic right-ear advantage. *Brain and Language*, 1975, *2*, 186-200.

Porter, R. J., Jr., Troendle, R., & Berlin, C. I. Effects of practice on the perception of dichotically presented stop-consonant-vowel syllables. *Journal of the Acoustical Society of America*, 1976, *59*(3), 679-682.

Roeser, R. J., & Daly, D. D. Auditory cortex disconnection associated with thalamic tumor. *Neurology*, 1974, *24*(5), 555-559.

Sobotka, K.  Neuropsychological and neurophysiological corre-
    lates of reading disability.  Unpublished master's thesis,
    Univ. of New Orleans, Department of Psychology, New
    Orleans, Louisiana.
Van Buren, J. M., & Borke, R. C.  Alterations in speech and the
    pulvinar:  A serial section study of cerebrothalamic rela-
    tionships in cases of acquired speech disorders.  *Brain*,
    1969, *92*, 255-284.
Witelson, S. F., & Pallie, W.  Left hemisphere specialization
    for language in the newborn:  Anatomical evidence of
    asymmetry.  *Brain*, 1973, *96*, 641-646.

# 18.
# Tachistoscopic and Dichotic-Listening Investigations of Laterality in Normal Human Subjects

*SALLY P. SPRINGER*

State University of New York at Stony Brook

LATERALIZING THE STIMULUS

In a standard lateralized tachistoscopic presentation procedure, the subject is required to fixate a point straight ahead while a stimulus is briefly flashed either to the left or to the right of the point of fixation. This procedure capitalizes on the anatomical fact that each visual half-field projects first to the contralateral hemisphere. The optic fibers from the nasal half of each retina cross at the optic chiasm and project contralaterally, whereas the temporal half of each retina projects ipsilaterally (see, e.g., Gross & Mishkin, this volume). Since the image of an object presented off midline falls upon the nasal portion of one retina and the temporal portion of the other, initial lateralization of input to the striate cortex of only one hemisphere occurs. Stimuli must be presented briefly, however, so saccadic eye movements, which could make the stimulus available to both hemispheres, do not have time to occur. Stimuli are usually presented one at a time in a random sequence in either the left or right visual field, permitting a comparison of performance for stimuli projected initially to the right or left cerebral hemisphere, respectively.

There is no simple auditory analogue to the lateralized tachistoscopic presentation procedure in vision. Each ear sends both contralateral and ipsilateral projections from the level of the superior olivary complex upward (Berlin, this volume) so that monaural presentation of material does not permit lateralization to one hemisphere.  A procedure that apparently does permit such initial lateralization, however, was discovered by Doreen Kimura (1961).  She observed that when two different spoken messages are presented simultaneously, one message to each ear, most subjects are better able to report the material presented to the right ear.  These results are interpreted as being due to suppression of the ipsilateral pathways under conditions of competition (cf. Heilman & Watson, this volume), leaving only the contralateral pathways functional; the right-ear advantage is hence due to language dominance of the left hemisphere.  Some support for the functional prepotency of the crossed auditory pathways comes from the work of Rosenzweig (1951) and Hall and Goldstein (1968) in cats.  Work with commissurotomy patients has further supported this interpretation.  Such patients experience no difficulty under monaural input conditions, but under dichotic presentation they are unable to report most of the left-ear inputs, presumably because these inputs project solely to the mute right hemisphere (Milner, Taylor, & Sperry, 1968).

THE NATURE OF LATERALIZED FUNCTIONS

The first major question to which researchers have directed their attention is this:  Just what is it that each hemisphere is specialized for?  Investigators working with neurologically intact subjects began with a legacy from clinical studies:  In most persons the left hemisphere is specialized for analytic processes, including the production and perception of speech and language, whereas the right hemisphere is superior in holistic processing tasks, including visual-spatial performance and music perception (see Milner, 1971).  Early behavioral research had emphasized the verbal or nonverbal nature of the input and sought to define hemispheric asymmetries of function in terms of the cortical loci for the processing of fundamentally different kinds of stimuli.  Thus, when work showed that right-handed subjects were better able to identify letters flashed in the right visual field, and hence to the left hemisphere, the finding was interpreted as reflecting the outcome of an interaction of a verbal processor with a verbal stimulus (Bryden, 1965; Kimura, 1966).  Stimuli revealing a right-hemisphere advantage proved more elusive:  A left-visual-field superiority has been reported for facial recognition (Rizzolatti, Umilta, & Berlucchi, 1971) and a left-ear advantage was obtained for recognition of dichotically presented melodies (Kimura, 1964).  These data were again interpreted as reflections of a match between stimulus and processor.

More recently, investigators have begun to emphasize less the nature of the stimulus in laterality studies and to place the primary stress instead on the type of task required of the subject.  Gibson, Dimond, and Gazzaniga (1972), for example, were

able to show a left-visual-field advantage in a word-matching
task when subjects could respond solely on the basis of the physical characteristics of the stimuli.  In this study, a subject
was presented with a single word displayed for 3 sec across both
visual fields, followed by a second word flashed for 40 msec on
the left or right of fixation.  The duration of the second stimulus was too brief to permit identification.  Subjects probably
performed the task of deciding whether or not the two letter
strings were identical on the basis of gross configurational
properties of the words rather than on the basis of their semantic content.

A similar reversal of the hemispheric effects that might be
predicted solely from the nature of the stimulus was obtained by
Klatzky and Atkinson (1971).  Pictures of common objects were the
stimuli and the subject's task was to determine the initial letter of the name of the object in order to compare it to a set of
letters previously presented.  The experiment yielded a right-
visual-field advantage.  The nature of the task, then, appears
to be a crucial determinant of the type of visual field advantage
to be found.

John Niederbuhl in our laboratory has provided additional
evidence of the importance of task variables.  His experiment
sought to produce opposite visual field effects using the same
stimuli solely as a function of instructions to the subject
(Niederbuhl, unpublished data).  The four letters *K*, *T*, *A*, and *Z*
were called the *positive set*.  On each trial, subjects were presented with the task of deciding as quickly as possible whether
a single letter flashed either to the left or right visual field
was a member of this positive set.  The *negative set* was defined
by exclusion, i.e., all letters that were not members of the
positive set could be members of the negative set.  One group of
subjects was initially presented with all four positive-set letters and told to rehearse them verbally between trials.  A second
group of subjects, who never saw the four members of the positive
set at once, was told to define positive-set membership in terms
of the physical properties of the letters; only letters composed
exclusively of straight lines were members of the set.  The letters *C*, *O*, *U*, and *S* formed the negative set for both groups of
subjects.

Results showed a significant hemisphere by instruction interaction ($p < .01$).  The right-visual-field/left-hemisphere
performance was faster under naming instructions, whereas the
left-visual-field/right-hemisphere system responded more quickly
under shape instructions.  Obtaining different results with the
same stimuli as a function of instructions is a powerful demonstration of the importance of task variables in determining the
outcome of laterality studies.  Niederbuhl has argued that many
experimental situations provide ambiguous instructions for subjects and hence promote great variability as each subject uses
his preferred strategy.  A conceivable consequence could be

experiments in which some subjects show a left-visual-field advantage and some a right-visual-field advantage, which may combine to produce a null result when averaged.

Before concluding, however, that stimulus characteristics per se are unimportant in laterality research, it should be noted that there are examples where certain properties of the stimulus seem to be crucial. In a dichotic listening experiment employing synthetic fricative-vowel syllables, Darwin (1971a) showed that fricatives synthesized with rapid frequency changes (called *formant transitions*) showed a right-ear advantage, whereas those synthesized without such transitions failed to reveal any asymmetry. Since subjects were required to identify the dichotic syllables on each trial with both types of material, task differences cannot explain the results.

One interpretation of these findings is that the left-hemisphere speech processor is specialized for the extraction of information in formant transitions, and that stimuli lacking such transitions may be processed in either hemisphere. The phonetic character of the stimuli would be irrelevant in this conception of the lateralized left-hemisphere mechanism, and from the model one would predict a right-ear advantage even for phonetically impossible stimuli as long as they contain formant transitions. Cutting (1974) has recently reported precisely this result. Additional complications arise, however, since speech stimuli without formant transitions often show a significant right-ear advantage as well. This has led Cutting (1974) to suggest that there may be two left-hemisphere mechanisms operating on incoming auditory information, one primarily phonetic and one primarily acoustic.

Although the key to the understanding of hemispheric asymmetry of function may lie primarily in processing strategy characteristics and secondarily in specific characteristics of the stimuli, the problem of the null result is still one that constantly plagues investigators. Should the failure to find a significant difference between visual fields or ears be taken as evidence for the absence of a lateralized mechanism for the task and/or stimulus involved? In general, the answer is no. In addition to the logical difficulties associated with affirming the null hypothesis, the position is assailable on at least two grounds for which corroborating data are available.

First, Niederbuhl has argued that failure to control for strategy may result in subjects' employing in the same task different strategies that engage one or the other hemisphere (cf. Gur & Gur, this volume), producing no differences when the data from all subjects are averaged. Real differences may be obscured, then, when subjects have available to them several optional approaches to a task.

Second, both tachistoscopic and dichotic listening experiments assume that visual field and ear effects exist because of an advantage that occurs when the stimulus to be processed and the processor meet directly, i.e., when the stimulus is initially presented to the hemisphere that will be responsible for its processing. A stimulus initially presented to the unspecialized hemisphere is presumed to be at a disadvantage since it is either handled in that hemisphere, but less efficiently, or must be transferred interhemispherically to the other side. It is easy to envision how less efficient processing might produce a performance decrement, and only slightly more difficult to imagine how information loss associated with interhemispheric transfer could be translated into poorer performance. However, these conditions need not necessarily be reflected in poorer performance (Darwin, 1974). Depending on the difficulty of the task, hemispheric differences in processing may or may not be observable. Less efficient processing or information loss could go undetected if the task did not require maximal utilization of information.

This analysis suggests that making tasks more difficult might produce asymmetries where none were previously found. Support for this notion comes from the work of Weiss and House (1973) with dichotically presented vowels. No ear advantage was observed under conditions of a favorable signal-to-noise ratio, but the right-ear superiority appeared with a lower signal-to-noise ratio. Presumably the use of a lower ratio moved the "observation" window to a region more sensitive to ear differences. A similar result has been reported with tachistoscopic presentation. A 20-msec presentation of single capital letters revealed a significant right-visual-field advantage in terms of percent correct identification, although a 25-msec exposure failed to produce any asymmetry (Bryden, 1965).

The use of reaction time (RT) has also been an important contribution to more sensitive observation. Its application is illustrated in a study of ear asymmetry when consonant-vowel (CV) syllables are opposed by contralateral noise. In this version of the dichotic paradigm, a single trial is composed of one of six CV syllables, /pa/, /ta/, /ka/, /ba/, /da/, /ga/, presented to one ear, while a burst of noise, aligned for onset and offset with the syllable, is presented to the other. Previous studies using percent correct identification as a dependent measure failed to reveal any ear asymmetries in this task (Corsi, 1967; Darwin, 1971b). Investigators have therefore concluded that items presented dichotically must be opposed by stimuli of the same class for "functional decussation" to occur (Darwin, 1971c).

To provide a nonverbal reaction time response measure, the basic paradigm was modified so that a CV syllable selected as the target occurred on 50% of the trials; the remaining 50% of the trials were composed of the other five CV syllables, each occurring equally often (Springer, 1973a, b). The subject's task was to decide on each trial whether or not the CV syllable presented was a token of the target syllable and to indicate that decision by moving a lever in one of two directions as quickly as possible. No percent correct differences as a function of ear were found, but the reaction time measure revealed a 14-msec advantage in favor of the right ear. Percent correct proved to be insensitive to a real difference between ears, which was revealed with reaction time. Reaction time has recently been extensively employed in tachistoscopic studies (Geffen, Bradshaw, & Wallace, 1971; Gross, 1972; Moscovitch, 1972) but only in a limited way in dichotic research (Springer, 1971a, b; 1973a, b; Kallman & Corballis, 1975). Use of reaction time paradigms in dichotic listening might reveal a pattern of asymmetries which has proven refractory with other dependent measures.


EXTENT OF LATERALIZATION

Although the primary thrust of most behavioral studies of hemispheric asymmetry has been the *direction*, left or right, of hemispheric asymmetries, a second important question is the *extent* of such asymmetries. If a hemisphere is specialized for a particular function, is it qualitatively different from its counterpart or is the difference basically a quantitative one? Research relevant to this question indicates that for most functions the differences are quantitative (Gazzaniga, Risse, Springer, Clark, & Wilson, 1975). Each hemisphere can perform almost any task, with the other half-brain superior in some and inferior in others.

The basic data for this contention come from studies of the so-called split-brain subjects. The generality of these findings, however, is limited, since one likely consequence of the intractable epileptic seizures requisite to the commissurotomy operation is a more equipotential representation of functions across the hemispheres than might be found in neurologically intact individuals. Moreover, because of the presence of intact interhemispheric pathways in normal subjects, standard laterality experiments cannot reveal whether the advantage of one visual field or ear over the other is due to loss associated with transfer to a single processor or loss resulting from processing by a less efficient mechanism. A variant of the dichotic listening paradigm employing reaction time as the dependent measure, however, has helped provide an answer to this question for normal speech processing (Springer, 1971a, 1973a).

Listening to a dichotic CV tape in which a particular syllable was designated as the target, subjects were required to respond to each occurrence of the target regardless of ear of presentation. Subjects responded with the right hand on half the trials in this go/no-go task; a verbal response (the name of the target) was required for the remaining half. Previous work had determined that right-ear targets are identified more quickly than left-ear targets for either left or right manual responses

(Springer, 1971b). If both left- and right-ear targets are processed in the left hemisphere, one would expect the RT difference
between ears to be the same for both manual and verbal responses,
since the left-ear item is available in the left hemisphere at
some point preceding output for either response mode. If, however, the left-ear items are processed in the right hemisphere,
the requirement of a verbal response should increase the time
difference between the two ears, since the right hemisphere cannot mediate a verbal response (Filbey & Gazzaniga, 1969). Transfer of information to the left hemisphere would be required,
thereby increasing the RT difference between the ears. Results
showed no difference in RT scores between the two ears as a
function of response mode. This suggests that all or at least
the terminal portion of the processing of these speech sounds
takes place in the left hemisphere.

Further support for a qualitative difference in speech-
processing capacity comes from dichotic testing of commissurotomy
patients. Patients whose sections included the region anterior
to the splenium and posterior to the first one-third to one-half
of the corpus callosum were unable to identify left-ear CV syllables under dichotic presentation, even with instructions to
attend to the left ear and a left-hand pointing response
(Springer & Gazzaniga, 1975). Both studies, then, converge upon
the conclusion that a qualitative difference in capacity for
speech processing exists between the hemispheres. The generality
of these findings for other kinds of processing remains to be
determined.


DEVELOPMENT OF LATERALIZATION

A third question of great interest concerning hemispheric
asymmetries of function is the issue of how these asymmetries
develop (see Gardiner & Walter; Sechzer, Folstein, Geiger &
Mervis; Stamm, Rosen, & Gadotti; Turkewitz, this volume). Are
they normally the result of the organism's interaction with the
environment in some fashion? Or, does the genetic blueprint
specify from the moment of conception the cerebral organization
of a given individual? One approach to this problem is to determine the earliest age at which behavioral manifestations of
hemispheric asymmetry may be found. If evidence of asymmetrical
functioning is found at birth, one might reasonably conclude
that the pattern of asymmetry is under genetic control. This
approach is limited, however, in that if the asymmetries are
first observed only later in life, one cannot conclude that
genetic factors were unimportant in their establishment. In
addition, behavioral techniques of the sort employed with adults
are not ideally suited to work with newborns because of the
infant's restricted response repertoire. Such techniques have
been employed, though, often with great ingenuity (Entus, 1975).

Another strategy is to obtain measures of cerebral organization for speech in adult monozygotic and dizygotic twins and to
compare the degree of intrapair similarity for the two groups.
If hemispheric organization is under genetic control, it would be
expected that genetically identical monozygotic twins would be
more similar in dichotic listening performance than dizygotic
twins who have, on the average, only half of their genes in common. Preliminary data show this to be the case (Springer &
Searleman, 1975). The twin paradigm, then, is useful in separa-
ting the two issues of genetic determination of cerebral asymmetries and the age at which such asymmetries become functional
(cf. Collins; Morgan, this volume).

## LIMITATIONS OF BEHAVIORAL PROCEDURES

The primary limitations upon the usefulness of tachistoscopic
and dichotic listening techniques in studying hemispheric asymmetry of function are a consequence of meeting the conditions
necessary to satisfy the assumptions of the procedures. Both
tachistoscopic presentation and dichotic listening designs require that stimuli be initially presented to one hemisphere.
This requirement is met in the visual case by capitalizing on
the anatomy of the visual pathways and the optical properties of
the lens. As long as a stimulus is presented sufficiently briefly and sufficiently far from fixation, lateralized input is
assured. Most researchers agree that stimulus presentation of
less than 200 msec is needed since the latency of saccadic eye
movements is in the 200-msec range (Woodworth & Schlosberg,
1954). Such brief, as well as nonfoveal, presentation severely
limits the complexity of the stimuli that can be presented, however. In addition, it is essential that subjects maintain fixation prior to stimulus presentation for lateralized input to be
achieved, a requirement that may not be met unless fixation is
monitored during the course of the experiment. Few studies attempt to monitor fixation, and many of those that do not are
probably rewarded with failure to observe visual field differences.

With the dichotic procedure, two inputs are presented simultaneously to a subject, one to each ear. Although each ear
sends projections both contralaterally and ipsilaterally from
the superior olivary complex upward, simultaneous presentation
seems to be effective in suppressing the ipsilateral inputs.
Split-brain subjects are able to report some left-ear material
presented dichotically (Milner, Taylor, & Sperry, 1968; Sparks
& Geschwind, 1968; Gazzaniga et al., 1975), however, suggesting
that suppression is not complete and hence that the dichotic
paradigm may in some instances not satisfy the initial requirement of lateralized input. Furthermore, Berlin (this volume)
has extensively explored a number of acoustic variables to determine their effects on the dichotic right-ear advantage for

speech. Intensity, spectral composition, and temporal variables each markedly affect the ear asymmetry. The mechanisms by which these variables operate must be understood if cerebral organization is to be inferred from dichotic studies.

Despite these difficulties, the dichotic listening and tachistoscopic paradigms have proven to be viable research tools for studying the main questions being asked about hemispheric specialization. Combining these with other behavioral and electrophysiological techniques as well as clinical observations, investigators are beginning to put together the pieces of the lateralization puzzle. Most research to date has sought to determine the nature of lateralized functions, the extent or degree of that lateralization, and the development of asymmetrical organization. Perhaps the next question to ask is how the brain exquisitely combines lateralized functions to produce behavior so well integrated that the experimenter has great difficulty isolating the components for study.

SUMMARY

Lateralized tachistoscopic presentation and dichotic listening are two paradigms widely used to study hemispheric asymmetry of function in the normal brain. They are utilized on the assumption that initial presentation of a stimulus to the hemisphere specialized for its processing will result in performance in some respect superior to that obtained when the stimulus is first projected to the unspecialized hemisphere.

Both the nature of the stimulus and the kind of processing to which the stimulus is subjected appear to be important determinants of the asymmetries to be observed. Support for the role of processing strategy comes from studies that hold stimuli constant as task requirements are manipulated; evidence pointing to the importance of stimulus properties may be found in work that varies stimulus characteristics within a fixed task.

Additional information concerning the nature and extent of hemispheric asymmetries can be obtained through the judicious selection of a dependent variable. Although most investigations have used percent correct as a measure of performance, reaction time has been employed increasingly as investigators become aware of its advantages. First, reaction time has been shown to be a more sensitive measure of hemispheric asymmetries, revealing asymmetries that percent correct fails to demonstrate. Second, reaction time is a useful analytical tool that can be used to test predictions regarding interhemispheric transfer of stimulus information and/or motor commands.

Developmental factors in cerebral organization constitute yet another line of behavioral investigation. One approach involves determining the earliest age at which asymmetries are observable, while another seeks to determine if patterns of asymmetry are

genetically determined.  The dichotic testing of monozygotic and
dizygotic twins has shown the performance of monozygotic pairs
to be less variable in terms of the magnitude and direction of
the ear advantage effect, suggesting that hemispheric specialization for speech perception is under some degree of genetic
control.

Dichotic listening and lateralized tachistoscopic presentation have contributed significantly to an understanding of
hemispheric asymmetries of function.  The complexity of the
questions that may be approached by these procedures is limited,
however, because of restrictions on stimulus presentation neces-
sitated by the requirements of the paradigms.  Nevertheless,
studies employing dichotic listening and lateralized tachistoscopic presentation are expected to continue to unravel parts
of the lateralization puzzle, and are perhaps most fruitfully
directed next to questions of how the brain combines lateralized
functions into integrated behavior.

REFERENCES

Bryden, M. P.  Tachistoscopic recognition, handedness, and cere-
    bral dominance.  *Neuropsychologia*, 1965, *3*, 1-8.
Corsi, P. M.  The effects of contralateral noise upon the per-
    ception and immediate recall of monaurally presented verbal
    material.  Unpublished master's thesis, McGill Univ., 1967.
Cutting, J. E.  Two left-hemisphere mechanisms in speech per-
    ception.  *Perception and Psychophysics*, 1974, *16*, 601-612.
Darwin, C. J.  Ear differences in the recall of fricatives and
    vowels.  *Quarterly Journal of Experimental Psychology*, 1971,
    *23*, 46-62.(a)
Darwin, C. J.  Dichotic forward and backward masking of speech
    and nonspeech sounds.  Paper presented to the Acoustical
    Society of America, Washington, D.C., 1971.(b)
Darwin, C. J.  Stimulus versus response competition and ear
    asymmetry in dichotic listening.  *Haskins Laboratories
    Status Report*, 1971, *25/26*, 29-33.(c)
Darwin, C. J.  Ear differences and hemispheric specialization.
    In F. O. Schmitt & F. G. Worden (Eds.), *The neurosciences -
    third study program*.  Cambridge, Massachusetts:  MIT Press,
    1974.  Pp. 57-63.
Entus, A.  Hemispheric asymmetry in processing of dichotically
    presented speech and nonspeech sounds by infants.  Paper
    presented to the Society for Research in Child Development,
    Denver, 1975.
Filbey, R. A., & Gazzaniga, M. S.  Splitting the normal brain
    with reaction time.  *Psychonomic Science*, 1969, *17*, 335-336.
Gazzaniga, M. S., Risse, G. L., Springer, S. P., Clark, E., &
    Wilson, D.  Psychologic and neurologic consequences of
    partial and complete cerebral commissurotomy.  *Neurology*,

1975, *25*, 10-15.

Geffen, G., Bradshaw, J., & Wallace, G. Interhemispheric effects on reaction time to verbal and nonverbal stimuli. *Journal of Experimental Psychology*, 1971, *87*, 415-422.

Gibson, A., Dimond, S., & Gazzaniga, M. S. Left visual field superiority for word matching. *Neuropsychologia*, 1972, *10*, 463-466.

Gross, M. M. Hemispheric specialization for processing of visually presented verbal and nonverbal stimuli. *Perception and Psychophysics*, 1972, *12*, 357-363.

Hall, J. L., & Goldstein, M. H. Representations of binaural stimuli by single units in primary auditory cortex of unanesthetized cats. *Journal of the Acoustical Society of America*, 1968, *43*, 456-461.

Kallman, H., & Corballis, M. Ear asymmetry in reaction time to musical sounds. *Perception and Psychophysics*, 1975, *17*, 368-370.

Kimura, D. Cerebral dominance and the perception of verbal stimuli. *Canadian Journal of Psychology*, 1966, *15*, 166-171.

Kimura, D. Left-right differences in the perception of melodies. *Quarterly Journal of Experimental Psychology*, 1964, *16*, 355-358.

Kimura, D. Dual functional asymmetry of the brain in visual perception. *Neuropsychologia*, 1961, *4*, 275-285.

Klatzky, R., & Atkinson, R. C. Specialization of the cerebral hemispheres for information in short term memory. *Perception and Psychophysics*, 1971, *10*, 335-338.

Milner, B. Interhemispheric differences in the localization of psychological processes in man. *British Medical Bulletin*, 1971, *27*, 272-277.

Milner, B., Taylor, L., & Sperry, R. Lateralized suppression of dichotically presented digits after commissural section in man. *Science*, 1968, *161*, 184-186.

Moscovitch, M. Choice reaction time study assessing the verbal behavior of the minor hemisphere in normal adult humans. *Journal of Comparative and Physiological Psychology*, 1972, *80*, 66-74.

Rizzolatti, G., Umilta, C., & Berlucchi, G. Opposite superiorities of the right and left cerebral hemispheres in discriminative reaction time to physiognomical and alphabetical material. *Brain*, 1971, *94*, 431-442.

Rosenzweig, M. R. Representations of the two ears at the auditory cortex. *American Journal of Physiology*, 1951, *167*, 147-158.

Sparks, R., & Geschwind, N. Dichotic listening in man after section of neocortical commissures. *Cortex*, 1968, *4*, 3-16.

Springer, S. P. Lateralization of phonological processing in a dichotic detection task. Unpublished doctoral dissertation, Stanford Univ., 1971.(a)

Springer, S. P. Ear asymmetry in a dichotic detection task.

*Perception and Psychophysics*, 1971, *10*, 239-241.(b)

Springer, S. P.  Reaction time measures of ear advantage in dichotic listening.  Paper presented to the Acoustical Society of America.  Boston, 1973.(a)

Springer, S. P.  Hemispheric specialization for speech opposed by contralateral noise. *Perception and Psychophysics*, 1973, *13*, 391-393.(b)

Springer, S. P., & Gazzaniga, M. S.  Dichotic testing of partial and complete split brain subjects. *Neuropsychologia*, 1975, *13*, 341-346.

Springer, S. P., & Searleman, A.  Genetic factors in cerebral organization:  A preliminary study of dichotic listening in twins.  Paper presented to the Acoustical Society of America, San Francisco, 1975.

Weiss, M., & House, A. S.  Perception of dichotically presented vowels. *Journal of the Acoustical Society of America*, 1973, *53*, 51-58.

Woodworth, R. S., & Schlosberg, H. *Experimental psychology*. New York:  Holt, 1954.

# Part VI

# SURFACE ELECTROCORTICAL INDICATERS OF LATERALIZATION I:

## Event-Related Potentials

# 19.
# Electrocortical Indices of Hemispheric Utilization

*EMANUEL DONCHIN, MARTA KUTAS AND GREGORY McCARTHY*

University of Illinois

It is well known that electroencephalographic (EEG) activity
recorded from widely spaced scalp electrodes is quite diverse; at
any instant the voltage at any site may be of a different amplitude or polarity than that recorded at other electrodes. When the
properties of the EEG as a time series are evaluated over extended
epochs, spectra of simultaneously recorded series vary considerably (Walter, Rhodes, Brown, & Adey, 1966). This variability is
due to the structural and functional differences between brain
sites underlying the electrodes. As brain tissue varies in its
activity patterns so do the manifestations of these activities on
the scalp.

The scalp distribution of EEG parameters, estimated from appropriately placed electrodes, has long served to support inferences
concerning intracranial electrophysiological events. The most
notable success and broadest application of these inferential
procedures has been in clinical neurology (Cooper, Osselton, &
Shaw, 1974). The scalp distribution of the EEG is widely used
in localizing epileptic foci (Gibbs, Lennox, & Gibbs, 1936),
tumors (Walter, 1936), focal lesions (Case & Bucy, 1938), and
other pathologies. The relative success of these procedures has

*This research was supported by the Advanced Research Projects
Agency (ARPA) of the Department of Defense under Contract No.
DAHC-15-73-C-0318 to E. Donchin managed by Dr. G. Lawrence of the
Human Research Resources Branch at ARPA. The contract is moni-
tored by the Defense Supply Agency. M. Kutas is supported by NIH
Training Grant 5 T01 MH 10715.

derived from the fact that the pathology may create localized electrical activity at the scalp (Cooper *et al.*, 1974). More recent attempts to identify the intracranial locus of the generators of components of time-locked, event-related potentials (ERPs) have also assumed that these generators represent spatially circumscribed entities (Vaughan, 1969, 1974; Goff, Matsumiya, Allison, & Goff, 1969). In the case of events generated early in the afferent sequence (events we shall label *exogenous*), such inferences seem to be well supported (Goff *et al.*, 1969; Jewett, Romano, & Williston, 1970).

This review is concerned with attempts to extend the use of EEG scalp distribution to the assessment of the differential utilization of distinct cortical areas under different circumstances. Our review is restricted to studies that compare the electrical activity recorded from homologous sites on the two hemispheres. The data collected in these studies are normally used to infer which of the two hemispheres is "utilized," or more actively engaged, during the performance of one task or another (cf. Gur & Gur, this volume).

The use of electrophysiological indices of hemispheric utilization has grown with the increasing interest in the study of the complementary specialization of the hemispheres. Much evidence, surveyed in other chapters of this volume, has accrued during the past two decades demonstrating that the two hemispheres are not functionally equivalent. A grossly oversimplified summary of these data would describe the left hemisphere, in dextrals, as supporting verbal, analytic processing, and the right hemisphere as specializing in spatial, holistic processing. Although the association between speech and the left hemisphere has been known since at least the mid-nineteenth century (Broca, 1861), the more extensive knowledge obtained during the past two decades has derived primarily from research on more recent populations of commissurotomized (Gazzaniga, 1970; Sperry, 1974), hemispherectomized (Smith, 1972), or lesioned patients (Milner, 1974). Extension of this work depends on complementary and more accessible sources of data. At present the most successful approach has been through the presentation of lateralized sensory inputs (Kimura, 1961; Bryden, 1965; see Berlin; Springer, this volume), which allow, through the use of the standard techniques of experimental psychology, an evaluation of differential hemispheric processing (Dimond & Beaumont, 1974).

Lateralization of sensory inputs, however, is not an easy procedure and imposes numerous restrictions on the range of paradigms in which hemispheric specialization can be studied. It is in this context that the use of electrophysiological techniques is of potential value. If indeed it is possible to infer hemispheric utilization from electrophysiological parameters, then this convenient, noninvasive technique would be available to complement the data obtained from commissurotomized patients.

This chapter is a review of past attempts to realize the

potential contribution of EEG lateralization studies (see also
Butler & Glass, 1974). As will become apparent, the literature
is replete with uncertain and conflicting results often due to
inadequate attention to methodology. The chapter concludes with
a description of work conducted in our laboratory.


A SURVEY OF CURRENT STUDIES

Virtually all studies reviewed in this chapter have employed
the same general paradigm. The independent variable is always
defined in terms of tasks assigned to the subject, some presumably involving the right, others the left hemisphere. The dependent variable is always some parameter of the scalp-recorded
EEG activity.

The term *parameter* is used in this paper in the following
sense: The primary data collected in all the reviewed studies
consist of the raw EEG recorded in either analog or digital form.
Any number of functions can be defined on these raw data. Such
statistics as the mean power, the frequency spectrum, the cross-
correlation function, or the ensemble average are all functions
of the raw data, and all estimate some *parameter* of the process
generating the data. Thus, investigators have wide freedom in
the choice of parameters. The specific choice they do make is
determined by their hypotheses on the nature of the EEG and EEG-
behavior relations. The choice, in turn, can determine the
import of the results.

The studies can be conveniently classified into two categories
according to the dependent variables used. In one category are
all studies that focus on the "ongoing" EEG activity and in which
frequency-domain parameters of the EEG are estimated (see
Gardiner & Walter; Nelsen, Phillips, & Goldstein; Webster, this
volume). Such parameters are usually measures of the power or
amplitude, of the EEG, integrated over some narrow or broad bandwidth. In the second category fall studies that analyze the EEG
in the time domain (see Anderson; Stamm, Rosen, & Gadotti;
Thatcher, this volume). These are exclusively concerned with the
waveforms of event-related potentials (ERPs) extracted from the
EEG by signal averaging. Within these two categories the studies
are classified in terms of the independent variables used by the
experimenter. An overview of the dependent variables follows.

Frequency-Domain Studies of the EEG

Many investigators have compared the distribution of the spectral power of the EEG at homologous hemispheric locations. Best
known are studies focusing on the activity in the 8-12 Hz band
(known as *alpha*). The interest in alpha activity derives from
the well-known inverse relationship between alpha power and mental effort (Adrian & Matthews, 1934; Berger, 1930). The assump-

tion is made that hemispheric involvement might be indexed by differential suppression of alpha in the two hemispheres (Galin & Ornstein, 1972). More recently, measures of intrahemispheric "coupling" have been used as indices of hemispheric utilization (Callaway & Harris, 1974). The assumption here is that hemispheric involvement leads to a greater degree of interaction between different intrahemispheric sites, which manifests itself in increased intrahemispheric coupling.

## Time-Domain Studies of Event-Related Potentials (ERPs)

With few exceptions, students of the ERP report their results in terms of amplitude or latency of the entire ERP waveform, or its features. It is important, however, to distinguish between three classes of ERP studies in terms of the components that are in fact analyzed. The ERP consists of a sequence of positive-negative potentials that either precede or follow the eliciting event. Post stimulus activity tends to subside after about 500 msec, though anticipatory processes are known to operate over several seconds. The early poststimulus components represent stages in the afferent stream (Buchwald & Huang, 1975) and are often referred to as exogenous. Exogenous components can only be recorded in association with some sensory stimulus. Their scalp distribution depends to a considerable extent on the modality of the stimulus (Goff *et al.*, 1969) and their morphology on the physical parameters of the stimulus.

By contrast, the later ERP components, those with latencies exceeding 150 msec, can be elicited in the absence of a stimulus (Sutton, Tueting, Zubin, & John, 1967; Klinke, Fruhstorfer, & Finkenzeller, 1968), are relatively insensitive to stimulus modality (Vaughan, 1969), and are enormously sensitive to task paramaters. We believe these components are manifestations of cortical information-processing activities engaged by task demands, and we shall refer to these as *endogenous* components (Donchin, 1975).

There are two classes of endogenous components, those appearing before and those appearing after the eliciting events. Of the postevent components, the best known is P300 (Sutton, Braren, Zubin, & John, 1965). The preevent components, such as the Contingent Negative Variation (CNV) or the Readiness Potential (RP), are apparently related to anticipatory or preparatory activities (Walter, Cooper, Aldridge, McCallum, & Winter, 1964; Kornhuber & Deecke, 1965).

The studies relating ERP components to hemispheric specialization have most often been concerned with endogenous components. However, data on the lateral distribution of exogenous components are available and will be reviewed.

*SURVEY OF FREQUENCY-DOMAIN STUDIES*

EEG Measures and Handedness

   This survey begins with an analysis of the relationship of EEG measures to manual preferences, followed by a discussion of task-induced changes in scalp distribution of EEG parameters.
   Early investigators of the EEG, although they noted occasional hemispheric asymmetries, stressed the similarity of EEG tracings recorded from the two hemispheres (Adrian & Matthews, 1934). Large differences between homologous recordings were considered abnormal and were used to localize focal disorders not character- ized by obvious dysrhythmias  (Aird & Bowditch, 1946; Aird & Zealear, 1951).  Much evidence, however, that the alpha rhythm is rarely symmetric in amplitude or in phase has accrued in the past few decades (Raney, 1939; Remond, Leservre, Joseph, Rieger, & Lairy, 1969; Liske, Hughes, & Stowe, 1967; Hoovey, Heinemann, & Creutzfeldt, 1972).  These asymmetries have sometimes been rela- ted to the subject's lateral preferences.  The alpha rhythm in the dominant hemisphere has been found to be of lower amplitude (Cornil & Gastaut, 1947; Raney, 1937), but this relationship is not universally reported (Butler & Glass, 1974a; Glanville & Antonitis, 1955; Liske *et al.*, 1967; Provins & Cunliffe, 1972; Remond *et al.*, 1969).  A relationship between interhemispheric EEG phase and laterality preferences has also been reported (Giannitrapani, 1967; Giannitrapani & Darrow, 1963; Giannitrapani, Darrow, & Sorkin, 1964; Giannitrapani, Sorkin, & Ennenstein, 1966).  However, the relationship appears to be quite complex and confused,  with the direction of the phase asymmetry changing with subject and state variables.
   In part, the confusion derives from difficulty in defining and validating a "resting" state in which to take baseline EEG measures.  The wide variations in measurement and analysis tech- niques also account for some of the confusion in the literature. Mostly, however, the relationship between EEG laterality and subjects' lateral preferences is *in fact* quite complex.  Inter- hemispheric alpha asynchrony has been reported to be more preva- lent in subjects with less established lateral preferences, such as the ambidextrous, or in those in whom lateral specialization may be weak, such as stutterers (Travis & Knott, 1937; Lindsley, 1940).  Similar asynchronies have also been found in children with disordered verbal-motor development (Lairy, Remond, Rieger, & Leserve, 1969).  Amplitude asymmetries, on the other hand, have been reported to be larger in subjects with clearly defined hand preferences (Lairy *et al.*, 1969; see Subirana, 1969).  EEG measures may, then, depend on the *degree* of lateral specializa- tion in individuals rather than on its *direction* (cf. Collins, this volume).  Such considerations must be kept in mind when evaluating the use of EEG measures to index functional asymmetry in the human brain.

## Interhemispheric EEG Asymmetries and Hemispheric Specialization

A number of recent studies have claimed that interhemispheric changes in alpha and total EEG power accompany the performance of functionally asymmetric tasks. Such investigations typically employ a paradigm in which a subject performs a task thought to engage primarily one hemisphere while bilateral samples of EEG are taken. Occipital (Dumas & Morgan, 1975; Morgan, Macdonald, & Hilgard, 1974; Morgan, McDonald, & Macdonald, 1971), temporal and parietal (Doyle, Ornstein, & Galin, 1974; Galin & Ornstein, 1972; McKee, Humphrey, & McAdam, 1973) electrode placements, referenced to the vertex ($C_z$) position, have been used. Intrahemispheric bipolar linkages have also been employed (Butler & Glass, 1974a).

Tasks presumed to utilize the left hemisphere differentially have included composing letters (Galin & Ornstein, 1972; Doyle *et al.*, 1974), word-search tasks (McKee *et al.*, 1973), mental arithmetic (Morgan *et al.*, 1971, 1974; Dumas & Morgan, 1975; Butler & Glass, 1974a), and verbal listening (Morgan *et al.*, 1971, 1974; Dumas & Morgan, 1975). Right-hemisphere tasks have included modified Kohs Blocks, Seashore tonal memory, and drawing tasks (Galin & Ornstein, 1972; Doyle *et al.*, 1974). They have also included spatial imagery tasks (Morgan *et al.*, 1971, 1974; Dumas & Morgan, 1975) and music listening tests (McKee *et al.*, 1973; Morgan *et al.*, 1971; see Gardiner & Walter, this volume). In addition, occupation (artist versus engineer) and hypnotic susceptibility have been used as independent variables (Morgan *et al.*, 1971, 1974; Dumas & Morgan, 1975).

Data have been analyzed in many different ways. Often, investigators have integrated the raw or filtered EEG (Dumas & Morgan, 1975; Galin & Ornstein, 1972; McKee *et al.*, 1973; Morgan *et al.*, 1971; Nelsen *et al.*; Webster, this volume). Others have computed amplitude histograms of the EEG (Butler & Glass, 1974a) or have used conventional spectral-analysis techniques (Doyle *et al.*, 1974; Gardiner & Walter, this volume). Despite the variety of methods for obtaining estimates of power, most researchers have then expressed their results in terms of right/left or left/right power ratios for homologous electrode sites (Doyle *et al.*, 1974; Galin & Ornstein, 1972; McKee *et al.*, 1973; Nelsen *et al.*; Webster, this volume) or as a laterality score expressing differences in power as a function of total power (Dumas & Morgan, 1975; Morgan *et al.*, 1974; Gardiner & Walter, this volume). Changes in these ratios are interpreted as evidence for differential hemispheric involvement. For example, Galin and Ornstein (1972) obtained the power of the total EEG at the right and left parietal electrodes. The right/left power ratio is 1.15 for the spatial Kohs Blocks task and 1.30 for the verbal letter-writing task. The increase in the power in the right hemisphere relative to the left hemisphere for the letter-writing task is presumed to reflect the greater involvement of the left hemisphere in that task (recall that increased power implies increased alpha activity and by inference implies a *lesser* degree of hemispheric involvement). Similar results were obtained in studies of activity in the alpha band (Dumas & Morgan, 1975; McKee *et al.*, 1973; Morgan *et al.*, 1971). Butler and Glass (1974a) found left-hemisphere suppression of alpha during mental arithmetic but only in their dextral subjects; unfortunately, no right-hemisphere tasks were used for comparison. A more sophisticated frequency analysis (Doyle *et al.*, 1974) revealed that the main locus of task-dependent distributional changes occurs in the alpha band. They reported minor interhemispheric differences in the beta and theta bands and no changes in the delta band (cf. Gardiner & Walter, this volume).

Although these studies may indicate that there are small task-dependent changes in the EEG spectrum, the implication that selective suppression in the dominant hemisphere for the task is the cause of the ratio changes cannot be supported on the evidence presented. It is not possible to tell if a ratio has been modified by changing the numerator, the denominator, or both when only the ratio figure is presented. Note also that in most of these studies the experimentally induced differences are superimposed upon a constant right/left hemisphere asymmetry and do not represent shifts from a symmetric baseline.

## Intrahemispheric EEG Measures and Hemispheric Specialization

To date, only one study has employed the intrahemispheric coupling approach to the study of hemispheric specialization (see Livanov, Gavrilova, & Aslanov, 1964, 1973 for related work). Callaway and Harris (1974) reported that appositional or spatial analysis of visual stimuli increases the relative amount of posterior right hemisphere coupling, and propositional examination of visual material (such as reading) increases posterior left hemisphere coupling. As yet unpublished data from the same laboratory tend to confirm and extend these observations (Callaway, personal communication).

*SURVEY OF TIME-DOMAIN STUDIES*

In this section we report on studies of event-related potentials (ERPs) extracted by signal averaging from the ongoing EEG. All the studies reviewed compared ERPs recorded at homologous hemispheric sites. As in the frequency-domain studies discussed in the previous section, the ERP investigators endeavored to demonstrate that task variables determine the relative amplitude of ERPs over the hemispheres. These differences were sometimes evaluated in terms of subjects' handedness and cerebral dominance.

## Studies of Exogenous Components

Very few of the studies reviewed in this section were motivated by an interest in hemispheric specialization. Rather, the investigators were seeking information on the scalp distribution of sensory evoked potentials. Their goal has usually been the elucidation of the intracranial sources of these exogenous components. Yet data were often collected from homologous hemispheric sites. These provide valuable baseline data on hemispheric asymmetries. Clearly, if ERPs associated with a given modality are asymmetric in the absence of any task inducement for such lateralization, such biases must be considered when testing hypotheses about hemispheric specialization. The results on hand, however, are equivocal. It would be difficult to develop, on the basis of the available literature, a specification of the lateralization biases for different stimulus modalities.

## Somatosensory ERPs

The data are scant. The consensus seems to be that the largest somatosensory responses are recorded from the scalp overlying the parietal cortex contralateral to the stimulation site (Calmes & Cracco, 1971; Goff, Rosner, & Allison, 1962; Manil, Desmedt, Debecker, & Chorazyna, 1967).

## Auditory ERPs

Considerable controversy exists regarding the lateral distribution of the various components of auditory ERPs. The maximal contralateral projection to the auditory cortex as well as the oft observed dominance of one ear over the other in dichotic-listening tasks (see Anderson; Berlin; Springer, this volume) suggest that, at least under certain conditions, different auditory ERPs should be recorded over the two hemispheres. Most investigators concur that right- and left-ear stimulation generate different scalp distributions, but there is no agreement on the specifics of these distributions. Most reports maintain that there is a general predominance of the contralateral response; some find differences in terms of a shorter latency response (Majkowski, Bochenek, Bochenek, Knapik-Fijalkowska, & Kopec, 1971), others in terms of a larger amplitude response (Andreassi, De Simone, Friend, & Grota, 1975; Peronnet, Michel, Echallier, & Girod, 1974; Price, Rosenblut, Goldstein, & Shepherd, 1966; Ruhm, 1971; Vaughan & Ritter, 1970), and a few in terms of both these measures (Butler, Keidel, & Spreng, 1969). Vaughan and Ritter (1970) reported a small but consistent tendency for larger responses to appear contralateral to the stimulated ear, but the effect was greater over the left hemisphere in response to right-ear stimulation. Other researchers (Peronnet *et al.*, 1974; Ruhm, 1971) report that the right-hemisphere response is consistently larger only for left-ear stimulation. Peters and Mendel (1974) failed to find such a consistent relationship between the ear stimulated and the latency and amplitude of early (less than 70 msec) ERP components. Given these contradictions, there seems to be little basis yet in trying to relate the lateral asymmetry of auditory ERPs to handedness, cerebral dominance, or ear perference.

## Visual ERPs

Similar inconsistencies appear in studies of the laterality of visual ERPs. Studies of interhemispheric differences in visual ERPs have been particularly hampered by the need to assure that the ERP elicited by stimulation of a retinal half-field is generated entirely within a single hemisphere. Whereas it has been well established that stimulation of different visual half-fields elicits different scalp distributions (see MacKay, 1969; Regan, 1972), the comparison of the hemispheric distributions of visual ERPs is not as straightforward. Several investigators (Kooi, Guvener, & Bagchi, 1965; Vaughan, Katzman, & Taylor, 1963; Harmony, Ricardo, Fernandez, & Valdes, 1973) have reported that visual ERPs recorded over homologous regions in normal subjects are symmetric. Other researchers, however, have maintained that visual ERPs recorded from the right hemisphere are larger than those recorded from the left hemisphere (Perry & Childers, 1969; Rhodes, Dustman, & Beck, 1969; Rhodes, Obitz, & Creel, 1975; Richlin, Weisinger, Weinstein, Giannini, & Morganstern, 1971; Schenkenberg & Dustman, 1970; Butler & Glass, 1972). A more recent report has indicated that retinal site of stimulation may induce latency asymmetries in ERP components (Andreassi, Okamura, & Stern, 1975).

The few investigations (Culver, Tanley, & Eason, 1970; Eason, Groves, White, & Oden, 1967; Gott & Boyarsky, 1972) concerned with the relations between handedness, cerebral dominance, eye dominance, and visual ERPs have yielded ambiguous results. Eason et al. (1967) originally reported that the visual ERPs were larger over the right than the left hemisphere for left-handers only. However, a subsequent report from the same laboratory (Culver et al., 1970) failed to confirm this finding. Rather, Culver et al. reported that visual ERP amplitudes were larger over the right than the left occipital lobe in response to left- but not right-visual-field stimulation. This failure to replicate previous results is attributed by Culver to confounding effects of sex and handedness (cf. Gur & Gur, this volume). Gott and Boyarsky (1972) reported that left-handers produced larger visual ERPs over the left hemisphere and that direct stimulation of the dominant hemisphere (generally right for sinistrals and left for dextrals) elicited ERPs with shorter latency than those elicited by stimulation of the opposite, nondominant hemisphere.

A report by Galin and Ellis (1975) indicates that the symmetry of the visual ERP is influenced by the spectral characteristics of the EEG at the time of stimulus presentation. They found that ERPs elicited during tasks inducing hemispheric asymmetries in alpha power were also asymmetric as determined by measures of peak-to-trough amplitude and power. Such results are provocative and suggest that baseline symmetry in ERPs may depend on variability in ongoing EEG activity, which may in turn depend on subject state variables.

## Studies of Endogenous Components

*Asymmetries in Movement-Related Potentials*

The most consistent observations of functionally interpretable lateralization have been obtained for slow potentials that are apparently associated with the control or the monitoring of movement.

1. *Readiness Potential.* There is now a general consensus that the slow negative shift preceding voluntary arm and hand movements, variously called the readiness potential (RP), Bereitschaftspotential (BSP), or N1 of the motor potential (MP), is a few microvolts larger over the pre-Rolandic area on the scalp contralateral to the responding limb (Gilden, Vaughan, & Costa, 1966; Kutas & Donchin, 1974a, 1974b; Vaughan, Costa, & Ritter, 1968). Kornhuber and his co-workers (Deecke, Scheid, & Kornhuber, 1969; Kornhuber & Deecke, 1965) maintain that this contralateral dominance is restricted to the abrupt negativity just preceding the movement, but Kutas and Donchin (1974a, 1974b) demonstrated that the hemispheric asymmetry can be observed hundreds of milliseconds prior to the response. The exact timing of the components of the motor potential immediately preceding the movement is, however, controversial. Gerbrandt, Goff, and Smith (1973) claimed that this negativity occurs after movement; Vaughan *et al.* (1968) found that the RP has a somatotopic distribution and clearly occurs prior to movement. Two reports (Gerbrandt *et al.*, 1973; Wilke & Lansing, 1973) reject the notion that these premovement potentials are associated with a motor command and claim that the potentials are manifestations of the activity of postresponse proprioceptive mechanisms. However this issue is resolved, there is no question that N1 precedes the movement. Thus, our demonstration that the N1 component of the MP is larger contralateral to the responding hand is a clear illustration of the manner in which EEG scalp distributions reflect hemispheric utilization (Kutas & Donchin, 1974a).

The absolute amplitude of the motor potentials depends on a number of variables such as force (Kutas & Donchin, 1974a, 1974b; Wilke & Lansing, 1973) and motivation (McAdam & Seales, 1969). The relevant parameters affecting the degree of N1 asymmetry, other than subject handedness and responding hand, have yet to be determined. A promising source of data is intracerebral recording from human patients (see McCallum & Papakostopoulos, 1974). These preliminary data suggest that subtle changes in timing and asymmetry of the RP may be obscured in scalp recordings.

2. *Response Variables and the Contingent Negative Variation.* Many investigators have noted the similarity of the CNV and N1. The suggestion that these two waveforms might represent identical processes is derived partly from the fact that most CNV studies have required a motor response to the imperative stimulus. Early mapping studies (Cohen, 1969; Low, Borda, Frost, & Kellaway, 1966) demonstrated that the CNV preceding a motor response in an RT paradigm is symmetrically distributed over the two hemispheres. Within the past few years it has been asserted that slightly larger CNVs appear over the hemisphere contralateral to the hand used for the response (Syndulko, 1969, 1972; Otto & Leifer, 1973). Syndulko (1972) reported that this response-related lateral asymmetry was specific to central as opposed to frontal, parietal, or occipital locations and developed only preceding unimanual response preparation. Otto and Leifer (1973), on the other hand, noted that a CNV laterality was statistically significant only when the data were pooled across their response and feedback conditions. It has been well established that CNVs can be generated in the absence of a motor response (Cohen & Walter, 1966; Donchin, Gerbrandt, Leifer, & Tucker, 1972; Donchin, Kubovy, Kutas, Johnson, & Herning, 1973; Low *et al.*, 1966) and must therefore represent more than mere motor preparation. The weak laterality of the slow negative wave in response-oriented CNV paradigms suggests that the negativity is multiply determined. It is conceivable that both a response-related lateralized negativity and a "cognitive" bilateral negativity are generated in the classical CNV paradigms. Such a two-component hypothesis has been suggested by Hillyard (1973; see also Gazzaniga & Hillyard, 1973). In one of our studies (Donchin, Kutas, & McCarthy, 1974, discussed in more detail later in this chapter), we were able to elicit in rapid succession a lateralized motor potential followed by a bilateral anticipatory potential. (See also Stamm *et al.*, this volume.)

*ERP asymmetries Associated with Cognitive Functions*

Very few studies have been designed specifically to seek concomitants of lateralized perceptual or cognitive functioning in such endogenous ERP components as P300 and CNV. It has been claimed that the lateral distribution of the CNV changes with task demands, but there is no consensus as to whether the engaged hemisphere has the larger or smaller CNV. Marsh and Thompson (1973) originally observed a symmetric CNV during preparation for a visuospatial discrimination, presumably a right-hemisphere task. When this nonverbal task was randomly interspersed among verbal stimuli and required a pointing (rather than a verbal) response, the hemisphere primary for that task had the smaller amplitude CNV. In contrast Butler and Glass (1974b) found a larger CNV over the dominant hemisphere during a warning interval in which subjects awaited numerical information. The CNV asymmetries took

the form of an earlier onset and greater amplitude potential over
the hemisphere contralateral to the preferred hand. Unfortunately, they had only one left-hander against whom to compare the
data of their right-handed subjects. The fact that in their
"control" condition large asymmetric CNVs were also generated
makes the results still more difficult to interpret. Care must
in general be exercised in the choice of stimulus modalities and
response requirements in designing such studies, as CNVs in different paradigms have distinct anterior-posterior scalp distributions, a central dominant CNV preceding tasks requiring motor
readiness (Jarvilehto & Fruhstorfer, 1970; Syndulko, 1972; Poon,
Thompson, Williams, & Marsh, 1975), a frontal dominant CNV
accompanying auditory discrimination (Jarvilehto & Fruhstorfer,
1970; Syndulko, 1972), and a parietal dominant CNV accompanying
similar visual tasks (Cohen, 1973; Syndulko, 1972). No definite
conclusions can be drawn at this time as to how CNV distribution
is related to cerebral dominance.

In summary, a start has been made toward using ERP methods to
investigate differences between the dominant and nondominant
hemispheres, but progress has been slow and somewhat hampered
by inadequate experimental design and analysis procedures.

*ERP Asymmetries in Linguistic Processing*

In this section we will review studies of the ERP relating
hemispheric asymmetries to linguistic functions. Given the
abundant evidence that verbal information is processed more efficiently by the left hemisphere, the search for ERP correlates
of linguistic processing has become increasingly energetic in
the past decade.

1. *Asymmetries in Language Reception: Visual Modality.* Results based on multiple electrode recordings have led to the
claim that asymmetric cerebral functions underlying evaluation of
visual stimuli are reflected in the ERP (see Thatcher, this
volume). Buchsbaum and Fedio (1969) have presented different
visual stimuli (words, dots, or designs) in a random sequence.
They reported that ERPs elicited by words can be differentiated
from ERPs elicited by nonlinguistic, patterned stimuli. They
also claimed that foveally presented verbal and nonverbal stimuli
elicit waveforms that are more differentiable when recorded at
the left than when recorded at the right hemisphere. They have
reported similar results in a study investigating interhemispheric differences in ERPs related to the perception of verbal
and nonverbal stimuli flashed to the left or right visual fields
(Buchsbaum & Fedio, 1970).

Marsh and Thompson (1973) investigated the possibility that
verbal sets would lead to differential right- and left-hemisphere
amplitudes of slow negative shifts by asking subjects to identify
their stimuli verbally. During the anticipation of flashed words,
symmetric CNVs were generated at the midtemporal and angular

gyrus placements. Preliminary data obtained when the two experimental conditions (verbal and nonverbal) were intermixed yielded asymmetries in the temporal and parietal sites. Other studies dealing with visually presented words have noted a striking lack of hemispheric asymmetry. Shelburne (1972, 1973) recorded visual evoked potentials to three individually flashed letters that comprised either a real or a nonsense word. A comparison of the responses elicited by these two different linguistic stimuli revealed no consistent differences between the visual ERPs to the words and to the nonsense syllables in either the left or right, parietal or occipital leads. In a similar paradigm, in which subjects were asked to report the key word in a visually presented sentence, no asymmetries in any of the components of the ERPs associated with words could be seen (Friedman, Simson, Ritter, & Rapin, 1975). Friedman and his associates present a trenchant critique of the studies reviewed in this section.

 2. *Asymmetries in Language Reception: Auditory Modality.* Although still contradictory and inconsistent, somewhat more promising results have been obtained with auditory stimuli (Brown, Marsh, & Smith, 1973; Cohn, 1971; Matsumiya, Tagliasco, Lombroso, & Goodglass, 1972; Molfese, Freeman, & Palermo, 1975; Morrell & Salamy, 1971; Neville, 1973; Teyler, Harrison, Roemer, & Thompson, 1973; Wood, Goff, & Day, 1971; Anderson, this volume). A number of studies have in fact supported the view that linguistic analysis occurs primarily in the left hemisphere. In a brief report, Cohn (1971) tells of a prominent, positive-going peak with a 14-msec latency elicited in the right hemisphere by click stimuli but not by single-syllable words. Morrell and Salamy (1971) found the N100 component elicited by nonsense words larger over the left than the right temporoparietal area. It is difficult to interpret their results, as they failed to use a nonlanguage control. Matsumiya *et al.* (1972) reported a hemispheric asymmetry in a "*W*-wave" (a positive response recorded bipolarly, peaking at 100 msec) elicited by real words and environmental sounds. They ascribe this hemispheric asymmetry to the significance of the auditory stimuli for the subject rather than to the linguistic features of the stimulus. Wood *et al.* (1971) reported differences in the ERPs recorded over the left hemisphere that appeared in the N100-P200 component, depending on whether the subject was required to perform a linguistic or an acoustic analysis of the stimulus (cf. Anderson, this volume). Molfese *et al.* (1975) found a similar enhancement in the amplitude of the *N1-P2* component of the ERP in the left relative to the right hemisphere for speech stimuli, even when the subject's task was merely to listen. On the other hand, nonspeech acoustic stimuli were found to produce larger amplitude responses in the right hemisphere. Although Molfese *et al.* found asymmetries in the auditory ERPs from infants, children, and adults, they noted that the lateral differences to both types of stimuli decreased with age. Neville (1974) reported lateral ERP amplitude and

latency differences elicited by digits but not by clicks in a dichotic listening paradigm.

Several investigators have attempted to evaluate the influence of linguistic meaning on scalp ERPs. Teyler *et al.* (1973) reported that different ERPs could be recorded from the same electrode site to the same click stimulus depending on the meaning of the verbal context (noun-verb) to which the stimulus was temporally related. Linguistic stimuli elicited responses of greater magnitude in the dominant hemisphere. In a similar study, Brown *et al.* (1973) recorded ERPs to the actual words rather than to coincidental clicks. The words they used were ambiguous and were disambiguated by their context. They reported (1) that the waveform of the ERPs evoked by a particular word differed according to its contextual meaning and (2) that these differences were significantly greater for left- than for right-hemisphere loci. It seems then that different investigators find in a variety of ERP parameters greater variability over the left than over the right hemisphere.

3. *Slow-Potential Asymmetries Preceding Language Production*. Whereas the studies just reviewed were primarily concerned with demonstrating different degrees of hemispheric asymmetry in response to verbal and nonverbal stimuli, others have tried to find the ERP concomitants of speech production. McAdam and Whitaker (1971) observed a small increase in the negativity over Broca's area (in the left hemisphere) preceding spontaneous spoken words but not preceding simple oral gestures. This report, however, has been attacked by Morrell and Huntington (1971) on several grounds. They questioned McAdam and Whitaker's procedures, analyses, and conclusions. Morrell and Huntington claim that when movement artifacts were monitored and the same measurements were made for all waveforms, no hemispheric asymmetries consistent with localization over Broca's area could be found (cf. Anderson, this volume). McAdam and Whitaker's findings, on the other hand, have been essentially confirmed by Low, Wada, and Fox (1974, 1976) who, in addition, found a significant correlation between hemispheric dominance as determined by the Wada sodium amytal test and dominance derived from the relative CNV amplitudes in the left and right motor speech area. Zimmerman and Knott (1974) applied similar procedures to an investigation of the physiological basis of stuttering. A comparison of CNVs in stutterers and normal speakers during speech and nonspeech tasks revealed that only 22% of the stutterers showed a left-greater-than-right asymmetry as opposed to 80% of the normal speakers. Thus, although a substantial amount of clinical data supports the theory of left-hemisphere superiority in language reception and production, the ERP data regarding this functional asymmetry are far from consistent. The methodological and statistical shortcomings existing in many of the studies cited render any decision about the efficacy of ERPs as indices of linguistic processing inconclusive.

METHODOLOGICAL CRITIQUE OF LATERALIZATION STUDIES

One need not be overly critical to conclude from the preceding review that it is premature to advocate the use of the EEG and ERP parameters as indices of hemispheric utilization; similar conclusions have recently been  adumbrated by Friedman *et al.* (1975) and by Galambos, Benson, Smith, Schulman-Galambos, and Osier (1975). Yet, within the welter of conflicting claims and apparent inconsistencies there is a thread of positive results that indicates the promise of the approach. The expectation that differential hemispheric utilization will manifest itself in scalp-recorded electrical activity is plausible.  Why then is the literature so confused? There are two related answers.  The functional significance of electrocortical "macro" potentials is, as yet, obscure. Although the evidence is strong that the EEG is a manifestation of "real" brain events, neither its general role nor the role of its many different parameters has been clarified. It is, therefore, the case that the studies reviewed earlier, as well as our own studies, are not guided by a specific theoretical view of the EEG. On the whole, investigators do not have a priori expectations regarding the direction of the differences they will observe. Until neurophysiologists supply a coherent view of the EEG, an empirical approach must predominate in this research. As long as it does, a measure of uncertainty will naturally pervade the literature.

The uncertainties and confusions deriving from our meager understanding of the EEG are exacerbated by inattention to proper methodology. Even within the constraints discussed previously, the issues could be clarified, were investigators to attend more carefully to methodological considerations. The following is a review of some of the more important points that should be considered in designing, conducting, and analyzing experiments in this field.

It would help to discuss first the formal structure of the experiments reviewed and to identify within that structure the major loci of methodological difficulty. The dependent variable in the reviewed literature is always the difference between a pair of values of some EEG or ERP parameter recorded at homologous bilateral sites. The independent variables are most often discussed in terms of the tasks the investigator has imposed on the subject. A class of tasks that is presumed, on previous data or intuitive grounds, to engage differentially one hemisphere or the other, is usually selected. The experimental conclusions can invariably be stated as a functional relationship between the sign and magnitude of the EEG parameter and task variables, which are in turn presumed to reflect basic features of human information processing.

Assume, for the sake of argument, that there really is a difference of the type sought. If the various experimental statements are in conflict or are not very convincing, any or all of the following reasons might be the cause:

1. The experimental design is not sufficiently sensitive to allow detection of the differences or is inadequate to support the conclusions.
2. The tasks assigned the subject may not in fact differentially engage the hemispheres.
3. The effects are range-restricted and the values of the independent variables are out of the relevant range.
4. Subject individual-difference variables are not considered.
5. The parameters of the EEG used as dependent variables were unwisely selected.
6. The measurement techniques used to obtain the parameters are inappropriate.
7. The data are improperly quantified and were inappropriately or insufficiently analyzed.

Design and analysis problems in recording scalp electrical activity in humans have been the topic of many comprehensive reviews (Donchin, 1973, 1975; Donchin & Lindsley, 1969; Thompson & Patterson, 1974). Our discussion is therefore limited to those problems specific to the use of the distribution of scalp potentials as an index of hemispheric functioning.

*SURVEY OF METHODOLOGICAL PROBLEMS*

Design Problems

If one point emerges with clarity from the studies reviewed, it is this: If there are any differences between the electrocortical activity of the two hemispheres, they will be minute. This implies that to reveal lateral dominance for study one must use techniques with the required high resolving power. The subtlety of the differences sought dictates the use of experimental designs of great sensitivity. Real but minute differences should not be ignored (type II errors), but at the same time artifactual sources of interhemispheric differences that may lead to type I errors should be avoided. The designs should minimize the chances of both types of errors. All too often the designs used in the reviewed studies were far from optimal.

In virtually all the reviewed studies, data were obtained from all subjects under all experimental conditions. For example, all subjects were challenged with spatial and verbal tasks. The investigators than chose between pooling the subjects' data, comparing group means, or using a repeated measurements design (with each subject serving as his own control). The last procedure is customarily preferred when large individual differences are expected in the data. The increased power of within-group designs aids in uncovering small-magnitude changes that would otherwise be obscured in between-group variance. Repeated-

measures designs are common in ERP work, but many of the widely
cited studies of frequency-domain parameters contain data that
were averaged over groups of subjects.

It is, of course, crucial to ensure that all experimental designs include proper control procedures. When lateral asymmetry
is attributed to the specific effects of a task, it is incumbent
upon the experimenter to demonstrate that the same parameter,
when estimated during some neutral task, does not display a similar asymmetry (see Thatcher, this volume). At the least, the
investigator should demonstrate that the lateral asymmetry can be
reversed or modulated with appropriate changes in the task
("double dissociation"); thus investigators should include tasks
designed to engage each hemisphere differentially. Unfortunately, many investigators fail to include such elementary controls.
It is sometimes difficult to determine whether asymmetries observed in the control conditions are a function of such variables
as handedness, cerebral dominance, ill-balanced electrode placements, or skull thickness. Again, this problem is especially
severe in studies of EEG spectra, although large CNV asymmetries
too have been reported in a presumably neutral task (Butler &
Glass, 1974b). More extensive baseline data should be collected.

## Validation of Task Variables

Common to a number of studies reviewed is the lack of attention directed toward the definition and validation of the task
variables presumed to be the independent variables. Too many
investigators (Brown et al., 1973; Doyle et al., 1974; Galin &
Ornstein, 1972; Morgan et al., 1971) merely ask their subjects
to imagine relationships or to perform mental operations without
objectively verifying that the subjects are in fact following
instructions. Even when measurable responses are required of the
subject, no systematic presentation or analysis of these behavioral measures is made (see for example Butler & Glass, 1974a;
McKee et al., 1973). Many studies leave the reader to wonder
whether the subject complied with task demands and, if so, to
what degree. The possible influence of task difficulty on these
results has often been ignored. The subjective estimates of
task difficulty that have been used are difficult to interpret
without performance measures (Dumas & Morgan, 1975; McKee et al.,
1973; Morgan et al., 1974).

Although negative results are notoriously difficult to interpret, confusion is compounded when EEG data are based on intui-
tively chosen tasks that have not been validated. Some advantages may be gained by selecting standard neuropsychological
paradigms for which differential hemispheric engagement has been
assessed (Neville, 1974). It is also important to avoid confounding psychological variables with varying physical parameters
of the task-related stimuli. Ample evidence in the literature
demonstrates that the characteristics of ERPs are grossly

affected by physical stimulus properties (see Regan, 1972).
Several investigators have devised clever strategies for holding
the physical parameters of the stimuli constant while varying
task variables (for examples, see Brown *et al.*, 1973; Wood *et al.*,
1971).

## Range of Operation of the Independent Variables

The subject's tasks are usually chosen with the assumption
that the manipulation of the independent variable will engage one
hemisphere or the other. If no interhemispheric differences are
found, the investigators tend to deduce that electrocortical activity is not related to hemispheric utilization. This may be a
rash deduction. It is, in fact, possible for the independent
variable to have a strong effect on the laterality of the EEG for
values of the independent variable other than those selected for
study. Consider, for example, the assertion that the N1 of the
MP displays no lateral asymmetry. This is in fact the case when
the subject merely presses a switch or makes a light movement
with his finger. If, however, the response requires a considerable degree of muscular involvement, lateral asymmetries appear
(Kutas & Donchin, 1974a). Similar results were obtained by
McCallum and Papakostopoulos (1974) with intracerebral recordings.

We describe, later, data that suggest that increasing cognitive demands likewise accentuate the lateral asymmetries in the
CNV. Within the same context, it is important to note that cognitive sets induced by the order in which experimental conditions
are presented can influence the range and direction of functional
asymmetries (for behavioral data, see Kimura & Durnford, 1974;
Kinsbourne, 1973; for application to ERP work, see Marsh &
Thompson, 1973).

## Subject Variables

It is a truism that one should know as much as is relevant
about the present state and past history of the subject. Yet,
such variables as age, sex, prior drug ingestion, and amount of
sleep, although known to alter the characteristics of brain activity (Perry & Childers, 1969; Shagass, 1972; Regan, 1972), are
sometimes ignored in EEG and ERP studies. Of critical importance in investigations of hemispheric specialization is the subject's history of handedness. Many reports concur that sinistrals differ from dextrals in their response to and recovery
from cortical damage and in their performance in a variety of
behavioral tasks (Hécaen & Ajuriaguerra, 1964; Levy, 1974).
Subject performance is affected not only by handedness but also
by familial history of handedness (for references see Levy,
1974). Apparently, the functional asymmetry in the recognition
of tachistoscopic material (Bryden, 1965; Springer, this volume)
and in dichotic listening (Zurif & Bryden, 1969; Berlin, this

volume) is appreciably smaller for individuals with left-handed relatives. Surprisingly, a number of studies of lateralization have failed to consider this aspect of the subjects' handedness (see Levy, this volume).

Assessing subjects' handedness should be the *sine qua non* of all investigations of laterality. However, subjective self-classification of handedness is inadequate as it correlates poorly with questionnaires and motor performance (Provins & Cunliffe, 1972; Satz, Achenbach, & Fennell, 1967). This is especially true for left-handers, who tend to form quite a heterogeneous population and often yield highly variable test results. Our own experience (Kutas, McCarthy, & Donchin, 1975) has been that handedness is difficult to classify and that, as a minimum requirement, self-reports should be supplemented with questionnaires.

## Paramaters of the Dependent Variable

Of critical importance is the selection of the proper parameters of EEG or ERP activity for the evaluation of task-induced changes. This is partly an empirical process as many parameters may need evaluation. These task-dependent changes may not always reveal themselves in gross measures of overall ERP amplitude or length, or in total EEG power spectra. They often, in fact, appear as small but consistent modulations of specific ERP components or EEG bandwidths (see Gardiner & Walter, this volume). It cannot be overemphasized that the ERP is not a unitary phenomenon, it is, rather, a sequence of independent components that react differentially to experimental variables (Donchin, 1969).

Care must be exercised in creating composite dependent variables based on various measures of EEG or ERP data. For example, interhemispheric ratios or laterality scores derived from power density spectra can provide a good summary statement descriptive of bilateral power relationships, but such ratios can be misused and are often misleading. Ratios presented independently of the data on which they are based (Doyle *et al.*, 1974; Galin & Ornstein, 1972; McKee *et al.*, 1973) leave the reader uncertain whether the changes are caused by differential engagement of the hemispheres by the tasks consistent with the functional asymmetry of the brain, or are due merely to changes in one hemisphere, perhaps reflecting task difficulty. Reassuring statements about the specific locus of change cannot be taken seriously unless supported by data from each hemisphere.

## Data Measurement

Whatever the procedure for measuring the parameters of the dependent variable, no interpretable results can be obtained if data are improperly recorded from the scalp. The necessity for a

EMANUEL DONCHIN *et al.*

common reference (either active or inactive) equidistant from the two electrodes being compared cannot be overemphasized. The use of a nonequidistant common reference, such as a single ear (Gott & Boyarsky, 1972), the use of equidistant but separate references such as $O_1$-A and $O_2$-$A_2$ (Buchsbaum & Fedio, 1969, 1970; Culver *et al.*, 1970; Fedio & Buchsbaum, 1971), and the use of intrahemispheric bipolar linkages without a common reference, such as $C_3$-$P_3$ and $C_4$-$P_4$ (Butler & Glass, 1974a; Matsymiya *et al.*, 1972) confound the assessment of hemispheric asymmetry. This problem is especially acute as the reported differences are often a microvolt or less.

A single nonequidistant reference should be avoided, as activity associated with the reference electrode will be unequally represented at the sites of comparison. Different unilateral reference electrodes allow for the possible introduction of systematic artifacts generated at a single reference but mistakenly identified as an asymmetric component. Intrahemispheric bipolar linkages, on the other hand, can mask existing interhemispheric differences, because of the common-mode-rejection characteristic of differential amplification. Although not without problems (Donchin, 1973), linked ears or mastoids and chin or active midline placements avoid most of the difficulties mentioned.

The number of conditions and electrode placements necessary for adequate examination of distributional effects of task variables on ERP components produce too much data to be easily handled by visual inspection or hand-measurement methods alone. Moreover, visual inspection is often inadequate for dealing with subtle differences between complex waveforms. As previously mentioned, marginal asymmetries, although consistent with experimental manipulations, can be washed out by larger, symmetric components (Hillyard, 1973). Also, experimental effects may not always be evident as a measurable peak or trough in the ERP waveform, but may rather be manifest as a modulation of another component.

We employ Principal Components Analysis (PCA) to identify the distinct components of the waveform and to assess their sensitivity to experimental effects (Donchin, 1966, 1969; Donchin, Tueting, Ritter, Kutas, & Heffley, 1975). This procedure provides an objective definition of ERP components and measures their contribution to each waveform with reference to the entire data set. A detailed treatment of the application of PCA to ERP research is beyond the scope of this paper (Chapman, 1973; Ruchkin, Villegas, & John, 1964). Briefly, the ERP waveform can be considered an estimate of the mean vector of a multivariate distribution. The PCA is one technique for decomposing this mean vector into its component vectors. The nature of this extraction procedure allows separate analyses of variance to be performed on derived factor scores to assess the sensitivity of the factors to the experimental variables. Thus, identification and quantification of the experimental effects can proceed in an objective manner. The use of the technique is illustrated later in this chapter.

## Data Analysis

It is commonly acknowledged that exacting data-analysis techniques are essential for the proper evaluation of the effect of experimental manipulations on measures of brain activity. There is certainly no lack of analysis procedures in the literature reviewed; unfortunately, however, the heterogeneity of quantification procedures makes comparisons between laboratories difficult. The ambiguous nature of many of the paradigms as well as the small magnitude of the experimental effects obtained in this type of research should discourage the more liberal approaches to data analysis, which often seem colored by the expectations of the investigator. Fundamental to the statistical evaluation of any data is the measurement of the magnitude and distribution of error variances. The use of grand averaging, qualitative analysis, and multiple univariate analyses can be criticized on several grounds, among them a disregard for the range of variability in the data.

Two forms of data reduction often employed in the analysis of ERPs, grand averaging (averaging waveforms across subjects and/or conditions) and qualitative analysis, give no indication of the real variability in the data. Grand averaging, although a useful means for visually summarizing a multitude of waveforms, should not be used as the sole method of analysis as no estimate of error variance is available. Purely qualitative analyses (e.g., Cohn, 1971) or visual scoring of asymmetry (Butler & Glass, 1974b) are too subject to experimenter bias to be the only method for assessing the influence of independent variables and, of course, do not allow for the evaluation of statistical significance.

Many of the statistical analysis procedures used in the determination of hemispheric asymmetries are not merely inadequate; they are often inappropriate. The comparison of ERP waveforms and EEG power ratios through multiple univariate procedures (Brown et al., 1973; Doyle et al., 1974; Wood et al., 1971) without adjustment for the number of tests being performed can result in misleading conclusions, since the probability of finding spuriously "significant" difference is underestimated (see the excellent paper by Friedman et al., 1975, for a discussion of the Bonferroni test). There are, moreover, multivariate techniques for the analysis of ERPs (such as those referred to previously) that take into account the interdependence of time points and are not subject to the aforementioned criticisms.

359

SLOW ERP COMPONENTS AND HEMISPHERIC INVOLVEMENT

We now describe studies from our laboratory that were designed to test the proposition that slow, preevent, "anticipatory" waves can be used to index hemispheric utilization. The data provide evidence that scalp-recorded EEG can be used in studies of hemispheric specialization.

These studies were conducted within the general framework of our interest in the endogenous components of ERPs (Donchin, 1975; Donchin *et al.*, 1973, 1975; Rohrbaugh, Donchin, & Ericksen, 1974). The CNV is one of the more prominent of these components (McCallum & Knott, 1973, 1976). There is no doubt that it is a manifestation of anticipatory processes, sensitive to a variety of behavioral manipulations; yet, it turns out to be strangely intractable to theoretical analysis. Various conflicting inter-pretations have been put forward (see, for example, McCallum & Knott, 1976). The crux is the degree to which the CNV represents generalized attentional variables (Karlin, 1970) or more specific preparatory processes (Tueting & Sutton, 1973). It has also been difficult to tease out the relative roles of motor and cognitive preparation. The evidence indicates that CNVs can be recorded in the absence of specific, overt, experimenter-directed motor activity (Donchin *et al.*, 1972; Irwin, Knott, McAdam, & Rebert, 1966), yet it is also clear that the CNV is larger when a motor response is required. If motor preparation is an important de-terminant of the slow potentials, then a lateralized response requirement should lead to a lateralization of the potentials, with larger amplitudes recorded contralateral to the responding hand.

We began by examining data collected for other purposes (Donchin *et al.*, 1973) in a choice reaction time paradigm. A warning tone preceded one of two possible flashes by 1500 msec; the subject was required to respond to one flash with the right hand and to the other with the left hand. In one series of trials, the two stimuli alternated; the subject, therefore, knew the hand with which to respond. In another series, the stimuli were presented in a random sequence and the subject could not predict the hand to be used. Data were recorded from laterally placed electrodes; thus differences in the lateral symmetry of the CNVs obtained in the random and the alternating sequences could be determined. If motor preparation affects these poten-tials, it should operate during the alternating sequence. A com-parison of the cortical activity preceding the subjects' re-sponses averaged separately for each responding hand failed to reveal any lateral asymmetry in either of the experimental con-ditions (Donchin, Kutas, & Johnson, 1974).

These data were puzzling. According to Kornhuber and Deecke (1965) and Gilden *et al.* (1966), asymmetric motor potentials pre-cede self-paced motor responses. A replication of these studies was attempted to determine whether a similar asymmetry could be

observed when the warning stimulus was eliminated from the sequence. This attempt also failed. When subjects pressed a button at a self-paced rate with one hand, the potentials recorded
from the two hemispheres were virtually identical.

A possible explanation for this failure to replicate came from
Otto (personal communication), who reported finding a lateral
asymmetry in potentials preceding a multiple finger response.
This was in accord with reports that the CNV was largest when
greater muscular effort was required (Low & McSherry, 1968;
Rebert, McAdam, Knott, & Irwin, 1967). These findings were originally interpreted in terms of the motivational state of the
subject, but it may be that response-force per se determines the
CNV (or RP) amplitude.

A systematic investigation of the effect of force on the RP
was therefore conducted. The lateral distribution of the RP over
the motor cortex in both right- and left-handed subjects squeezing a dynamometer with either hand at three levels of force were
compared. The force levels were calibrated in terms of the subject's capabilities rather than in absolute terms. In right-
handed subjects, the premovement RPs (N1) were larger over the
hemisphere contralateral to the responding hand. Left-handed
subjects showed contralateral dominance only when responding
with their right hands (see Figure 1). An analysis of the N1
magnitude revealed that although response-force does accentuate
the motor asymmetry, the absolute right-left asymmetry does not
change with increasing force levels (for a more detailed account,
see Kutas & Donchin, 1974b).

It turns out, then, that past failures to demonstrate conclu-
sively the hemispheric asymmetry of the RP may have been due to
the range of the independent variable (response-force, in this
case) and to an inattention to subject variables. Many reports
concerning the RP have failed to mention subjects' handedness,
and the few that did mention it failed to consider it in evaluating the data.

*A COMPARISON OF READINESS POTENTIAL AND CNVs*

The results described previously led to an investigation of
the relationship between the lateral asymmetry of the RP and
the CNV (Donchin *et al.*, 1974). Again, subjects were required
to squeeze a dynamometer with one hand or the other. In addition, various tests of each subject's lateral preference were
administered. After a detailed examination of various tests for
handedness (Kutas *et al.*, 1975), we selected the Edinburgh questionnaire (Oldfield, 1971) as an instrument of choice.

In order to make the dynamometer squeeze less tiresome to the
subjects, scenic slide presentations were made contingent on
dynamometer squeezes that attained a specified force level.
Figure 2 presents the sequence of events in an experimental trial.
A self-paced squeeze, if "correct," was followed after 1800 msec

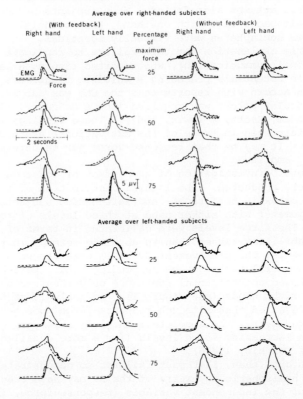

Fig. 1. *A comparison of event-related potentials (ERPs) recorded
at electrodes placed at left-central (C₃, solid line) and right-
central (C₄, dashed line) loci during voluntary squeezes. Under
each pair of superimposed ERPs we have plotted the integrated
electromyogram (EMG) (dashed line) and the output of the force
transducer (solid line) averaged over the same trials over which
the ERP was averaged. Comparisons are presented as a function of
subject's handedness (right versus left), nominal force output
(25, 50, and 75% of subject's maximal force), responding hand
(right versus left) and feedback (presence or absence of visual
signal indicating force level). Averages were obtained over all
subjects, after the elimination of trials in which the EEG was
contaminated by electrooculogram (EGO) activity. Number of
trials per ERP ranges between 600 and 1050. The polarity convention is negative up. Hatching in two areas of the comparisons
illustrates the areas measured for the purpose of the quantitative data analysis. From Kutas and Donchin, 1974a.*

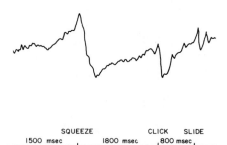

SQUEEZE                CLICK    SLIDE

1500 msec        1800 msec    800 msec

*Fig. 2. The sequence of events in an experimental trial. Trial duration was 4500 msec. The waveform drawn above the time line is of the ERP obtained by averaging the entire data set collected from left-handed subjects at a central position. It serves merely to indicate the time of occurrence of the various ERP components.*

by an audible click (generated by the mechanism of the slide projector) which was followed after 800 msec by the presentation of the slide. Thus, each trial consisted of three distinct phases: a preresponse interval over which an RP could be recorded, a post response interval, and finally the click-slide interval during which a measurable CNV could be recorded. This paradigm enabled a comparison of the hemispheric asymmetry of the premovement RP, which we expected to vary as a function of the responding hand, with the hemispheric symmetry of the CNV. This design thus permitted an examination of the degree to which the asymmetries observed by Kutas and Donchin (1974a) were specific to the premotor interval, or were extended over a long interval. This also allowed for an examination of the possibility that, although the RP is asymmetric, the CNV is symmetric.

In Figure 3 are grand averages for the right- and left-handed subjects, recorded at the frontal, central, and parietal locations. The ERPs recorded at homologous hemispheric sites are superimposed. These averages were obtained by triggering the computer on the dynamometer squeeze. Several aspects of the data are immediately apparent. Clearly, the squeeze is preceded by an RP, which is asymmetric. Moreover, the asymmetry reverses with the responding hand. Following the squeeze, a long-lasting asymmetric slow wave appears, which displays a polarity opposite that of the presqueeze potential. The CNV that follows the click is symmetric, though superimposed on the slow wave. There are substantial differences between the scalp distribution of the CNV and the RP. The CNV is equally large at the frontal and central sites, but the RP is largest centrally. Note also the sharper resolution of the CNV in the parietal sites.

A more detailed look at the data is provided in Figure 4, where waveforms are shown for five individual subjects. The

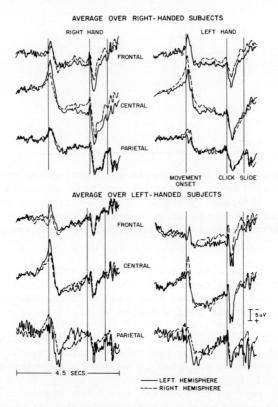

*Fig. 3. ERP waveforms recorded from frontal, central, and parietal positions. Data obtained simultaneously from homologous sites are superimposed. There were approximately 75 trials per subject per condition.*

curves displayed were obtained by element-to-element subtraction of the ERPs at the right and left central electrodes (these then are equivalent to a "bipolar" recording between the two central electrodes). For each subject, data obtained with right- and left-hand squeezes were superimposed. When the premotor interval is examined, a strong measure of asymmetry is observed. For each subject the potential difference reverses polarity with the responding hand. It is important to note that the degree of polarity reversal is far more evident when intrasubject rather than intersubject comparisons are made. The specific difference waveforms vary considerably from subject to subject, yet within subjects the potentials are of opposite polarity, suggesting a change in the direction of laterality.

No such asymmetries are observable for the CNV. Whereas the postresponse slow potential is quite prominent and seems to

DIFFERENCE CURVES FOR ERPS OBTAINED
WITH RIGHT AND LEFT HAND RESPONDING

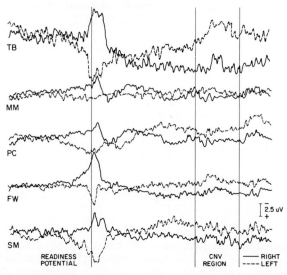

*Fig. 4. All waveforms shown in this figure were obtained by
point-to-point subtraction of ERPs recorded at the left-central
electrode from ERPs recorded at the right-central electrode.
This difference will be negative if the left-hemisphere potential
is larger, and positive if the right-hemisphere potentials are
larger. For five subjects (three dextral and two sinistral) we
superimposed data obtained when subjects were squeezing a dynamometer with the right hand (solid line) and the left hand (dashed
line). Each waveform represents an average of 75-80 trials.
The first vertical line separates pre- from postsqueeze activity;
the second and third lines delineate the click-slide interval
(CNV).*

extend over the entire recorded epoch and probably beyond it, the
click-flash CNV is apparently equal in amplitude at both sites.
A quantitative statement of this trend is shown in Figure 5. We
have fitted a quadratic function to the RP and to the CNV segments of the curve. In Figure 5 is a plot of the coefficients
of the quadratic terms that were computed for ERPs associated
with right-hand squeezes against coefficients associated with the
left-hand squeezes. If the two curves show opposite polarity,
the coefficients should be of opposite sign. For the RP, the coefficients are large, and for most subjects the magnitudes of
the two coefficients are reasonably similar, but the signs are
different. For the CNV, the coefficients are clustered around
the origin and show no tendency toward opposite polarity.
    These data provide support for the idea that lateral asymmetry
can be used as an index of hemispheric utilization. Shifts in

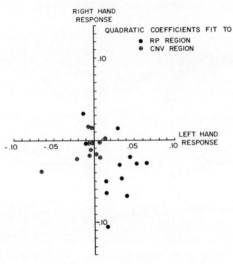

*Fig. 5. Regression coefficients of the quadratic term obtained from a polynomial fit to the premovement (full circles) and CNV (crossed circles) region of the difference waveforms illustrated in Figure 4. Coefficients computed on the basis of right-hand response data are plotted against coefficients obtained when subjects were squeezing with their left hands.*

asymmetry appear to be quite rapid and are finely tuned to shifts in the subject's tasks. The nature and significance of the long, slow, postresponse wave is not clear, yet it is obvious that the more rapid shifts in asymmetry can be detected when they are superimposed on such long-term trends. Thus, these data lend plausibility to the "two-factor hypothesis," which views antici-patory negative shifts as a mixture of motor and cognitive pre-paratory processes (Hillyard, 1973).

*LATERAL ASYMMETRIES IN A CNV PARADIGM*

Although the data presented in the preceding section demon-strate the differential anterior-posterior and interhemispheric distribution of the RP and CNV, it remains to be determined if the CNV is always symmetric or perhaps, with proper choice of tasks, can be lateralized. Conceivably, just as a forceful squeeze was required to demonstrate the asymmetry of the RP, a stronger cognitive "squeeze" might be required to demonstrate the lateralization of the CNV. An experiment was designed, therefore, to manipulate task variables that might contribute to the forma-tion of an asymmetric CNV.

The task chosen was patterned after the Structure-Function matching task developed by Levy (1974) in her work with commis-surotomized patients. One of two warning tones (1000 Hz or 2000

Hz) preceded, by 1000 msec, a brief (50 msec) presentation of a slide. Each slide contained three figures, two of which formed a structural or "look-alike" match (right-hemisphere dominant task) and two of which formed a functional or conceptual match (left-hemisphere dominant task). Both types of matches could be made from each slide with one figure common to the two matches (see Figure 6). Subjects responded by pressing one of three

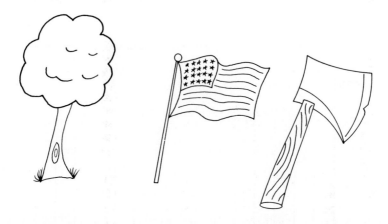

*Fig. 6. One of the 42 slides used in the study. The ax and the tree are functionally matched; the ax and the flag are structurally matched. If cued to make a functional match, the subject would respond by pressing a button with the second finger of his right hand. For a structural match, the subject would press a button with the third finger.*

buttons (with one of three fingers of the right hand) coded for the three possible figure combinations. Subjects were instructed to respond as quickly as possible following the slide presentation. Reaction time (RT) and the subject's choice were recorded for each trial along with 2000 msec of EEG from a nine-electrode montage ($F_3$, $F_4$, $C_3$, $C_4$, $P_3$, $P_4$, $F_z$, $C_z$, $P_z$ --according to the 10-20 system for electrode placement). The vertical electrooculogram (EOG) was recorded on a separate channel. Trials associated with eye movements were excluded from analysis. Recording of the EEG data began 200 msec prior to the warning stimulus. (For data-acquisition procedures see Donchin & Heffley, 1975.)

Two general experimental conditions were used. In *fixed-match* series the warning tone was the same on all trials in a run, the subject making the same match on each trial. In *mixed-match* series, the tones varied randomly from trial to trial, and the required match varied accordingly. For each subject each tone pitch was always associated with one match type. An additional series was used in which the subject was instructed to respond by using a single response button to all slides. Results were obtained in a pilot study of five female subjects, all dextral (as verified by the Edinburgh Inventory, Oldfield, 1971) and all without sinistral relatives.

The reaction times and matching errors are presented in Figure 7. It is apparent that both measures differ significantly as a function of task. These data establish that the two tasks placed different demands on the subjects. This does not, of course, prove that the two tasks engaged the hemispheres differentially.

PERFORMANCE DATA FOR EACH EXPERIMENTAL CONDITION

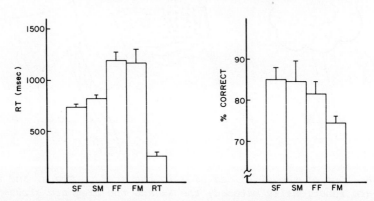

*Fig. 7. Performance data (mean and standard error). Differences in reaction time (p < .0005, F = 21.66, df = 1,16) and in percentage correct (p < .048, F = 4.57, df = 1,16) between structural and functional matching are significant. Abbreviations: SD, structural/fixed-match condition; SM, structural/mixed-match; FF, functional/fixed-match; FM, functional/mixed-match; RT, baseline reaction time to signal with no match required.*

Hemispheric engagement was assayed by spectral analysis of the single-trial EEG data. It was necessary to determine if changes in the distribution of power within the delta (1-3.5 Hz), theta (4-7.5 Hz), and alpha (8-12 Hz) bandwidths accompanied performance of the tasks. The data analyzed were the 2000-msec epoch, which included 1200 msec of preslide EEG as well as 800 msec of data taken while the subject was actively performing the task. Figure 8 (top frame) presents the distribution of power within each frequency band. An analysis of variance of power measures at each band was performed to determine if the nature of the matching task affected the scalp distribution of the power. Our data indicated that, within the alpha bandwidth only, the tasks differentially affected the distribution of power, primarily at the parietal electrode sites (p < .03; F = 2.97, df = 5,20). There is relatively less alpha activity (see Figure 8, bottom

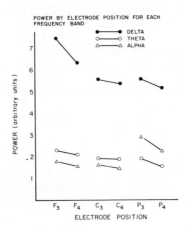

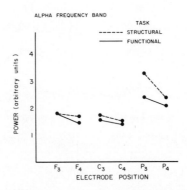

Fig. 8. Top: *distribution of the mean power for the delta (1-3.5 Hz), theta (4-7.5 Hz), and alpha (8-12 Hz) bands is shown for left and right frontal ($F_3$, $F_4$), central ($C_3$, $C_4$), and parietal ($P_3$, $P_4$) electrode sites. The data for analysis were obtained from the fixed-structural or functional-match conditions. Data from 15 trials in which the subject responded correctly were used for each analysis. Bottom: the task by electrode interaction for power and the alpha band. The power associated with functional matching is lower at all electrode positions than the power associated with structural matches. The difference, however, is accentuated at the left parietal position.*

frame) at the left parietal ($P_3$) during functional matching than during the structural matching. Our data are too preliminary to permit a strong statement concerning the relationship of these differences to hemispheric specialization; it is conceivable that the changes at $P_3$ are related to task difficulty--recall that functional matching was performed more slowly and less accurately than structural matching. Figure 8 (bottom) shows that the functional match power is smaller than structural match power at all electrode sites. Nonetheless, the differences are interesting and provide suggestive evidence of the efficacy of our tasks in differentially engaging the hemispheres.

Of central concern in the design of this experiment was the extent to which preparation to perform different analyses, presumed to engage the hemispheres differentially, would result in the formation of asymmetric CNVs prior to slide presentation.

Grand averaged waveforms (Figure 9) for all experimental conditions reveal large asymmetries in the CNVs for all match conditions relative to the RT conditions. The most consistent asymmetries appear in the mixed conditions. Note that, when asymmetric, the left-hemisphere potential amplitudes always exceed the right-hemisphere potentials. In the mixed series, a prominent positive component appears 450 msec after the warning stimulus.

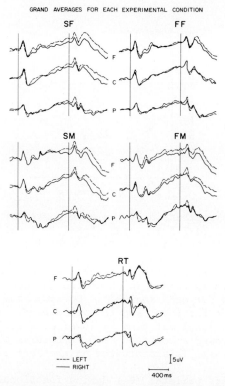

Fig. 9. *Grand-averaged waveforms for frontal, central, and parietal electrode positions for all experimental conditions for all trials in which the subject responded correctly. Right (solid line) and left (dashed line) lateral positions are superimposed. The vertical lines indicate the occurrences of the warning tone (S1) and slide (s2).*

To illustrate the variability in the data, averaged waveforms from individual subjects for the mixed series are presented in Figure 10. For a more objective analysis, the waveforms from

WAVE FORMS FROM INDIVIDUAL SUBJECTS

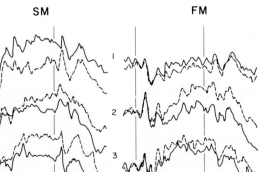

Fig. 10.  *ERP from five subjects for left (dashed line) and right (solid line) frontal electrode positions (superimposed) are shown for the mixed-match condition.*

each subject, electrode, and condition were submitted as a data matrix to a Principal Components Analysis followed by Varimax rotation. Six orthogonal factors were extracted from the data, accounting for 78% of the experimental variance. A plot of the factor loadings, representing the degree of association of each time point with each factor, is presented in Figure 11. Such a plot identifies the temporal locus of activity for each of the factors. Factor scores, derived from these factor loadings, measure the degree to which each factor contributes to the waveforms for each condition and electrode placement. Thus, it is possible to assess the degree to which each factor is affected by the experimental conditions and to evaluate the relationships statistically. Space does not permit a full discussion of the behavior of each factor; attention will therefore be restricted to the two factors (1 and 2) clearly within the CNV region.

The time course of factor 1 is similar to that of a CNV, peak-

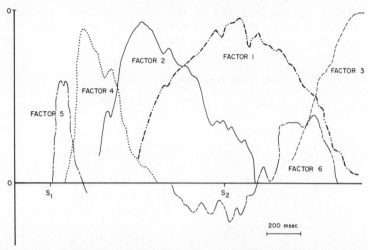

*Fig. 11. Factor loadings for six orthogonal factors extracted by Principal Component Analysis and rotated by the Varimax procedure. The loadings represent the temporal locus of activity for each of the six factors.*

ing just after the slide (S2). The factor scores indicate that this factor is maximal at the central electrodes declining in amplitude in the frontal and parietal electrodes ($p < .001$, $F = 20.44$, $df = 7,28$). The decline is steeper toward the parietal than frontal sites. This scalp distribution has often been reported for the CNV. These scores also indicate that this component, which we identify with the CNV, is laterally asymmetric; it is more negative at the left hemisphere for all homologous pairs. This asymmetry appears to be affected by mode, appearing to be more marked for the mixed than the fixed series ($p < .025$, $F = 2.77$, $df = 7,28$). The three-way interaction, electrode position X matching task X mode ($p < .007$, $F = 3.51$, $df = 7,28$), indicates that this factor is largest for the two mixed conditions and indicates that the asymmetry is least pronounced in the functional fixed condition.

Factor 2 peaks approximately 475 msec after the warning tone (S1). Its latency suggests that this factor may be the same as the early component of the CNV described by Loveless and Sanford (1974, 1975) and heretofore only seen with very long interstimulus intervals. Mode has a very pronounced effect upon the anterior-posterior distribution of this factor ($p < .001$, $F = 8.05$, $df = 7,28$). When S1 conveys no information about the task to the subject (as in the fixed series), this factor is negative at all electrode sites, appearing largest frontally. When S1 is task relevant (as in the mixed series), this component becomes positive in the parietal regions and marginally more negative frontally. The effect of matching tasks on this component is not statistically significant ($p < .066$, $F = 2.18$, $df = 7,28$) but nonetheless intriguing. At the frontal sites, this component appears to change its lateral distribution as a function of task; appearing larger over the left hemisphere for functional tasks and larger over the right hemisphere for structural matching.

The data just described demonstrate that CNVs of different amplitudes can be simultaneously recorded from homologous electrodes. The CNV is asymmetric when the matching mode varies randomly from trial to trial. The evidence also indicates that when the mode of matching is uniform over a block of trials (as in the fixed condition) the CNV is more symmetric. It seems then that the extent to which the asymmetry is observable may depend on the strategies the experimental situation permits the subject to adopt.

It is noteworthy that the direction of asymmetry is independent of the match required (structural versus functional). Clearly, the CNV does not *reverse* asymmetry in preparation for tasks that presumably engage one or the other hemispheres. A detailed replication of the experiment is now underway, using a larger sample and a richer set of control conditions. Although the new data seem to corroborate the data presented here, the nature of the observed asymmetry must be more fully elucidated in relation to the response requirements of the task.

Not directly related to the asymmetry question, yet a theoretically important aspect of these data, is the support they lend to the reports (Weerts & Lang, 1973; Loveless & Sanford, 1974, 1975), that two distinct components may operate in the CNV interval. These components vary in scalp distribution and in their sensitivity to task demands.

## SUMMARY

We have reviewed the evidence for the proposition that differences between the electrical activity recorded at homologous scalp locations over the left and right hemispheres can be used to index hemispheric utilization. There seems to be adequate support for the assertion that the ratio of EEG power over the hemispheres is sensitive to task variables. The direction of the difference is to some extent consistent with predictions derived from contemporary ideas about hemispheric specializations. Of the various ERP parameters studied, the sturdiest results come from investigations of anticipatory potentials that appear to be asymmetric, again, in the predicted direction.

These trends are far from conclusive. Some methodological problems were reviewed. Attention should be paid to the independent validation of the behavioral effects of experimental instructions, to the greater sensitivity of within-group repeated-measures designs, to the choice of EEG parameters for study, and to the measurement and analysis of data.

We have presented data that demonstrate that (1) slow potentials preceding a voluntary self-paced motor response are largest
over the hemisphere contralateral to the responding hand (at
least in dextrals); (2) the preresponse asymmetry can coexist
with cognitive anticipations which are symmetric; (3) the preresponse asymmetric readiness potentials appear to be followed
by a prolonged potential shift with a polarity apparently inverse
to that of the motor potential; (4) when the information-processing load is increased, some lateralization effects seem to occur
in the CNV; and (5) both this CNV negativity and task-related
shifts in power in the alpha band appear mostly as modulation of
left-hemisphere activity rather than as reciprocal changes in
hemispheric activities.

REFERENCES

Adrian, E. D., & Matthews, B. H. C.   The Berger rhythm:  Potential changes from the occipital lobes in man.  *Brain*, 1934,
*57*, 355-385.
Aird, R. B., & Bowditch, S.   Cortical localization by electroencephalography.  *Journal of Neurosurgery*, 1946, *1*, 245-261.
Aird, R. B., & Zealear, D. S.   The localizing value of asymmetrical electroencephalographic tracings obtained simultaneously
by homologous recording.  *Electroencephalography and
Clinical Neurophysiology*, 1951, *3*, 487-495.
Andreassi, J. L., De Simone, J. J., Friend, M. A., & Grota, P. A.
Hemispheric amplitude asymmetries in the auditory evoked
potential with monaural and binaural stimulation.
*Physiological Psychology*, 1975, *3*, 169-171.
Andreassi, J. L., Okamura, H., & Stern, M.   Hemispheric asymme-
tries in the visual cortical evoked potential as a function
of stimulus location.  *Psychophysiology*, 1975, *12*, 541-546.
Berger, H.   " er das Elektrenkephalogramm des Menschen.  Sweite
Mitteilung.  *Journal für Psychologie und Neurologie*, 1930,
*40*, 160-179.
Broca, P.   Remarques sur le siège de la faculté du langage
articulé suivi d'une observation d'aphemie.  *Bulletin
Societé Anatomie*, 1861, *6*, 330-357.
Brown, W. S., Marsh, J. T., & Smith, J. C.   Contextual meaning
effects on speech evoked potentials.  *Behavioral Biology*,
1973, *9*, 755-761.
Bryden, M. P.   Tachistoscopic recognition, handedness and cerebral dominance.  *Neuropsychologia*, 1965, *3*, 1-8.
Buchsbaum, M., & Fedio, P.   Visual information and evoked responses from the left and right hemisphere.  *Electroencephalography and Clinical Neurophysiology*, 1969, *36*, 266-272.
Buchsbaum, M., & Fedio, P.   Hemispheric differences in evoked
potentials to verbal and nonverbal stimuli in the left and
right visual fields.  *Physiology and Behavior*, 1970, *5*,

207-210.

Buchwald, J. S., & Huang, C. M. Far-field acoustic response: Origins in the cat. *Science*, 1975, *189*, 382-384.

Butler, S. R., & Glass, A. Asymmetries in the electroencephalogram associated with cerebral dominance. *Electroencephalography and Clinical Neurophysiology*, 1974, *36*, 481-491.(a)

Butler, S. R., & Glass, A. Asymmetries in the CNV over left and right hemispheres while subjects await numeric information. *Biological Psychology*, 1974, *2*, 1-16.(b)

Butler, S. R., & Glass, A. EEG correlates of cerebral dominance. In *Advances in psychobiology*. New York: *Wiley*, 1974.

Butler, R. A., Keidel, W. D., & Spreng, M. An investigation of the human cortical evoked potential under conditions of manaural and binaural stimulation. *Acta oto-laryngolica*, Stockholm, 1969, *68*, 317-326.

Callaway, E., & Harris, P. R. Coupling between cortical potentials from different areas. *Science*, 1974, *183*, 873-875.

Calmes, R. L., & Cracco, R. Q. Comparison of somatosensory and somatomotor evoked responses to median nerve and digital nerve stimulation. *Electroencephalography and Clinical Neurophysiology*, 1971, *31*, 547-562.

Case, T. J., & Bucy, P. C. Localization of cerebral lesions by electroencephalography. *Journal of Neurophysiology*, 1938, *1*, 245-261.

Chapman, R. M. Evoked potentials of the brain related to thinking. In F. J. McGuigan & R. A. Schoonover (Eds.), *The psychophysiology of thinking: Studies of covert processes*. New York: Academic Press, 1973. Pp. 69-108.

Cohen, J. Very slow brain potentials relating to expectancy: The CNV. In E. Donchin & D. B. Lindsley (Eds.), *Average evoked potentials, methods, results, and evaluation*. Washington, D.C.: NASA-191, U.S. Government Printing Office, 1969. Pp. 143-198.

Cohen, J. CNV and visual recognition. In W. C. McCallum & J. R. Knott (Eds.), *Event related slow potentials of the brain*. New York: Elsevier, 1973. Pp. 201-204.

Cohen, J., & Walter, W. G. The interaction of responses in the brain to semantic stimuli. *Psychophysiology*, 1966, *2*, 187-196.

Cohn, R. Differential cerebral processing of noise and verbal stimuli. *Science*, 1971, *172*, 599-601.

Cooper, R., Osselton, J. W., & Shaw, J. C. *EEG technology*. (2nd ed.) London: Butterworths, 1974.

Cornil, L., & Gastaut, H. Étude electroencéphalographique de la dominance sensorielle d'un hemisphere cerebral. *La Presse Medicale*, 1947, *37*, 421-422.

Culver, C. M., Tanley, J. C., & Eason, R. G. Evoked cortical potentials: Relation to hand dominance and eye dominance. *Perceptual and Motor Skills*, 1970, *30*, 407-414.

Deecke, L., Scheid, P., & Kornhuber, H. H.  Distribution of readiness potential, pre-motion positivity, and motor potential of the human cerebral cortex preceding voluntary finger movements. *Experimental Brain Research*, 1969, *7*, 158-168.

Dimond, S. J., & Beaumont, J. G. (Eds.)  *Hemisphere function in the human brain*. London:  Paul Elek Ltd., 1974.

Donchin, E.  A multivariate approach to the analysis of average evoked potentials. *IEEE Transactions Biomedical Engineering*, 1966, *BME-13*, 131-139.

Donchin, E.  Data analysis techniques in evoked potential research.  In E. Donchin & D. B. Lindsley (Eds.), *Average evoked potentials, methods, results, and evaluations*. Washington, D. C.:  NASA-191, U.S. Government Printing Office, 1969.  Pp. 199-236.

Donchin, E.  Methodological issues in CNV research.  A review. In W. C. McCallum & J. R. Knott (Eds.), *Event related slow potentials of the brain*. New York:  Elsevier, 1973.  Pp. 1-17.

Donchin, E.  Brain electrical correlates of pattern recognition. In G. F. Inbar (Ed.), *Signal analysis and pattern recognition in biomedical engineering*. New York:  John Wiley, 1975.  Pp. 199-218.

Donchin, E., Gerbrandt, L., Leifer, L., & Tucker, L.  Is the contingent negative variation contingent on a motor response? *Psychophysiology*, 1972, *9*, 178-188.

Donchin, E., Kubovy, M., Kutas, M., Johnson, R. Jr., & Herning, R. I.  Graded changes in evoked response (P300) amplitude as a function of cognitive activity. *Perception and Psychophysics*, 1973, *14*, 319-324.

Donchin, E., & Heffley, E.  Minicomputers in the signal-averaging laboratory. *American Psychologist*, 1975, *30*(3), 299-312.

Donchin, E., Kutas, M., & Johnson, R. Jr.  The CNV does not behave like a "motor" potential. *Electroencephalography and Clinical Neurophysiology*, 1974, *37*, 434.

Donchin, E., Kutas, M., & McCarthy, G.  Comparison of the hemispheric asymmetries of the readiness potential and CNV. Paper read before the Psychonomic Society 15th Annual Meeting, Boston, 1974.

Donchin, E., & Lindsley, D. G. (Eds.)  *Average evoked potentials, methods, results, evaluations*. Washington, D.C.:  NASA-191, U.S. Government Printing Office, 1969.

Donchin, E., Tueting, P., Ritter, W., Kutas, M., & Heffley, E. On the independence of the CNV and P300 components of the human averaged evoked potential. *Electroencephalography and Clinical Neurophysiology*, 1975, *38*, 449-461.

Doyle, J. C., Ornstein, R., & Galin, D.  Lateral specialization of cognitive mode:  II.  EEG frequency analysis. *Psychophysiology*, 1974, *11*, 567-578.

Dumas, R., & Morgan, A.  EEG asymmetry as a function of occupation, task, and task difficulty. *Neuropsychologia*, 1975, *13*, 219-228.

Eason, R. G., Groves, P., White, C. T., & Oden, D. Evoked cortical potentials: Relation to visual field and handedness. *Science*, 1967, *156*, 1643-1646.

Fedio, P., & Buchsbaum, M. Unilateral temporal lobectomy and changes in evoked responses during recognition of verbal and nonverbal material in the left and right visual fields. *Neuropsychologia*, 1971, *9*, 261-271.

Friedman, D., Simson, R., Ritter, W., & Rapin, I. Cortical evoked potentials elicited by real speech words and human sounds. *Electroencephalography and Clinical Neurophysiology*, 1975, *38*, 13-19.

Galambos, R., Benson, P., Smith, T.S., Schulman-Galambos, C., & Osier, H. On hemispheric differences in evoked potentials to speech stimuli. *Electroencephalography and Clinical Neurophysiology*, 1975, *39*, 279-283.

Galin, D., & Ellis, R. R. Asymmetry in evoked potentials as an index of lateralized cognitive processes: Relation to EEG alpha asymmetry. *Psychophysiology*, 1975, *13*, 45-50.

Galin, D., & Ornstein, R. Lateral specialization of cognitive mode: An EEG study. *Psychophysiology*, 1972, *9*, 412-418.

Gazzaniga, M. S. *The bisected brain*. New York: Appleton, 1970.

Gazzaniga, M. S., & Hillyard, S. A. Attention mechanisms following brain bisection. In S. Kornblum (Ed.), *Attention and performance IV*. New York: Academic Press, 1973. Pp. 221-238.

Gerbrandt, L. K., Goff, W. R., & Smith, D. B. Distribution of the human average movement potential. *Electroencephalography and Clinical Neurophysiology*, 1973, *34*, 461-474.

Giannitrapani, D. Developing concepts of lateralization of cerebral functions. *Cortex*, 1967, *3*, 353-370.

Giannitrapani, D., & Darrow, C. W. Differences in EEG time relationships in right and left handed individuals. *Electroencephalography and Clinical Neurophysiology*, 1963, *15*, 721P.

Giannitrapani, D., Darrow, C. W., & Sorkin, A. Asleep and awake interhemispheric EEG phase relationships in left- and right-handed subjects. *American Psychologist*, 1964, *19*, 480-481.

Giannitrapani, D., Sorkin, A. I., & Ennenstein, J. Laterality preference of children and adults as related to inter-hemispheric EEG phase activity. *Journal of Neurological Science*, 1966, *3*, 139-150.

Gibbs, F. A., Lennox, W. G., & Gibbs, E. L. The electro-encephalogram in diagnosis and in localization of epileptic seizures. *Archives of Neurology and Psychiatry*, 1936, *36*, 1225-1235.

Gilden, L., Vaughan, H. G., & Costa, L. D. Summated human EEG potentials associated with voluntary movement. *Electroencephalography and Clinical Neurophysiology*, 1966, *20*, 433-438.

Glanville, A. D., & Antonitis, J. J. The relationship between occipital alpha activity and laterality. *Journal of Experimental Psychology*, 1955, *49*, 294-299.

Goff, W. R., Matsumiya, Y., Allison, T., & Goff, G. D. Cross-modality comparisons of averaged evoked potentials. In E. Donchin & D. B. Lindsley (Eds.), *Average evoked potentials, methods, results, and evaluations*. Washington, D.C.: NASA-191, U.S. Government Printing Office, 1969. Pp. 143-198.

Goff, W. R., Rosner, B. S., & Allison, T. Distribution of cerebral somatosensory evoked responses in normal man. *Electroencephalography and Clinical Neurophysiology*, 1962, *14*, 697-713.

Gott, P. S., & Boyarsky, L. L. The relation of cerebral dominance and handedness to visual evoked potentials. *Journal of Neurobiology*, 1972, *3*, 65-77.

Harmony, J., Ricardo, G. O., Fernandez, S., & Valdes, P. Symmetry of the visual evoked potential in normal subjects. *Electroencephalography and Clinical Neurophysiology*, 1973, *35*, 237-240.

Hécaen, H., & Ajuriaguerra, J. de. *Left-handedness: Manual superiority and cerebral dominance*. New York: Grune & Stratton, 1964.

Hillyard, S. A. The CNV and human behavior: A review. In W. C. McCallum & J. R. Knott (Eds.), *Event related slow potentials of the brain*. New York: Elsevier, 1973. Pp. 162-172.

Hoovey, Z. B., Heinemann, U., & Creutzfeldt, O. D. Inter-hemispheric "synchrony" of alpha waves. *Electroencephalography and Clinical Neurophysiology*, 1972, *32*, 337-347.

Irwin, D. A., Knott, J. R., McAdam, D. W., & Rebert, C. S. Motivational determinants of the "contingent negative variation". *Electroencephalography and Clinical Neurophysiology*, 1966, *21*, 538-541.

Jarvilehto, T., & Fruhstorfer, H. Differentiation between slow cortical potentials associated with motor and mental acts in man. *Experimental Brain Research*, 1970, *11*, 309-317.

Jewett, D., Romano, H. N., & Williston, J. S. Human auditory evoked responses: Possible brain stem components detected on the scalp. *Science*, 1970, *167*, 1517-1518.

Karlin, L. Cognition, preparation, and sensory-evoked potentials. *Psychological Bulletin*, 1970, *73*, 122-136.

Kimura, D. Cerebral dominance and the perception of verbal stimuli. *Canadian Journal of Psychology*, 1961, *15*, 166-171.

Kimura, D., & Durnford, M. Normal studies of hemisphere functions of the right hemisphere in vision. In S. J. Dimond & J. G. Beaumont (Eds.), *Hemisphere function in the human brain*. London: Paul Elek Ltd., 1974. Pp. 25-47.

Kinsbourne, M. The control of attention by interaction between the cerebral hemispheres. In S. Kornblum (Ed.), *Attention and human performance IV*. New York: Academic Press, 1973. Pp. 239-256.

Klinke, R., Fruhstorfer, H., & Finkenzeller, P. Evoked responses as a function of external and stored information. *Electroencephalography and Clinical Neurophysiology*, 1968, *25*, 119-122.

Kooi, K. A., Guvener, A. M., & Bagchi, B. K. Visual evoked responses in lesions of the optic pathways. *Electroencephalography and Clinical Neurophysiology*, 1965, *18*, 524.

Kornhuber, H. H., & Deecke, L. Hirnpotentialanderungen bei Willkurbewegungen und passiven Bewegungen des Menschen: Bereitschaftspotential und reafferente Potentiale. *Pflugers Archiv fur die gesamte Physiologie des Menschen und der Tiere*, 1965, *284*, 1-17.

Kutas, M., & Donchin, E. Studies of squeezing: Handedness, responding hand, response force, and asymmetry of readiness porential. *Science*, 1974, *186*, 545-548.(a)

Kutas, M., & Donchin, E. Motor potentials, force of response and handedness. In *Proceedings of the International Symposium on Cerebral Evoked Potentials in Man*, Brussels, 1975.(b)

Kutas, M., McCarthy, G., & Donchin, E. Differences between sinistrals and dextrals in inferring a whole from its parts: A failure to replicate. *Neuropsychologia*, 1975, *13*, 455-464.

Lairy, G. C., Remond, A., Rieger, H., & Lesevre, N. The alpha average. III. Clinical application in children. *Electroencephalography and Clinical Neurophysiology*, 1969, *26*, 453-467.

Levy, J. Psychobiological implications of bilateral asymmetry. In S. J. Dimond & J. G. Beaumont (Eds.), *Hemispheric function in the human brain*. London: Paul Elek Ltd., 1974. Pp. 121-183.

Lindsley, D. B. Bilateral differences in brain potentials from the two cerebral hemispheres in relation to laterality and stuttering. *Journal of Experimental Psychology*, 1940, *26*, 211-225.

Liske, E., Hughes, H. M., & Stowe, D. E. Cross-correlation of human alpha activity: Normative data. *Electroencephalography and Clinical Neurophysiology*, 1967, *22*, 429-426.

Livanov, M. N., Gavrilova, N. A., & Aslanov, A. S. Intercorrelations between different cortical regions of human brain during mental activity. *Neuropsychologia*, 1964, *2*, 281-289.

Livanov, M. N., Gavrilova, N. A., & Aslanov, A. S. Correlations of biopotentials in the frontal parts of the human brain. In K. H. Pribram & A. R. Luria (Eds.), *Psychophysiology of the frontal lobes*. New York: Academic Press, 1973. Pp. 91-107.

Loveless, N. E., & Sanford, A. J. Slow potential correlates of preparatory sets. *Biological Psychology*, 1974, *1*, 303-314.

Loveless, N. E., & Sanford, A. J. The impact of warning signal intensity on reaction time and components of the contingent negative variation. *Biological Psychology*, 1975, *2*, 217-226.

Low, M. D., Borda, R. P., Frost Jr., J. D., & Kellaway, P. Surface-negative slow-potential shift associated with conditioning in man. *Neurology* (Minneapolis), 1966, *16*, 771-782.

Low, M. D., & McSherry, J. W. Further observations of psychological factors involved in CNV genesis. *Electroencephalography and Clinical Neurophysiology*, 1968, *35*, 203-207.

Low, M. D., Wada, J. A., & Fox, M. Hemispheric specialization for language production: Some electrophysiological evidence. *Proceedings of the International Symposium on Cerebral Evoked Potentials in Man*, Brussels, 1974.

Low, M. D., Wada, J. A., & Fox, M. Electroencephalographic localization of the conative aspects of language production in the human brain. In W. C. McCallum & J. R. Knott (Eds.), *The responsive brain*. Bristol: John Wright, 1976. Pp. 165-168.

MacKay, D. M. Evoked brain potentials as indicators of sensory information processing. *Neurosciences Research Program Bulletin*, 1969, *7*(3), 181-276.

Majkowski, J., Bochenek, Z., Bochenek, W., Knapik-Fijalkowska, D., & Kopec, J. Latency of averaged evoked potentials to contralateral and ipsilateral auditory stimulation in normal subjects. *Brain Research*, 1971, *25*, 416-419.

Manil, J., Desmedt, J. E., Debecker, J., & Chorazyna, H. Les potentiels cerebraux évoques par la stimulation de la main chez le nouveau-né normal. *Revue Neurologique*, 1967, *117*, 53-61.

Marsh, G. R., & Thompson, L. W. Effect of verbal and non-verbal psychological set on hemispheric asymmetries in the CNV. In W. C. McCallum & J. R. Knott (Eds.), *Event related slow potentials of the brain*. New York: Elsevier, 1973. Pp. 195-200.

Matsumiya, Y., Tagliasco, V. L., Lombroso, C. T., & Goodglass, H. Auditory evoked response: Meaningfulness of stimuli and interhemispheric asymmetry. *Science*, 1972, *175*, 790-792.

McAdam, D. W., & Seales, D. M. Bereitschaftspotential enhancement with increased level of motivation. *Electroencephalography and Clinical Neurophysiology*, 1969, *27*, 73-75.

McAdam, D. W., & Whitaker, H. A. Language production: Electroencephalographic localization in the normal human brain. *Science*, 1971, *172*, 499-502.

McCallum, W. C., & Knott, J. R. (Eds.) *Event related slow potentials of the brain*. New York: Elsevier, 1973.

McCallum, W. C., & Knott, J. R. (Eds.), *The responsive brain*. Bristol: John Wright, 1976.

McCallum, W. C., & Papakostopoulos, D. Slow potential changes in human brainstem associated with preparation for decision or action. *Proceedings of the International Symposium on Cerebral Evoked Potentials in Man*, Brussels, 1974.

McKee, G., Humphrey, B., & McAdam, D. W. Scaled lateralization of alpha activity during linguistic and musical tasks.

*Psychophysiology*, 1973, *10*, 441-443.

Milner, B. Hemispheric specialization: Scope and limits. In F. O. Schmitt & F. G. Worden (Eds.), *The neurosciences third study program*. Cambridge, Massachusetts: MIT Press, 1974. Pp. 75-89.

Molfese, D. L., Freeman, R. B. Jr., & Palermo, D. S. The ontogeny of brain lateralization for speech and nonspeech stimuli. *Brain and Language*, 1975, *2*, 356-368.

Morgan, A. H., Macdonald, H., & Hilgard, E. R. EEG alpha: Lateral asymmetry related to task and hypnotizability. *Psychophysiology*, 1974, *11*, 275-282.

Morgan, A. H., McDonald, P. J., & Macdonald, H. Differences in bilateral alpha activity as a function of experimental task with a note on lateral eye movements and hypnotizability. *Neuropsychologia*, 1971, *9*, 459-469.

Morrell, L. K., & Huntington, D. A. Electrocortical cortical localization of language production. *Science*, 1971, *174*, 1359-1360.

Morrell, L. K., & Salamy, J. G. Hemispheric asymmetry of electrocortical response to speech stimuli. *Science*, 1971, *174*, 164-166.

Neville, H. Electrographic correlates of lateral asymmetry in the processing of verbal and nonverbal auditory stimuli. *Journal of Psycholinguistic Research*, 1974, *3*, 151-163.

Oldfield, R. C. The assessment and analysis of handedness: The Edinburgh Inventory. *Neuropsychologia*, 1971, *9*, 97-113.

Otto, D. A., & Leifer, L. J. The effect of modifying response and performance on the CNV in humans. In W. C. McCallum & J. R. Knott (Eds.), *Event related slow potentials of the brain*. New York: Elsevier, 1973. Pp. 29-37.

Peronnet, F., Michel, F., Echallier, J. F., & Girod, J. Coronal topography of human auditory evoked responses. *Electroencephalography and Clinical Neurophysiology*, 1974, *37*, 225-230.

Perry Jr., N. W., & Childers, D. G. *The human visual evoked response: Method and theory*. Springfield, Illinois: C. C. Thomas, 1969.

Peters, J. F., & Mendel, M. I. Early components of the averaged electroencephalic response to monaural and binaural stimulation. *Audiology*, 1974, *13*, 195-204.

Poon, L. W., Thompson, L. W., Williams Jr., R. B., & Marsh, G. Changes of antero-posterior distribution of CNV and late positive component as a function of information processing demands. *Psychophysiology*, 1974, *11*, 660-673.

Price, L. L., Rosenblut, B., Goldstein, R., & Shepherd, D. C. The averaged evoked response to auditory stimulation. *Journal of Speech and Hearing Research*, 1966, *9*, 361-370.

Provins, K. A., & Cunliffe, P. The relationship between EEG activity and handedness. *Cortex*, 1972, *8*, 136-146.

Raney, E. T. Brain potentials and lateral dominance in identical twins. *Journal of Experimental Psychology*, 1939, *24*, 21-39.

Rebert, C. S., McAdam, P. W., Knott, J. R., & Irwin, D. A. Slow potential changes in human brain related to level of motivation. *Journal of Comparative and Physiological Psychology* 1967, *63*, 20-23.

Regan, D. *Evoked potentials in psychology, sensory physiology, and clinical medicine.* London: Chapman & Hall, 1972.

Remond, A., Lesevre, N., Joseph, J. P., Rieger, H., & Lairy, G.C. The alpha average. I. Methodology and description. *Electroencephalography and Clinical Neurophysiology*, 1969, *26*, 245-265.

Rhodes, L. E., Dustman, R. E., & Beck, E. C. The visual evoked response: A comparison of bright and dull children. *Electroencephalography and Clinical Neurophysiology*, 1969, *27*, 364-372.

Rhodes, L. E., Obitz, F. W., & Creel, D. Effect of alcohol and task on hemsipheric asymmetry of visually evoked potentials in man. *Electroencephalography and Clinical Neurophysiology*, 1975, *38*, 561-568.

Richlin, M., Weisinger, M., Weinstein, S., Giannini, M., & Morganstern, M. Interhemispheric asymmetries of evoked cortical responses in retarded and normal children. *Cortex*, 1971, *7*, 98-104.

Rohrbaugh, J., Donchin, E., & Ericksen, C. W. Decision making and the P300 component of the cortical evoked response. *Perception and Psychophysics*, 1974, *15*, 368-374.

Ruchkin, D. S., Villegas, J., & John, E. R. An analysis of averaged evoked potentials making use of least mean squares techniques. *Annals of the New York Academy of Sciences*, 1964, *115*, 799-826.

Ruhm, H. B. Lateral specificity of acoustically evoked EEG responses. I. Non-verbal, non-meaningful stimuli. *Journal of Auditory Research*, 1971, *11*, 1-8.

Satz, P., Achenbach, K., & Fennell, E. Correlations between assessed manual laterality and predicted speech laterality in a normal population. *Neuropsychologia*, 1967, *5*, 295-310.

Schenkenberg, T., & Dustman, R. E. Visual, auditory, and somatosensory evoked response changes related to age, hemisphere and sex. *Proceedings of the 78th Annual Convention of the American Psychological Association*, 1970, 183-184.

Shagass, C. *Evoked brain potentials in psychiatry.* New York: Plenum Press, 1972.

Shelburne Jr., S. A. Visual evoked responses to word and nonsense syllable stimuli. *Electroencephalography and Clinical Neurophysiology*, 1972, *32*, 17-25.

Shelburne Jr., S. A. Visual evoked responses to language stimuli in normal children. *Electroencephalography and Clinical Neurophysiology*, 1973, 135-143.

Smith, A. Dominant and nondominant hemispherectomy. In W. L. Smith (Ed.), *Drugs, development and cerebral function.* Springfield, Illinois: C. C. Thomas, 1972.

Sperry, R. W. Lateral specialization in the surgically separated hemispheres. In F. O. Schmitt & F. G. Worden (Eds.), *The neurosciences third study program*. Cambridge, Massachusetts: MIT Press, 1974. Pp. 5-19.

Dubirana, A. Handedness and cerebral dominance. In P. J. Vinken & G. W. Bruyn (Eds.), *Handbook of Clinical neurology*, Vol. 4. Amsterdam: North-Holland Pub., 1969. Pp. 248-272.

Sutton, S., Braren, N., Zubin, J., & John, E. R. Evoked-potential correlates of stimulus uncertainty. *Science*, 1965, *155*, 1187-1188.

Sutton, S., Tueting, P., Zubin, J., & John, E. R. Information delivery and the sensory evoked potential. *Science*, 1967, *155*, 1436-1439.

Syndulko, K. Relationships between motor potentials and CNV. *Electroencephalography and Clinical Neurophysiology*, 1969, *27*, 706.

Syndulko, K. Cortical slow potential shifts in humans during sensory and motor tasks. Unpublished doctoral dissertation, Univ. of California, Los Angeles, 1972.

Teyler, T., Harrison, T., Roemer, R., & Thompson, R. Human scalp recorded evoked potential correlates of linguistic stimuli. *Journal of the Psychonomic Society Bulletin*, 1973, *1*, 333-334.

Thompson, R. F., & Patterson, M. M. (Eds.) *Bioelectric recording techniques. Part B: Electroencephalography and human brain potentials*. New York: Academic Press, 1974.

Travis, L. E., & Knott, J. R. Bilaterally recorded brain potentials from normal speakers and stutterers. *Journal of Speech Disorders*, 1937, *2*, 239-241.

Tueting, P., & Sutton, S. The relationship between pre-stimulus negative shifts and post-stimulus components of the averaged evoked potential. In S. Kornblum (Ed.), *Attention and performance IV*. New York: Academic Press, 1973. Pp. 185-207.

Vaughan, H. G. The relationship of brain activity to scalp recording of event-related potentials. In E. Donchin & D. B. Lindsley (Eds.), *Average evoked potentials, ethods, results, and evaluation*. Washington, D.C.: NASA-191, U.S. Government Printing Office, 1969. Pp. 143-198.

Vaughan, H. G., Jr. The analysis of scalp-recorded brain potentials. In R. F. Thompson & M. M. Patterson (Eds.), *Bioelectrical recording techniques. Part B: Electroencephalography and human brain potentials*. New York: Academic Press, 1974. Pp. 157-207.

Vaughan, H. G., Costa, L. D., & Ritter, W. Topography of the human motor potential. *Electroencephalography and Clinical Neurophysiology*, 1968, *25*, 1-10.

Vaughan, H. G., Katzman, R., & Taylor, J. Alterations of visual evoked response in the presence of homonymous visual defects. *Electroencephalography and Clinical Neurophysiology*, 1963, *15*, 737-746.

Vaughan, H. G., & Ritter, W. The sources of auditory evoked responses recorded from the human scalp. *Electroencephalography and Clinical Neurophysiology*, 1970, *28*, 360-367.

Vella, E. J., Butler, S. R., & Glass, A. Electrical correlates of right hemisphere function. *Nature*, 1972, *236*, 125-126.

Walter, W. G. The location of cerebral tumors by electro-encephalography. *Lancet*, 1936, *2*, 305-312.

Walter, W. G., Cooper, R., Aldridge, V. J., McCallum, W. C., & Winter, A. L. Contingent negative variation: An electric sign of sensorimotor association and expectancy in the human brain. *Nature*, 1964, *203*, 380-384.

Walter, D. O., Rhodes, J. M., Brown, D., & Adey, W. R. Comprehensive spectral analysis of human EEG generators in posterior cerebral regions. *Electroencephalography and Clinical Neurophysiology*, 1966, *20*, 224-237.

Weerts, T. C., & Lang, P. J. The effects of eye fixation and stimulus and response location on the contingent negative variation (CNV). *Biological Psychology*, 1973, *1*, 1-19.

Wilke, J. T., & Lansing, R. W. Variations in the motor potential with force exerted during voluntary arm movements in man. *Electroencephalography and Clinical Neurophysiology*, 1973, *35*, 259-265.

Wood, C. C., Goff, W. R., & Day, R. S. Auditory evoked potentials during speech perception. *Science*, 1971, *173*, 1248-1251.

Zimmermann, G. N., & Knott, J. R. Slow potentials of the brain related to speech processing in normal speakers and stutterers. *Electroencephalography and Clinical Neurophysiology*, 1974, *37*, 599-607.

Zurif, E. B., & Bryden, M. P. Familial handedness in left-right difference in auditory and visual perception. *Neuropsychologia*, 1969, *7*, 179-187.

# 20.
# Lateralization of Functions in the Monkey's Frontal Cortex

*JOHN S. STAMM, STEVEN C. ROSEN AND ALCIDES GADOTTI*

State University of New York at Stony Brook

The broad aim of the research in our laboratory has been to obtain electrophysiological measures that would express the involvement of specific cortical areas in the solution of complex tasks by monkeys with intact brains. The experiments conducted thus far have been concerned primarily with functions of dorsolateral prefrontal cortex during performance of delayed-response (DR) tasks. This paradigm was selected because ablation studies have demonstrated that this area, particularly cortex in the principal sulcus, constitutes the cortical focus for DR performance (Goldman, Rosvold, Vest, & Galkin, 1971; Stamm, & Weber-Levine, 1971). The electrophysiological measures were macropotentials, recorded with nonpolarizable electrodes that were chronically implanted bilaterally in prefrontal, precentral, and occipital areas. This method appeared most suitable for our research, because it permitted simultaneous recordings to be obtained from several cortical sites throughout many months of behavioral testing. The experimental procedure consisted of systematically varying task parameters and testing conditions while monitoring concomitant changes in event-related cortical macropotentials from the various electrode locations (see also Douchin, Kutas, & McCarthy, this volume). This approach has resulted in the delineation of functional dissociations among cortical areas and among several identifiable components of the averaged potentials in each area. The findings have led to inferences with regard to the sensory, mnemonic, and motor (response selection) functions of prefrontal cortex during short-term memory tasks.

This report will first describe the general procedures and findings concerning prefrontal involvement in DR performance. Then results will be presented from recent experiments more specifically designed for the determination of possible functional asymmetries between the monkey's cerebral hemispheres.

GENERAL METHOD AND PROCEDURES

*TESTING APPARATUS*

The experimental animals were stumptail monkeys (*Macaca speciosa*) weighing 3-4 kg. Before each testing session the monkey was placed in a restraining chair that restricted its body and head movements. During preliminary adaptation sessions single peanut-kernels were presented to each monkey from different directions in order to assess its hand preference in reaching for the peanut (see Warren, this volume). For the formal testing sessions, one of the monkey's arms was restrained by a wrist-cuff bolted to the shelf of the restraining chair.

The chair was placed securely in front of a vertical testing panel that contained two circular display windows (3.3 cm in diameter) at the monkey's eye level, with 12 cm between their centers. The chair placement was arranged so that a shift in gaze between the centers of the two display windows required eye rotations of approximately $36^{\circ}$. Below each display window was a plastic cup into which food rewards (45-mg sucrose pellets) could be delivered. Colored lights could be projected from the rear onto each window. In front of each window was a transparent plastic disk, which, when pressed lightly, activated a microswitch.

The DR trial (Figure 1, *A* and *B*) started with presentation of

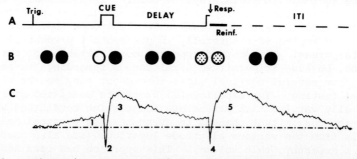

*Fig. 1. Schematic representations of the delayed-response (DR) task. (A) Sequence of component events during the trial and (B) concurrent illumination of the display windows. During cue presentation either the left or right window was illuminated with white light (1 or 2 sec) and at the end of the delay both windows*

the cue, consisting of either the left or right display window receiving white illumination for a predetermined period. Both windows were then darkened during the intratrial delay, at the end of which they were illuminated with blue light. The monkey's press on either disk at that time (the choice response) extinguished both lights for the intertrial interval. A correct response (to the cue window) was followed by delivery of a sugar pellet to the appropriate food cup and 0.5-sec white-light illumination of the cup. The testing chamber was dimly illuminated throughout the experimental session.

The training procedure consisted of 120-trial sessions. The intratrial delay was initially zero and then was increased in steps to 8 sec. The response criterion for each delay setting was 90% correct for at least two consecutive sessions. The durations of cue presentation and the intertrial interval (ITI) differed in the various experiments, but were generally in the ranges of 1 to 2 sec, and 8 to 24 sec, respectively.

*RECORDING ELECTRODES AND PROCEDURES*

Prior to behavioral training, each monkey, under pentobarbital anesthesia, received chronic implantations of pairs of capillary pore Ag-AgCl nonpolarizable electrodes in the left and right prefrontal, precentral, and occipital areas. Solid miniature nonpolarizable electrodes were placed subcutaneously across one eye for recordings of lateral eye movements. For the prefrontal placements, the surface electrode was on cortex in the depth of the posterior segment of the principal sulcus and the reference electrode was in subjacent white matter of the bank inferior to this sulcus. The precentral surface electrode was placed approximately midway between the central sulcus and the prefrontal dimple, and the occipital surface electrode was between the lunate sulcus and the occipital pole, approximately 2 cm lateral to the midline of the brain. Corresponding depth electrodes were implanted in subjacent white matter. All electrode leads were soldered to points on an Amphenol connector, which was cemented to the skull. Fascia and skin were then sutured around the cement mound. In several experiments some of the monkeys were not implanted with the complete array of precentral and

*were blue-illuminated. The monkey's choice response (Resp.) extinguished the illumination for the intertrial interval (ITI) and a correct response was rewarded with a sugar pellet and a 2-sec illumination of the food cup (Reinf.). A trigger pulse (Trig.) was generated for computer averaging. (C) Components of averaged potentials that have been recorded from the surface of prefrontal cortex. Components 2 (CEP) and 4 (REP) are evoked responses to onset of disk illumination; the other components represent surface-negative steady-potential (SP) shifts.*

occipital electrodes; also, a few precentral electrodes were placed on superjacent dura.

During recording sessions the Amphenol plug was connected by shielded, low-noise cables to dc preamplifiers of a Grass polygraph. Output from the power amplifiers led to a seven-channel FM magnetic tape recorder, which also recorded a trigger pulse six sec before cue onset. Each session's data were averaged in 40-trial blocks with an analysis sweep of 32 sec. With the Catacal averaging program for a PDP-12A (*Digital Corp.*) computer several features of the cortical potentials could be measured. The magnitude of surface-negative steady-potential (SP) shifts were computed as the area between 6-sec averaged shifts following cue onset and a baseline determined by the 6-sec SP level immediately preceding cue onset. It should be noted that the magnitude of an averaged SP shift is a function of both the amplitude of the shift and the degree of time-locking of individual shifts.

## CORTICAL MACROPOTENTIALS DURING DR PERFORMANCE

Averaged prefrontal recordings revealed five distinct components during the course of the DR trial (Figure 1C), of which two were evoked potentials to the onset of the cue (CEP) and the response lights (REP), respectively, and the others were slow surface-negative SP shifts. The first negative SP shift started toward the end of the ITI in some of the monkeys and attained maximum amplitude at cue onset. The magnitude of this shift was found to increase gradually during the course of testing with a constant ITI, and to subside with the introduction of variable ITIs. This finding suggests that this SP shift reflects neuronal processes similar to those underlying the *contingent negative variation* (Donchin, Otto, Gerbrant, & Pribram, 1971; Walter, Cooper, Aldridge, McCallom, & Winter, 1964; Donchin *et al.*, this volume) and is therefore designated as an *expectancy* potential.

The final SP shift is seen after delivery of the sugar pellet, and its magnitude was affected by experimental variations in reinforcement contingencies. This SP shift declined during testing conditions when the food reward and cup illumination were omitted, while the monkey continued to respond at 90% correct, and it appeared again with reinstitution of the reinforcement contingencies. The occurrence of this shift seems to correspond to the SP shifts that have been recorded from many cortical areas in relation to consummatory behavior (Rowland, 1968). Consequently, this potential has been designated as a *reinforcement* SP shift. Since concomitant SP changes were recorded from all electrode locations during the periods of both the expectancy and the reinforcement SP shifts, we interpret these as reflections of processes of general neuronal activation, associated with behavioral arousal.

Of particular relevance to the aims of the research was the

occurrence of the second surface-negative SP shift during the cue
and delay periods (Figure 1C). This shift started toward the end
of cue presentation, reached maximum amplitude after the start of
the delay, and then declined to baseline level. The time course
appears to correspond to patterns of activation of single prefrontal units that have been obtained during performance by
monkeys on a similar DR task (Fuster, 1973). In the present experiments the magnitudes of the SP shifts remained unaffected by
variations in duration of either the cue (between .06 and 8 sec)
or of the delay period (between 4 and 20 sec). However, as shown
in Figure 2, the SP shift magnitudes appear positively related to
the level of the monkey's correct performance. Correlations

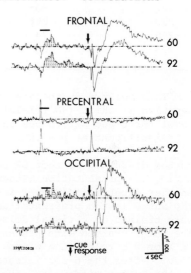

*Fig. 2. Averaged electrocorti-
cal potentials (40-trial blocks)
from prefrontal (Frontal), precentral, and occipital areas
during 8-sec DR performance by
monkey 229. Scores of choice-
responses are 60% and 92% correct, as indicated. Stippled
areas indicate magnitudes of
SP shifts. Horizontal bars
indicate presentation of the cue
light, and arrows indicate
illumination of both windows for
the monkey's choice response.*

between integrated measures of SP shifts from prefrontal cortex
for four monkeys during training on 8-sec DR with correct performance scores, ranging from 60% to 95% correct, resulted in
substantial and significant product-moment correlation coefficients (Table 1). These correlations are in contrast to those
obtained for concurrent precentral and occipital SP shifts,
which were variable and insignificant. The findings indicate
that the SP shifts reflect localized involvement of principalis
cortex in mediation of the transient memory required for DR
performance.

Furthermore, other experiments with brief electrocortical
stimulation during task performance have provided evidence of
the specific involvement of prefrontal cortex in spatial transient memories. When stimulation was applied during different
portions of the DR trial the monkeys' correct performance on
this task became markedly disrupted only with stimulus applications across the principal sulcus during the early portion of
the intratrial delay, whereas stimulation of inferotemporal

TABLE 1

*Correlation Coefficients between SP Shift Magnitudes[a] and Correct Performance on Eight-Second Delayed-Response Task*

| | Cortical area | | |
| Monkey no. | Prefrontal | Precentral | Occipital |
|---|---|---|---|
| 221 | .90* | .16 | .41 |
| 223 | .89* | .20 | -.42 |
| 226 | .74 | .74 | -.56 |
| 229 | .86* | .14 | .54 |

[a]This measure is the area between 6-sec averaged surface-negative SP shift (40 trials) following cue onset and SP baseline level for 6-sec before cue onset.
*Significant at $p < .01$.

cortex disrupted correct DR performance only with application during cue presentation (Stamm, 1969; Stamm & Rosen, 1973). In another experiment (Kovner & Stamm, 1972) monkeys with electrodes implanted in the prefrontal and inferotemporal cortical areas were trained on a visual delayed matching-to-sample task (DMS). The trial started with presentation of the sample pattern (either an X or a circle) in a window located above the two choice windows. After the 6-sec intratrial delay, both patterns appeared in the bottom windows and the monkey's response to the sample pattern was rewarded. The monkey's performance became impaired only with inferotemporal stimulation applied toward the end of the intratrial delay or matching (choice-response) periods; it remained unaffected by prefrontal stimulation during any portion of the DMS trial. In a different experiment (Cohen, 1972) the monkeys' performance on a delayed successive visual discrimination task was disrupted by electrical stimulation of either prefrontal cortex during the early intratrial delay or of inferotemporal cortex during presentation of the visual patterns. These findings indicate a dissociation between spatial and visual transient memories, with the former mediated by dorsolateral prefrontal, and the latter by inferotemporal cortical structures. Additional support for modality-specific cortical functions has been obtained in recordings of SP shifts in monkeys tested concurrently on DR and DMS tasks (Rosen and Stamm, 1973). The resulting averaged SP shift magnitudes were larger on the DR trials for the prefrontal, and on the DMS trials for the occipital electrode locations.

The findings that have thus far been presented provide evidence that the prefrontal cortical SP shift that occurs during the early intratrial delay of DR reflects a specific function of this region. The high correlation between the magnitude of the SP shift and the measure for correctness of the subsequently occurring choice response suggests that the SP shift may be considered as a neuronal expression of the underlying mnemonic processes. Moreover, this SP shift seems to reflect a modality-specific function, i.e., spatial transient memory.

## THE CUE-EVOKED RESPONSE

In a different experiment with four monkeys trained on 8-sec DR, cortical potentials were averaged separately for the left and the right cue presentations. The results (Figure 3) indicate

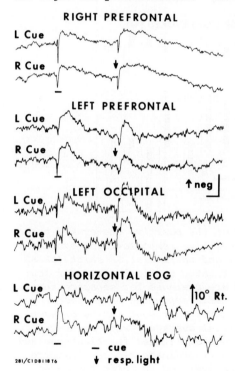

Fig. 3. Averaged prefrontal and occipital electrocortical potentials and horizontal electrooculograms (EOGs) for monkey 281 during 8-sec DR performance for trials with left-cue and right-cue presentations. Each average is for 40 trials. Horizontal bars indicate cue presentation and arrows onset of the response lights. Calibrations: vertical bar, 100 µV; horizontal bar, 2 sec. EOG calibration as shown. Upward deflections indicate cortical surface negativity or eye deviation to the right. Note: The amplitudes of the positive components of the cue-evoked response are larger in the prefrontal area contralateral to the location of the light.

that the amplitude of the positive component of the evoked response to onset of the cue light (CEP) was related to cue position, with greater amplitudes in the right prefrontal area to the left cue, and in the left prefrontal area to the right cue. The results for the four monkeys, who were tested on separate days with the right and left responding hand, are shown in

Figure 4. The CEP amplitude in the left and right prefrontal
area was consistently larger to the contralateral than to the
ipsilateral cue light, but no such systematic relationship was
obtained for either the response-light evoked potentials or for
the magnitude of the mnemonic SP shift. The amplitude of the

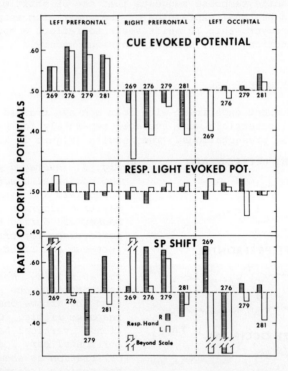

Fig. 4. *Effect of cue position on the positive cue-evoked potential (CEP, upper section), the positive response-light evoked
potential (REP, middle section), and intratrial SP shift (SP shift,
lower section). The data are for three cortical areas for four
monkeys (numbered as shown) and are averages for separate testing with the right and with the left responding hand (each 10
sessions). The CEP and REP ordinates represent ratios of each
mean EP amplitude (based on 40-trial averages) with right-cue
presentation to the sum of the mean amplitudes for right-cue and
left-cue presentation. The SP-shift ordinate represents corresponding ratios, computed for the averaged SP shift for 6-sec
epochs following cue onset, with reference to the 6-sec epoch
preceding the cue. Ratios above .50 indicate greater potentials
for right- and than left-cue presentation, and vice versa.
Note: Greater CEPs resulted for every monkey from left prefrontal area with right cues and from right prefrontal area for
left cues, but there were no consistent results for occipital
CEPs or for REPs and SP shifts from any electrode location.*

EPs did not seem to be appreciably affected by the changes in the responding hand.

Of further interest are the findings from the left occipital cortex (electrodes had not been implanted in the right occipital area), which showed no consistent differences in CEPs to left and right cue lights. It is unlikely that the latter results can be attributed to inappropriate electrode placements, because it was found in other experiments (Rosen & Stamm, 1973) that the magnitude of SP shifts from similarly placed electrodes was affected by the nature of the task, i.e., it was greater for DMS than for DR tasks. The occipital SP shift magnitude was also found to vary as a function of cue duration (Stamm & Rosen, 1972).

Furthermore, there were systematic differences in terms of CEP latency, which was 75 to 115 msec for the occipital and 85 to 115 msec for the prefrontal electrodes; the latency of the initial deflection in the electrooculogram (EOG) was 185 to 235 msec. Figure 3 indicates a coincidence of the start of eye deviations with the negative rise of the SP shift in prefrontal, but not in occipital, cortex. This observation has been confirmed by the results from other experiments that suggest that the intratrial prefrontal potentials may reflect not only sensory processes, but also oculomotor functions (see Anderson, this volume).

EFFECTS OF INTERMANUAL TRANSFER ON SP SHIFTS

In the early experiments the testing procedure was standardized by training all monkeys with the right hand (regardless of their preferences in reaching for peanuts) and by systematic data analyses for potentials from only the left hemisphere. Examination of the recordings from the right hemisphere indicated only negligible SP shifts from both the prefrontal and precentral areas. The marked discrepancies between the left and right prefrontal SP shift magnitude suggested the need for further experimentation (Stamm, Gadotti, & Rosen, 1975). Four monkeys that had learned 8-sec DR with the right hand and had been extensively overtrained (mean of 24,500 trials) were retrained on the task. After 10 sessions of additional right-hand training they were tested with their left hands. Although they continued to respond above 90% correct, the intermanual transfer tests had negligible effects on SP shift magnitude in either left or right prefrontal areas, as illustrated by Figure 5.

Further training with the left hand (Figure 6A) also revealed little changes in SP shift magnitudes and the right prefrontal SP shifts remained near baseline levels for each of the four monkeys. Only one of these monkeys (monkey 267) showed a transitory decrease in the left and a concomitant increase in the right prefrontal SP shift magnitude, but both of these returned to their pretransfer levels by the seventh session with the left hand.

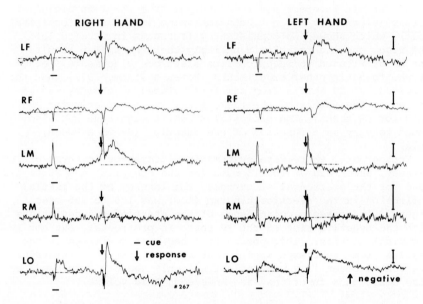

*Fig. 5. Averaged electrocortical potentials for monkey 267, recorded with transcortical electrodes from prefrontal, precentral, and occipital areas during 8-sec DR performance. Electrodes were implanted in pairs--one on the cortical surface (except RM, on dura), the other in subjacent white matter. Each trace represents an average of 40 trials and is of 32-sec duration. The monkey was trained extensively with the right hand and then given intermanual transfer tests to the left hand. Abbreviations: L, left; R, right; F, prefrontal (principalis); M, precentral (motor); O, occipital area. Horizontal bars indicate cue presentation and arrows indicate onset of response lights. Calibrations: vertical bars, 25 µV. Cue duration, 1 sec. Surface negativity upward. Note: There are no systematic differences for LF and RF potentials between the responding hands, and the SP shifts appear greater in the LF than in the RF traces.*

The results suggest that transient spatial memory was mediated by only one hemisphere in these highly overtrained monkeys and that it did not seem to be affected by transfer of the responding hand (cf. Collins; Glick, Jerussi & Zimmerberg, this volume). This interpretation appears consonant with the finding obtained by brief disruptive electrical stimulation of prefrontal cortex (Stamm & Rosen, 1973). Disruption in correct DR performance resulted only from stimulation of the prefrontal area contralateral to the trained responding hand (cf. Doty & Overman, this volume) and no changes in the effects of stimulation after intermanual

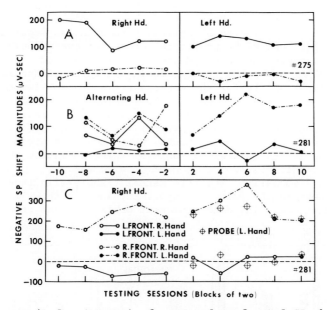

*Fig. 6. Magnitudes (µV-sec) of averaged prefrontal SP shifts
during 8-sec DR performance with intermanual transfer. Each
point in the graphs represents the averages for the first 40
trials of two consecutive 120-trial sessions that were computed
for 6-sec epochs following cue onset, with reference to 6-sec
epochs preceding the cue. (A) Monkey 275, which had been extensively trained with the right hand and then tested with the
left hand. The data are for the final sessions preceding, and
the sessions following, intermanual transfer. (B) Monkey 281,
which was trained with the left and right hand during successive
sessions and then tested only with the left hand. (C) Continued
testing of this monkey with the right hand. The breaks in the
graphs indicate 10 right-hand sessions that were not recorded.
The probes are single sessions with the left hand that were
interspersed during right-hand overtraining. Note the substantial differences in SP shift magnitudes between left and right
prefrontal areas, regardless of responding hands (A and C), and
(B) divergence between SP shift magnitudes with left-hand training.*

transfer were observed.

The hemispheric asymmetry in prefrontal SP shifts appears related to the monkey's responding hand during acquisition of the
DR task and may also be a function of the extensive overtraining.
In order to assess the effects of these conditions an additional
experiment was conducted. Four naive monkeys were trained to
90% criterion on 8-sec DR, two with only their left hands and two

with their left and right hands during alternate testing sessions. The averaged cortical recordings obtained during testing on 8-sec DR revealed SP shifts of substantial magnitude from both the left and right prefrontal areas for every monkey. For the left-hand-trained monkeys the SP shift magnitude was consistently larger in the right than in the left hemisphere. The prefrontal SP shifts for the monkeys trained with alternate hands (Figure 6*B*) showed session-to-session fluctuations, which may be reflections of the changing testing conditions, but overall the magnitudes were also greater in the right prefrontal area. Intermanual transfer tests, which could be given to only one of the left-hand-trained monkeys, revealed little change in SP shift magnitudes from both prefrontal areas.

Figure 7 summarizes the intermanual transfer findings for the four monkeys in the previous experiment and the three monkeys in the present one. The data represent prefrontal and precentral

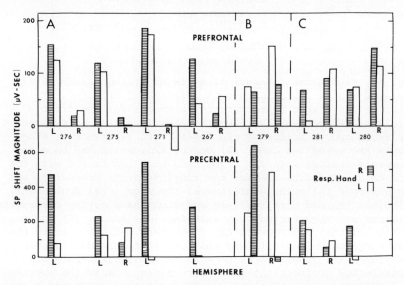

Fig. 7. *Magnitudes (µV-sec) of averaged SP shifts during 8-sec DR performance, recorded from the left (L) and right (R) prefrontal (upper section) and precentral (lower section) cortical areas for seven monkeys (numbered as shown). Each bar represents the average SP shift for the first 40 trials in two consecutive 120-trial sessions with the right or left responding hand, immediately before and after intermanual transfer. The prefrontal SP shifts were computed for 6-sec epochs following cue onset, and the precentral shifts for 6-sec epochs preceding onset of the response lights, both with reference to 6-sec epochs preceding the cue. (A) Four monekys that had been trained only with the right hand; (B) one monkey that had been trained only with the*

averaged SP shift magnitudes before and after intermanual transfer by five monkeys trained with one hand, and SP shift magnitudes obtained during left- and right-hand testing of two monkeys
trained with both hands.  (Right precentral electrodes were not
implanted in every monkey.)  The precentral SP shifts were computed for 6-sec epochs preceding onset of the response lights,
because the shifts appeared time-locked to the choice response.
These data show consistent effects of intermanual transfer tests
for every monkey, namely marked dissociations between prefrontal
and precentral function.  The SP shifts from the right and left
precentral areas changed substantially in the expected direction,
with greater magnitudes in the hemisphere contralateral to the
responding hand.  The prefrontal SP shifts were hardly affected
by intermanual transfer, with magnitudes remaining larger in one
hemisphere for each monkey.


THE TIME COURSE OF THE ESTABLISHMENT OF PREFRONTAL ASYMMETRY

One aim of the prior experiment was to assess the effects of
overtraining on the asymmetry of prefrontal SP shifts.  Unfortunately, extensive overtraining could be given to only one
monkey, but the results seem impressive.  After this monkey had
been trained under the alternate-hand procedure  (Figure 6B) it
was given 10 consecutive sessions with the left hand.  During
this procedure a marked divergence developed between the magnitudes of the two prefrontal SP shifts, with a substantial increase in the right, and a decrease to baseline level in the
left SP shift.  Subsequent transfer to the right hand and continued overtraining for 30 sessions revealed no substantial
changes in the magnitudes of the prefrontal SP shifts (Figure 6C),
which also remained unaffected by periodic single-session tests
(probes) with the left hand.  The final data for overtraining
revealed prefrontal SP shifts whose magnitudes resembled those
that had been found with the four original monkeys, except that
the greater shifts occurred in the right hemisphere.
The averaged EOGs for several monkeys were also evaluated.
Recordings for two of the three monkeys for which systematic data
were available indicate that their visual orientation prior to
cue presentation was toward only one of the display windows, so
lateral eye movements occurred only with cue presentation in the
opposite window.  These findings are illustrated by the averaged
EOG in Figure 3, which shows substantial eye deviations only

*left hand; (C) two monkeys that were trained on successive ses-
sions with the left and right hands (the SP shift averages are
for the training sessions with each hand).  Note:  Intermanual
transfer had relatively little effect on the L or R prefrontal,
but marked effects on precentral SP shift magnitudes.  (In four
monkeys R precentral electrodes were not implanted.)*

397

when the right cue was presented, but little eye movements to the left cue. In the third monkey appropriate lateral eye movements were recorded to cues in either position. The leftward orientation bias of two of the monkeys is also indicated by their error responses, which occurred predominantly when the right cue had been presented, as well as by the incidence of interresponse presses that were predominantly to the left window. Both these monkeys had substantially larger prefrontal SP shifts in the right than in the left hemisphere.


DISCUSSION

The findings concerning averaged cortical macropotentials during DR task performance by monkeys have suggested several functional dissociations among cortical areas and among component potentials in each area. For recordings from dorsolateral cortex (principal sulcus) two components appear to be of special significance, namely the cue-evoked response (CEP) and the SP shift that occurs during the early portion of the intratrial delay.

Interhemispheric differences were found for the CEP in relation to the spatial location of the cue lights, with larger amplitude positive waves in each prefrontal area in response to presentation of the contralateral cue. Differential effects of left and right cues during DR performance have also been reported for discharge patterns of single prefrontal neurons (Niki, 1974). These findings appear consistent with reports of contralateral visual receptive fields of neurons in the prefrontal eye field (Mohler, Goldberg, & Wurtz, 1973) and of prefrontal neuronal discharges during saccadic eye movements (Bizzi, 1968; Bizzi & Schiller, 1970). These reports, as well as our finding of long latencies for the CEPs, support the interpretation that this electrocortical potential reflects neuronal processes involved in the visuospatial or oculomotor functions required for formation of the transient spatial memory during DR performance.

With regard to the mnemonic prefrontal SP shift, an important finding is the high correlation between its magnitude and the correctness of choice responses made after the shift has subsided. This SP shift is therefore considered to be an expression of the neuronal processes in the transient memory. The prefrontal SP shifts can be dissociated from concurrent SP shifts in the precentral areas, whose magnitudes are affected by changes in the responding hand; furthermore, the prefrontal SP shift becomes dominant in only one hemisphere.

Hemispheric asymmetries in prefrontal SP shifts do not imply unilateral localization of the transient engram (Doty & Overman, this volume). The evidence indicating bilateral formation of engrams for acquired tasks has received extensive support from ablation experiments, as well as from recent findings obtained with commissurectomized monkeys (Hamilton, this volume). The correspondence in time course between prefrontal SP shifts and activation patterns of underlying neurons (Fuster, 1973; Niki, 1974) would indicate that these cortical potentials reflect similar mnemonic functions. The most appropriate interpretation for the asymmetrical SP shifts is that the monkey utilizes only one prefrontal segment for mediation of the transient memory required by the task.

The important question remains as to the processes that determine the localization of the prefrontal SP shift in the monkey's left or right hemisphere. There is no evidence in support of the concept of innate processes, analogous to those of cerebral dominance in the human brain (cf. Dawson; Rubens, this volume). Furthermore, no evidence has been obtained for a relationship between hemispheric localization and the monkey's hand preference in reaching for peanuts. As has been described by Warren (this volume) such tests appear inadequate for evaluation of possible hemispheric dominance for motor responses in the monkey.

Our investigations suggest two possible behavioral functions that may account for the hemispheric asymmetry--namely the hand that is available for the choice response, and the monkey's preference for spatial orientation. In every one of the six monkeys trained on the DR task with only one hand, the prefrontal SP shift became dominant and stable in the hemisphere contralateral to that hand. Moreover, the monkey that had been trained on DR with the alternate-hand procedure showed a substantial divergence in the prefrontal SP shift magnitudes during the subsequent sessions with only left-handed training, with the right prefrontal potential becoming large and stable.

The present evidence for the importance of spatial orientation preferences is less substantial. With the alternate-hand training procedure, which was instituted in order to avoid the effects of extensive unimanual performance, greater magnitude SP shifts were found from the right than from the left prefrontal area for both monkeys. These monkeys' errors and interresponse presses, as well as their oculograms, indicate orientation bias toward the left window, a spatial preference that is contralateral to the dominant hemispheric prefrontal SP shift.

At this time one can only speculate with regard to the importance of spatial orientation preferences in affecting both behavioral strategies and possible hemispheric differences (cf. Anderson; Glick, Jerussi & Zimmerberg; Gur & Gur; Heilman & Watson, this volume). During the acquisition of behavioral tasks many monkeys have been found to respond predominantly to the location of one of the spatially separated choice objects. Many observations have also indicated that most monkeys prefer to look and turn their heads toward one side. It is entirely possible that these spatial preferences are acquired during the early life of the animals (cf. Turkewitz, this volume), such as during their suckling periods. Thus, the conclusion of our investigations points to the importance of the ontogeny of spatial orientation preferences. This appears to be a productive area for further research.

SUMMARY

A series of experiments was conducted in which monkeys with chronically implanted electrodes were tested on a two-choice visual delayed-response (DR) task. Pairs of nonpolarizable electrodes were placed bilaterally in prefrontal (principal sulcus), precentral, and lateral occipital areas, with one electrode of each pair on the cortical surface and the other (reference) in subjacent white matter. Electrodes were also implanted across the eyes for electrooculogram (EOG) recordings.

Computer averages of macropotentials, recorded during DR performance, with differing parameters of the task, revealed five distinct components during the course of the trial. Two of these seemed to reflect specific prefrontal functions; namely the evoked potential to onset of the cue light (CEP) and a surface-negative steady-potential (SP) shift that occurred at the end of cue presentation and the early intratrial delay. The magnitude of the latter was unaffected by changes in duration of cue presentation or of the delay period, but was highly correlated with the scores of correct choice responses. Functional dissociations between hemispheres and among cortical areas are indicated by the following findings, obtained during correct performance of DR: (1) The positive component of the prefrontal CEP was a function of the location of the cue lights, with greater amplitudes on the side contralateral to the hemifield in which the cue was presented; corresponding differences were not found for the occipital CEPs, or for prefrontal SP shifts. (2) For monkeys trained to respond with one hand the magnitudes of the SP shifts were appreciably larger in the contralateral prefrontal area; ipsilateral prefrontal SP shifts were near baseline. (3) Intermanual transfer had no consistent effects on SP shift magnitudes from either prefrontal area but resulted in substantial changes in precentral SP shifts preceding the choice response. These were larger in the hemisphere contralateral to the responding hand. (4) For monkeys trained on DR alternatively with left and right hands, SP shifts of substantial magnitudes were recorded from both prefrontal areas. (5) Subsequent training of these monkeys with one responding hand resulted in increased magnitude of the contralateral prefrontal SP shift with a corresponding decrease in ipsilateral magnitude. (6) EOGs indicated that before cue presentation most monkeys tended to orient their eyes toward the display window contralateral to the hemisphere exhibiting the larger prefrontal SP shift.

The present findings provide evidence for functional asymmetry in the monkeys' frontal lobes. Overtrained monkeys seem to uti-

lize only one prefrontal area for mediation of the transient
memory required by the DR task.  The establishment of this hemispheric specialization appears related to two processes, namely
the hand that is involved in task acquisition and more general
spatial orientation preferences.

ACKNOWLEDGMENTS

This investigation was supported by NSF Grant BO 35735-X01.
We wish to express our appreciation to Richard Reeder for his
technical assistance and to Oscar Gillespie, Michele Parker, and
Barry Sandrew for their help in various phases of this research.

REFERENCES

Bizzi, E.  Discharge of frontal eye field neurons during saccadic
    and following eye movements in unanesthetized monkeys.
    *Experimental Brain Research*, 1968, *6*, 69-80.
Bizzi, E., & Schiller, P. H.  Single unit activity in the frontal
    eye fields of unanesthetized monkeys during eye and head
    movement.  *Experimental Brain Research*, 1970, *10*, 151-158.
Cohen, S. M.  Electrical stimulation of cortical-caudate pairs
    during delayed successive visual discrimination in monkeys.
    *Acta Neurobiologiae Experimentalis*, 1972, *32*, 211-233.
Donchin, E., Otto, D. A., Gerbrant, L. K., & Pribram, K. H.
    While a monkey waits:  Electrocortical events recorded
    during the foreperiod of a reaction time study.  *Electroen-
    cephalography & Clinical Neurophysiology*, 1971, *31*, 115-127.
Fuster, J. M.  Unit activity in prefrontal cortex during delayed-
    response performance:  Neuronal correlates of transient
    memory.  *Journal of Neurophysiology*, 1973, *36*, 61-78.
Goldman, P. S., Rosvold, H. E., Vest, B., & Galkin, T. W.
    Analysis of the delayed-alternation deficit produced by
    dorsolateral prefrontal lesions in the rhesus monkey.
    *Journal of Comparative & Physiological Psychology*, 1971, *77*,
    212-220.
Kovner, R., & Stamm, J. S.  Disruption of short-term visual
    memory by electrical stimulation of inferotemporal cortex
    in the monkey.  *Journal of Comparative & Physiological
    Psychology*, 1972, *81*, 163-172.
Mohler, C. W., Goldberg, M. E., & Wurtz, R. H.  Visual receptive
    fields of frontal eye field neurons.  *Brain Research*, 1973,
    *61*, 385-389.
Niki, H.  Differential activity of prefrontal units during right
    and left delayed response trials.  *Brain Research*, 1974,
    *70*, 346-349.
Rosen, S. C., & Stamm, J. S.  Attention or Memory?  An analysis
    of prefrontal cortical activity in delayed response tasks.

*Federation Proceedings,* 1973, *32,* 367.

Rowland, V.   Cortical steady potentials in reinforcement and learning.   In E. Stellar & J. M. Sprague (Eds.), *Progress in physiological psychology.* New York:  Academic Press, 1968.

Stamm, J. S.   Electrical stimulation of monkey's prefrontal cortex during delayed response performance. *Journal of Comparative & Physiological Psychology,* 1969, *67,* 535-546.

Stamm, J. S., Gadotti, A., & Rosen, S. C.   Interhemispheric functional differences in prefrontal cortex of monkeys. *Journal of Neurobiology,* 1975, *6,* 39-49.

Stamm, J. S., & Rosen, S. C.   Cortical steady potential shifts and anodal polarization during delayed response performance. *Acta Neurobiologiae Experimentalis,* 1972, *32,* 193-209.

Stamm, J.S., & Rosen, S. C.   The locus and crucial time of implication of prefrontal cortex in the delayed response task. In K. H. Pribram & A. R. Luria (Eds.), *Psychophysiology of the frontal lobes.*   New York:  Academic Press, 1973.

Stamm, J. S., & Weber-Levine, M.   Delayed alternation impairments following selective prefrontal cortical ablations in monkeys. *Experimental Neurology,* 1971, *33,* 263-278.

Walter, W. G., Cooper, R., Aldridge, V. J., McCallum, W. C., & Winter, A. L.   Contingent negative variation:  An electrical sign of sensorimotor association and expectancy in the human brain. *Nature,* 1964, *203,* 380-384.

# 21.
# Language-Related Asymmetries of Eye-Movement and Evoked Potentials

SAMUEL W. ANDERSON

New York State Psychiatric Institute

Although the speech-related auditory evoked potential (AEP) does not always show lateral amplitude asymmetries, there are certain characteristic patterns often reported. This chapter will review findings indicating that at least one of these patterns, replicated in this study, is directly correlated with the electrooculographic pattern (EOG) of an eye-movement bias associated with verbal function.

Three proposed sources for the common pattern are discussed: retinal, occipital, and frontal. Although the case appears strongest in favor of a frontal origin, it remains to be shown convincingly that the cortex generates an asymmetric speech-related potential in the absence of any lateral eye movement.

## ASYMMETRIES REPORTED IN SPEECH-RELATED AEP STUDIES

Since language is differentially affected by electrical stimulation of corresponding regions on opposite sides of the human brain, it has often been proposed that the relation may hold the other way too: There should be some distinctive, natural electrical activity occurring only in the speech-dominant hemisphere during normal language behavior. By use of the highly sensitive technique of signal averaging, so goes the argument, this special electrical activity should be detectable in the form of an AEP difference between a pair of electrodes, one placed over the speech cortex, the other over its homologue in the minor hemi-

403

sphere. That such an asymmetry was language-specific would be
demonstrable by showing that it appeared only when averaging was
triggered on a linguistic event, such as perceiving a syllable
or speaking a word.

Numerous investigations of evoked potentials have now carried
the argument to this point, often but not invariably revealing
speech-related asymmetries. It should be possible by now to ask
whether evoked potentials can show distinct asymmetric loci for
speech perception and production. Yet, it is not, largely because of an important difficulty: AEPs have a special sensitivity for events associated in time with systematic eye movements,
which are seen to have electrical consequences of various kinds
over much of the head (cf. Stamm, Rosen, & Gadotti, this volume).

Electroencephalographers have only lately begun to overcome
years of bedevilment by unwanted eye-movement effects. They have
done it as much by carefully measuring and evaluating electrical
phenomena associated with the active EOG as by attempting to im-
mobilize the wandering eye. Similar care is called for in work
on speech potentials, particularly because the ordinary, natural
functions of talking and listening to speech appear to involve
systematic eye-movement effects (Kinsbourne, 1972; Gur & Gur,
this volume).

There are three types of language-evoked electrocortical asymmetries that have been replicated regularly. Although they are
logically consistent with one another, all three have never been
reported together.* All three asymmetries are in terms of amplitude and, as each involves differences between AEP components
$N_1$ and $P_2$, they are distinguished as asymmetries of type A, B,
and C in Figure 1; studies obtaining each type of effect are
listed in Table 1.

Type A consists of a greater difference between $N_1$ and $P_2$ on
the left than on the right; type B consists of a larger $N_1$ on the
left; type C consists of a larger $P_2$ on the right. The entries
in Table 1 are derived from any available information in the report of each study, both from the text and the figures. Cohn,
for example, stated only that "seventeen subjects showed a greater amplitude of output over the left brain when presented with
verbal stimuli [1971, p. 600]" but a type A asymmetry is exhibited in the figure shown. Molfese (1972) also reported type A
only, although he presented data on no other aspect of his results; his more recent findings have been type B or C rather

---

*There are numerous other findings of asymmetry not mentioned
here, either because they have not been replicated or because
they differ enough from studies in Table 1 in terms of design
that they cannot be usefully compared. Visual evoked potentials,
for example, involve successive fixation or pursuit eye movements
that are not found in auditory studies; the result of Matsumiya,
et al., 1972, is excluded simply because of their unusual "W-
wave" asymmetry, probably the result of unusual electrode locations, which appears to obscure standard AEP components.

TABLE 1

Outcomes and design of auditory-evoked potential studies employing speech stimuli, classified by type[a]

| Study | Outcome type | Stimuli[b] | Active electrodes[c] | Reference | EOG |
|---|---|---|---|---|---|
| Cohn (1971) | A | cat, bar, rat | $C_1$-$C_2$ | ear | "about the eyes" |
| Morrell & Salamy (1971) | B | /pi/, /pa/, /əpik/, /əpak/ | $F_7$-$F_8$, $C_7$-$C_8$, $TP_1$[d] | linked ears | |
| Wood et al. (1971) | B, C[e] | /ba/, /da/ | $C_3$-$C_4$, $T_3$-$T_4$ | linked ears | |
| Molfese (1972) | A | boy, dog | $T_3$-$T_4$ | ears | |
| Neville (1974) | B[f] | monosyllabic digits | $C_5$-$C_6$ | linked mastoids | "forehead" |
| Haaland (1974) | C | CVC[g] monosyllables | $F_7$-$F_8$, $T_3$-$T_4$ | linked mastoids | above, below eye |
| Friedman, Simson, Ritter, & Rapin (1975) | B | kick, cake, pint, bowl, dive | Midway between $P_z$ and mastoids | nose | above right eye |
| Galambos et al. (1975) | B, C | /pa/, /ba/ | $TP_2$[h] | linked mastoids | |

[a]See Figure 1.

[b]Slashes indicate phonetic symbols.

[c]Except where otherwise noted, loci in 10-20 system (Jasper, 1958).

[d]Temporal-parietal pair, midway between $P_3$, $T_5$-$P_4$, $T_6$

[e]Relative to lateral differences on a nonspeech task.

[f]Measured from component $P_1$.

[g]Consonant-vowel-consonant.

[h]Temporal-parietal pair, between $T_3$, $T_5$-$T_4$, $T_6$

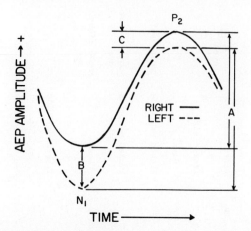

*Fig. 1. Schematic characterization of three types of asymmetry in potentials evoked by speech. In type A, $P_2$-$N_1$ is greater on the left; in type B, /$N_1$/ is greater on the left; in type C, $P_2$ is greater on the right.*

than A.

Morrell and Salamy (1971) obtained results of type B from frontal, central, and parietal electrode pairs, the asymmetry increasing toward the more posterior locations (cf. Thatcher, this volume). Observations on A and C effects were made, but only the difference in $N_1$ was statistically significant (p. 166). Haaland (1974) reported only type C, but Wood, Goff, and Day (1971) observed both B and C asymmetries provided comparisons were made with baselines taken from performance on a nonlanguage task employing the same syllabic stimuli. Neville (1974) computed $N_1$ shifts from $P_1$ rather than from the usual prestimulus baseline, and obtained only a type B amplitude effect,* as did Friedman et al. (1975) in averages for signal words (i.e., words to which the subject was set to respond selectively). Friedman found a slight $P_3$ difference in terms of the averages, but only the type B result reached statistical significance by the conservative Bonferroni criterion employed in this study. In a similar design, Galambos, Benson, Smith, Schulman, Galambos, and Osier (1975) failed to find any significant amplitude asymmetries in a series of repeated measures analyses of variance (p. 280), although the Wilcoxon test (used by Wood, Goff, & Day, 1971) implicated asymmetries principally at $P_3$ but also at $N_1$ for target syllables versus tones (p. 281). A $P_3$ asymmetry has yet to be replicated convincingly in an auditory evoked potential speech study,

---

*Neville's main finding was an asymmetry of latencies for components $N_1$, $P_2$, and $N_2$ (shorter on the left).

although it has been found in a visual task (Thatcher, this volume). (See also Tueting and Sutton, 1973.) In their published figure Galambos *et al.* showed both type B and type C effects for nontarget syllables (1975, p. 380), although they did not report having tested them for significance. Across the eight studies in Table 1, type A appears in two, type B in five and type C in three.

Eye movements were monitored in only half these studies, and when done, served mainly as a means of identifying and rejecting trials containing evidence of gross eye movement. It is known, however, that on single trials the EOG is not reliably sensitive to eye shifts of less than approximately $5^0$ and during fixation the eye undergoes a continuous process of involuntary drift and correction that results in movements seldom reaching $1^0$; with visual inattention there are apparently aimless oscillatory movements that are considerably smaller than $5^0$ (Gaarder, 1966; Gaarder, Krauskopf, Graf, Kropfl, & Arnington, 1964). If these small motions contained a language-related lateral bias, this would be too small to be evident in the EOG on any single trial, yet might be systematically added to the signal by the averaging technique.

Neville (1974) and Haaland (1974) did average their EOG records, Haaland doing so after rejecting trials containing as much as a 25 μV shift (p. 340). In spite of this, the averaged EOGs still show what is obviously a high correlation with the AEPs, especially within the epoch containing $N_1$ and $P_2$ (p. 342, Figure 1). These averaged EOGs are inconclusive, however, as both Neville and Haaland located their EOG electrodes in positions that maximize sensitivity to vertical eye movements, whereas it is the lateral component that would be reflected directly in lateral asymmetries of the evoked potential.

This detailed discussion of eye-movement control methods certainly does not demonstrate that there must be lateral eye-movement biases at work whenever brain differences are reported, but it does indicate that this possibility has seldom, if ever, been ruled out.


EYE-MOVEMENT LATERALITY DURING VERBAL COGNITION

Other experiments, however, suggest that right-biased lateral eye movement does occur. Simultaneously, Kinsbourne (1972) and Kocel, Galin, Ornstein, and Merrin (1972) discovered a rightward lateral eye movement bias that occurs after a subject is asked a question requiring verbal, as opposed to spatial, reasoning.

The procedure is simple: The experimenter asks a question and then observes the direction of the first lateral eye movement. The method was developed by Teitelbaum (1954) and Day (1967), who had used it to find consistent individual differences between persons responding exclusively as left-movers or right-movers

when asked any question whatever (see also Harnad, 1972). This
seeming contradiction of the Kinsbourne-Kocel phenomenon has recently been resolved: Apparently the personality-trait bias is
elicited if the experimenter questions the subject face to face,
but the verbal cognitive mode bias occurs if the experimenter
positions himself outside of the subject's visual field (Gur &
Gur, this volume).

Hiscock (1975) has looked at the EOG correlates of each of
these phenomena and has found an additional difference in the
character of the movements. The Teitelbaum-Day eye movement consists of a pair of lateral saccades, one sharply to the right or
left, the other back to center. The Kinsbourne-Kocel movement,
on the other hand, is a more gradual shift to the right, upon
which is superimposed a ragged jitter, persisting over several
seconds between onset of question and response (see Figure 2).
It appears that the former is a voluntary gaze aversion, perhaps
containing a brief reflective excursion between the breaking and
restoring of eye contact with the experimenter; in contrast, the
latter gives the appearance of a more involuntary series of
movements.

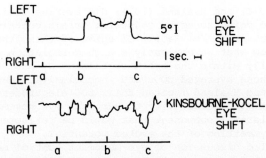

*Fig. 2. Diagram of EOGs purporting to show eye biases due to per-
sonality trait (Day) and verbal cognitive mode (kinsbourne-Kocel).
The beginning of the question is marked by a; end of question, b;
subject's verbal response, c. After Hiscock (1975).*

Hiscock's temporal analysis of the verbal eye-movement bias
not only reveals rightward movement while listening to speech,
but may also indicate an even greater rightward movement just
prior to speaking. It happens that an asymmetry in brain potentials has been reported for this particular epoch too. McAdam
and Whitaker (1971) found a relative left-negative asymmetry between inferior frontal and precentral electrode pairs during the
course of a slowly developing negative shift. Prior to spontaneously uttered words beginning with *p* or *k*, this slow potential
showed a time course of 1.5 sec, which matches the Hiscock analysis rather well. Subjects were instructed to maintain gaze upon

a fixation stimulus, but fine eye movements were not monitored. Grozinger, Kornhuber, and Kriebel (1975) have replicated the McAdam and Whitaker asymmetry. They systematically examined and rejected a number of possible artifactual explanations and concluded that the effect is generated intracortically and has something to do with respiration (pp. 266-267). The EOG was monitored for rejection of trials with gross eye movement, but not averaged, so it is again possible to ask whether a subtle involuntary eye-movement bias had not occurred. In the present study an attempt was made to answer this rather neglected question, with respect to both listening and speaking.

## EXPERIMENTAL COMPARISON OF AEP ASYMMETRY AND LATERAL EYE-MOVEMENT BIAS

Subjects were selected from a group of 28 volunteer medical, dental, and nursing students and technicians between the ages of 18 and 40. (See Anderson & Jaffe, 1973.) All 28 were given the Harris Test of Lateral Dominance (Harris, 1955) and a dichotic-listening test similar to that of Dirks (1964; see Berlin; Springer, this volume) with the following modifications: The subject was presented with dichotic pairings of the CV (consonant-vowel) monosyllables /ba/, /da/, and /ga/ and asked to write after each pair the one CV he was "most confident he had heard" on each trial. Forty-seven dichotic trials were randomly dispersed among another 47 on which the same CV pair was presented to both ears. The interstimulus interval was 4 sec. Correctly reported CVs on dichotic trials were classified by ear, and an ear-preference score calculated by the familiar formula, $D = (R - L)/(R + L)$.

To avoid having to contend with the generally reported unpredictability and complexity of speech-lateralization findings among left-handers (Dee, 1971), all subjects showing any degree of sinistral or mixed manual dominance on the Harris test were excluded from this study. Also excluded as unclearly or insufficiently lateralized were subjects who had $D$ scores within $\pm$ .100 of zero. This yielded only three remaining subjects showing left-ear preferences ($D$ negative), so the three subjects with the highest positive $D$ scores were selected so as to constitute a total balanced set of six dextral subjects, three inferred to be left-hemisphere dominant for speech perception, and three right-hemisphere dominant. All were males but one. The mean $D$ score for the right-eared group was + .431, and for the left-eared group, - .345. Henceforth, they are referred to as the $D+$ and $D-$ groups. Note that both groups were right-handed.

The highest positive $D$ score was + .787, the most negative was - .512. The two subjects obtaining these scores are referred to as the polar $D+$ and polar $D-$ subjects, respectively.

None of the three $D+$ subjects reported any left-handedness or ambidexterity whatever in family background on the Harris test. The polar *D-* subject reported a left-handed cousin and an ambidextrous grandfather, and one of the others, whose family was Chinese, reported that her brother was required to switch from the left to the right hand when he was 2 years old. The remaining *D-* subject reported only a dextral family background.

Relative speech reception thresholds (SRT) were determined for each subject, one ear at a time, by taking the average of ascending and descending limits with a pair of Hewlett-Packard Model 350D matched attenuators, while the subject attempted to identify two CV stimuli as presented in the listening task (discussed later). Among the six subjects, maximum SRT difference between left and right ears was 5.5 dB; the average difference was 3.7 dB for the *D-* group and 2.0 dB for the *D+* group. There appeared to be no systematic relationship between SRT discrepancy and ear preference.

*PROCEDURE*

After pretesting as described earlier, Beckman nonpolarizing disk electrodes were placed at the left and right inferior frontal locations (LIF and RIF) specified by McAdam and Whitaker (1971, p. 500) and also at each outer canthus (LOC and ROC) to record the EOG.

All four active electrodes were referenced to linked mastoids. Interelectrode resistances were always below 10,000 ohms, and differences between bilateral homotopic pairs were below 1000 ohms. The subject was given three tasks: a *listening* task, which was a close approximation to the "stop consonant" task of Wood, Goff, and Day (1971) and what we shall call the *speaking* task, which was the "P-word" condition of McAdam and Whitaker (1971) together with a nonspeech control task similar to theirs. A 15-min rest period separated the first and second tasks.

*LISTENING TASK*

A stimulus tape was prepared containing random occurrences of the CVs /ba/ and /ga/, spoken by an American male. The CV syllables were presented binaurally at 12 dB above background noise through a stereo headset. They varied between 120 and 150 msec in duration, with a pseudorandom distribution of ISI (interstimulus intervals) ranging from 3 to 10 sec, averaging 7 sec between stimuli. EEG and EOG channels were amplified by four Grass 7PI preamplifiers and drivers with a bandpass width of .20 to 15.0 Hz. All channels were equalized at a gain of 10,000 for an effective range of $\pm100$ µV, and continuously recorded on four channels of a Sangamo model 3562 tape recorder at 19.05 cm/sec. After a tape head-separation lag of 750 msec, the signals were played back into analog channels of a PDP-12 computer. On each trial a 1-sec sweep was digitized every 4 msec and stored on PEC magnetic tape for averaging off-line. Instead of triggering on stimulus onset, the PDP-12 monitored the vocalic rise time of each syllable and triggered on the vocalic peak (Anderson & Jaffe, 1972; Jaffe, Anderson, & Rieber, 1973) about 28 dB above onset level.

After the attachment of electrodes and calibration of the apparatus, the subject was instructed to remain motionless and relaxed with his eyes open, but he was given no further instruction about fixation so as to permit involuntary eye movement if it should occur. He sat facing a white wall and clasping a button box in one hand with which he was told to respond to the two stimuli by pressing with either his middle or index finger. After 50 trials the button box was switched to the opposite hand; this order was counterbalanced across subjects. Altogether, 100 CVs were presented binaurally, delivered to each ear at 20 dB above its own SRT.

## SPEAKING TASK

At the outset each subject was asked to practice by spontaneously uttering different words beginning with the letter *t*. After producing 20 such words, during which time the subject's speech-onset level was calibrated for the purpose of triggering upon articulatory release of a voiceless stop consonant (McAdam & Whitaker, 1971; Morell & Huntington, 1971), the subject was given the main task instructions, to utter 50 different freely selected words beginning with the letter *p*. The Sangamo tape delay was employed for the purpose of initiating each trial record at 750 msec prior to response onset.

An attempt was made to control the motoric, nonlinguistic characteristics of the speaking task, as did McAdam and Whitaker (1971), by eliciting from the subject a "spitting gesture." In pretesting, we had found that most persons, when asked simply to produce this gesture, emit unvoiced sounds; however, others give voiced ones. In order to eliminate voicing (and possibly other articulatory factors) as an irrelevant source of signal variance, a *nonspeech oromotor response* (NOR) was arbitrarily defined; an unvoiced, bilabially released air puff, executed with the tongue pre-positioned to protrude slightly from between the lips. This gesture, not unlike one sometimes spontaneously produced to expel a hair adhering to the tip of the tongue, was described and demonstrated to the subject, who quickly adopted it. Again, 50 trials were run, sampling was triggered on voiceless bilabial release and the data were recorced in the same manner as in the speaking task.

The records from the four active electrodes for each subject in each condition were averaged separately, then the results were combined and averaged across the three subjects in each group. Averaged cortical records and their asymmetries appear in Figure 3. The cortical asymmetries and corresponding EOG differences are shown in Figure 4. For statistical treatment, each record was quantized into 30 points (every 33.3 msec). Pearson Product-

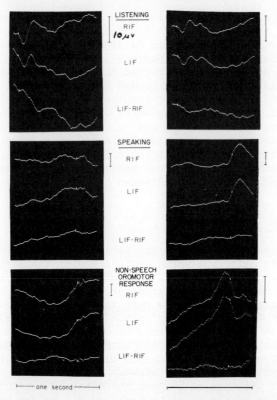

*Fig. 3. AEPs and EOGs in left- and right-eared groups, during listening, speaking, and nonspeech tasks. Left column, left-eared subjects (D-); right column, right-eared subjects (D+). Abbreviations: LIF, left, and RIF, right, inferior frontal electrodes. Polarity convention is positive up; sweep, 1 sec; calibration, 10 μV.*

Moment correlations were calculated for the corresponding eye and brain records of Figure 4 over three epochs: the entire 1-sec record (Table 2), 733-msec poststimulus in the listening condition, and 733-msec preresponse in the other two conditions, and 167 msec in the other two conditions (Table 2). Detailed results follow, according to experimental condition.

*LISTENING RESULTS*

Correlations between eye-movement and inferior frontal asymmetries are significant at the .01 level across the entire record, for both *D-* and *D+* groups (Table 2, A). Restricting the correlated epoch to the first 733 msec after the stimulus attenuates the correlations, especially in the *D+* group, but both

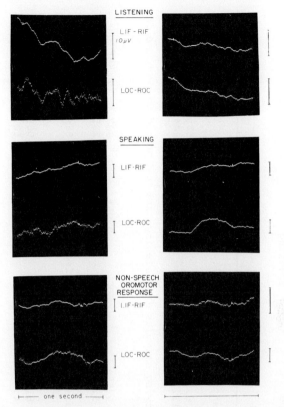

Fig. 4. AEP asymmetries (left minus right) of the records shown in Figure 3, and corresponding EOG asymmetries. Abbreviations: LOC, left, and ROC, right, outer canthal electrodes.

remain significant at .01 (Table 2, B). During the first 167 msec after the trigger, EOG frontal correlations are significant at .01 in both groups (Table 2, C).

*SPEAKING AND NONSPEECH OROMOTOR RESPONSE (NOR)*

For epochs of 1 sec and 733 msec, EOG frontal asymmetry correlations are significant ($p < .01$) on the speaking task in both groups, but only in the *D*- group on the NOR task (Table 2). Correlations over the last 167 msec prior to response fail to reach significance in both groups for either task (Table 2, C). The two most highly lateralized left- and right-dominant subjects, polar *D*+ and polar *D*-, are compared in Figure 5.

TABLE 2

Correlations between EOG and frontal AEP asymmetries[a]

| | Listening | | Speaking | | NOR[b] | |
|---|---|---|---|---|---|---|
| | r | t | r | t | r | t |
| A. Correlations during length of entire record (1 sec). df = 28. | | | | | | |
| Group D− | .788 | 6.77* | .828 | 7.80* | .585 | 3.82* |
| Group D+ | .904 | 11.22* | .736 | 5.75* | .244 | 1.33 |
| B. Correlations on 733 msec, following stimulus in listening task and preceding response in speaking and NOR tasks. df = 20. | | | | | | |
| Group D− | .779 | 5.55* | .800 | 5.96* | .887 | 8.58* |
| Group D+ | .793 | 5.82* | .946 | 13.01* | .235 | 1.08 |
| C. Correlations on 167 msec, immediately following stimulus in listening task and preceding response in speaking and NOR. df = 3. | | | | | | |
| Group D− | .980 | 8.61* | −.173 | .30 | −.609 | 1.33 |
| Group D+ | .932 | 4.46** | .453 | .88 | .527 | 1.07 |

[a] 33-msec epochs.

[b] Nonspeech oromotor response.

*p <.01.

**p <.05.

414

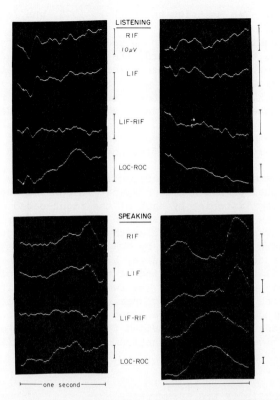

*Fig. 5. AEP and EOG asymmetries in the two subjects scoring largest left- and right-ear preferences in dichotic listening. Left column, polar D-; right column, polar D+.*

## EYE MOVEMENT

First, it should be noted that the *D-* group showed a large amount of jitter, especially during listening, and a slow "eyes right" in the EOG matched by a corresponding frontal shift (Figure 4). A similar slow "eyes right" occurred in the *D+* group, but the groups contrast sharply in the presence of a quick and early "eyes left," beginning before termination of the stimulus, and exhibited only by the *D-* group (cf. Stamm *et al.*, this volume). This initial, quick "eyes left" was present in each of the subjects in the *D-* group, and in none of the *D+* subjects (e.g., Figure 5). Assuming that the probability of this shift is one-half in the population as sampled, it is significantly related to speech dominance at the .02 level. The slow "eyes right" shift was not uniform in the *D-* group; in fact, the polar *D-* subject showed an "eyes left" over the entire record that is a near mirror-opposite of the "eyes right" in the polar *D+* subject

415

(Figure 5) (cf. Van Mastrigt and Sutker, 1975, who found no
secondary shift at all).

During speaking the *D-* group showed an "eyes left" that increased across the entire record; the *D+* group had a distinct
early "eyes left" about 400 msec prior to speech onset followed
by an "eyes right" immediately prior to speech onset (Figure 4).
On the NOR task, both groups showed seemingly random right-left-
right-left patterns, the individual shifts occurring at slightly
different times. Thus, the two groups are distinguished by eye-
movement patterns on the two speech tasks, but not on the nonspeech task, although these differences are not found to be
statistically significant.

An eye-movement bias in the direction predicted by the
Kinsbourne-Kocel phenomenon does appear in the EOG records
averaged during listening by each of the right-eared subjects,
but a late bias in the same direction is suggested prior to
speaking. Perhaps if a 1.5-sec epoch had been averaged in advance of speech onset, as done by McAdam and Whitaker, our result
might have better resembled theirs, although the present averages
look rather flat at the beginning of the sweep, especially in the
crucial right-eared subjects. The two facts--that different eye-
movement biases appear in the groups showing opposite receptive
speech dominance and that these group biases are distinct only
on the two language tasks--provided further support for the
verbal-cognitive-mode interpretation of these lateralization
effects.

SPECTRAL ANALYSIS OF EEG ASYMMETRIES

Of possible help in clarifying some of these results is another electrophysiological correlate of the verbal cognitive mode,
reported by Galin and Ornstein (1972). Obtaining average power
ratios from the ongoing EEG in 1-sec epochs from temporal ($T_4/T_3$)
and parietal ($P_4/P_3$) locations, they compared the verbal tasks of
writing a letter or mentally composing one with two spatial tasks,
the Kohs Blocks and Minnesota Paper Form Board tests. Ratios
were significantly larger, especially in the temporal electrodes,
on the verbal tasks (pp. 415-416). As might be expected, there
was an attempt to assess this asymmetry independently of eye
movement. After the usual editing to eliminate trials containing
gross movement artifacts, the analysis was performed both with
and without inclusion of trials on which the EOG indicated eye
movements greater than $6°$. Since these analyses did not differ
significantly (the $6°$-edited results are not shown), it was concluded that there was no important influence of eye bias on the
main result (p. 416).

This outcome was later replicated by Doyle, Ornstein, and
Galin (1974). A more sophisticated power spectrum analysis was
employed, but the trials with eye movements greater than $6°$ were

retained. (It is not reported in either study how many of these occurred.) This time, a speech listening task was included, which lateralized in the same way as did the other verbal tasks. The verbal versus spatial difference was found to be focused in the alpha region of the spectrum and consisted of a relatively larger alpha component on the left in the spatial tasks, at least those with motor performance requirements (written letter and Kohs Blocks tasks; see Doyle *et al.*, 1974, p. 571). No task resulted in a correspondingly larger alpha on the right. In neither report was there any indication that the authors believed that the eye-movement bias associated with verbal activity could be accounted for in any way by this power ratio asymmetry.

Kinsbourne, however, has speculated that the eye-movement bias may indeed be due to some kind of asymmetry in cortical activation. He proposed that verbal activation is effectively restricted to the left hemisphere but not restricted to the language areas within it: ". . . when subjects await a verbal stimulus and must also look centrally, the verbal activation overflows into the left-sided orientation center, driving attentional balance off center and to the right [Kinsbourne, 1972, p. 539]." Kinsbourne cited Robinson and Fuchs' (1969) finding that direct electrical stimulation of a frontal eye field produces a contralaterally directed conjugate deviation of the eyes. The expected time course of such a putative overflow process is not clear, and it is difficult to link it to the event-related eye-movement bias of the AEP and response-related potential; clearly, the eye cannot move continuously to the right for very long, and the eye-movement bias is necessarily a discontinuous phenomenon.

Galin and Ellis (1975) have attempted to bridge the gap between power spectrum and evoked potential measures of cognitive mode. Sweeps were triggered on flashes presented sporadically throughout task performance, whereupon averaged amplitudes were found to be directly related to integrated power; the power spectrum showed the clearer contrasts between verbal and spatial task conditions.

This evoked potential result is atypical. Although both EEG and AEP amplitudes are sensitive to the effectiveness of task performance, they are usually inversely related to one another: AEPs increase and EEGs decrease with attentiveness to the task. However, it is also usual to trigger evoked potentials on task-related events, and, as Galin and Ellis have stated, "When the stimulus is task relevant, the evoked potential amplitude increases as a function of increasing attention or involvement, . . . conditions usually associated with decreasing background EEG alpha [1975, p. 49]." Since their flashes were task-irrelevant, they were probably not well attended, suggesting that their AEPs are not comparable to AEPs from task-relevant stimuli, responses, or oculomotor biases associated with with verbal activity.

## OCCIPITAL POSTINHIBITORY REBOUND

There is reason to believe that eye movement is not independent of alpha. Gaarder *et al.* (1964) found an eye movement evoked potential (EMEP) between inion and midline occipital electrodes during steady illumination. (Recall that even auditory-evoked-potential studies are usually not conducted in the dark.) This potential, resembling an ordinary VEP, occurred just after the eyes underwent saccadic movements (even very fine ones), which were monitored for triggering by the highly sensitive photoelectric method (p. 1482). The EMEP has been explained as a consequence of the reflex inhibition of visual input to prevent blurring during a saccade. As soon as the eye stops moving, the visual cortex gives an "on" discharge due to postinhibitory rebound (Gross, Vaughan, & Valenstein, 1967). Now, saccades have also been found to be phase-locked to the alpha cycle (Gaarder, Koresko, & Kropfl, 1966), although the rate of saccadic movement itself seems not to exceed about 3 per sec (measured to within 10' of arc (see Gaarder, 1966, p. 84). Nevertheless, saccades and evoked potentials might have a common generator that is alpha-locked. Future investigation of this point would be desirable, as the rate of polarity alternation in AEP components $N_1$, $P_2$, $N_2$, $P_3$ is usually within the alpha range (see also Mulholland and Evans, 1966; Mulholland and Peper, 1971; Rémond and Lesèvre, 1967; Wertheim, 1974).

But there are two difficulties in attempting to explain the speech-related AEPs as instances of visual postinhibitory rebound: First, the AEPs are most prominent in frontal and central electrodes. Second, rebound would not show hemispheric asymmetry, regardless of how often the eyes moved in each direction.

## PASSIVE SPREAD OF THE CORNEORETINAL POTENTIAL (CRP)

Both of these difficulties are easily handled by the traditional interpretation of all EOG-like waveforms in the EEG or AEP as artifactual "surface fields generated by eye movement," (Peters, 1967) and "distribution of eye movement potentials over the scalp" (Overton & Shagass, 1969). (See also Mowrer, Ruch, & Miller, 1935; Vaughan and Koren, 1975.) Logically pursued, this view leads to more than a haunting doubt that no genuine brain asymmetry has occurred in any of the event-related-potential studies reported in this chapter, since eye-movement patterns can be conceived that would yield EOG asymmetries of types A, B, and C, if they were arranged to occur in phase with the appropriate components ($N_1$ and $P_2$). Simplistic reasoning of this kind has been dubbed *electrophrenology* by McAdam (1973, p. 85). I propose two fundamental axioms:

1. Each chunk of cortex signals its unique electrical

activity directly to the nearest flap of scalp.
2.  Similarities in surface-potential waveforms at
    different loci are due to passive spread.

These axioms entail the postulate that if different surface loci
show the same waveform at different amplitudes, the site of the
largest amplitude locates a generator, and the matching activity
at secondary sites is artifact.  Of course, the axioms and postulate must apply without prejudice both to brain and eye-movement
potentials.  That this line of reasoning leads to problems is
shown by the finding of unchanged secondary activity after removal of a generator located in this way.

Perhaps the most dramatic form of the eye-movement-artifact
hypothesis is Lippold's (1970) claim that the occipital alpha is
a passively spreading waveform, possibly conveyed through ocular
muscles, which is generated by small shifts in orientation of the
eye potential dipole due to tremor of the orbit (see also Lippold
& Shaw, 1971).  Indeed, Barlow (1964) found an occipital-evoked-
potential correlation with the averaged EOG (pp. 451-452).
Lippold's most direct demonstration is the induction of a lateral
asymmetry in the right/left alpha amplitude ratio when the corneo-
retinal potential (CRP) is reduced in the right eye by depriving
it of light (1970).  This experiment, with some changes, was
replicated by Leisman (1974) in both normal and hemiplegic subjects.

A CRP dipole *magnitude* asymmetry is not, of course, an eye-
*movement* asymmetry (see Arden & Kelsey, 1962), but if magnitude
fluctuations do propagate passively along the head, then rotational asymmetries of a constant magnitude CRP dipole would do so
as well.  Also, if the asymmetries appear as far from the eye as
the occiput, they might be expected also at frontal, central,
and parietal sites.  Neither Lippold nor Leisman showed any EOG
records containing lateral tremor at alpha frequencies, nor, as
we have seen, did Gaarder (1966).

But the CRP passive spread alpha hypothesis met no small dis-
aster when normal alpha was found, both frontally and occipitally,
in subjects whose eyes had both been totally removed (Armington
& Chapman, 1959; Chapman, Cavonius, & Ernest, 1971; see also
Abbott & Dymond, 1970).  It was decided to attempt this crucial
test of the CRP hypothesis with respect to the slow potential
shifts of laterally biased eye movement.  Specifically, the following observations were performed to examine the effect of CRP
magnitude on slow frontal potentials.

Two adult male volunteers were recruited, one normal (subject
X), the other a former patient who had recovered from surgery for
enucleation and prosthetic restoration of one eye (subject Y).  A
monocular patient was sought who had normal motion in the prosthetic eye, but since this is rare, it was necessary to select a
man who exhibited the largest lateral range available.  Upon
direct observation, his prosthetic left eye was seen to move in

conjugate fashion with his normal right eye in both directions, but with angular displacements reduced by about 50%.

Electrodes, amplifier settings, and data-processing methods were employed exactly as in the experiment to record frontal AEP and lateral EOG. The subject sat facing a white metal wall at a distance of 1.5 m from the wall. A steel magnetic marker, placed on the wall directly ahead at eye level, served as intertrial fixation point. Another marker was placed 38 cm away, either to the left or right. The subject was instructed to look straight ahead until hearing a tone, at which time he was to shift his eyes promptly to the other marker (an angle of 14°). Fifty trials were run on each of the two marker positions "eyes left" and "eyes right."

Tones (2500 Hz) were presented binaurally at 12 dB above background noise through a stereo headset. Their duration varied between 120 and 150 msec and they occurred pseudorandomly in the same sequence as that employed for the syllable stimuli. On each trial the computer was triggered at tone onset, with sampling delayed to match the Sangamo tape head separation lag. (Although not needed here, the tape lag was retained and compensated for in order to match our original technical procedure.) As before, 1-sec sweeps were digitized every 4 msec and stored on PEC magnetic tape for averaging off-line.

Results for the normal subject (X) are shown in Figure 6.

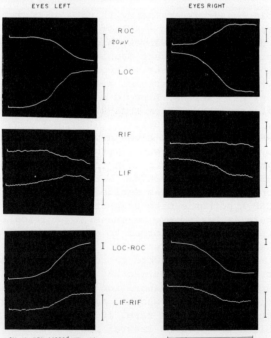

*Figure 6. AEPs and EOGs during tone-cued boluntary eye movement; normal subject (X). Sweep, 1 sec; calibration, 20 μV.*

420

It is seen that left-negative asymmetry occurs in both canthal and frontal electrodes on "eyes right," and right-negative asymmetry in both pairs of electrodes on "eyes left." EOG asymmetry is about eight times greater than frontal, and the two are noticeably conjointly time-locked throughout the record.

In the monocular subject (Y) the absence of a CRP on the left is seen in the EOG, which is normal on the right and essentially nil on the left. However, inferior frontal responses appear equal and opposite (Figure 7). EOG asymmetry is approximately four times greater than the frontal. Interpreting this result as CRP passive spread is anomalous: A large lateral difference in CRP dipole magnitude fails to propagate to produce a corresponding frontal amplitude difference. The anomaly is highlighted by the fact that each frontal electrode *alone* decodes the direction of eye movement, and does so equally in both subjects. It has been suggested that since the EOG on the left in subject Y shows a wave resembling that found at the left frontal, perhaps both electrodes are responding to ipsilateral motor potentials associated with the lateral rectus muscle.

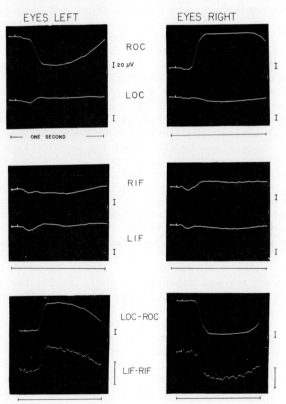

*Fig. 7. AEPs and EOGs during tone-cued voluntary eye movement; monocular subject (Y).*

Although that interpretation cannot be specifically ruled out for this subject, it should be noted that Bizzi (1968) found that the oculomotor EMG did not contain continuous eye position information (pp. 75-76), yet in my experiments there are repeated indications that the frontal evoked potential does. Thus, slowly developing frontal asymmetries, even though they match the pattern of the rotated CRP in the EOG, are apparently not passive followers of the retinal potential. This leaves only the hypothesis of active following, which will be taken up after consideration of one other interpretation found in the literature (see also Kurtzberg & Vaughan, 1970).

## ASYMMETRICAL SLOW POTENTIALS IN BRAIN

McAdam and Whitaker (1971) interpreted their frontal asymmetry result as a difference in *readiness potential* (RP)(Kornblum, 1973; McAdam, 1973; Deeke, Becker, Grozinger, Scheid, & Kornhuber, 1973; Stamm *et al*, this volume) over the speech motor area in comparison with its homologue. The frontal focus and time course are both consistent with this view, since readiness potentials are often observed during a period of about 1 sec prior to voluntary movement and yield appropriately localized amplitude asymmetries when measured over the central fissure during such tasks as squeezing a dynamometer with one hand (Donchin *et al.*, this volume). But if these shifts are speech RPs (and indeed, they *are* speech-anticipatory), then they accompany rather than precede eye movements. Only if frontal asymmetry had preceded the occurrence of lateral gaze deviation by many milliseconds could the AEP-EOG correlation be accounted for by "overflow" of a single RP between speech and oculomotor centers in the left hemisphere. Becker, Hoehne, Iwase, and Kornhuber (1973) reported an RP prior to saccades, finding it larger when the subject was given a pattern-recognition task (p. 101). Presumably it is absent in studies of AEPs and response-related potentials reviewed here because they involve no visual recognition task. In any case, if it is held to be present it does not meet the usual definition of RP.

There are other problems as well. There is no known unique cortical center for eye movement as there is for the spinally innervated motor functions localized along the primary motor strip; eye movement can be produced by stimulating either the frontal eye field or visual cortex (see, e.g., Lindsley, 1952). Inferior frontal electrodes are close enough to both the eye fields and the third frontal convolution so that potentials from either locus can be picked up in the detected surface wave. But the eye fields would be identified as a source, if it were shown that they were differentially activated during laterally biased orbital rotations.

Bizzi (1968) has shown, in the primate frontal eye field, the

422

existence of cells (Group II) that frequency-code horizontal eye position. Group II cells are further implicated in that they do not anticipate eye movement but track the changes in orientation with a negligible latency (see also Bizzi & Evarts, 1971). All that is missing in this explanation is a demonstration that single-unit frequency shifts in Brodmann area 8 due to eye tracking are accompanied by frontally propagating surface shifts. Yet Bizzi's discovery already confirms that the frontal cortex receives neurally coded continuous eye position information. If there were an overflow of verbal RP from speech cortex into the left eye field, it might well result in momentary distortions of the eye orientation code as though the eye had moved; this could lead quickly to an involuntary corrective eye movement or a distortion of the code for the midpoint of eye position, leading to a biased drift. The timing of such distortions, given that they were induced periodically by phonological events originating in the speech cortex, would be expected to coincide, as do the observed eye and brain asymmetries, with the perception of syllables and the speaking of words.

## SUMMARY

After reviewing of speech-event-related potential studies, I reported an experiment in which two groups of normal subjects showing opposite ear preferences for monosyllables in dichotic listening were given a speaking task and a listening task.

On the listening task, all three subjects in the group showing left-ear preference responded at syllabic peak with a brief and rapid eye movement to the left. The three subjects in the right-eared group responded with a slow deflection to the right, which continued throughout the period between the presentation of the syllable and the end of a 1-sec sweep. This slow shift was found in some of the left-eared subjects as well (following the early leftward deflection). On the speaking task, both groups exhibited similar eye-movement patterns; these patterns appeared to differ from movements on a nonspeech control task.

AEPs correlated significantly in amplitude with simultaneously averaged EOGs for each group on both tasks. EOG and frontal electrodes both displayed the greatest asymmetries for the listening task, small asymmetries for the speaking task and negligible asymmetries for the control task.

The interpretation of this relationship between purported speech dominance and eye-movement directionality was discussed in connection with theories of postinhibitory and retinal potential generators; it was tentatively concluded that since the relationship follows the time course of the eye-movement bias accompanying verbal activities, the frontal AEP asymmetry is probably due to distortion of the frontal eye field orientation code during verbal activation.

ACKNOWLEDGMENTS

Research supported by the Department of Mental Hygiene of New
York State, a General Research Support Grant to the Research
Foundation for Mental Hygiene, Inc., and N.I.H. Grant No.
MH-17240.  Acknowledgments are due to the following persons:
William R. Goff and Thomas Fisher of the Veterans Hospital, West
Haven, Conn., for use of their dichotic stimulus tape, and
Merrill Hiscock of the Hospital for Sick Children, Toronto, for
permission to reprint the data in Figure 2.  I am indebted to my
colleagues and co-workers at the New York Psychiatric Institute,
among whom the following deserve special mention:  Paul Redlin,
for assistance in computer programming; Michael Tobin and Benoni
Djoleto for help with instrumentation.  Most of all I would like
to thank Marcel Kinsbourne, W. Crawford Clark, and Samuel Sutton
for their valuable suggestions and comments on the manuscript.

REFERENCES

Abbott, M., & Dymond, A. M.  Alpha rhythm and extraocular muscles.
    *Lancet*, 1970, *II*, 933.
Anderson, S. W., & Jaffe, J.  *The definition, detection and
    timing of vocalic syllables in speech signals*.  Scientific
    Rep. No. *12*, Dept. of Communication Sciences, N. Y. S.
    Psychiatric Institute, 1972.
Anderson, S. W., & Jaffe, J.  *Eye movement bias and ear prefer-
    ence as indices of speech lateralization in brain*.  Scienti-
    fic Rep. No. 15, N. Y. S. Psychiatric Institute, 1973.
Arden, G. B., & Kelsey, J. H.  Changes produced by light in the
    standing potential of the human eye.  *Journal of Physiology*,
    1962, *161*, 189-204.
Armington, J. C., & Chapman, R. M.  Temporal potentials and eye
    movements.  *Electroencephalography and Clinical Neurophysi-
    ology*, 1959, *11*, 346-348.
Barlow, J. S.  Evoked responses in relation to visual perception
    and oculomotor reaction times in man.  In R. Katzman (Ed.),
    *Sensory evoked response in man*.  Annals of the New York
    Academy of Sciences, 1964, *112*, 432-467.
Becker, W., Hoehne, O., Iwase, K., & Kornhuber, H. H.  Cerebral
    and ocular muscle potentials preceding voluntary eye move-
    ments in man.  In W. C. McCallum & J. R. Knott (Eds.),
    Event related slow potentials in brain.  *Electroencephalo-
    graphy & Clinical Neurophysiology*, 1973, Supplement No. 33,
    99-104.
Bizzi, E.  Discharge of frontal eye field neurons during saccadic
    and following movements in unanesthetized monkeys.  *Experi-
    mental Brain Research*, 1968, *6*, 69-80.
Bizzi, E., & Evarts, E. V.  Translational mechanisms between in-
    put and output.  In E. V. Evarts, E. Bizzi, R. E. Burke,

M. DeLong, & W. T. Thach, Jr. (Eds.), Central control of movement. *Neurosciences Research Program Bulletin*, 1971, *9*(1), 31-59.

Chapman, R. M., Cavonius, C. R., & Ernest, J. T. Alpha and kappa electroencephalogram activity in eyeless subjects. *Science*, 1971, *171*, 1159-1161.

Cohn, R. Differential cerebral processing of noise and verbal stimuli. *Science*, 1971, *172*, 599-601.

Day, M. E. An eye-movement indicator of individual differences in the psychological organization of attentional processes and anxiety. *Journal of Psychology*, 1967, *66*, 51-62.

Dee, H. L. Auditory asymmetry and strength of manual preference. *Cortex*, 1971, *7*, 236-245.

Deeke, L., Becker, W., Grozinger, B., Scheid, P., & Kornhuber, H. H. Human brain potentials preceding voluntary limb movements. In W. C. McCallum & J. R. Knott (Eds.), Event related slow potentials in brain. *Electroencephalography and Clinical Neurophysiology*, 1973, Supplement No. 33.

Dirks, D. Perception of dichotic and monaural verbal material and cerebral dominance for speech. *Acta Otolaryngologica*, 1964, *58*, 73-80.

Dorman, M. *Auditory evoked potential correlates of speech perception.* (Doctoral dissertation, Univ. of Connecticut) Ann Arbor, Michigan: University Microfilms, 1971, No. 72-14.

Doyle, J. C., Ornstein, R., & Galin, D. Lateral specialization of cognitive mode: II. EEG frequency analysis. *Psychophysiology*, 1974, *11*, 567-578.

Friedman, D., Simson, R., Ritter, W., & Rapin, I. Cortical evoked potentials elicited by real speech words and human sounds. *Electroencephalography and Clinical Neurophysiology*, 1975, *38*, 13-19.

Gaarder, K. Fine eye movements during inattention. *Nature*, 1966, *209*, 83-84.

Gaarder, K., Koresko, R., & Kropfl, W. The phasic relation of a component of alpha rhythm to fixation saccadic eye movements. *Electroencephalography and Clinical Neurophysiology*, 1966, *21*, 544-551.

Gaarder, K., Krauskopf, J., Graf, V., Kropfl, W., & Armington, J. C. Averaged brain activity following saccadic eye movement. *Science*, 1964, *146*, 1481-1483.

Galambos, R., Benson, P., Smith, T. S., Schulman-Galambos, C., & Osier, H. On hemispheric differences in evoked potentials to speech stimuli. *Electroencephalography and Clinical Neurophysiology*, 1975, *39*, 279-283.

Galin, D., & Ellis, R. R. Asymmetry in evoked potentials as an index of lateralized cognitive processes: Relation to EEG alpha asymmetry. *Neuropsychologia*, 1975, *13*, 45-50.

Galin, D., & Ornstein, R. Lateral specialization of cognitive mode: An EEG study. *Psychophysiology*, 1972, *9*, 412-418.

Galin, D., & Ornstein, R. Individual differences in cognitive style: I. Reflective eye movements. *Neuropsychologia*,

1974, *12*, 367-376.
Girton, D. G., & Kamiya, J.  A simple on line technique for removing eye movement artifact from the EEG. *Electroencephalography and Clinical Neurophysiology,* 1973, *34*, 212-216.
Gross, E. G., Vaughan, H. G., Jr., & Valenstein, E.  Inhibition of visual evoked responses to patterned stimuli during voluntary eye movements. *Electroencephalography and Clinical Neurophysiology,* 1967, *22*, 204-209.
Grözinger, B., Kornhuber, H. H., & Kriebel, J.  Methodological problems in the investigation of cerebral potentials preceding speech. *Neuropsychologia,* 1975, *13*, 263-270.
Haaland, K. Y.  The effect of dichotic, monaural and diotic verbal stimuli on auditory evoked potentials. *Neuropsychologia,* 1974, *12*, 339-345.
Harnad, S. R.  Creativity, lateral saccades and the nondominant hemisphere. *Perceptual and Motor Skills,* 1972, *34*, 653-654.
Harris, A. J.  *The Harris test of lateral dominance.*  (2nd ed.) New York: Psychological Corp., 1955.
Hiscock, M.  Some situational antecedents and dispositional correlates of lateral eye movement direction.  Unpublished doctoral dissertation, Univ. of Texas, 1975.
Jaffe, J., Anderson, S. W., & Rieber, R. W.  Research and clinical approaches to disorders of speech rate. *Journal of Communication Disorders,* 1973, *6*, 225-246.
Jasper, H. H.  The ten-twenty electrode system of the International Federation. *Electroencephalography and Clinical Neurophysiology,* 1958, *10*, 371-375.
Kinsbourne, M.  Eye and head turning indicate cerebral lateralization. *Science,* 1972, *176*, 539-541.
Kocel, K., Galin, D., Ornstein, R., & Merrin, E.  Lateral eye movement and cognitive mode. *Psychonomic Science,* 1972, *27*, 223-224.
Kornblum, S. (Ed.) *Attention and performance IV.*  New York: Academic Press, 1973.
Kurtzberg, D., & Vaughan, H. G., Jr.  Electrocortical potentials associated with eye movement. In V. Zikmund (Ed.), The oculomotor system and brain functions. *Proceedings of the International Colloquium,* Smolenice, October 1970.  Pp. 135-145.
Leisman, G.  The relationship between saccadic eye movements and the alpha rhythm in attentionally handicapped patients. *Neuropsychologia,* 1974, *12*, 209-218.
Lindsley, D. B.  Psychological phenomena and the electroencephalogram. *Electroencephalography and Clinical Neurophysiology,* 1952, *4*, 443-456.
Lippold, O.  Origin of the alpha rhythm. *Nature,* 1970, *226*, 616-618.
Lippold, O. C., & Shaw, J. C.  Alpha rhythm in the blind. *Nature,* 1971, *232*, 134.
Matsumiya, Y., Tagliasco, V., Lombroso, C. T., & Goodglass, H.

Auditory evoked response:  Meaningfulness of stimuli and interhemispheric asymmetry.  *Science*, 1972, *175*, 790-792.

McAdam, D. W.  Physiological mechanisms.  In W. C. McCallum & J. R. Knott (Eds.), Event related slow potentials in brain. *Electroencephalography and Clinical Neurophysiology*, 1973, Supplement No. 33.

McAdam, D. W., & Whitaker, H.  Language production:  Electroencephalographic localization in the normal human brain. *Science*, 1971, *172*, 499-502.

Molfese, D. L.  Cerebral asymmetry in infants, children and adults:  Auditory evoked responses to speech and music stimuli.  Paper presented at the Eighty-fourth Meeting of the Acoustical Society of America, Miami, Florida, December 1972.

Morrell, L. K., & Huntington, D.  Electrocortical localization of language production. *Science*, 1971, *174*, 3159-1360.

Morrell, L. K., & Salamy, J. G.  Hemispheric asymmetry of electrocortical responses to speech stimuli. *Science*, 1971, *174*, 164-166.

Mowrer, O. H., Ruch, T. C., & Miller, N. E.  The corneo-retinal potential difference as the basis of the galvanometric method of recording eye movements. *Psychological Bulletin*, 1935, *32*, 423-428.

Mulholland, T., & Evans, C. R.  Oculomotor function and the alpha activation cycle. *Nature*, 1966, *211*, 1278-1279.

Mulholland, T., & Peper, E.  Occipital alpha and accommodative vergence, pursuit tracking and fast eye movements. *Psychophysiology*, 1971, *8*, 556-575.

Neville, H.  Electrographic correlates of lateral asymmetry in the processing of verbal and nonverbal auditory stimuli. *Journal of Psycholinguistic Research*, 1974, *3*, 151-163.

Overton, D. A., & Shagass, C.  Distribution of eye movement and eyeblink potentials over the scalp. *Electroencephalography and Clinical Neurophysiology*, 1969, *27*, 544-549.

Peters, J. F.  Surface electrical fields generated by eye-movements. *American Journal of EEG Technology*, 1967, *7*, 27-40.

Rémond, A., & Lesèvre, N.  Variations in averaged visual evoked potential as a function of the alpha rhythm phase ("Autostimulation"). *Electroencephalography and Clinical Neurophysiology*, 1967, *26* (Supplement), 42-52.

Robinson, D., & Fuchs, A.  Eye-movements evoked by stimulation of frontal eye fields. *Journal of Neurophysiology*, 1969, *32*, 637-648.

Teitelbaum, H. A.  Spontaneous rhythmic ocular movements. Their possible relationship to mental activity. *Neurology* 1954, *4*, 350-354.

Tueting, P., & Sutton, S.  The relationship between pre-stimulus negative shifts and post-stimulus components of the averaged evoked potential.  In S. Kornblum (Ed.), *Attention and performance IV*. New York: Academic Press, 1973. Pp. 185-205.

Van Mastrigt, R. L. & Sutker, L. W.  Lateral eye movement in response to presentation of dichotic words, and questions differing in degree of rated vividness. *Bulletin of International Neuropsychology Society*, November 1975, p. 7.

Vaughan, H. G., Jr., & Korey, S. R.  The analysis of scalp recorded brain potentials.  In R. F. Thompson & M. M. Patterson (Eds.), *Methods in physiological psychology*.  Vol. 2. *Bioelectric recording technique*.  New York: Academic Press, 1975.  Pp. 157-206.

Wertheim, A. H.  Oculomotor control and occipital alpha activity: A review and a hypothesis. *Acta Psychologica*, 1974, *38*, 235-256.

Wood, C. C., Goff, W. R., & Day, R. S.  Auditory evoked potentials during speech perception. *Science*, 1971, *173*, 1248-1251.

# 22.
# Evoked-Potential Correlates of Hemispheric Lateralization During Semantic Information-Processing

*ROBERT W. THATCHER*
New York Medical College

Many studies have reported hemispheric asymmetries of the averaged evoked potential (AEP) during linguistic information-processing using visual and auditory stimuli (Brown, Marsh, & Smith, 1973; Buchsbaum & Fedio, 1969, 1970; Cohn, 1971; Galin & Ellis, 1975; McAdam & Whitaker, 1971; Morrell & Morrell, 1965; Morrell & Salamy, 1971; Neville, 1974; Teyler, Harrison, Roemer, & Thompson, 1973; Wood, Goff, & Day, 1971). However, AEP hemispheric asymmetries also occur to clicks, blank flashes, and other meaningless stimuli (Beck & Dustman, 1975; Davis & Wada, 1974; Lewis, Dustman, & Beck, 1970), and other studies have failed to observe any asymmetries (Shelburn, 1972; Harmony, Ricardo, Otero, Fernandez, & Valdes, 1973; Friedman, Simson, Ritter, & Rapin, 1975; Galambos, Benson, Smith, Schulman, & Osier, 1975; see also Anderson, this volume; and for a review, Donchin, Kutas, & McCarthy, this volume).

The fact that left-right AEP asymmetries have been observed is indisputable. However, their functional significance is currently poorly understood. For example, AEP component amplitude is generally larger over the right hemisphere than the left (Beck & Dustman, 1975; Cohn, 1971; Davis & Wada, 1974; Lewis *et al.*, 1970; Vella, Butler, & Glass, 1972). However, the presentation of verbal stimuli often results in enhanced AEP amplitude on the left hemisphere in comparison to the right (Buchsbaum & Fedio, 1969, 1970; Morrell & Morrell, 1965; Morrell & Salamy, 1971; Teyler *et al.*, 1973; Wood *et al.*, 1971). No clear explanation for this shift has been offered. Some studies demonstrate

only AEP amplitude asymmetries (Morrell & Morrell, 1965; Morrell
& Salamy, 1971; Teyler et al., 1973), whereas others show asymmetries of the waveform or its components (Brown et al., 1973;
Buchsbaum & Fedio, 1969, 1970; Cohn, 1971). Amplitude asymmetries independent of a change in waveform suggest bilateral and
synchronous information processing. Amplitude differences alone
may only reflect a quantitative and not a qualitative difference
in function between the two hemispheres (cf. Riklan & Cooper,
this volume). Waveform asymmetries, on the other hand, may represent unique or localized processes occurring in one hemisphere.
However, waveform or morphology asymmetries appear to be extremely sensitive to task demands and occur inconsistently across
subjects.


BACKGROUND INFORMATION PROBE (BIP) PARADIGM

There are two broad categories of approach to the study of the
evoked potential (EP). One involves eliciting EPs by presenting
task-irrelevant stimuli in one sense modality while subjects are
processing information in the same or a different sense modality
(Hudspeth & Jones, 1975; Khachaturian & Kluck, 1969; Kitai, Cohen,
& Moren, 1965; Morrell & Morrell, 1965). With this method, EPs
elicited by the irrelevant stimulus reflect baseline neural excitability changes preceding and following information processing. The second approach is to present task-relevant information
in the evoking stimulus itself. This method can reveal EP changes
specific to the feature content of the evoking stimulus. For instance, visual EP experiments have demonstrated AEP changes due
to stimulus intensity (Armington, 1964; Rietveld, 1963), contour
density (Harter & White, 1968, 1970; Karmel, Miller, Dettweiler,
& Anderson, 1970), and spatial frequencies (Campbell & Kulikowski,
1972).
Both approaches offer advantages and disadvantages. Evoked
responses to the information stimuli are often confounded by nonspecific excitability changes, whereas EPs elicited by the irrelevant stimulus do not necessarily reflect the information content of the evoking stimulus.
The Background Information Probe (BIP) paradigm was developed
to incorporate both approaches to EP analysis. Examples of AEP
correlates of hemispheric lateralization using the BIP paradigm
will be presented here. The goal is to describe a general procedure that optimizes on the principles of evoked-potential genesis and experimental design. The complete details of the AEP
phenomena described in this chapter are presented elsewhere
(Thatcher, in press).


Delayed Letter Matching

The procedure involved the presentation of brief (20-msec)

computer-generated displays to human subjects. The displays were usually presented at a repetition frequency of one per sec and, within an experiment, were equated for total luminance and retinal area subtended. An example of a one-trial series of displays in a delayed-letter-matching paradigm is shown in Figure 1.

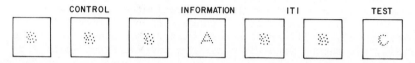

*Fig. 1. Trial sequence of computer-generated displays in a delayed-letter-matching paradigm. The number of control and ITI (intertest interval) displays before and after the first letter (information) was variable. All displays were 20 msec in duration and were presented at a repetition-frequency of 1 Hz. Total luminance and retinal area subtended (1.5°) were the same for all displays.*

This experiment (nine subjects: seven right-handed and two left-handed) involved presenting a variable number (two to six) of random dot displays (pre-letter controls), then a letter (information display)--either A, B, or C--then another series of from two to six random dot displays (intertest interval displays, ITIs), then a second letter that either matched or did not match the first letter. There were 24 trials per session and a 5-sec delay between sessions; the content of the first letter, the number of random dot stimuli, and the match and mismatch conditions were counterbalanced across trials. Subjects were instructed to delay 1 sec and then move a lever to the left when the second letter was a match and to the right when it was a mismatch. The direction of lever movement was counterbalanced across sessions. The procedure is short in duration, requiring about 5 min per session; the subjects cannot predict the exact time of letter presentation and therefore must attend to all stimuli. With this method, AEPs elicited by the random dot displays preceding the first letters can be compared to AEPs elicited by identical displays following the first letters. In addition, identical first and second letters can be compared, as well as matching versus mismatching second letters. In this way, AEPs elicited by identical physical stimuli can be compared before and after information delivery, under conditions in which different cognitive operations are required and when memory is being matched or mismatched.

A number of experiments using this general procedure have been designed to investigate neurolinguistic functioning, including form match-mismatch, cross-modal match-mismatch, word match-mismatch, semantic match-mismatch, and mathematical operations (see Thatcher, 1976).

## Delayed Semantic Matching

The application of the BIP paradigm to semantic information-
processing is shown in Figure 2. As in the delayed-letter-
matching paradigm, two to six random dot displays precede and
follow information presentation. In this experiment there were
36 trials per session. Subjects (*n* = 8, all right-handed) were
tested in at least two sessions (approximately 6 min per
session). In a given session, there were 36 different first
words by only 12 different second words. For one-third of the
trials, the second word was a synonym for the first word; for
one-third of the trials, the two words were antonyms; and for one-
third of the trials, the second word was semantically neutral
with respect to the first word. In this way the group of 12

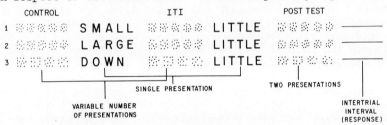

Fig. 2. *Trial sequences and experimental design. Within a
session of trials the total number of illuminated dots and the
average retinal area subtended were the same for all display conditions. Displays were 20 msec in duration and were presented
at 1 Hz.*

physically identical second words occurred in three different
semantic categories. After a delay period (approximately
3 sec), the subjects moved a lever to signal which of the three
semantic relationships occurred on that trial. All conditions,
including the semantic relationships and the number of random dot
displays, were counterbalanced across trials. Direction of lever
movement was counterbalanced across sessions and average luminance and retinal area subtended were equated for all stimuli.

Only one of the subjects participated in both experiments and
no effort was made to select or use experimentally "good" subjects. Recordings in both the delayed-letter-matching experiment
and the delayed-semantic-matching experiment were monopolar.
Linked earlobes were used as a reference and eye movements were
monitored either by using a transorbital eye electrode or the $F_{p_1}$
and $F_{p_2}$ derivations.

RESULTS: DELAYED LETTER MATCHING

An example of AEPs from a subject participating in the
delayed-letter-matching experiment is shown in Figure 3. The

EVOKED-POTENTIAL CORRELATES OF LATERALIZATION

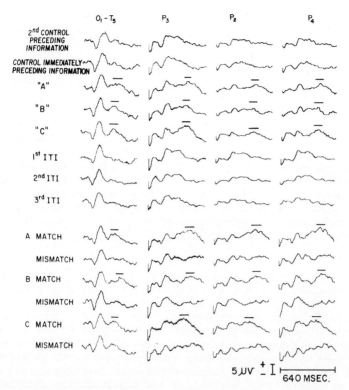

Fig. 3. Examples of AEPs (n = 24 for controls and ITIs; n = 16 for letters) from a subject (J.G.) performing in the letter-matching experiment. Bars denote enhanced positivity to first letters and matching second letters. Positive is up in this and the other figures.

important features are that waveform and amplitude are stable in the control condition and exhibit distinct changes when information is delivered in both the first and second letter position. AEP correlates of letter features and match and mismatch conditions are discussed elsewhere (Thatcher, 1974, 1976; Thatcher & John, 1975). Figure 4 shows examples of AEPs from another subject in the delayed-letter-matching experiment. In this subject (right-handed), hemispheric asymmetries were present to the pre-letter control stimuli and to the ITI stimuli. The asymmetries were most pronounced in temporal derivations ($T_5$ and $T_6$; $T_3$ and $T_4$) to the first letters and the first ITI (see arrows). Note the lateralized persistance of a negative component (320 msec) to the first ITI. Waveform and amplitude changes to the first ITI were observed in eight of the nine subjects. Figure 5 shows an example of temporal lobe AEP asymmetries in the delayed-letter-matching experiment in a left-handed subject (P.E.). Amplitude

433

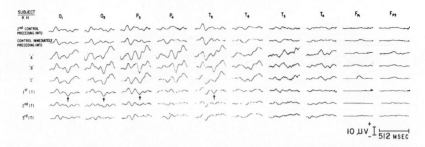

*Fig. 4. Examples of AEPs to controls, first letters, and ITIs*
*(n = 24 for controls and ITIs; n = 16 for letters) for a subject*
*(K.H.) performing in the letter match-mismatch experiment.*
*Arrows point to a persistent negative peak to the first ITI fol-*
*lowing information. Hemispheric asymmetries are evident, par-*
*ticularly in $P_3$ versus $P_4$ and $T_5$ versus $T_6$. Analysis epoch is*
*512 msec.*

and waveform asymmetries were present in both the control and the
letter conditions. In this subject asymmetries were absent in
occipital derivations and only moderately present in parietal and
posterior temporal derivations.

As mentioned previously, there are two types of AEP asymmetry:
(1) amplitude asymmetry, in which overall waveform is the same
(see Figure 4) and (2) waveform component asymmetry in which the
overall amplitude of the AEPs are the same (see Figure 9).
Often, of course, both morphology and amplitude are different
(see Figures 5 and 6) although these two aspects of AEP asymmetry
can be differentiated.

For example, Varimax factor analysis of amplitude normalized
waves (in which the total area of each of a group of AEPs is
equated) can result in waves of different morphology loadong on
orthogonally different factors (see Thatcher & John, 1975 for
methodology and factor interpretation). Table 1 shows an example
from another subject (D.D.) of a within-condition (controls, information, ITI) Varimax factor analysis. In this analysis,
amplitude-normalized AEPs from 12 different derivations were submitted to the Varimax factor analysis in each of five separate
conditions. Because the analyses are independent, the order of
the factors is irrelevant. In the control-2 and control-1 conditions, AEPs from the posterior derivations ($O_1$, $O_2$, $P_3$, $P_4$, $T_5$,
$T_6$) load on one factor while the AEPs from the anterior derivations ($T_3$, $T_4$, $F_7$, $F_8$) load on a different factor. A waveform
asymmetry independent of amplitude is noted in $T_3$ and $T_4$ in which
AEPs from these derivations exhibit different factor structures.
The presentation of the first letter resulted in a marked change
in factor structure in comparison to the controls. In this case,
the anterior-posterior distinction was reduced, with left-side

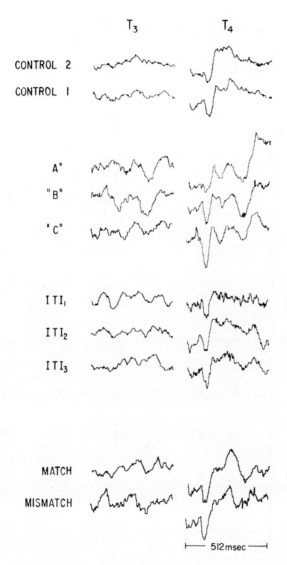

Fig. 5. *Average EPs (n = 24) to control, ITI, and letter stimuli from a left-handed subject (P.E.) performing in the delayed-letter-matching experiment. Both early and late component asymmetries persistently occurred in $T_3$ versus $T_4$ derivations.*

derivations ($P_3$, $T_5$, $T_3$, $F_7$) loading on one factor independent of the anterior-posterior plane. Hemispheric asymmetries are observed in which left- and right-side derivations ($P_3$, $P_4$; $T_5$, $T_6$,

TABLE 1

*Within-Condition Varimax Factor Analysis (Subject D.D.)*

| Factors | Derivations[a] | | | | | | | | | | | |
|---|---|---|---|---|---|---|---|---|---|---|---|---|
| | $O_1$ | $O_2$ | $P_3$ | $P_4$ | $T_5$ | $T_6$ | $T_3$ | $T_4$ | $F_7$ | $F_8$ | eye | $F_z$ |
| | Control-2 | | | | | | | | | | | |
| 1 | .89 | .88 | .65 | .85 | .67 | .46 | .06 | .40 | .06 | .06 | .00 | .06 |
| 2 | .06 | .04 | .15 | .07 | .11 | .05 | .63 | .44 | .91 | .83 | .34 | .67 |
| 3 | .00 | .00 | .00 | .00 | .06 | .03 | .29 | .02 | .00 | .02 | .00 | .10 |
| 4 | .00 | .00 | .01 | .00 | .02 | .06 | .01 | .00 | .00 | .01 | .65 | .01 |
| Total | .95 | .92 | .81 | .92 | .86 | .60 | .99 | .86 | .97 | .92 | .99 | .84 |
| | Control-2 | | | | | | | | | | | |
| 1 | .94 | .92 | .85 | .88 | .73 | .41 | .30 | .13 | .02 | .01 | .00 | .20 |
| 2 | .00 | .00 | .01 | .01 | .04 | .09 | .07 | .71 | .57 | .82 | .09 | .00 |
| 3 | .00 | .00 | .00 | .00 | .00 | .00 | .62 | .00 | .29 | .06 | .02 | .01 |
| 4 | .01 | .00 | .07 | .02 | .00 | .17 | .00 | .01 | .01 | .00 | .08 | .78 |
| Total | .95 | .92 | .93 | .91 | .77 | .67 | .99 | .85 | .89 | .89 | .19 | .99 |
| | First letter | | | | | | | | | | | |
| 1 | .90 | .96 | .42 | .57 | .22 | .17 | .02 | .08 | .01 | .01 | .00 | .11 |
| 2 | .04 | .00 | .35 | .10 | .54 | .18 | .95 | .35 | .90 | .04 | .00 | .28 |
| 3 | .01 | .02 | .00 | .07 | .06 | .10 | .00 | .42 | .04 | .95 | .08 | .17 |
| 4 | .00 | .00 | .15 | .16 | .07 | .52 | .00 | .06 | .00 | .00 | .14 | .32 |
| 5 | .00 | .00 | .00 | .01 | .00 | .00 | .00 | .00 | .00 | .00 | .77 | .00 |
| Total | .95 | .98 | .92 | .91 | .89 | .97 | .97 | .91 | .95 | 1.00 | .99 | .88 |

ITI-2

| | | | | | | | | | | | | |
|---|---|---|---|---|---|---|---|---|---|---|---|---|
| 1 | .84 | .85 | .81 | .96 | .83 | .57 | .77 | .03 | .05 | .10 | .12 | .00 |
| 2 | .00 | .00 | .00 | .00 | .00 | .00 | .00 | .89 | .21 | .68 | .11 | .24 |
| 3 | .03 | .02 | .02 | .00 | .01 | .02 | .07 | .00 | .63 | .00 | .08 | .00 |
| 4 | .04 | .07 | .08 | .00 | .03 | .01 | .03 | .00 | .11 | .00 | .20 | .76 |
| Total | .91 | .94 | .91 | .96 | .87 | .60 | .87 | .92 | 1.00 | .78 | .51 | 1.00 |

Second letter (match)

| | | | | | | | | | | | | |
|---|---|---|---|---|---|---|---|---|---|---|---|---|
| 1 | .59 | .85 | .08 | .36 | .00 | .00 | .03 | .00 | .15 | .01 | .00 | .01 |
| 2 | .32 | .13 | .66 | .25 | .96 | .36 | .71 | .01 | .12 | .00 | .07 | .19 |
| 3 | .00 | .00 | .12 | .14 | .01 | .15 | .11 | .96 | .39 | .93 | .02 | .47 |
| 4 | .00 | .00 | .01 | .09 | .01 | .49 | .05 | .00 | .00 | .00 | .00 | .01 |
| Total | .91 | .98 | .87 | .84 | .98 | .90 | .90 | .97 | .66 | .94 | .09 | .68 |

<sup></sup>

a
Odd numbers left, even numbers right.

Legend Table 1:

Varimax factor analyses on amplitude-normalized AEPs from 12 derivations for each of five conditions in subject D.D. Each row represents the loading of AEPs from different anatomical derivations on a single factor. Each column represents the factor structure for a given derivation. Results show that anterior brain regions $(T_3, T_4, F_7, F_8, F_z)$ load on different factors than do the posterior brain regions $(O_1, O_2, P_3, P_4, T_5, T_6)$. Also, left-right AEP asymmetries can be seen to emerge when information is presented. Underlined numbers represent maximum factor loading for at least 60% of the variance. Except for the eye-movement monitor four factors account for at least 60% of the variance. When five factors are represented then at least 88% of the variance is accounted for. In all cases, however, the waves recorded from the eye-movement monitor loaded strongly on a different factor than the AEPs. See Thatcher and John (1975) for a description of factor-analysis methodology and interpretation of the factors.

437

$T_3$, $T_4$; $F_7$, $F_8$) exhibit different factor structures. Note that $O_1$, $O_2$ derivations fail to exhibit a waveform asymmetry. In this subject the asymmetries persisted to the first ITI display but then slowly decayed to the control condition. Also observe in Table 1 that the waves recorded from the eye-movement monitor load on a different factor than do the AEPs. Generally, the AEP lateralization effects were stronger in the posterior derivations than in the frontal derivations (see Table 2 and Figure 9). This is further evidence that eye-movement potentials are not involved in these effects (cf. Andersen, this volume).

Not all subjects in the delayed-letter-matching experiment showed clear hemispheric asymmetries. In seven of the nine subjects AEP asymmetries were demonstrated by the factor analysis; for five of these subjects these asymmetries were evident to visual inspection of the averaged tracings. The two remaining subjects showed no evidence of AEP asymmetry. Asymmetries were most pronounced when information was presented and occurred most consistently in temporal derivations ($T_5$, $T_6$; $T_3$, $T_4$).

RESULTS: DELAYED SEMANTIC MATCHING

Examples of AEPs elicited from one subject by first words, controls, and synonyms and antonyms are shown in Figure 6. An enhanced late positive component (440 msec to synonyms and 460 msec to antonyms) occurred only to second words (see arrows). Hemispheric asymmetries (see $T_5$ versus $T_6$ and $T_3$ versus $T_4$, in Figure 6B) occurred in the second word condition but not in the first word condition or the control and ITI conditions. These asymmetries were of both the amplitude and component type. Note that the late positive component to second words (which was absent in the other conditions) was widely distributed, appearing even in frontal derivations ($F_7$, $F_8$). AEP differences between the first word condition and the second word condition are explained by the fact that retrieval of the meaning of the first word and a comparison with the meaning of the second word occurred only in the second word condition.

Average evoked potentials elicited during the synonym, antonym, and neutral-word experiment were also submitted to Varimax factor analysis. Figure 7 shows an example from one subject of a Varimax factor analysis of control, ITI, and first- and second-word AEPs. The first row of waves are AEPs from the various conditions of the experiment. The factors are the first column of waves on the left. The factor loadings of each of the four factors on the AEPs are represented by scaling the amplitude of the factors by their appropriate weighting coefficients. It can be seen that the control, ITI, and neutral-word AEPs load on factors 1 and 2. Because of their nonspecificity, factors 1 and 2 are called *nonspecific control factors*. The synonym (S) (factor loading = .49) and antonym (A) (factor loading = .66) AEPs load

TABLE 2

*Proportion of Left versus Right Amplitude Asymmetries of P-4(00)[a]*

| | Occipital ($O_1$ vs. $O_2$) | Parietal ($P_3$ vs. $P_4$) | Posterior temporal ($T_5$ vs. $T_6$) | Anterior temporal ($T_3$ vs. $T_4$) | Frontal ($F_7$ vs. $F_8$) |
|---|---|---|---|---|---|
| Control (1 + 2) | .57 | .39 | .41 | .46 | .43 |
| ITI (1 + 2 + 3) | .72* | .76* | .41 | .44 | .43 |
| Word (second) | 1.00** | .86** | .75* | .52 | .50 |

[a] Each number = $\dfrac{\text{no. L greater than R cases}}{\text{total no. of cases}}$

\*$p < .03$.

\*\*$p < .01$.

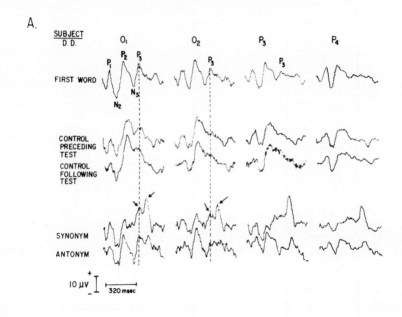

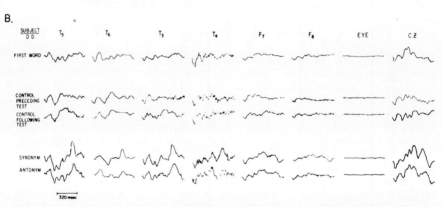

Fig. 6. *Averaged EPs (n = 24 for synonym and antonym; n = 48 for the other conditions) to words and random dot controls in one subject. (A) P-300 in occipital regions (dotted line) to both first and second words. Arrows show the P-400 process to synonyms and antonyms, which is anatomically and temporally differentiable from the P-300. (B) Same as A but showing AEPs from anterior derivations. Note difference between first word and second word responses in $T_5$, $T_6$ and $T_3$, $T_4$. Note also asymmetries in the temporal lobe to second words, which are not present in control or first-word AEPs.*

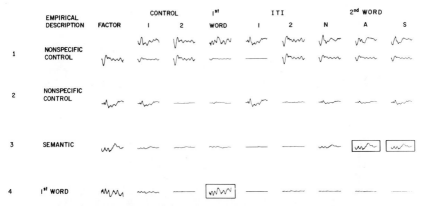

*Fig. 7. Varimax factor analyses of AEPs from P₃, in a subject (L.F.) performing in the synonym, antonym, and neutral-word experiment. AEPs (n = 24), in the top row of waves, are normalized for amplitude. Four orthogonal factors (which account for 87% of the total variance) are in the column of waves on the left. Factor loadings are represented as the factor waveshapes multiplied by the appropriate weighting coefficients. The factors were given empirical descriptions based upon their relative loadings. Note that control and ITI AEPs load on orthogonally different factors than the word AEPs and that synonym (S) and antonym (A) AEPs load on a different factor than the neutral (N) AEP.*

more heavily on factor 3 than the neutral (N) AEP (factor loading = .18). Because of this differential loading, factor 3 is called a *semantic factor*. Factor 4 accounts almost exclusively for the AEP elicited by the first word (factor loading = .89). The results of this Varimax factor analysis further demonstrate that overall AEP waveform, independent of amplitude, can change as a function of the various conditions of the experiment. The results of the factor analysis in Figure 7 are presented primarily to emphasize the utility of applying multivariate statistics to complex data such as that derived from linguistic paradigms. As noted earlier, such methods can help simplify interpretations as well as isolate and quantify AEP changes related to the critical variables of an experiment.

In order to analyze the late positive component, referred to here as the $P$-4(00), the absolute amplitude (in $\mu v$) of the maximum late positive peak between 400 and 500 msec was measured with respect to a prestimulus baseline for each condition and each derivation. This measure has been used in Figure 8, which shows mean $P$-4(00) amplitude to random dot displays and words. A repeated measures analysis of variance demonstrated significant differences between synonym and neutral conditions ($F = 80.7$, $df = 1/146$, $p < .001$), as well as between antonym and neutral

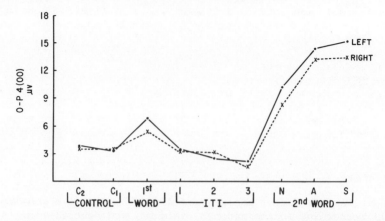

*Fig. 8. Mean baseline to P-4(00) amplitude for left and right electrode sites for the various conditions of the experiment.*

conditions ($F$ = 49.3, $df$ = 1/146; $p$ <.001). No significant differences in mean P-4(00) amplitude were noted between synonyms and antonyms ($F$ = .28; $df$ = 1/146; $p$, not significant). All the second-word conditions were significantly different from the first-word condition ($p$ <.01). Also, the first word P-4(00) was significantly different from the control, $C_1$ ($F$ = 16.7, $df$ = 1/146, $p$ <.001). There were no significant differences between C and ITI ($F$ = 2.8; $df$ = 1/146; $p$, not significant), or between left and right derivations when all leads were averaged ($F$ = 3.45; $df$ = 1/7; $p$, not significant). However, there was a significant side X derivation interaction ($F$ = 2.34, $df$ = 9/63, $p$ <.05). The last finding indicates that hemispheric asymmetries are not uniform across posterior-anterior derivations. This finding justified additional analyses, which showed significant left-right differences ($F$ = 6.57, $df$ = 1/71, $p$ <.05) in posterior derivations ($O_1$ + $P_3$ + $T_5$ versus $O_2$ + $P_4$ + $T_6$) in the second word contition. No significant left-right differences were noted in anterior derivations ($T_3$ + $F_7$ versus $T_4$ + $F_8$) to either the first or second word, nor was a significant difference noted in posterior derivations to the first word alone.

Since several workers have reported only rather small AEP asymmetries, i.e., 1 to 3 $\mu V$ (Buchsbaum & Fedio, 1969; Morrell & Salamy, 1971; Wood et al., 1971), a sign test for the side of greatest late positive component (LPC) amplitude for each subject for control, ITI, and second-word conditions was conducted. Table 2 shows the results of binary sign tests (Hays, 1963), which reveal clear asymmetries in posterior derivations (occipital, parietal, and posterior temporal) during the ITI and first- and second-word conditions (combined) but not during the control. Significant asymmetries always involved left side greater than

right (100% of the subjects exhibited left > right in occipital
derivations in the word condition).  It is interesting that asymmetries are not present to random dot stimuli that precede the
first word but emerge to random dot stimuli that follow the first
word.  This suggests that lateralized operations were active
during the ITI or so-called rehearsal period.

Another example of a relatively localized asymmetry occurring
to second words in a linguistic paradigm is shown in Figure 9.
The subject participated in an experiment similar to the synonym-
antonym experiment illustrated in Figure 2.  However, in this
paradigm, semantic comparisons sometimes required a Spanish to
English or an English to Spanish translation.  That is, the words
*azul, rojo, red,* and *blue* were presented, counterbalanced so that
in one-half of the trials a language translation was required for
the subject to determine whether the second word had a meaning
the same as or different than the first word.  All combinations
of words were presented.  Figure 9 shows that AEPs from the left
posterior temporal derivation ($T_5$) changed only slightly between
the first and second word conditions as compared to the right
homologous derivation ($T_6$) which changed markedly.  The same
words were presented in the first and second word positions, the
difference being that the subject had to make a semantic comparison following the second word presentation.  This figures shows
(see also Figure 6) a relative absence of asymmetries in occipital and frontal derivations, and a gradient of maximal asymmetries in the temporal lobes ($T_5$ versus $T_6$ and $T_3$ versus $T_4$).
The waves from $T_5$ and $T_6$ derivations show a clear example of a
component or waveform asymmetry.  That is, there is an attenuation of a negative component (294 msec) in $T_6$ that occurs only to
the second word.  However, although AEP hemispheric asymmetries
are consistently and reproducibly present in this subject, their
precise significance is currently unknown.


DISCUSSION

The present studies demonstrate asymmetry of AEPs elicited by
linguistic stimuli.  Asymmetries are generally absent to random
dot control stimuli and emerge most clearly to the second words
in the synonym, antonym, neutral comparison paradigm.  These
findings are consistent with those of studies showing AEP asymmetries with visual and auditory stimuli (Buchsbaum & Fedio, 1969,
1970; Morrell & Salamy, 1971; Wood et al., 1971; Davis & Wada,
1974; Lewis et al., 1970; Galin & Ellis, 1975).  Lewis et al.
(1970) and Davis and Wada (1974) demonstrated that AEP asymmetries can occur to nonverbal blank flashes and click and somatic
stimuli.  Thus AEP asymmetries may reflect more general sources
than cognitive information-processing, e.g., anatomical and inherent physiological asymmetries (cf. Rubens, this volume).
Some support for this is provided by the presence of AEP

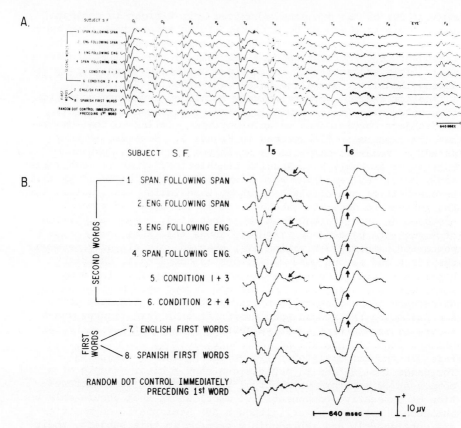

Fig. 9. Averaged evoked potentials (n = 24) from 12 scalp derivations (including a transorbital eye monitor) to random dot control displays and words in a semantic matching task requiring a
language translation. Spanish and English words (rojo, red,
azul, blue) were presented in all combinations. Top six AEPs (in
A and B) represent responses to second words (numbers 1 thru 6).
Conditions 1 and 3 represent responses to second words when no
translation is required. Conditions 2 and 4 represent responses
to second words when they followed words in the other language.
Second and third AEPs from the bottom (numbers 7 and 8) represent responses to first words. Intensity and retinal area (2.2°)
are the same in all conditions (including the control). Note
enhanced hemispheric asymmetries to second words in comparison
to first words (see arrows, $T_6$). B shows $T_5$ and $T_6$ derivations.

asymmetries to random dot stimuli in some subjects. These asymmetries are weak and infrequently seen in comparison to the AEP
asymmetries that occur following the first word and, particularly, the second word in the synonym, antonym, neutral experiment.
This indicates that AEP asymmetries are maximized by engaging

subjects in difficult cognitive tasks (cf. Donchin *et al.*, this volume).

It is currently difficult to assess the precise meaning of the laterality results observed in these studies. For example, it is unclear whether the AEP asymmetries to second words are due to lateralization of verbal functions or to lateralization of comparison operations such as required in the delayed matching paradigm. This question is currently under study in linguistic and nonlinguistic delayed matching experiments. The idea underlying the latter experiments is to maintain the general operation of comparison while varying the linguistic versus nonlinguistic content of those comparisons.

The latter experiments are designed to explore the possibility that AEP correlates of hemispheric lateralization reflect localization of a general cognitive operation, for example, a comparison operation or a symbolic match-mismatch operation, and not linguistic function per se. According to the latter view, the content of a comparison (linguistic material versus nonlinguistic material) does not uniquely determine AEP laterality. Preliminary results from delayed-form-matching experiments, in which no verbal labels are involved, have demonstrated left-hemisphere AEP enhancement in occipital and parietal derivations and not in temporal derivations. In the latter experiments, the relative absence of asymmetries in temporal derivations indicates that the anterior-posterior location of the asymmetry may reflect the stage or level of serial information-processing at which symbolic or representational comparisons occur.

SUMMARY

I have presented the results of a series of experiments that involved computer-generated displays, very specific information loading, and the simultaneous recording of evoked potentials from a relatively large number of scalp electrodes in humans. These experiments involved presenting two delayed information displays that were embedded within a series of random dot displays. All the displays were equated for average size and luminance, and the exact time of presentation and the exact content of the information displays were unpredictable. One experiment used a delayed-letter-matching procedure, another experiment used a delayed-semantic-matching procedure involving synonym, antonym, and neutral-word paris. These experiments demonstrated that physically identical stimuli elicit different evoked responses depending on whether they match or mismatch the first information stimulus. Evoked potential hemispheric asymmetries were observed to occur most strongly to the second information stimulus in the delayed information pair. Hemispheric evoked potential asymmetries were also observed to occur to the random dot displays that immediately followed the first information stimulus. These asym-

metries were interpreted as possible correlates of a rehearsal
process. Factor analyses of amplitude-normalized evoked potentials demonstrated waveshape asymmetries, which occurred independent of amplitude asymmetries. These asymmetries were maximal in posterior regions of the brain (occipital, parietal, and
posterior temporal) and were shown not to involve lateralized
eye movements. The precise meaning or significance of the asymmetries in terms of language processing is currently unknown.
The major purpose in presenting the data was to emphasize methodological and data-analysis procedures and to show that language
information-processing is correlated to evoked potential hemispheric asymmetries.


ACKNOWLEDGMENTS

I would like to thank Kim Hopper, Alice Adelson, Marie
Cordova, and Eileen Maisal for helping in the collection of the
data and the data analysis. Thanks are also due to Dr. Bernard
Karmel for help with statistics and Dr. E. Roy John for his
support and advice.


REFERENCES

Armington, J. C. Relations between electroretinograms and occipi-
    tal potentials elicited by flickering stimuli. *Documenta
    Ophthalmologica*, 1964, *18*, 194-206.
Beck, E. C., & Dustman, R. E. Changes in evoked responses during
    maturation and aging in man and Macaque. In N. Burch &
    H. I. Altshuler (Eds.), *Behavior and brain electrical
    activity*. New York: Plenum Press, 1975. Pp. 431-472.
Brown, W. S., Marsh, J. T., & Smith, J. C. Contextual meaning
    effects on speech evoked potentials. *Behavioral Biology*,
    1973, *9*, 755-761.
Buchsbaum, M., & Fedio, P. Visual information and evoked re-
    sponses from the left and right hemisphere. *Electroence-
    phalography and Clinical Neurophysiology*, 1969, *36*, 266-272.
Buchsbaum, M., & Fedio, P. Hemispheric differences in evoked
    potentials to verbal and nonverbal stimuli in the left and
    right visual fields. *Physiology and Behavior*, 1970, *5*,
    207-210.
Campbell, F. W., & Kulikowski, J. J. The visual evoked potential
    as a function of contrast of a grating pattern. *Journal of
    Physiology*, 1972, *222*, 345-356.
Chapman, R. M. Evoked potentials of the brain related to think-
    ing. In F. J. McGuigan & R. A. Schoonover (Eds.), *The
    psychophysiology of thinking: Studies of covert processes*.
    New York: Academic Press, 1973. Pp. 69-108.
Chapman, R. M., Bragdon, H. R., Chapman, J. A., & McCrary, J. W.

Semantic meaning of words and average evoked potentials. In J. E. Desmedt (Ed.), *Recent developments in the psychobiology of language: The cerebral evoked potential approach.* London: Oxford Univ. Press, 1976.

Cohn, R. Differential cerebral processing of noise and verbal stimuli. *Science,* 1971, *172,* 599-601.

Cooper, R., Winter, A. L., Crow, H. J., & Walter, W. G. Comparison of subcortical, cortical and scalp activity using chronically indwelling electrodes in man. *Electroencephalography and Clinical Neurophysiology,* 1965, *18,* 217-228.

Davis, A. E., & Wada, J. A. Hemispheric asymmetry: Frequency analysis of visual and auditory evoked responses to nonverbal stimuli. *Electroencephalography and Clinical Neurophysiology,* 1974, *37,* 1-9.

Friedman, D., Simson, R., Ritter, W., & Rapin, I. The late positive component (P-300) and information processing in sentences. *Electroencephalography and Clinical Neurophysiology,* 1975, *38,* 255-262.

Galambos, R., Benson, P., Smith, T. S., Schulman-Galambos, C., & Osier, H. On hemispheric differences in evoked potentials to speech stimuli. *Electroencephalography and Clinical Neurophysiology,* 1975, *39,* 279-283.

Galin, D., & Ellis, R. R. Asymmetry in evoked potentials as an index of lateralized cognitive processes: Relation to EEG alpha asymmetry. *Neuropsychologia,* 1975, *13,* 45-50.

Harmony, J., Ricardo, G., Otero, Fernandez, S., & Valdes, P. Symmetry of the visual evoked potential in normal subjects. *Electroencephalography and Clinical Neurophysiology,* 1973, *35,* 237-240.

Harter, M. R., & White, C. T. Effects of contour sharpness and check-size on visually evoked cortical potentials. *Vision Research,* 1968, *8,* 701-711.

Harter, M. R., & White, C. T. Evoked cortical responses to checkerboard patterns: Effect of check-size as a function of visual acuity. *Electroencephalography and Clinical Neurophysiology,* 1970, *28,* 48-54.

Hays, W. L. *Statistics for psychologists.* New York: Holt, 1963.

Hudspeth, W. J., & Jones, G. B. Stability of neural interference patterns. In P. Greguss (Ed.), *Holography in medicine: Proceedings of the International Symposium on Holography in Biomedical Sciences.* London: IPC Science and Technology Press, 1975.

Karmel, B. Z., Miller, P. N., Dettweiler, L., & Anderson, G. Texture density and normal development of visual depth avoidance. *Developmental Psychobiology,* 1970, *3,* 73-90.

Khachaturian, Z. S., & Gluch, H. The effects of arousal on the amplitude of evoked potentials. *Brain Research,* 1969, 589-606.

Kitai, S. T., Cohen, B., & Morin, F. Changes in the amplitude of photically evoked potentials by a conditioned stimulus.

*Electroencephalography and Clinical Neurophysiology,* 1965, *19,* 344-349.

Lewis, E. G., Dustman, R. E., & Beck, E. C. The effects of alcohol on visual and somato-sensory evoked responses. *Electroencephalography and Clinical Neurophysiology,* 1970, *28,* 202-205.

McAdam, D. W., & Whitaker, H. A. Language production: Electroencephalographic localization in the normal human brain. *Science,* 1971, *172,* 499-502.

Morrell, F. & Morrell, L. Computer aided analysis of brain electrical activity. In L. D. Proctor & W. R. Adey (Eds.), *The analysis of central nervous system and cardiovascular data using computer methods.* Washington, D.C.: NASA, U.S. Government Printing Office, 1965. Pp. 441-478.

Morrell, L. K., & Salamy, J. G. Hemispheric asymmetry of electrocortical response to speech stimuli. *Science,* 1971, *174,* 164-166.

Neville, H. Electrographic correlates of lateral asymmetry in the processing of verbal and nonverbal auditory atimuli. *Journal of Psycholinguistic Research,* 1974, *3,* 151-163.

Rietveld, W. J. The occipitocortical response to light flashes in man. *Acta Physiologica et Pharmacologica Neerlandica,* 1963, *12,* 373-407.

Shelburne, S. A. Jr. Visual evoked responses to word and nonsense syllable stimuli. *Electroencephalography and Clinical Neurophysiology,* 1972, *32,* 17-25.

Teyler, T., Harrison, T., Roemer, R., & Thompson, R. Human scalp recorded evoked potential correlates of linguistic stimuli. *Journal of the Psychonomic Society Bulletin,* 1973, *1,* 333-334.

Thatcher, R. W. Evoked potential correlates of human short-term memory. *Annual Neurosciences Convention,* 1974, 450 (abstract).

Thatcher, R. W. Electrophysiological correlates of animal and human memory. In R. D. Terry & S. Gershon (Eds.), *The neurobiology of aging.* New York: Raven Press, 1976. Pp. 42-102.

Thatcher, R. W., & John, E. R. Information and mathematical quantification of brain states. In N. Burch & H. L. Altschuler (Eds.), *Behavior and brain electrical activity.* New York: Plenum, 1975. Pp. 303-324.

Thatcher, R. W. Evoked potential correlates of delayed letter matching. *Behavioral Biology* (in press).

Vella, E. J., Butler, S. R., & Glass, A. Electrical correlates of right hemisphere function. *Nature* (Lond.), 1972, *236,* 125-126.

Wood, C. C., Goff, W. R., & Day, R. S. Auditory evoked potentials during speech perception. *Science,* 1971, *173,* 1248-1251.

# Part VII

# SURFACE ELECTROCORTICAL INDICATORS OF LATERALIZATION II:

# EEG

# 23.
# Interhemispheric EEG Laterality Relationships Following Psychoactive Agents and During Operant Performance in Rabbits

*JUDITH M. NELSON, RUTH PHILLIPS, AND LEONIDE GOLDSTEIN*

College of Medicine and Dentistry of New Jersey and Rutgers Medical School

Differences in patterns of hemispheric electrical activity in man under certain behavioral conditions have been interpreted as being due to lateral specialization of cognitive mode (Galin & Ornstein, 1972; Donchin, Kutas, & McCarthy; Gardiner & Walter; Thatcher, this volume). Although the opinion has been widely held that there is no functional lateralization in nonhuman species, evidence of the existence of cerebral asymmetries in lower mammals is growing (Goldstein, Stoltzfus, & Gardocki, 1972; Dewson; Glick, Jerussi, & Zimmerberg; Webster, this volume). We will describe recent investigations of functional laterality in rabbits as indicated by electroencephalographic (EEG) activity. Specifically, shifts in hemispheric electrocorticographic relationships that accompany spontaneous and drug-induced changes in arousal states, as well as shifts accompanying changes in behavioral states during performance of an operant task, will be examined.

GENERAL METHODS

Subjects

All experiments were performed on adult male New Zealand rabbits weighing 3-4 kg. Four gold-plated, self-tapping screws (3.0 mm in length of threaded shaft; 1.25 mm in diameter at widest point of shaft) served as electrodes. They were inserted in the cranium 5 mm anterior and posterior to the coronal suture and 5 mm lateral to the sagittal suture, and were thus positioned over the anterior and posterior parietal cortices. A fifth screw, inserted in the nasal bone, served as the ground electrode. Leads from the screw-electrodes were soldered to a female Winchester multisocket connector, which was fixed permanently to the skull with polyacrylic dental cement.

## EEG Recording and Analysis

Electrical activity was recorded in the bipolar mode utilizing the pair of electrodes over the left and right hemispheres, respectively, with a Beckman Dynograph, Model RP. The nominal lower and upper cutoff values for the EEG frequency band analyzed were 1.6 Hz and 32 Hz. EEG analysis and quantification were performed using amplitude integration techniques. (See Goldstein and Beck, 1965.) The EEG signals were analyzed on-line by solid state analog-to-digital integrators that performed continuous full-wave rectification and integration of the resulting waveforms. The integrators operated such that whenever a predetermined voltage (proportional to an area subtended by the EEG waves) was reached, a pulse was produced. The pulses from the integrator were automatically accumulated and printed out as a digital value on a paper tape every 5 sec or every 15 sec, depending on the particular study. These quantified data were used to produce time-effect curves representing the ongoing electrical activity on either side of the brain and to develop indices of the interhemispheric relationships.

## LEFT-RIGHT ASYMMETRIES IN EEG AMPLITUDES ACCOMPANYING CHANGES IN STATE OF CONSCIOUSNESS

Much of the recent work described herein grew out of the findings of Goldstein et al. (1972), who examined EEG amplitude characteristics during sleep. They reported well-defined shifts in the relationship of the EEG amplitudes from the two hemispheres (parietal areas) during REM and non-REM sleep periods not only in man, but also in the cat and the rabbit. Illustrated in Figure 1 are the amplitude patterns of brain electrical activity during sleep, including both REM and non-REM periods, and the deviation of the amplitude ratio of left and right EEG activity (for each successive 2-min epoch) from the overall mean left over right amplitude ratio for the total recording period. The results of this study indicated that shifts from REM to non-REM sleep (and vice versa) are accompanied by consistent, though small, changes in the relationship between left and right EEG activity. Hence, it could be concluded that two states of consciousness (REM and non-REM sleep states) are characterized by and can be differentiated by their interhemispheric patterns of electrical activity. These findings have been confirmed by

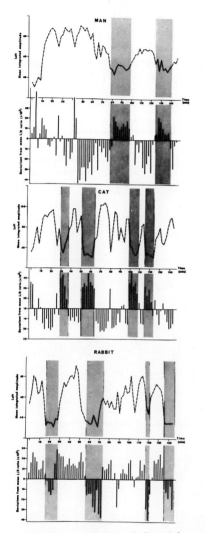

Fig. 1. Sample plots of the
mean integrated amplitudes and
interhemispheric amplitude relationships versus time, during
sleep in the three species
studied. For each species, the
successive levels of the EEG
amplitudes (in terms of arbitrary units) from the left hemisphere are represented by the
broken lines. The deviations
of the successive ratios of
amplitudes from the left (L) and
right (R) hemispheres from the
overall mean L/R ratio (x $10^3$)
for the whole period of recording are represented by the solid
bars (positive deviations up and
negative deviations down). The
shaded areas correspond to REM
episodes and the nonshaded areas
to slow-wave sleep. Redrawn
from data presented by
Goldstein, Stoltzfus, &
Gardocki, 1972.

Webster as reported in this volume.
    In a new series of studies of brain electrical activity in the
rabbit, we have found that the relationship between left and
right amplitudes during a baseline state of wakefulness is stable
and reproducible across sessions for an individual animal. In
other words, there is a characteristic left to right amplitude
relationship for an individual when in the waking state. It
should be noted that the behavior of the rabbits was continuously
observed and recorded during all experimental sessions. Behavioral indices of states of consciousness were compared and
correlated with the electroencephalographic recordings. Sleep
was differentiated from wakefulness behaviorally on the basis of
the presence of postural changes (muscle relaxation), ear droop,

ptosis, and respiratory rate. The EEG concomitants of arousal
levels in rabbits have been well described (cf. Longo, 1962).
To summarize briefly, the waking, aroused, or activated state is
characterized by a predominance of low-amplitude, high-frequency
brain waves (LVF); the sleeping state is characterized by high-
amplitude, low-frequency waves (HVS). The latter description
refers to slow-wave sleep. Because of specific experimental conditions, REM sleep was not manifested in these experiments.
Thus, there were both behavioral and EEG criteria for assessing
the relative state of alertness of the subjects in these studies.

Illustrated in the left half of Figure 2 is the integrated
amplitude of EEG activity from the left and the right hemisphere
during a 46-min control recording session. The rabbit was awake

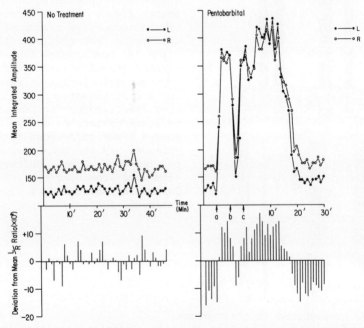

*Fig. 2. Mean integrated amplitudes from the left and right hemi-
spheres and the interhemispheric amplitude relationships versus
time, for two recording sessions with a rabbit whose right
amplitudes were consistently higher than left during normal wakefulness. Throughout the no-treatment session shown on the left,
the rabbit was awake. Hemispheric activity patterns after sodium pentobarbital-induced (total of 8 mg/kg) sleep are shown on
the right with a on the time axis indicating a 4-mg/kg injection
of pentobarbital; b, an injection of saline; and c, a second injection of 4-mg/kg pentobarbital, all given via a catheter inserted in a marginal ear vein.*

throughout the session and, as indicated, the amplitude levels of left ($L$) and right ($R$) hemisphere activity represented in terms of integration units varied within a rather limited range (mean $\pm$ SD: 127.52 $\pm$ 7.34 for left and 167.52 $\pm$ 9.32 for right). As has been generally found, the successive left- and right-amplitude values were significantly correlated with each other ($r$ = .673, $p$ <.001). In the serial recordings collected from this rabbit for a period of more than a year, a characteristic baseline left-right amplitude relationship (right amplitude being higher than left in this subject) was always exhibited during normal, control states of wakefulness. The deviations of the $L/R$ ratio for successive minutes from the overall mean $L/R$ ratio appeared to be distributed unsystematically in positive and negative directions. The "one-sample runs test" (Siegel, 1956, pp. 52 ff.) confirmed that the distribution was not significantly different from a random one. However, during sleep (HVS) states (either spontaneous or pentobarbital-induced), the left-right relationship underwent a marked alteration. As shown on the right half of Figure 2, sedation produced by pentobarbital resulted in the expected increase in amplitude (HVS), but also in a decrease in the relative difference between left and right amplitudes. In fact, during periods of peak sedation, the amplitude laterality relationship was reversed with the left amplitude becoming higher than the right. The phenomenon is well illustrated by the pattern of successive deviations from the mean left over right ratio represented in the lower right of Figure 2. The periods of relative arousal (wakefulness during the preinjection period and from Minute 18 on, after the sedative effect was dissipated) were characterized by negative deviations and the periods of sedation by positive deviations reflecting the relatively greater increase in the left amplitude compared to the increase on the right during sedation.

Some animals were found to have a baseline hemispheric amplitude relationship opposite to the one just described (i.e., left amplitude higher than the right during wakefulness) as was the case for the rabbit whose data are represented in Figure 3. The animal exhibited two periods of deep, spontaneous sleep during the control recording session, the results of which are illustrated on the left of the figure. During wakefulness, left amplitudes were greater than right, but during the peak periods of HVS activity (sleep), the absolute amplitude on the right was greater than that on the left. The pattern of successive deviations from the mean left over right ratio clearly showed the characteristic laterality relationships manifested by this animal during two states of consciousness: The deviations were positive during wakefulness and negative during sedation, indicating a reversal of amplitude relationships when the animal went from wakefulness to sleep. The same pattern was obtained when sedation was induced by intravenous administration of sodium pentobarbital (Figure 3). The period of sedation was marked by a relative shift

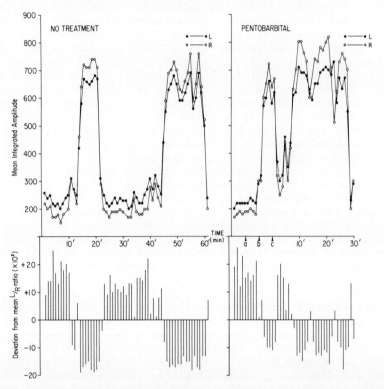

*Fig. 3. Mean integrated amplitudes from the left and right hemi-spheres and the interhemispheric amplitude relationships versus time, for two recording sessions with a rabbit whose left ampli-tudes were higher than right during normal wakefulness. During the no-treatment session shown on the left, two periods of spon-taneous slow-wave sleep occurred. These can be compared with the pentobarbital-induced sleep represented on the right. The treat-ment was the same as that described for Figure 2.*

(and, in fact, an absolute shift during peak sedation) toward higher amplitudes on the right, again the reversal of the rela-tionship holding during wakefulness.

This reversal of laterality relationships was not the case for every rabbit in terms of *absolute* amplitude values. However, of 11 rabbits examined extensively, 10 consistently showed the same pattern illustrated by the two preceding examples: When the amplitude relationships are expressed in terms of successive de-viations from the mean left over right ratio for the session, the polarity of the deviations during sedation is the opposite of that which holds during the waking state. The sole rabbit whose EEG responses did not conform to the pattern described was considered an unreliable subject before data analysis was performed: It exhibited behavioral and physiological signs of sustained hyperarousal extending over a period of months, and it failed to adapt to experimental procedures.

The results of studies with the 10 rabbits just described indicate that the side of the brain that has the lower amplitude during normal wakefulness undergoes the more marked change (increase in amplitude) when the arousal state shifts from wakefulness to HVS sleep either spontaneously or as a result of pentobarbital administration. It has been suggested that more activated central and behavioral states are accompanied by EEG waves of low amplitude, e.g., the EEG patterns have been described as *desynchronization* (Adrian & Matthews, 1934), *activation* (Rheinberger & Jasper, 1937), and *arousal* (Moruzzi & Magoun, 1949; see also Heilman & Watson, this volume). If the hemisphere with the lower integrated amplitude is the more activated (and, for the moment, is designated the *dominant* hemisphere in the rabbit), then a link between these findings and certain clinical findings suggests itself. Clinical investigations of the effects of intracarotid administration of sodium amobarbital have been suggestive of a hemisphere dominance for the control of consciousness in man (Serafetinides, Driver, & Hoare, 1965a; Serafetinides, Hoare, & Driver, 1965b; Hommes & Panhuysen, 1970). Differential effects on consciousness (duration of loss, and consistency of occurrence of loss of consciousness) were observed when the barbiturate was administered unilaterally on one side or the other. These effects were interpreted as indicating that the control of consciousness is linked primarily to the hemisphere that is dominant for speech. Serafetinides *et al.* (1965b, pp. 128-129) have suggested that parallel studies should be done in "animal subjects where no cerebral dominance is believed to exist. . .". Lack of differences in responsivity would support the argument for lack of lateral specialization but "consistent differences between the two sides in terms of responsiveness should throw new light on what we know about cerebral organization in the absence of speech." The results from the studies with the rabbit are not inconsistent with a concept of selective hemispheric contributions to the maintenance of consciousness. However, at this point, they can be considered only suggestive of the existence of a phenomenon in rabbits that reflects some parallels to that found in man. However, the data do give clear evidence that differential lateral asymmetries of cortical activity accompany various states of consciousness, i.e., normal wakefulness, REM sleep, and non-REM (HVS) sleep.

## PATTERNS OF HEMISPHERIC EEG AMPLITUDES DURING OPERANT TASK PERFORMANCE

The systematic differences in hemispheric amplitude asymmetries found to accompany widely divergent arousal states prompted the initiation of an examination of laterality relationships within a more confined range of the arousal spectrum. It was hypothesized that the central arousal state of an animal performing on a behavioral task would vary depending on the stimulus and reinforcement contingencies of the task and that amplitude asymmetries might reflect shifts within the waking state.

Rabbits were trained to perform a simple discrimination task. The experimental chamber (Figure 4) was designed to provide a bilaterally symmetrical environment. The manipulandum (a disk

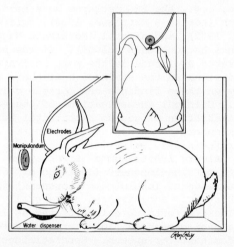

*Fig. 4. A representation of the experimental chamber used for the water-reinforced discrimination task.*

attached to an omnidirectional lever) was fixed at the horizontal midpoint of the front panel of the chamber as was the receptacle into which the reinforcement was delivered. Both were positioned to allow the (symmetrical) operant response (a nose press) and the consummatory behavior (drinking) to be executed by the subject with minimal movement. Rabbits were deprived of water and then trained to press the disk for water reinforcement in the presence of a continuous buzzer sound. The use of water as the reward greatly reduced the consummatory artifact generated in the EEG recordings, which has been a confounding factor in previous studies of EEG correlates of behavioral performance in the rabbit (Sadowski & Longo, 1962; McGaugh, de Baran, & Longo,1963; Baran & Longo, 1964). Following initial training, the schedule was modified so that 30-sec periods with the buzzer sounding were alternated with 30-sec periods with the buzzer silenced. Only presses made while the buzzer sounded were reinforced. Rabbits were trained in daily sessions until they had learned the discrimination. Session lengths were controlled by the individual subject: The rabbit was allowed to continue working for water

(*performance phase*) until it became satiated, but EEG recording
was extended for at least 15 min after the rabbit had ceased
responding (*satiation phase*).

We have collected data from eight rabbits that underwent extensive training for this task. The results indicate different
states of electrocortical activity when an animal is making reinforced responses as opposed to periods when responses are not
reinforced or during satiation. Figure 5 illustrates the EEG and
behavioral results from a test session. The rabbit pressed consistently at a high rate during the buzzer-on periods relative to
the rate during the buzzer-off periods. Mean number of reinforced presses per 30-sec period during the performance phase was
19.65; mean number of nonreinforced presses during the same
phase of the session was 2.33. Visual inspection did not reveal
obvious differences in mean integrated amplitude $[(L+R)/2]$ between buzzer-on and buzzer-off periods. In the performance
phase, the mean amplitude level was slightly but significantly
higher (3.48 units, $t = 5.16$, $df = 59$) during buzzer-on periods
than during silent periods. In the satiation phase, amplitudes
during buzzer-on and buzzer-off periods did not differ significantly. However, when the amplitude relationships between the
two hemispheres were considered by means of the transformation of
the data to successive deviations from the overall mean $L/R$
amplitude for the total session, differences in patterns of brain
electrical activity during the various periods of the session
were revealed. A systematic pattern of positive deviations ($L/R$
ratios higher than the overall mean $L/R$ ratio for the entire
session) emerged during the performance phase when responses were
reinforced. In comparison, during the nonreinforced periods
(buzzer-off) of the performance phase, the distribution of positive and negative deviations was unsystematic. "One-sample runs
tests" (Siegel, 1956, pp. 52 ff.) confirmed that the pattern of
positive deviations during reinforced performance was not random
(2 $p = .008$) and that the corresponding distribution during nonreinforced periods was not significantly different from a random
one. The deviations during the satiation phase tended to be in
the negative direction (statistically significant according to
the one-sample runs test for the buzzer-on period).

The pattern of the EEG interhemispheric amplitude relationships for this animal during a separate recording session is
shown as an inset in the right portion of Figure 5. This was a
session during which EEG recordings were taken while the animal
was in an alert, waking state, but no behavioral performance was
required and no manipulandum, buzzer sounds, or reinforcements
were presented. It should be noted that this pattern of left-
right relationships was random, as was that exhibited during the
nonreinforced periods of the behavioral performance phase.

Just as in the previously described studies of background EEG
in the absence of any task, during behavioral sessions some individuals characteristically exhibited shifts in the directionality

JUDITH M. NELSON *et al.*

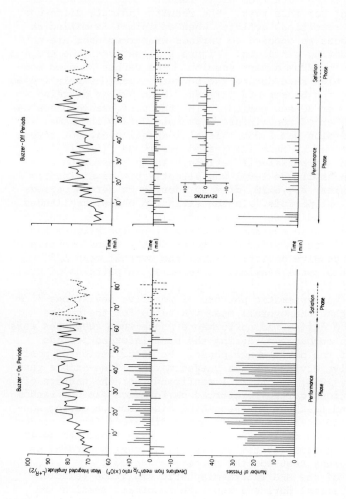

*Fig. 5. Patterns of integrated EEG activity* [(L+R)/2], *interhemispheric amplitude relationships (deviations from the mean L/R ratio) and operant responding (lever presses) from one session with a rabbit well trained on the instrumental reward discrimination task. During the first 30 sec of each minute, the buzzer sounded and presses were reinforced; during the second 30 sec, the buzzer was silent and presses were not reinforced. Thus, successive data points under the "Buzzer-on Periods" heading represent, respectively, amplitude, deviations, and reinforced presses for alternate 30-sec periods. Data from the intervening 30-sec periods (when presses were not reinforced) are shown under the "Buzzer-off Periods" heading. The inset on the right shows the successive deviations from*

460

of the deviations from the mean $L/R$ ratio which were the reverse
of those in the preceding example. Nevertheless, the general
pattern of the relationships held: Deviations were primarily in
one direction during reinforced periods of performance phases, in
the opposite direction during satiation, and distributed randomly
in either direction during the buzzer-off (nonreinforced) periods
of the performance phase.

Administration of psychoactive drugs can alter EEG amplitude
relationships as well as behavior; however, even when the conscious state and behavior of an animal were temporarily modified
by administration of a psychoactive drug, the general pattern of
relationships between amplitude asymmetries and task performance
tended to be maintained. That is, with the recovery of discriminative performance following any drug-induced disruption, the
pattern of amplitude laterality relationships observed during
normal, non-drug-altered test sessions was reestablished. This
was the case whether the drug was amphetamine, which altered the
lateral asymmetries in one direction, or pentobarbital, which
altered the hemispheric asymmetries in the opposite direction
during the initial disruption of discriminated performance.

The phenomenon is illustrated in Figure 6 for a rabbit that in
nondrug, control test sessions exhibited an amplitude laterality

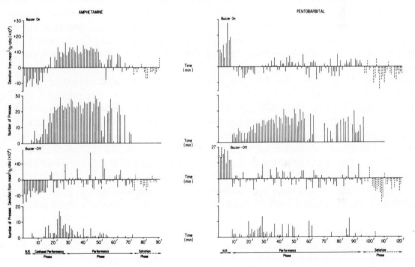

*Fig. 6. Patterns of integrated EEG activity, interhemispheric
amplitude relationships and operant responding on the instrumental reward discrimination tasks. Shown on the left are the patterns following administration of* d-*amphetamine sulfate (1.5
mg/kg, i.v.) and on the right, the patterns following sodium pentobarbital (6 mg/kg, i.v.). The "N.R." notation indicates the
phase of behavioral silence (no operant responses) following drug
administration.*

pattern of positive deviations from the mean $L/R$ amplitude ratio during the reinforced performance phase, negative deviations during satiation, and positive and negative deviations distributed unsystematically during the nonreinforced performance phase. Represented in the left portion of the figure are the interhemispheric amplitude relationships and patterns of operant responding from the rabbit after intravenous administration of $d$-amphetamine sulfate (1.5 mg/kg). The initial response to amphetamine was a block of operant responding followed by a period of confused or nondiscriminating behavior. However, about 28 min after injection, discriminated performance was established. From this point in the session, the relationships between the hemisphere asymmetries and behavioral conditions corresponded to those identified in nondrug, control sessions. The response to sodium pentobarbital (6 mg/kg, intravenous) was similarly characterized by an initial block of responding followed by confused, nondiscriminating responding until about 29 min after administration of the drug (Figure 6, right side). After that time, performance stabilized somewhat, but was more variable and marked by more inappropriate responding than the amphetamine session, indicating a more sustained period of confusion with pentobarbital.

With regard to the correspondence of the amplitude asymmetries with the behavioral conditions, pentobarbital produced very high $L/R$ amplitude ratios (those accompanying the initial behavioral silence) whose contributions to the mean $L/R$ ratio tended to dilute the expression of the relatively high $L/R$ ratios (positive deviations) during the reinforced performance phase. However, careful examination of the hemispheric amplitude relationships indicates that they do distinguish reinforced and nonreinforced performance phases in the fashion predicted. A chi-square analysis of the 30-sec periods of the reinforced performance phase (starting at Minute 30) indicated that there was a significant relationship between the occurrence of a positive deviation and the occurrence of presses within a 30-sec period ($\chi^2 = 7.19$, $p < .01$). The chi-square for the 30-sec periods of nonreinforced performance phase was not statistically significant, indicating no systematic relationship between the occurrence of positive and negative deviations and the occurrence and nonoccurrence of operant responses. During the satiation period, the deviations were almost exclusively negative. Hence the EEG asymmetry was predictive of the disruption and recovery of discriminative performance (cf. Stamm, Rosen, & Gadotti, this volume).

These data suggest that lateral asymmetries differ systematically during the three arousal states related to task contingencies: (1) the one predominant during reinforced performance, when the animal was motivated to respond and did respond; (2) the one during nonreinforced performance, when the animal was motivated to seek water but inhibited responding; and (3) the one during satiation, when it was not motivated to seek water and did not respond. The symmetry of the behavioral paradigm and the

differences between the amplitude relations during satiation and
during the nonreinforced performance phases argue against accounting for the changes in interhemispheric relationships on the
basis of motor activity levels per se.

POSSIBLE IMPLICATIONS OF HEMISPHERIC AMPLITUDE ASYMMETRIES AFTER
ADMINISTRATION OF PSYCHOACTIVE DRUGS

Analyses so far have transformed successive interhemispheric
amplitude ratios across several states or experimental conditions into successive deviations from the overall mean $L/R$ amplitude ratio for the entire session.  This has been a useful tool
for the characterization of relative changes in the lateral asymmetries accompanying shifts in arousal states and/or behavioral
conditions.  However, large changes in amplitude during short segments of the session may bias the mean $L/R$ ratio and reduce the
informational value of this index.  This was the case for experiments in which pentobarbital administration preceded testing of
discrimination performance.  Several alternative indices of interhemispheric amplitude relationships may have potential usefulness.  One rather elementary one has been applied to the analysis
of lateral asymmetries after drug administration.  It is the
simple arithmetic difference between left and right integrated
amplitude values for each epoch of the recording session.

The data to be discussed indicate that the $L$ minus $R$ index
correlates well with the relative state of EEG arousal as assessed
by brain-wave amplitude levels (low amplitude indicative of the
alert, waking state and high amplitude indicative of sleep).
Further, these data suggest that patterns of laterality relations
may reveal other features relevant to the state of arousal and
the functional state of the organism.

Background EEG recorded during 23 experiments with nine rabbits was examined.  These were sessions during which substantial
changes in arousal state were exhibited, including periods of
either spontaneous or pentobarbital-induced HVS activity.  The
analyses indicated that in addition to the characteristic $L/R$
amplitude relationship existing in each individual during the
normal waking state (as described earlier), there was a characteristic continuum formed by the $L$ to $R$ indices (in this case,
$L - R$) in relation to points on a spectrum of arousal that ranged
from waking through deep-sleep states.  For each experiment, the
relationship between the EEG arousal state $[(L+R)/2]$ and the
hemispheric amplitude asymmetry ($L - R$) across successive minutes
of the session was statistically significant as indicated by the
product-moment correlation coefficient.  The orderliness of the
continuum was maintained even when an individual exhibited a
crossover in terms of which hemisphere had the higher amplitude
during a particular arousal state.  The results to be described
suggest that exceptions or deviations from the orderly relation-

ship between overall amplitude levels and the interhemispheric
amplitude states may be of particular value for understanding
hemispheric asymmetries in terms of their behavioral and functional significance.

In the upper half of Figure 7 are represented the time-effect
curves for mean EEG amplitude $[(L+R)/2]$ and the corresponding
plot of successive *L-R* amplitudes following intravenous administration of sodium pentobarbital (8 mg/kg). The predrug control

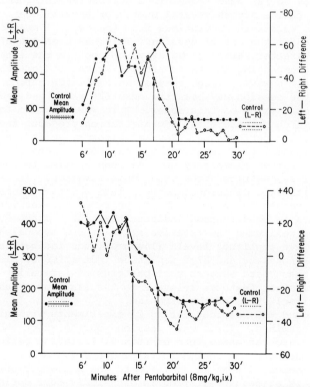

*Fig. 7. Time-effect curves for the mean EEG amplitudes* $[(L+R)/2]$
*and the chronologically related plots of successive left minus
right integrated amplitudes following administration of sodium
pentobarbital (8 mg/kg, i.v.) to two rabbits. The solid line indicates the mean EEG amplitudes and the dashed line the left
minus right index of interhemispheric relationships. The first
arrow on each time axis indicates the "signal" for an awakening
and the second, the time of full EEG and behavioral awakening.
The pretreatment, control mean integrated amplitude ± s.d. and
mean L - R hemispheric amplitude difference ± s.d. are shown on
the left and right, respectively, of each pair of time-effect
curves.*

levels (mean $\pm$ SD) of $(L+R)/2$ and $L - R$ amplitude are indicated.
The curve generated by the successive mean EEG amplitudes
$[(L+R)/2]$ indicates (in order of occurrence) the shifting states
of arousal through the session: onset of the sedative effect
(increasing amplitude), the period of sustained pentobarbital-
induced sleep (high amplitude), the trend toward reestablishment
of the wakeful state (decreasing amplitude), and the period of
fully expressed EEG and behavioral wakefulness indicated by the
presence of EEG activation and the return of mean amplitudes to
the predrug levels.

The curve generated by the successive $L - R$ differences was
almost a duplication of the mean amplitude curve. The correlation coefficient between the amplitudes and the differences was
significant ($r = -.75$, $p < .001$, $df = 23$). Thus, the asymmetry
was strongly correlated with the relative state of EEG arousal.
But, additionally, the $L - R$ difference scores seem to provide
information not readily derivable from the patterns of left,
right, or mean $[(L+R)/2]$ amplitudes alone. The changes in the
$L - R$ index of lateral asymmetry in fact *precede* the shift in
arousal state.

Starting at Minute 17 following the injection (Figure 7), the
mean amplitude indicated sedation (in fact, deepening sedation,
in that amplitude was increasing), while the left-right index
began to move in the direction expected for an awakening or activation. After a 3-min latency, the mean amplitude began to decrease, indicating the beginning of a shift toward arousal which
was not fully expressed until 4 min after the $L - R$ index had
"signaled" that the change in state was to occur. In the lower
half of Figure 7, the results of the same treatment and analysis
for a test session with another rabbit are represented. The correlation coefficient between EEG arousal state and the lateral
asymmetries index was significant ($r = .934$, $p < .001$, $df = 23$).
At 14 min after pentobarbital administration, the $L - R$ chrono-
gram indicated a shift toward hemispheric relationships that
normally accompany the waking state. The arithmetic sign of the
left-right difference became negative for the first time, the
lateral asymmetry normally consistent with wakefulness or EEG activation. This signal for an oncoming awakening occurred 4 min
before a full expression of arousal occurred in terms of the
mean EEG amplitude and behavior of the rabbit.

Speculatively, one might consider the period between the signal provided by the laterality index and the full establishment
of the awake state to represent a discordance between the EEG
arousal state and the relative hemispheric amplitude states. If
the same discordance is manifested in man during similar drug
states, the relationship between this electrophysiological pattern and the functional impairment (confusional state) that commonly accompanies recovery from barbiturate anesthesia might be
worthy of investigation.

Recently, data from some rather complicated experiments have

JUDITH M. NELSON *et al.*

been reexamined. In these studies, either saline or small doses
of chlorpromazine hydrochloride (CPZ) were administered to five
rabbits while the animals were in a state of pentobarbital-induced
sedation. (Four mg/kg of pentobarbital were administered intravenously; next, 5 min later, either saline or .1 mg/kg CPZ was
injected; after another 5 min, an additional 4 mg/kg injection of
pentobarbital was given.) During normal wakefulness, three of
the rabbits consistently exhibited *R* amplitudes higher than *L* and
two rabbits, *L* higher than *R*. The results indicated that CPZ produced a disruption or breakdown of the orderly continuum of interhemispheric relationships across EEG arousal states. Intriguingly, the disturbance appeared to be more marked for one hemisphere than for the other, and which hemisphere was affected predominantly depended on the direction of the baseline hemispheric
amplitude asymmetries.

The results of product-moment correlations are summarized in
Table 1. The data at the top of the table are from the three
rabbits that, under control conditions, had *R* amplitudes higher
than *L*. (*L* - *R* amplitude scores were used as indices of hemispheric asymmetries.) During the pentibarbital control sessions,
correlations between *L* - *R* and (*L*+*R*)/2, *L*, and *R* respectively
were all statistically significant. When CPZ was given, all
three amplitude relationships were weakened for all animals, with
the more predominent effect being on the relationship between
*L* - *R* and *R*. For the two rabbits whose *L* amplitude was higher
than *R* during control, the more prominent hemispheric effect of
CPZ was seen in the relationship between *L* - *R* and *L*. In some
cases the CPZ effect was expressed as a weakening of the correlation between the critical variables. In others, it was expressed as a reversal of the direction of the correlation. In
all cases the lateralized effect involved predominantly the hemisphere that had the higher baseline amplitude.

Some recent data from nine rabbits support the notion that CPZ
disturbs the relationship of the continuum of hemispheric asymmetries to normal EEG arousal states. EEG was recorded following
the administration of CPZ alone (2 mg/kg, intravenously). This
dose produced only moderate sedation in terms of EEG amplitude
levels. Although full quantitative analyses of the data are not
complete, examination of the hemispheric amplitude chronograms
(plots of amplitude levels for successive minutes) revealed that
reversals of hemispheric asymmetries occurred at relatively low
amplitude levels. These were amplitude levels below those at
which reversals of asymmetries due to either spontaneous or pentobarbital-induced HVS activity had been observed.

In view of these findings, it is tempting to consider the possible relationships between hemispheric EEG phenomena and the now
classical finding that CPZ will disrupt avoidance behavior selectively (in a shock escape-avoidance operant procedure) at a dose
that does not impair escape behavior (Courvoisier, Fournel,
Duerot, Kolsky, & Koetschet, 1953; Cook & Weidley, 1957). In

TABLE 1

*Correlation coefficients and student's t values[a] for the relationship between hemispheric amplitude patterns*

| Rabbit no. | Saline (L+R)/2 vs. (L-R) | Saline L vs. (L-R) | Saline R vs. (L-R) | Chlorpromazine (L+R)/2 vs. (L-R) | Chlorpromazine L vs. (L-R) | Chlorpromazine R vs. (L-R) |
|---|---|---|---|---|---|---|
| *Rabbits with Right Amplitude Higher than Left Amplitude* | | | | | | |
| RP15  r | 0.937 | 0.948 | 0.920 | 0.252 | 0.422 | 0.055 |
|       t | 14.163 | 15.792 | 12.454 | 1.380 | 2.466 | 0.293 |
| RP35  r | 0.533 | 0.622 | 0.422 | -0.345 | -0.174 | -0.487 |
|       t | 3.335 | 4.210 | 2.460 | -1.943 | -0.936 | -2.950 |
| RP42  r | 0.940 | 0.957 | 0.911 | 0.646 | 0.771 | 0.484 |
|       t | 14.535 | 17.050 | 11.724 | 4.481 | 6.412 | 2.928 |
| *Rabbits with Left Amplitude Higher than Right Amplitude* | | | | | | |
| RP33  r | -0.863 | -0.814 | -0.896 | -0.354 | -0.164 | -0.508 |
|       t | -9.054 | -7.415 | -10.685 | -2.002 | -0.882 | -3.121 |
| RP46  r | -0.539 | -0.472 | -0.597 | -0.335 | -0.223 | -0.434 |
|       t | -3.386 | -2.837 | -3.935 | -1.882 | -1.210 | -2.553 |

[a]The critical t value (.05 level of significance, $df = 28$, two-tailed test) is 3.05.

467

contrast, pentobarbital, at a dose that impairs avoidance, also impairs escape behavior. It may be that the selective functional impairment after CPZ is not related to an overt sedative effect, but to a mechanism that may involve an alteration of hemispheric relationships inducing a state normally existing during deep sedation, although the CPZ-treated organism is not deeply sedated in terms of absolute EEG amplitude levels. It should be recalled that with pentobarbital, which has nonspecific effects on escape-avoidance behavior, the manifestation of lateral asymmetries similar to those observed after CPZ was limited to phases of deep sedation. In terms of clinical effects, these results suggest that the dysphoria and behavioral impairment that normals suffer after receiving chlorpromazine should be considered in relation to a possible discordance between EEG arousal state and the hemispheric asymmetries accompanying it.


CONCLUDING COMMENTS

The experiments described represent a first step in the attempt to elucidate the characteristics and significance of EEG amplitude asymmetries between homologous areas of the hemispheres of the rabbit. The existence and possible functional significance of asymmetries in neural activity between intrahemispheric loci on either the horizontal or vertical brain axis may well be related issues and deserve examination (see Webster, this volume). The present findings suggest that interhemispheric amplitude relationships depend systematically on the arousal and/or behavioral state of the organism. Full understanding of our results concerning base-state EEG asymmetries and the apparent hemispheric selectivity of action of pentobarbital and chlorpromazine and how these phenomena may relate to lateral specialization or dominance in nonverbal species invites and awaits further investigation. The findings of Webster (this volume), that the direction of the shift in EEG amplitude relationships occurring when cats passed from non-REM to REM sleep did not appear to be related to paw preference, might suggest that paw preference is not an indication of cerebral dominance as is handedness in man (see Collins; Warren, this volume). However, the findings do not preclude the existence of organized lateral organization in nonverbal animals.

In conclusion, it might be suggested that the concept of the uniqueness of man with regard to hemispheric differentiation may prove to be more apparent than real. Certainly, the development of Broca's and Wernicke's area (see Gardiner & Walter; Rubens, this volume) represents a decisive advantage in terms of evolutionary mechanisms. However, the use that animals may be making of a primitive homologue of man's major hemisphere is largely unexplored. It may be that the lateral specialization exemplified by the central organization for speech in man has not been a sudden development; rather, it may represent the result of the

gradual enhancement of a long-established lateralization not yet
fully recognized in nonverbal species.

## SUMMARY

Analyses of data collected from rabbits gave evidence that
differential lateral amplitude asymmetries of electrocortical
activity accompany various states of consciousness, i.e., normal
wakefulness, REM sleep, and non-REM (high voltage, slow wave)
sleep. An orderly function was generated relating the overall
level of cortical activation and hemispheric amplitude asymmetries when shifts in the level of arousal occurred spontaneously
and when they were induced with pentobarbital. However, administration of chlorpromazine appeared to disrupt the orderliness of
the relationship between the level of cortical activation and
underlying functional asymmetries. Further examinations of the
EEG during the performance of an operant task by rabbits also
revealed relative shifts in hemispheric asymmetries. These shifts
were dependent on the stimulus and reinforcement contingencies
of the task and hence, presumably, on the nature of the central
arousal state. The base-state EEG asymmetries, apparent hemispheric selectivity of action of certain drugs, and selectivity
of focus of change for certain behavioral states suggests the existence of lateral specialization in the rabbit.

## ACKNOWLEDGMENTS

The authors are grateful to Zoltan Sisko for his technical
assistance, to Kathleen Pelley and Florence Szymanski for their
aid in the preparation of this manuscript, and to the editors
for their thoughtful comments.

## REFERENCES

Adrian, E. D., & Matthews, B. H. C. Berger rhythm, potential
    changes from the occipital lobes in the human brain.
    *Brain*, 1934, *57*, 355-367.
Baran, L., & Longo, V. G. Instrumental reward discrimination in
    rabbits. Electroencephalographic and behavioral effects of
    a series of lysergic acid derivatives. *Acta Physiologica
    Latino americana*, 1964, *14*, 125-137.
Cook, L., & Weidley, E. Behavioral effects of some psychopharma-
    cological agents. *Annals of the New York Academy of
    Sciences*, 1957, *66*, 740-752.
Courvoisier, S., Fournel, J., Ducrot, R., Kolsky, M., &
    Koetschet, P. Properties pharmacodynamiques du chlorhydrate
    de chloro-3(dimethylamino-3' propyl)-10 phenothiazine

(4560RP). Archives internationales de Pharmacodynamie et de Therapie, 1953, 92, 305-361.

Galin, D., & Ornstein, R. Lateral specialization of cognitive mode: An EEG study. Psychophysiology, 1972, 9, 412-418.

Goldstein, L., & Beck, R. Amplitude analysis of the electroencephalogram. Review of the information obtained with the integrated method. International Review of Neurobiology, 1965, 8, 265-312.

Goldstein, L., Stoltzfus, N. W., & Gardocki, J. F. Changes in interhemispheric amplitude relationships in the EEG during sleep. Physiology and Behavior, 1972, 8, 811-815.

Hommes, O. R., & Panhuysen, L. H. H. M. Bilateral intracarotid amytal injection: A study of dysphasia, disturbance of consciousness and paresis. Psychiatria, Neurologia, Neurochirurgia, 1970, 73, 447-459.

Longo, V. G. Rabbit brain research. Vol. II. Electroencephalographic atlas for pharmacological research: Effect of drugs on the electrical activity of the rabbit brain. New York: Elsevier, 1962.

McGaugh, J. L., de Baran, L., & Longo, V. G. Electroencephalographic and behavioral analysis of drug effects on an instrumental reward discrimination in rabbits. Psychopharmacologia, 1963, 4, 126-138.

Moruzzi, G., & Magoun, H. W. Brainstem reticular formation and the activation of the EEG. Electroencephalography and Clinical Neurophysiology, 1949, 1, 455-473.

Rheinberger, M. B., & Jasper, H. H. Electrical activity of the cerebral cortex in the unanesthetized cat. American Journal of Physiology, 1937, 119, 186-198.

Sadowski, B., & Longo, V. G. Electroencephalographic and behavioral correlates of an instrumental reward conditioned response in rabbits. A physiological and pharmacological study. Electroencephalography and Clinical Neurophysiology, 1962, 14, 465-476.

Serafetinides, E. A., Driver, M. V., & Hoare, R. D. EEG patterns induced by intracarotid injection of sodium amytal. Electroencephalography and Clinical Neurophysiology, 1965, 18, 170-175.(a)

Serafetinides, E. A., Hoare, R. D., & Driver, M. V. Intracarotid sodium amylobarbitone and cerebral dominance for speech and consciousness. Brain, 1965, 88, 107-130.(b)

Siegel, S. Nonparametric statistics for the behavioral sciences. New York: McGraw-Hill, 1956.

# 24.
# Hemispheric Asymmetry in Cats

*WILLIAM G. WEBSTER*

Carleton University

## A SPLIT-BRAIN APPROACH TO ANIMAL BRAIN ASYMMETRY

My work on hemispheric asymmetry in cats began several years ago under the guidance of J. M. Warren and P. R. Cornwell at the Pennsylvania State University. The approach adopted was similar to that involved in testing human split-brain patients (Sperry, 1974): Cats were trained preoperatively on a variety of visual discrimination problems. The corpus callosum and optic chiasm were then sectioned in the midline and each hemisphere was tested for retention of the discrimination (Webster, 1972). A small plastic cup, molded to the approximate curvature of the cornea, was placed on one or the other eye after application of a local anesthetic, thus limiting visual input to the contralateral hemisphere. Most of the discrimination testing was carried out in a Wisconsin General Test Apparatus (WGTA) similar to that described by Harlow (1949). The animal must make a unimanual response in order to displace the correct discriminandum and receive a food reward. The other testing was in a two-choice Grice Box (Hirayoshi & Warren, 1967), an apparatus with an enclosed start box opening into a choice compartment that fans out to form two

---
*The research reported in the first part of this chapter was supported by Grant MH04726 from the National Institute of Mental Health, U. S. Public Health Service, awarded to Dr. J. M. Warren, and that in the latter part by Grant APA-0399 from the National Research Council of Canada, awarded to the author.

response compartments containing the stimulus objects. On each trial, the animal must leave the start box and approach one of two objects, the correct one concealing a food reward.

Before training began on the discriminations, the paw preference of each of the eight cats was assessed by paw use in reaching for pieces of food (see Warren, Abplanalp, & Warren, 1967). Throughout pre- and postoperative training in the WGTA, the paw used to displace the discriminanda was noted. All animals showed highly consistent paw preferences throughout the study, irrespective of the eye used in postoperative testing.

The visual discrimination problems on which the cats were trained included four pattern and two form discriminations administered in the WGTA, and one form discrimination administered in the Grice Box. The positive and negative stimuli were present on each trial. Training continued until the animal achieved a criterion of 10 consecutive correct responses on two consecutive test sessions. The animals were also trained in the WGTA on a go/no-go discrimination. The stimuli were three-dimensional forms: a white triangle and a cylinder painted in a checkerboard pattern. Stimuli were presented one at a time and the animal had to respond within 15 sec to the positive stimulus and withhold response for 15 sec to the negative stimulus.

As already indicated, each hemisphere was tested for retention of these discriminations following the sectioning of the optic chiasm and corpus callosum. To determine whether paw preference was related to hemispheric asymmetry, the performance of the hemisphere contralateral to the preferred paw was compared to that of the ipsilateral hemisphere. In the first two figures to follow, these are for convenience referred to as the *dominant* and *nondominant* hemispheres, respectively.

On the go/no-go discrimination, 300 postoperative trials were administered to each hemisphere. There was a highly consistent performance difference in favor of the hemisphere ipsilateral to the preferred paw. As Figure 1 indicates, performance by the nondominant hemisphere was superior in terms of withheld responses to the negative stimulus on all six blocks of 50 trials. Consistent with this finding was the fact that within the 300 postoperative trials the nondominant hemisphere of six of the eight cats reattained preoperative criterion performance, whereas in only two of the eight cats did the dominant hemisphere do so. The asymmetry was also displayed in terms of response latencies to the positive stimulus (Figure 2). On all six blocks of 50 trials, responses were faster with the nondominant than the dominant hemisphere. These response latency data indicate that the withheld-response results cannot be accounted for by motivational differences.

On the simultaneous discriminations, there were mixed results. On three of the pattern discriminations, there were no consistent differences, but on the fourth (three smaller circles versus one larger circle), there was a consistent and statistical-

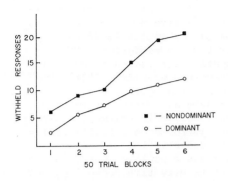

*Fig. 1. Median number of with-held responses to negative stimulus on each of the six blocks of 50 trials of go/no-go postoperative testing of the hemisphere contralateral to the preferred paw (dominant hemisphere) and of the hemisphere ipsilateral to the preferred paw (nondominant hemisphere). The maximum number of correctly withheld responses in each block is 25. From Webster, 1972.*

*Fig. 2. Median latency of response (in seconds) to the positive stimulus on each of the six blocks of 50 trials of go/no-go postoperative testing of the hemisphere contralateral to the preferred paw (dominant hemisphere) and of the hemisphere ipsilateral to the preferred paw (nondominant hemisphere). From Webster, 1972.*

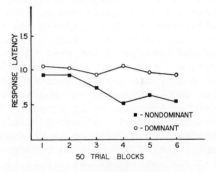

ly reliable difference favoring the hemisphere ipsilateral to the preferred paw. Similarly, on the form discrimination administered in the Grice Box, all cats showed better retention with the nondominant hemisphere.

These data seem to point to a hemispheric asymmetry in cats, an asymmetry related to paw preference. In my earlier discussion of these data (Webster, 1972), I suggested that the asymmetry might be related to spatial processes of either perception of response such that the hemisphere ipsilateral to the preferred paw is superior to the contralateral hemisphere. A comment is in order, however, since two of the pattern discriminations on which no consistent differences were detected involved stimulus orientation: horizontal lines versus vertical lines, and an upright versus inverted arrowhead shape. Although these can be classified as spatial problems, such is probably not the point of view of the cat. Animals are notorious for attending only to those aspects of the stimulus configuration that are close to the locus of response (Cowey, 1968; Meyer, Treichler, & Meyer, 1965). In the WGTA, the cat's response is directed toward the base of the stimulus objects, near where the reward is located, and it is likely that the animals attended only to the lower part of the stimulus configuration. This would transform these two apparent-ly spatial problems into nonspatial pattern discriminations on which the hemispheres may perhaps not be functionally asymmetric (cf. Hamilton, this volume). Numerous investigators have re-ported that animals may use nonspatial strategies on spatial tasks (Beale & Corballis, 1968; Lehman & Spencer, 1973). The question of attentional and response strategies impinges upon one of the central problems in the behavioral testing of animals (and probably of man as well --cf. Gur & Gur, this volume): that of assessing the extent to which task performance actually reflects the kinds of processing assumed to underlie it.

The split-brain approach is not one I would encourage anyone to follow, at least with cats. It is very time consuming, very expensive, and is a very inefficient paradigm in terms of the amount of information gained for effort expended. In subsequent work that attempted to apply this paradigm to the study of hemi-spheric differences on more complex perceptual and learning tasks, the separated hemispheres were found to require substanti-ally more trials to relearn the problems postoperatively than for initial preoperative acquisition. The poor learning capability of one hemisphere compared to both is certainly not a new obser-vation (Sechzer, Folstun, Geiger, & Mervis, this volume), but it does raise serious questions about differential retention by the two hemispheres and poses serious problems in the interpreta-tion of hemispheric differences (or their absence) on difficult discriminations. A second problem is that the paradigm requires the two hemispheres to be treated as similarly as possible post-operatively, but it then becomes difficult to study more than one discrimination per cat. This raises serious practical and eco-nomic problems, as well as difficulties in studying groups of tasks on which there are consistent hemispheric differences *within* cats. The restrictedness of the visual field (one-sixth the normal visual field) and poor unihemispheric learning in split-brain cats also raise questions as to the comparability of their discrimination learning with that of normal cats. For all these reasons, and because of the possibility that cutting the callosum may attenuate interesting hemispheric differences (if indeed there is, as Kinsbourne, 1972, suggests, reciprocal inhi-bition between the hemispheres mediated by the collosum; cf. Glick, Jerussi, & Zimmerberg; Heilman & Watson; Sechzer *et al.*, this volume), my recent efforts have been directed more toward the study of hemispheric differences in normal, surgically intact cats.


ELECTROPHYSIOLOGICAL APPROACHES TO BRAIN ASYMMETRY

Reports in the human literature indicate that differential hemispheric involvement in task performance is reflected in amplitude and frequency differences in the EEG recorded from symmetrical points on the two hemispheres during problem solving (e.g., Galin & Ornstein, 1972; see also Donchin, Kutas, & McCarthy; Gardiner & Walter, this volume). An attempt is currently underway to apply an analogue of this work to cats, that is, to record EEG from symmetrical points on the two hemispheres of normal, surgically intact cats during different phases of discrimination performance.

Our interest in this approach was stimulated by a most provocative study (Goldstein, Stoltzfus, & Gardocki, 1972) reporting that in human subjects there occurred during shifts from REM (Rapid Eye Movement) to non-REM phases of sleep a shift in the relative activity of the two hemispheres (see also Nelsen, Phillips, & Goldstein, this volume). During non-REM sleep, all seven of the right-handed subjects showed a more active left than right hemisphere, but during periods of REM sleep, the right hemisphere increased its relative activity. What was exciting was that these same shifts were also found in rabbits and cats, and in fact were in these organisms of even greater magnitude than those in man. In three of five rabbits and in three of four cats, the shift was in the same direction as man, and in the other animals the shift was in the opposite direction. This raised the possibility that these shifts might represent an interhemispheric phenomenon reflecting some dimension of hemispheric differentiation.

We first replicated in six adult cats the basic findings of Goldstein *et al.* (1972). Included in the study (Webster, Howitt, & LeBlanc, 1976) were three right-pawed and three left-pawed animals. Epidural electrodes were symmetrically placed on the middle suprasylvian and middle marginal gyri. Analysis of the EEG employed an integrator for each channel that generated an analogue voltage proportional to the average amplitude of the signal (Figure 3). This voltage drove a voltage-to-frequency converter that emitted pulses with a frequency proportional to the voltage. The pulses were then counted over a fixed time interval and these counts were used to form ratios of the EEG amplitude between homologous points on the two hemispheres as well as between points within the two hemispheres. For reasons discussed by Goldstein *et al.* (1972), data analysis is with respect to deviation of each recording epoch from the mean interhemispheric ratio. The whole system is shown schematically in Figure 4.

Preliminary analysis confirmed the basic findings of Goldstein *et al.* (1972). All six cats showed significant interhemispheric shifts in relative activity corresponding to shifts from REM to NREM phases of sleep. This was the case for the EEG recorded both from the suprasylvian and the marginal gyrus electrodes. There was, however, no obvious relationship between the direction of the shift at either site and paw preference. Because of the recent work of Glick *et al.* (this volume), we also recorded the predominant direction of rotation during each recording session

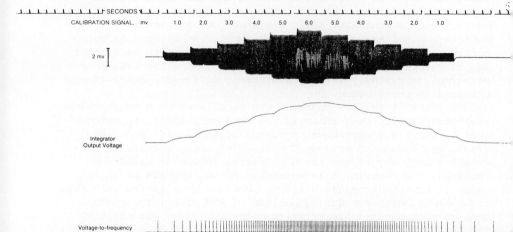

Fig. 3. *Illustration of EEG analysis system. Top trace: time-marker. Second trace: square-wave calibration signal. Third trace: analogue voltage output of integrator, the amplitude of which is proportional to average signal amplitude. Fourth trace: output from voltage-to-frequency converter (divided by 100), pulses whose frequency is proportional to the integrator analogue voltage.*

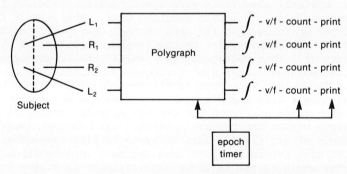

Fig. 4. *Schematic drawing of data-collection system. At the end of each epoch, the epoch timer activates a polygraph event marker, activates the printer, and resets the counters.* !

by simply noting at the end of the session the direction in which the recording cables had become twisted. Despite a finding of a consistent direction of rotation within each animal across recording sessions (in five of six animals, the rotation direction was ipsilateral to the paw preference), this too failed to be

476

related to the direction of shifts in interhemispheric activity. In two kittens implanted with cortical electrodes at ·3 weeks of age, EEG was recorded at 4 and 6 weeks of age respectively, and the same shifts were seen as in the adult animals.

The interpretation of these shifts is, I believe, far more complex than one might expect. The data were analyzed for between-hemisphere ratios (that is, the amplitude of the EEG recorded from the left hemisphere relative to that from the same point on the right hemisphere), and also for within-hemisphere ratios (that is, for the ratio of suprasylvian to marginal gyrus amplitude within each hemisphere). If indeed this is an interhemispheric phenomenon, there should be little or no systematic intrahemispheric shifts. In fact, however, we found the intra- and interhemispheric changes were of the same order of magnitude. There thus seemed to be a diagonal shift in activity corresponding to shifts from REM to NREM sleep, rather than a strictly left-right or strictly anterior-posterior shift. Also suggesting that this is not a purely interhemispheric phenomenon of the sort anticipated (i.e., mediated through the corpus callosum) is the fact that in two additional adult cats with a sectioned corpus callosum, the pattern of intra- and interhemispheric shifts was indistinguishable from that of the six cats with the callosum intact.

This certainly leaves very unclear the appropriate interpretation for this fascinating phenomenon, but further research into its interhemispheric aspects is warranted.

Research presently in progress focuses on variations in interhemispheric EEG amplitude ratios as a function of variations in stimulus and response parameters of visual discrimination learning in cats. We have developed a technique combining delayed response (Warren, Warren, & Akert, 1962) with behavioral titration (Weiskrantz & Cowey, 1963) to achieve good stimulus control and to ensure that the subjects are attending to the stimuli during the EEG recording epoch. This is conceptually similar to the work of Stamm, Rosen and Gadotti (this volume). The primary objective of the work at this stage is to provide a description of behavioral tasks with which hemispheric differences can be reliably demonstrated in the cat, and to evaluate the appropriateness of various subject variables in characterizing the polarity of hemispheric differences. These variables include left versus right hemisphere, paw preference, spatial preferences, patterns of interhemispheric amplitude shifts during REM and NREM sleep, anatomical asymmetry in the visual cortex, and nigrostriatal dopamine asymmetry (Glick *et al.*, this volume).

Most EEG recording is undertaken on an assumption of anatomical symmetry between homologous regions on the left and right. Recently, an anatomical asymmetry has been noted in the visual area of a large proportion of cats (Webster & Webster, 1975). Thus, despite recording electrodes being placed symmetrically with respect to sutures of the skull, it may be questionable as to whe-

ther in fact the recording actually samples from symmetrical
brain areas (cf. Rubens, this volume).

ANATOMICAL ASYMMETRY IN THE CAT BRAIN

When maps of the cortex were constructed with reference to the
sutures of the skull for use in implanting cortical EEG electrodes an anatomical asymmetry was noted. Thirty-nine intact
cat brains were analyzed for symmetry or asymmetry. Each hemisphere of each brain was classified according to the scheme of
Otsuka and Hassler (1962) who identified four types of sulcus
patterns in cats (Figure 5). These types differ with respect to

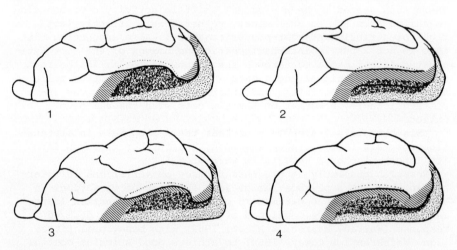

*Fig. 5. Four fissure-pattern types found in the cat brain as
described by Otsuka and Hassler (1962). Note the continuity and
discontinuity between the lateral and posterolateral sulci and/or
between the lateral ansate sulcus and the coronal sulcus. The
area in light cray corresponds to area 17, that in drak gray to
area 18, and that in lines to area 19. Adapted from Otsuka &
Hassler, 1962.*

the continuity of the lateral with the posterolateral sulci and/or
with respect to continuity of the lateral ansate sulcus with the
coronal sulcus. Of the 33 brains for which there was no ambiguity of classification for either hemisphere, 18 had a symmetrical
fissure pattern and 15 had asymmetrical patterns. Included in
the symmetrical cases were two brains that had symmetrical fissure pattern types but were asymmetrical with respect to their
being, in the left marginal gyrus, a distinct entolateral sulcus.
Included among the asymmetrical brains was one of three newborn
kittens, indicating that the asymmetry was inborn. So far, the

asymmetry does not appear to be related to paw preference.
According to the classification scheme used, a brain could be asymmetrical with respect to anterior and/or posterior features. Of the 15 brains comprising the asymmetrical group, 3 were asymmetrical with respect to both anterior and posterior features, 2 were asymmetrical with respect to anterior but not posterior features, and the remaining 10 were asymmetrical with respect to posterior but not anterior features. This predominance of a posterior asymmetry in the visual area, seen in 13 of the 15 asymmetrical brains, as well as in the 2 symmetrical brains with an entolateral sulcus in the left marginal gyrus, suggests that this might form the substrate of a functional asymmetry in visual processes. This suggestion is, of course, based on the assumption that cortical surface features such as sulci, dimples, and spurs delimit functionally distinct areas. Such an assumption seems reasonably well supported by the anatomical work of Sarⁱdes (1972) and by the physiological work of Welker and Campos (1963) but remains to be examined in the specific case of asymmetry.


CONCLUSIONS

Just 10 or 15 years ago, it was not at all unreasonable to accept the proposition that a difference between human and nonhuman brains, perhaps even a defining difference, lay in the symmetry or asymmetry of the hemispheres. In the past few years, there have been several demonstrations of a functional asymmetry in animals, and some of these are discussed in other chapters of this volume (see e.g. Nottebohm; Dewson; cf. Hamilton). However, there are no data yet to indicate convincingly that the asymmetry is more than just quantitative (cf. Riklan, this volume) and there are no data that indicate convincingly that the asymmetry is more than a rough analogue of that found in the human brain. What the data do indicate, and what the changing conceptual climate allows, is that nonhuman species may yet be found to display some degree of lateralization and that this in turn may be of relevance to that found in man.


REFERENCES                          REFEREN

Beale, I. L., & Corballis, M. C. Beak shift: An explanation for interocular mirror-image reversal in pigeons. *Nature*, 1968, *220*, 82-83.
Cowey, A. Discrimination. In L. Weiskrantz (Ed.), *Analysis of behavioral change*. New York: Harper & Row, 1968.
Galin, D., & Ornstein, R. Lateral specialization of cognitive mode: An EEG study. *Psychophysiology*, 1972, *9*, 412-418.
Goldstein, L., Stoltzfus, N. W., & Gardocki, J. F. Changes in interhemispheric amplitude relationships in the EEG during

sleep. *Physiology and Behavior*, 1972, *8*, 811-815.

Harlow, H. F. The formation of learning sets. *Psychological Review*, 1949, *56*, 51-65.

Hirayoshi, I., & Warren, J. M. Overtraining and reversal learning by experimentally naive kittens. *Journal of Comparative and Physiological Psychology*, 1967, *64*, 507-510.

Kinsbourne, M. Eye and head turning indicates cerebral lateralization. *Science*, 1972, *176*, 539-541.

Lehman, R. A. W., & Spencer, D. D. Mirror-image shape discrimination: Interocular reversal of responses in the optic chiasm sectioned monkey. *Brain Research*, 1973, *52*, 233-241.

Meyer, D. R., Treichler, F. R., & Meyer, P. M. Discrete-trial training techniques and stimulus variables. In A. M. Schrier, H. F. Harlow, & F. Stollnitz (Eds.), *Behavior of nonhuman primates*. Vol. 1. New York: Academic Press, 1965.

Otsuka, R., & Hassler, R. Uber Aufbau und Gliederung der corticalen Sehsphäre bei der Katze. *Archiv für Psychiatrie und Zeitschrift f.d.ges. Neurologie*, 1962, *203*, 212-234.

Sanides, F. Representation in the cerebral cortex and its areal lamination patterns. In G. H. Bourne (Ed.), *The structure and function of nervous tissue*. Vol. 5. New York: Academic Press, 1972.

Sperry, R. W. Lateral specialization in the surgically separated hemispheres. In F. O. Schmitt & F. G. Worden (Eds.), *The neurosciences: Third study program*. Cambridge: Massachusetts: MIT Press, 1974.

Warren, J. M., Abplanalp, J. M., & Warren, H. B. The development of handedness in cats and rhesus monkeys. In H. W. Stevenson, E. H. Hess, & H. L. Rheingold (Eds.), *Early behavior: Comparative and developmental approaches*. New York: Wiley, 1967.

Warren, J. M., Warren, H. B., & Akert, K. Orbitofrontal cortical lesions and learning in cats. *Journal of Comparative Neurology*, 1962, *118*, 17-41.

Webster, W. G. Functional asymmetry between the cerebral hemispheres of the cat. *Neuropsychologia*, 1972, *10*, 75-87.

Webster, W. G., Howitt, M. J., & LeBlanc, R. Inter- and intrahemispheric EEG amplitude shifts during sleep in the cat. In preparation, 1976.

Webster, W. G., & Webster, I. H. Anatomical asymmetry of the cerebral hemispheres of the cat brain. *Physiology and Behavior*, 1975, *14* (in press).

Weiskrantz, L., & Cowey, A. Striate cortex lesions and visual acuity of the rhesus monkey. *Journal of Comparative and Physiological Psychology*, 1963, *56*, 225-231.

Welker, W. I., & Campos, G. B. Physiological significance of sulci in somatic sensory cerebral cortex in mammals of the family *procyonidae*. *Journal of Comparative Neurology*, 1963, *120*, 19-36.

# 25.
# Evidence of Hemispheric Specialization from Infant EEG

*MARTIN F. GARDINER*

Harvard Medical School

*DONALD O. WALTER*

University of California, Los Angeles

Until recently, information concerning the development of
adult functional lateralization has been obtained almost exclusively from clinical data. Considerable plasticity in the development of language lateralization has been observed following
early brain injury. Both hemispheres seem to have the capacity
to develop speech at birth since if unilateral brain injury
occurs at a sufficiently early age, language will develop in the
uninjured hemisphere (Basser, 1962; Rasmussen, 1964; cf. Nottebohm, this volume). In addition, some disruption of language
development has been reported to occur following injury to *either*
hemisphere if it occurs within the first 2 years of life (Basser,
1962), although the equipotentiality of such disruption has recently been questioned (Annett, 1973; Kohn & Dennis, 1975). In
1967 Lenneberg reviewed the available clinical literature and
concluded that language was probably equally represented in both
hemispheres up to about 2 years of age, and that lateralization
for language was not fully completed until adolescence.

However, as Kinsbourne (1975) has emphasized, the observed
plasticity of language specialization following brain damage does
not necessarily imply equal hemispheric representation for
language at birth. Many examples of the capacity of the immature
nervous system to shift from the normal developmental course to
compensate for early brain damage are known, and the dynamics of
such compensation are of interest in their right (Bach-y-Rita,
1972; Geschwind, 1974; Rosen, & Butters, 1974). In clinical
material such potent compensating mechanisms could well obscure

evidence of factors associated with a normal course of development.

Work that has appeared since Lenneberg's review has in fact provided increasing evidence that hemisphere differences in the processing of linguistic and nonlinguistic stimuli may already normally exist very early in infancy and perhaps at birth. The clinical evidence on which Lenneberg based his conclusions has been criticized (Kinsbourne, 1975) and new clinical data have appeared that fail to support the view that there is complete equipotentiality for language development after early injury to either hemisphere (Annett, 1973; Kohn & Dennis, 1975). Corresponding findings have also been reported concerning nonlinguistic visuospatial functions (Kohn & Dennis, 1974). These studies reveal that the asymptotic capacities of the right and left hemisphere differ regardless of the age of injury: The right has a lower asymptote for verbal functions and the left for visuospatial functions.

There is also evidence of anatomical asymmetries between left and right temporal cortex favoring a region on the left (Wernicke's area) that appears to play an important role in language functions in the adult (Geschwind, 1970; Luria, 1970; Rubens, this volume). This asymmetry was first demonstrated in adult brains (Geschwind & Levitsky, 1968) and has recently been shown to be present already in newborns (Wada, 1973; Wada, Clarke, & Hamme, 1975; Witelson & Pallie, 1973). Wada and his colleagues also found an asymmetry at the frontal operculum and reported that both temporal and frontal asymmetries can be seen by the twenty-ninth week of gestation.

Other evidence has come from studies on normal infants. Molfese, Freeman and Palermo (1975) have reported that in a group of 10 infants ranging in age from 1 week to 10 months a late component of the averaged auditory evoked potential was larger over the left hemisphere for verbal stimuli (CV--consonant-vowel-- sounds or spoken words), but larger over the right hemisphere for nonverbal stimuli (noises or tones). Employing a method that had already revealed that preverbal infants exhibit categorical perception of speech sounds (Eimas, Siqueland, Jusezyk, & Vigorito, 1971), Entus (1975) presented dichotic stimuli to very young infants. She reported a right-ear advantage for discrimination with verbal (CV) stimuli, but a left-ear advantage with nonverbal stimuli in infants who were only a few weeks old. (See also: Anderson; Berlin; Springer; Turkewitz, this volume.)

Another approach to the study of lateralization of functions during early infancy was taken by Gardiner, Schulman, and Walter (1973). In an initial analysis of pilot data from four 6-month-old infants, they found interhemispheric differences in EEG activity during the presentation of verbal and nonverbal stimuli. Similar effects in a higher frequency band (alpha) in the EEG of adults have been taken to reflect differences in lateralization of mental processing (e.g., Morgan, McDonald, & MacDonald, 1971;

Galin & Ornstein, 1972; Gardiner *et al.*, 1973). In this chapter
we will report and discuss the results of further analysis of
these pilot recordings by a new method that supports and clari-
fies our earlier observations and will then propose a hypothesis
for interpreting these data.


DATA COLLECTION

The data-collection procedure was suggested by Dr. Carol
Schulman based on her previous observations and was refined
during the pilot study (Gardiner *et al.*, 1973). EEG was recorded
from each infant during a series of brief presentations of continuous natural stimulus material. Some of the material was
verbal (investigator or mother speaking, or playback of taped
speech), and some nonverbal (episodes of eye contact between investigator and infant, times when infant was allowed to look
around the room, playback of music from radio or tape). The total
duration of the recording session was 10-15 min and the order of
stimulus presentations was varied across infants to compensate
for possible order effects. Short periods of lack of movement,
if they occurred shortly after a stimulus presentation began,
were taken as indication of attention to stimulus materials, as
the infants were otherwise very active (Eisenberg, 1969;
Kearsley, 1973; Wolff, 1965. An investigator present in the room
with the infant during the stimulus presentation periods shifted
to a new stimulus as soon as the infant showed signs of loss of
interest in the material (restlessness, crying, and pulling of
the EEG cables).
The recordings with the first infant were made at the University of California, San Diego, and were intended to test the
feasibility of the procedure. Subsequently, three more infants
were recorded under somewhat different, and more controlled conditions at the University of California, Los Angeles. We will
consider each infant's records individually. All four gave
essentially the same result.
In the feasibility study, the recordings were obtained while
the infant was supine. In the later studies each of the infants
was recorded while seated, either in a feeding chair or on its
mother's lap. Auditory stimuli were presented from a position
several feet away from the infant. In the UCLA experiments this
position was centered directly in front of the infant. During
the collection of all data discussed here room lights were
kept at low intensity. EEG electrodes were attached by
electrode paste at $C_3$, $C_4$, $P_3$, $P_4$, $O_1$ and $O_2$ according to the
10-20 system (Jasper, 1958). In the UCLA experiments, an electrode was also positioned over Wernicke's area in the left hemisphere (Morrell and Salamy, 1971)($W_1$), and over the homologous
region of the right hemisphere ($W_2$). EEG from each electrode
was recorded against a linked mastoid reference, and some bipolar

TABLE 1

*Description of data epochs that were analyzed*

| Infant no. | Age (months) | Sex | Type of presentation | Description | Length of eopch available for analysis (seconds) |
|---|---|---|---|---|---|
| 1 | 6 | F | Music | Music from radio | 42 |
| | | | Speech | Investigator talks to baby whose head is covered | 62 |
| 2 | 6 | F | Music | Tape playback of classical music | 40 |
| | | | Speech | Tape playback of woman reading | 50 |
| 3 | 6 | F | Music | Tape playback of music box | 38 |
| | | | Speech | Tape playback of baby doll speech | 40 |
| 4 | 6 | M | Music | Tape playback of music box | 23 |
| | | | Speech | Tape playback of baby doll speech | 58 |

pairs were also recorded for each infant. A computer program permitted simulation of additional bipolar channels by subtraction of properly scaled monopolar channels. EEG tracings, together with an event timing code, were recorded simultaneously on paper and on magnetic tape for later analysis.

In this chapter we will deal only with the auditory presentations, and only those during which the baby could not see the individual speaking (in the case of speech) or a musical instrument or music-producing individuals (in the case of music). In all but one case, such presentations were from tape or radio (Table 1). One verbal and one musical presentation of this type was included for each infant and was repeated if the infant did not give indication of interest the first time. Repeated presentations proved to be necessary with only one infant (infant 3).


DATA ANALYSIS

The EEG records were initially digitized using a DEC PDP-12 computer at the University of California, Los Angeles, Brain Research Institute Data Processing Lab (DPL), and were then analyzed with an IBM 360/91 computer at the UCLA Health Sciences computer facility. Those portions (epochs) of EEG records that were to be analyzed were, with the aid of the paper records, selected to begin at the first moment after stimulus initiation when movement artifact was no longer apparent in the records, and to continue until movement artifact resumed, or the stimulus material ended. This produced analyzable epochs of 38 sec or more in all infants, and for all conditions except the music condition for infant 4, where only 24 sec were available (Table 1).

Continuous plots of laterality ratio versus time $[L(\Delta f, c, e, T)$, where $\Delta f$ is a selected frequency band, $c$ indexes a particular symmetrical pair of EEG channels, $e$ is a particular epoch, and $T$ is time] were then calculated by the method that will now be described. Complex demodulation (Walter, 1969) followed by squaring and smoothing was first used to obtain estimates of power in the selected frequency band ($\Delta f$) versus time ($T$) in both the left (L) and right (R) members of the $c$th channel pair ($c_L$ and $c_R$) (Otnes & Enochson, 1972; Otnes, 1973). Then $L(\Delta f, c, e, T) = \{P(\Delta f, c_L, e, T)/[P(\Delta f, c_L, e, T) + P(\Delta f, c_R, e, T)]\} - .5$ was calculated and stored for plotting. That is $L$ measures as a function of time the proportion of the total power across both channels that is in the left channel, corrected so that $L = 0$ when the two channels have equal power. The $L$ ratio can also be calculated according to the formula,

$$L = \tfrac{1}{2}\ \frac{P(\Delta f, c_L, e, T) - P(\Delta f, c_R, e, T)}{P(\Delta f, c_L, e, T) + P(\Delta f, c_R, e, T)}$$

Positive values of $L$ indicate that power is lower in the right channel than in the left. Thus, shifts in a positive direction indicate a decrease on the right or an increase on the left, or both.

Smoothing was used partly to bring out average trends in the index, and also to improve the stability of the running power estimates (Otnes & Enochson, 1972). The moment-to-moment changes in the index reflect the dynamics of the power shifts being measured as seen through those of the analyzing system. The present report is based on an exponential smoothing window whose equivalent width (Otnes, 1973) was 2.7 sec. The principal data will be mean values of the $L$ functions obtained from each analysis epoch. However, in most cases we will omit the first 2.7 sec of the $L$ function from each mean value reported, as this early portion is influenced by power buildup in the analyzing system and thus contains somewhat less reliable laterality estimates than later portions of the curve. Averages using entire epochs, or omitting the first 5.5 sec, appeared to give basically similar results.

RESULTS

Our major finding from the analysis of these epochs is given in Figure 1. This figure shows mean values for laterality ratios based on a 3.0-5.0 Hz frequency band for the W1, W2 pair in the three infants where that pair was available, and for the P3, P4 pair in all four infants. For this frequency band, the average value for $L$ was found to be lower during the speech samples than during the music samples in all comparisons. In five of the seven comparisons, the mean value of $L$ was positive for music samples and negative for speech samples, and in the remaining two comparisons, less negative for music than for speech.

It will be argued below that such differences in the proportion of left hemisphere activity to the total activity across left and right hemisphere channels can be related to differences in the interhemispheric distribution of alpha-band activity which have been reported recently for adults during verbal or analytical and music tasks (Gardiner, 1976; Gardiner et al., 1973; Herron, 1975; McKee, Humphrey & McAdam, 1973; Schwartz, Davidson, Maer, & Bromfield, 1974).

Repeating the analysis for these same channel pairs, but narrowing the band on which the laterality ratio was calculated to 3.5-4.5 Hz, increased the differences between the means for speech and music conditions, and now six of the seven comparisons showed mean values of $L$ that were negative for music and positive for speech (Figure 2). On the other hand, enlarging the band to 2.0-6.0 Hz reduced the differences between the means, and in one infant the mean value for $L$ from the music condition was now more negative than from the speech condition (Figure 2).

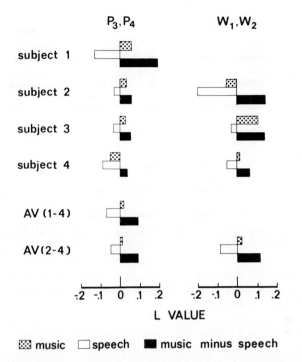

Fig. 1. *Individual and group-averaged mean values for L for two electrode pairs and two classes of stimuli, calculated from the epochs described in Table 1 using an analysis band of 3.0-5.0 Hz. As described in the text, $L(\Delta f, c_L, e, T) = \{P(\Delta f, c_L, e, T)/ [p(\Delta f, c_L, e, T) + P(\Delta f, c_R, e, T)]\} - .5$, where $\Delta f$ is a selected analysis band, $c_L$ and $c_R$ are the left-hemisphere and right-hemisphere members of a symmetric pair of EEG channels, e indexes the epoch, and T is time. $P(\Delta f, c_L, e, T)$ and $P(\Delta f, c_R, e, T)$ are then smoothed estimates of EEG power versus time in the left and right channels respectively, within the selected analysis band. Music - Speech is obtained by subtracting the mean value for the speech condition from that for the music condition.*

Differences between the $L$ functions from the speech and music conditions tended to be larger during the earlier portions of the epochs (Figure 3), though they often could also be seen at later times in the epochs.

We did not carry out a complete survey of the frequency dependence of $L(T)$ with these data. However, $L(T)$ functions were calculated for parietal and Wernicke pairs using a 1-Hz bandwidth analysis at one lower center frequency and one higher center frequency in order to make a comparison with results obtained with the 3.5-4.5 Hz band. As shown in Figure 4, interhemispheric differences in both the lower and higher bands

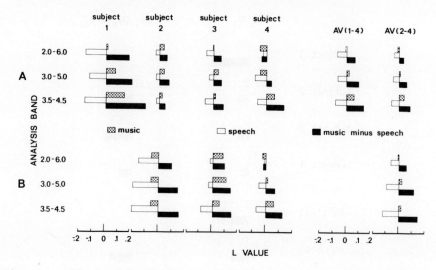

Fig. 2.  Effect of bandwidth on indices from bands centered on
4.0 Hz.  L was calculated as in Figure 1, for (A) the $P_3$, $P_4$ pair
and (B) the $W_1$, $W_2$ pair.

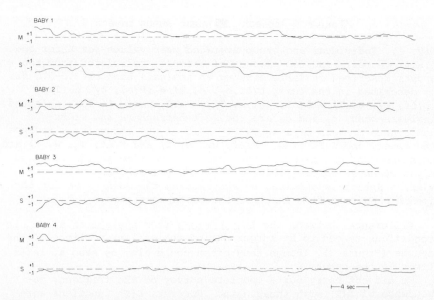

Fig. 3.  Plots of L(T) defined as in Figure 2, for the speech
and music epochs for each infant, based on 2.7-sec smoothing
window with an analysis bandwidth of 3.0-5.0 Hz.  Electrode pair
$P_3$, $P_4$ was used for infant 1, and pair $W_1$, $W_2$ for infants 2-4.

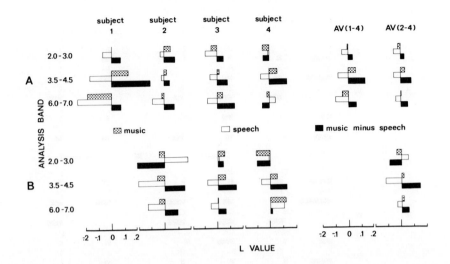

Fig. 4. Comparison of indices from three bands of 1-Hz bandwidth
L was calculated as in Figure 1 for (A) the $P_3$, $P_4$ pair and (B)
the $W_1$, $W_2$ pair.

often tended to be in the same direction as those seen in the
3.5-4.5 Hz band, but were not of the same magnitude, nor as
consistent across subjects, as those found in the band centered
on 4.0 Hz. This contrast was particularly clear for the $W_1$, $W_2$
electrode pair.

Laterality indices calculated with 3.0-5.0 and 3.5-4.5 Hz
analysis bands usually showed larger differences between speech
and music conditions at $W_1$, $W_2$ than at $P_3$, $P_4$, in the three
infants where both pairs were available (Figures 2 and 5).
Using these analysis bands, indices obtained from Wernicke and
parietal pairs were also compared to those obtained with a more
anterior monopolar pair ($C_3$, $C_4$), a more posterior monopolar
pair ($O_1$, $O_2$), and a bipolar pair ($P_3$-$O_1$, $P_4$-$O_2$) (Figure 5).
The anterior and posterior monopolar pairs as well as the bipolar pair tended to show weaker and less consistent effects,
but in the same general direction as the parietal and Wernicke
pairs.

DISCUSSION

A number of recent studies with normal adults have compared
the interhemispheric distribution of alpha-band (8-13 Hz) EEG
activity during various lateralized tasks (cf. Donchin, this
volume; Galin & Ornstein, 1973). To encouarge greater left

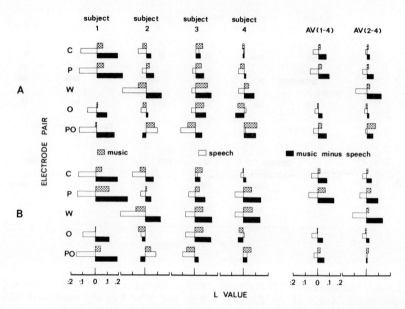

Fig. 5. Comparison of indices from five pairs of electrode channels. L was calculated as in Figure 1, except that the first 2.7
sec of each epoch were not deleted. Comparison with Figure 1
indicates that these mean values from the P and W pairs were not
substantially different from those calculated when the first 2.7
sec of the epochs was included. (A) 3.0-5.0 Hz analysis band,
and (B) 3.5-4.5 Hz analysis band. Abbreviations: C, the $C_3$, $C_4$
channel pair; P, the $P_3$, $P_4$ pair; W, the $W_1$, $W_2$ pair; O, the $O_1$,
$O_2$ pair; and PO, the $P_3$-$O_1$, $P_4$-$O_2$ pair.

hemisphere involvement, verbal or analytical tasks have been
used; to increase right hemisphere involvement, visuo-spatial
tasks (Morgan et al., 1971; Morgan et al., 1974; Dumas & Morgan,
1975; Galin & Ornstein, 1972; Doyle et al., 1973; Robbins et al.,
1974), musical tasks (Gardiner et al., 1973; McKee et al., 1973;
Schwartz et al., 1974; Herron, 1974) or recordings with the
subject at rest (Butler & Glass, 1973; Doyle et al., 1974) were
used.

In spite of considerable differences among these studies in
terms of experimental design, electrode placement, and method
of EEG quantification, they report generally similar results.
The average balance of alpha-band activity in a chosen left and
right hemisphere channel pair is reported to be different for
verbal or analytical compared to visuo-spatial or musical tasks,
or compared to a baseline with the subject at rest. Verbal or
analytical tasks are associated with relative decrease in the
proportion of alpha band activity in the left hemisphere

channel; visuo-spatial, musical or resting baseline conditions with a shift in the balance towards decrease in the right hemisphere channel. That is, the alpha band balance is reported to shift in a direction such that a predicted increase in processing for a particular hemisphere is associated with a relative decrease in alpha band activity recorded from leads above that hemisphere.

The experimental paradigm in the present study was comparable to corresponding investigations with adult subjects but with certain necessary adaptations to the special problems of recording from a young infant. Instructions and cognitive tasks have typically been used in the adult studies to elicit the kind of information processing that was the object of investigation. It was of course impossible to use such instructions or tasks with infants. However, previous observations by Dr. Schulman had suggested a way to select certain critical times during the session when there was behavioral evidence indicating that the infants were paying attention to the stimulus material. She had noticed that the infants would sometimes become quiet shortly after the presentation of a stimulus and would tend to remain so during the entire presentations. It was inferred that such periods of quiescence were caused by attentiveness to the stimuli.

A review of the literature reveals that such transient quieting shortly after the onset of sensory stimulation has been observed even in the neonate (Pratt, 1955) where it has been interpreted as indicative of a primitive type of orienting response (Eisenberg, 1969; Kearsley, 1973; cf. Heilman & Watson; Turkewitz, this volume). Aversive stimuli, in contrast, elicit a different reaction (Kearsley, 1973). Wolff (1965) finds quieting, which he calls *alert inactivity*, to be present at times when the young infant is paying attention to novel stimuli, and Kagan and Lewis (1965) have used quieting as an indicator of attention in the 6-month-old infant. Quieting has also been used as an indicator of perception in hearing tests on infants (DiCarlo & Bradley, 1961; Sheridan, 1958). In the present study, analysis has been limited to epochs that meet this behavioral criterion. In practice, these periods were easily detectable in the EEG record itself because they were devoid of the usual movement artifacts characteristic of most of the waking record in infants.

Activity outside the alpha band has usually not been examined in adult EEG studies concerned with functional asymmetry. Thus it has not been possible to tell whether activity in other frequency bands might have shown variations comparable to those seen in the alpha band. However, two adult studies that did not limit data processing specifically to the alpha band do indicate that alpha activity may well be more informative than activity in other frequency bands for detecting shifts in the lateralization of information processing in adults. Galin and Ornstein (1972) examined power integrated over the whole 0-32 Hz band and reported shifts in the ratios of EEG power between left- and right-hemisphere electrodes, which they interpreted as reflecting changes in the lateralization of information processing in their subjects. They commented that visual inspection of their records suggested that the major EEG activity contributing to these shifts emanated from within the alpha range. A second study from the same laboratory (Doyle, Ornstein, & Galin, 1973) replicated Galin and Ornstein's original finding and confirmed, by a more comprehensive frequency analysis, that the major contribution to the shifts they had reported was indeed from within the alpha band.

Our analysis of EEG activity from 6-month-old infants has initially focused on frequency bands in the vicinity of 4 Hz, rather than on the alpha band. Rhythmic activity first appears in occipital EEG approximately 3 months after birth at a frequency of about 4 Hz(Ellingson, 1967). Its appearance has been interpreted as signaling an important developmental advance (Dreyfus-Brisac, 1958). The existence of such rhythmic activity at this stage of development has been repeatedly confirmed in later studies (Eichorn, 1970; Ellingson, 1967). Such activity was originally interpreted (Lindsley, 1939; Smith, 1941) on the basis of longitudinal developmental studies as an immature version of adult alpha, and though this interpretation has been disputed (Walter, 1959), similarities between this activity and adult alpha have been noted (Lindsley, 1938). Many electroencephalographers have accepted the view of Lindsley and Smith (Eichorn, 1970; Ellingson, 1967). Rhythmic activity near this frequency can be demonstrated with monopolar recordings not only from occipital but also from parietal and temporal placements (Gibbs & Gibbs, 1950). The importance of the alpha band in the corresponding EEG studies in adults, therefore, suggested an examination of activity near 4.0 Hz in the search for comparable effects in 6-month-old infants.

In all four infants, parietal and Wernicke pairs (where available) exhibited reduction in the proportion of left hemisphere to total bihemispheric power for speech relative to music, in the activity near 4.0 Hz. When the analysis band was broadened, the speech-music difference reversed its direction in one infant. This reversal had already been noted in our earlier analysis with the 2.0-6.0 Hz band (Gardiner et al., 1973). The infant in whom the reversal was seen was the only male, and was also the only infant who was classified as "possibly left-handed" by his mother (positive signs of handedness had not yet developed in any of the babies, cf. Collins, this volume). Gardiner et al. (1973) suggested that the potential left-handedness indicated by the mother might account for the anomalous finding in this infant. A more likely explanation is suggested by Figures 2 and 4. These show that in these infants the laterality information was most consistent in narrow bands near 4.0 Hz. Thus the results in infant 4 may have been contaminated by noise when the widest analysis band was used.

We have reported that the Wernicke and parietal pairs generally showed the largest and most consistent speech-music differences

in our data.  The majority of the corresponding adult studies
have used electrodes near these same locations (Gardiner, 1975;
Gardiner et al., 1973; Herron, 1975; McKee et al., 1973).  In
this study, more posterior or more anterior pairs have yielded
smaller or less consistent speech-music differences than those
obtained in these pairs.  The left hemisphere $W_1$ and $P_3$ electrodes are both relatively near Wernicke's area, which is particularly involved in human language functions (Geschwind, 1970;
Luria, 1970); an early anatomical asymmetry associated with this
region has been noted (Wada et al., 1975; Witelson & Pallie,
1973; cf. Rubens, this volume).  On the other hand, the right-
hemisphere electrodes could be picking up activity from regions
of the right temporal lobe where lesions have been associated
with sensory amusia in adults (McFie, 1969).

Neither the lower nor the higher frequency band we examined
showed the speech-music shifts with the same magnitude or consistency as did the band centered on 4.0 Hz.  As a working hypothesis, we suggest that the shifts in activity near 4.0 Hz that we
have observed are  homologous to the alpha-band shifts detected
in adults.  This interpretation must be advanced with caution
until the frequency dependence of these shifts has been studied
more extensively and such shifts have been demonstrated not only
in additional infants of the same age, but also at appropriate
intermediate frequencies at intermediate stages of development.

We noted indications of true power decreases over the right
hemisphere in three of the four infants during the music condition.  Should this finding be confirmed (see e.g., Molfese et al.,
1976) it would contrast with the findings reported in most adult
studies, where a prevailing bias toward a relatively lower degree
of left-hemisphere as compared to right-hemisphere alpha activity is rarely overcome.  The relative immaturity of the corpus
callosum (Hewitt, 1962; Sechzer et al., this volume) could be involved.  Another type of explanation comes from the suggestion
that the decreased left-hemisphere alpha activity observed in
many adult studies reflects a cognitive bias during the experiment (Butler & Glass, 1974).  Butler and Glass suggest that such
a bias may be due to an analytical emphasis within the experimental protocols.  Whether or not reaction to the experiment is the
actual cause of such a bias, it could help to account for the
results in the adult experiments if it exists.  The absence of
systematic asymmetry in the infantile records we have examined,
then, could indicate that a cognitive bias favoring left-hemisphere processing was not yet consistently present in these
infants.

Although comparisons with previous work must be made cautiously because of differences in methodology, it can be argued
Butler & Glass, 1974; Gardiner, 1975; Gardiner et al., 1973;
Herron, 1975; Morgan et al., 1971) that the findings in the
adult studies may be related to earlier observations that "a
problem which claims the whole attention [Adrian & Matthews,

1934]" will block alpha activity (Pollen & Trachtenberg, 1972; Kreitman & Shaw, 1965; Chapman et al., 1962; Lorens & Darrow, 1962; Glass, 1964, 1967; Mundy Castle, 1957; Adrian & Matthews, 1934; Berger, 1929, 1930). Viewed from the perspective of this earlier work, the recent adult series could be accounted for by the hypothesis that alpha activity is disrupted asymmetrically during asymmetrical hemispheric involvement in mental processing (cf. Anderson; Watson & Heilman, this volume). Thus a shift in the lateralization of information processing would cause an opposite shift in the relative laterality of ongoing alpha activity.

A more localized model of alpha suppression would be needed to accommodate the fact that we obtain stronger indications of lateralization from parietal and Wernicke pairs than from more anterior or posterior pairs. Most studies have only analyzed one bilateral pair of sites at a time, but Butler and Glass (1974) have examined interhemispheric alpha shifts simultaneously in occipital-parietal and more anterior (parietal-central) channels and also report local alpha-blocking. They compared alpha distribution during a rest condition and during mental arithmetic and reported significant alpha suppression over the left hemisphere for arithmetic compared to rest in parietal-central pairs, but not in occipital-parietal pairs. They comment that their more anterior channels are perhaps particularly favorably located to detect task-related EEG activity in their experiment, as the electrodes of the left hemisphere channel bridge the left angular gyrus, an area where a lesion is associated with acalculia (Grewel, 1969). They comment that "while as strictly topistic view of cerebral function is not currently favored, the present findings seem to be in accord with some degree of localization for this type of cognitive activity." Another study in adults (Gardiner & Walter, 1975) has provided further evidence that changes in the distribution of alpha activity along the antero-posterior axis may well be a useful indicator of changes in the organization of mental activity in man (Gardiner, 1976; cf. Webster, this volume).

Although our data suggest differential hemispheric involvement during attentiveness to speech and music, we cannot exclude the possibility that both hemispheres contribute (though perhaps differently) to the processing of both types of stimuli. Molfese et al. (1976) have recently reported results from a factor analysis of auditory potentials evoked by several types of speech sounds and one tonal stimulus in newborn infants. Their results, although still difficult to interpret, appear to point to the existence of interactions between both hemispheres for all the stimuli. A comparable analysis would appear desirable for the types of results presented here.

SUMMARY

Electroencephalographic (EEG) power distributions from four
normal 6-month-old infants were recorded from homologous sites
over left and right hemispheres during the presentations of
samples of normal speech and music. Periods of transient behavioral quiescence during the presentations were used to index
attentiveness to the material presented. In all four infants,
the EEG at these critical times displayed interhemispheric differences between speech and music in terms of the distribution
of power within a frequency band centered at 4.0 Hz. In adults
comparable differences in a higher frequency band (alpha) have
been interpreted as reflecting lateralized differences in information processing. We propose that these EEG asymmetries in infants are homologous to those observed in adults, and that they
indicate early differences in lateralization for the processing
of speech and music signals. Our results fail to support
Lenneberg's (1967) theory of gradual development of lateralization of function but instead give added support to recent findings, both from patients and normal subjects, that suggest that
some functional asymmetries may already be present in the normal
human brain at, or soon after birth.

ACKNOWLEDGMENTS

The preparation of this chapter was supported in part by funds
from NSI-EP 1 POI NS 09704-01, NSPA HD, National Institute of
Neurological Diseases and Stroke, and from the Boston Children's
Hospital Medical Center Mental Retardation and Human Development
Research Program (HDO3-0773) National Institute of Child Health
and Development. We are indebted to Dr. C. Schulman for bringing the problem to our attention, and for providing some of the
support for the development of the method of analysis. We are
also grateful to Dr. Peter Tanguay, University of California,
Los Angeles, for providing some additional support for the study
of the method.
    The research described here was based on work carried out
while Dr. Gardiner was at the University of California, Los
Angeles. Some of the results reported here were presented at
the Hemisphere Differences Session of the Bucke Society Conference on Transformations of Consciousness, Montreal, Canada,
November 1973.

REFERENCES

Adrian, E. C., & B. H. C. Matthews. The Berger rhythm: Poten-
    tial changes from the occipital lobes of man. *Brain*, 1934,
    *57*, 355-384.

Annest, M.  Laterality of childhood hemiplegia and the growth of apeech and intelligence. *Cortex*, 1973, *9*, 4-33.

Bach-y-Rita, P.  *Brain mechanisms in sensory substitution*. New York: Academic Press, 1972.

Basser, L. S.  Hemiplegia of early onset and the faculty of speech with special reference to the effects of hemispherectomy. *Brain*, 1962, *85*, 427-460.

Berger, H.  Über das Electrenkephalogram des Menschen. Zweite Mitteilung. In P. Gloor (Translater and Ed.), *Electroencephalography and Clinical Neurophysiology*, 1969, Supplement, *28*, 75-93.

Butler, S. R., & Glass, A.  Asymmetries in the electroencephalogram associated with cerebral dominance. *Electroencephalography and Clinical Neurophysiology*, 1974, *36*, 481-491.

Chapman, R. M., Armington, J. C., & Braedon, H. R.  A quantitative survey of kappa and alpha EEG activity. *Electroencephalography and Clinical Neurophysiology*, 1962, *14*, 885-868.

DiCarlo, L. M., & Bradley, W. M.  A simplified auditory test for infants and young children. *Laryngoscope*, 1961, *71*, 628-646.

Doyle, J. C., Ornstein, R., & Galin, D.  Lateral specialization of cognitive mode: II. EEG Frequency Analysis. *Psychophysiology*, 1973, *11*, 567-578.

Dreyfuss-Brisac, C., Samson, D., Blanc, C., & Monod, N.  L'electroencéphalogramme de l'enfant normal de moins de 3 ans. *Études Neo-Natales*, 1958, *7*, 143-175.

Dumas, R., & Morgan, A.  EEG asymmetry as a function of occupation, task and task difficulty. *Neuropsychologia*, 1975, *13*, 219-228.

Eichorn, D.  Physiological development. In P. Mussen (Ed.), *Carmichael's manual of child psychology*. (3rd ed.) New York: Wiley, 1970.

Eimas, P. D., Siqueland, E. R., Jusezyk, P., & Vigorito, J.  Speech perception in infants. *Science*, 1971, *171*, 303-306.

Eisenberg, R. B.  Auditory behavior in the human neonate: functional properties of sound and their ontogenic implications. *International Audiology*, 1969, *8*, 34-45.

Eisenberg, R. B., Griffith, E. J., Coursin, D. B., & Hunter, M.A.  Auditory behavior in the human neonate: A preliminary report. *Journal of Speech Hearing Research*, 1964, *7*, 245.

Ellingson, R. J.  The study of brain electrical activity in infants. *Advances in Child Development and Behavior*, 1967, *3*, 53-97.

Entus, A. R.  Hemispheric asymmetry in processing of dichotically presented speech and nonspeech stimuli by infants. Paper presented at biennial meeting of the Society for Research in Child Development, Denver, Colorado, April, 1975.

Galin, D., & Ornstein, R.  Lateral specialization of cognitive mode: An EEG study. *Psychophysiology*, 1972, *9*, 412-418.

Galin, D., & Ornstein, R.  Hemispheric specialization and the duality of consciousness. In H. Widrow (Ed.), *Human behavior and brain function*. Springfield, Illinois: C. C. Thomas, 1973.

Gardiner, M. F. Changes in evoked electrical activity at the scalp of man associated with change in a stimulus analysis task. Unpublished doctoral dissertation, Univ. of California, Los Angeles, 1969.

Gardiner, M. F. Alpha suppression and localization of function. In preparation, 1976.

Gardiner, M. F., Schulman, C., & Walter, D. O. Facultative EEG asymmetries in infants and adults. In *Cerebral dominance*. *BIS Conference Report* #34, 1973, 37-40.

Gardiner, M. F., & Walter, D. O. Differences between human evoked potentials elicited by the same stimuli during loudness and pitch discrimination tasks. In E. Donchin & D. B. Lindsley (Eds.), *Average evoked potentials: Methods, results and evaluations*. Washington, D.C.: NASA SP-191, U.S. Government Printing Office, 1969.

Gardiner, M. F., & Walter, D. O. Differences between EEGs recorded from individuals at different stages of a psychological treatment. In D. O. Walter (Ed.), *Human brain function*. Brain Information Service, Univ. of California, 1975.

Geschwind, N. The organization of language and the brain. *Science*, 1970, *27*, 940-945.

Geschwind, N. Late changes in the nervous system: An overview. In D. G. Stein, J. J. Rosen, & N. Butter (Eds.), *Plasticity and recovery of function in the central nervous system*. New York: Academic Press, 1974. Pp. 467-508.

Geschwind, N., & Levitsky, W. Human brain; left-right asymmetries in temporal speech region. *Science*, 1968, *161*, 186-187.

Gibbs, F. A., & Gibbs, E. L. *Atlas of electroencephalography*. Vol. I. Reading, Massachusetts: Addison-Wesley, 1950.

Glass, A. Mental arithmetic and blocking of the occipital alpha rhythm. *Electroencephalography and Clinical Neurophysiology*, 1964, *16*, 595-603.

Glass, A. Changes in the prevalence of alpha activity associated with the repetition, performance and magnitude of arithmetical calculations. *Psychologisches Forschungen*, 1967, *30*, 250-272.

Glass, A. Factors influencing changes in the amplitude histogram of the normal EEG during eye opening and mental arithmetic. *Electroencephalography and Clinical Neurophysiology*, 1970, *28*, 429.

Grewel, F. The acalculias. In P. J. Vinken & G. W. Bruyn (Eds.), *Handbook of clinical neurology*. Vol. IV. New York: Wiley, 1969. Pp. 181-194.

Herron, J. EEG alpha asymmetry and dichotic listing in stutterers. Unpublished manuscript, 1975.

Hewitt, W. The development of the human corpus callosum. *Journal of Anatomy*, 1962, *96*, 355-358.

Jasper, H. The ten twenty system of the international federation. *Electroencephalography and Clinical Neurophysiology*, 1968, *10*, 371-375.

Kagan, J., & Lewis, M. Studies of attention in the human infant. *Merrill-Palmer Quarterly*, 1965, *11*, 95-128.

Kearsley, R. B. The newborn's response to auditory stimulation: A demonstration of orienting and defensive behavior. *Child Development*, 1973, *44*, 582-590.

Kinsbourne, M. The ontogony of cerebral dominance. In D. Aaronson & R. Rieber (Eds.), Developmental psycholinguistics and communication disorders. *Anals of the New York Academy of Sciences*, 1975, *263*, 244-250.

Kohn, B., & Dennis, M. Selective impairments of visuo-spatial abilities in infantile hemiplegics after right cerebral hemidecortication. *Neuropsychologia*, 1974, *12*, 505-512.

Kohn, B., & Dennis, M. Comprehension of syntax in infantile hemiplegia after cerebral hemidecortication: Left hemisphere superiority. *Brain and Language*, 1975, in press.

Kreitman, N., & Shaw, J. C. Experimental enhancement of alpha activity. *Electroencephalography and Clinical Neurophysiology*, 1965, *18*, 147-155.

Lenneberg, E. H. *Biological foundations of language*. New York: Wiley, 1967.

Lindsley, D. B. Electrical potentials of the brain in children and adults. *Journal of General Psychology*, 1938, *19*, 285-306.

Lindsley, D. B. A longitudinal study of the occipital alpha rhythm in normal children: Frequency and amplitude standards. *Journal of Genetic Psychology*, 1939, *55*, 197.

Lorens, S. A., & Darow, C. W. Eye movements, EEG, GSR and EKG during mental multiplication. *Electroencephalography and Clinical Neurophysiology*, 1962, *14*, 739-746.

Luria, A. R. *Traumatic aphasia*. The Hague: Mouton, 1970.

McFie, J. The diagnostic significance of disorders of higher nervous activity: Syndromes related to frontal, temporal, parietal, and occipital lesions. In P. J. Vinken & G. W. Bruyn (Eds.), *Handbook of Clinical Neurology*. Vol. IV. New York: Wiley, 1969. Pp. 1-12.

McKee, G., Humphrey, B., & McAdam, D. Scaled lateralization of alpha during linguistic and musical tasks. *Psychophysiology*, 1973, *10*, 441-443.

Molfese, D. L., Freeman, Jr., R. B., & Palermo, D. S. The ontogeny of brain lateralization for speech and nonspeech stimuli. *Brain and Language*, 1975, *2*, 356-368.

Molfese, D. L., Nunez, U., Seibert, S. M., & Ramanaiah, N. V. Cerebral asymmetry: Changes in factors affecting its development. In Origins and evolution of language and speech.

*Annals of the New York Academy of Sciences*, 1976, in press.
Morgan, A. H., MacDonald, H., & Hilgard, E. R.  EEG alpha:
Lateral asymmetry related to task and hypnotizability.
*Psychophysiology*, 1974, *1*, 275-282.
Morgan, A. H., McDonald, P. J., & MacDonald, H.  Differences in
bilateral alpha activity as a function of experimental
task, with a note on lateral eye movements and hypnotiza-
bility. *Neuropsychologia*, 1971, *9*, 459-469.
Morrell, L., & Salamy, J.  Hemsipheric asymmetry of electro-
cortical responses to speech stimuli. *Science*, 1971, *174*,
164-166.
Mundy-Castle, A. C.  The electroencephalogram and mental activity. *Electroencephalography and Clinical Neurophysiology*,
1957, *9*, 643-655.
Otnes, R. K., Coherence computation on a small computer.  Unpublished manuscript, 1973.
Otnes, R. K., & Enochson, L.  *Digital time series analysis*.  New
York:  Wiley, 1972.
Pollen, D. A., & Trachtenberg, M. C.  Some problems of occipital
alpha block in man. *Brain Research*, 1972, *41*, 303-314.
Pratt, K. C.  The Neonate.  In L. Carmichael (Ed.), *Manual of
child psychology*. (2nd ed.)  New York:  Wiley, 1955.
Rasmussen, T.  Discussion on the current status of cerebral
dominance. *Research Publications of the Association for
Research on Nervous and Mental Disorders*, 1964, *42*, 113-115.
Russell, W., & Espir, M.  *Traumatic aphasia. A study of
aphasia in war wounds of the brain*. London:  Oxford Univ.
Press, 1961.
Robbins, K. I., & McAdams, D.  Interhemispheric asymmetry and
imagery mode. *Brain and language*, 1974, *1*, 189-193.
Schwartz, G. E., Davidson, R., Maer, F., & Bromfield, F.
Patterns of hemispheric dominance during musical, verbal,
and spatial tasks. *Psychophysiology*, 1974, *11*, 227P.
Sheridan, M. D. C.  Simple hearing tests for very young or mentally retarded children. *British Medical Journal*, 1958,
*10*, 999-1004.
Smith, J. R.  The frequency growth of the human alpha rhythms
during normal infancy and childhood. *Journal of Psychology*,
1941, *11*, 177.
Stein, D. G., Rosen, J. J., & Butters, N. (Eds.) *Plasticity and
recovery of function in the central nervous system*.  New
York:  Academic Press, 1974.
Trehub, S. E., & Rabinovitch, M. S.  Auditory-linguistic sensitivity in early infancy. *Developmental Psychology*, 1972,
*6*, 74-77.
Vella, E. J., Butler, S. R., & Glass, A.  Electrical correlate
of right hemisphere function. *Nature*, 1972, *236*, 125-126.
Wada, J.  Sharing and shift of cerebral speech dominance and
morphological hemispheral asymmetry. *Excerpta Medica
International Congress Series*, 1973, *296*, 252.

Wada, J. A., Clarke, R., & Hamme, A. Cerebral hemisphere asymmetry in humans. *Archives of Neurology*, 1975, *32*, 234-246.

Walter, D. O. The method of complex demodulation. *Electroencephalography and Clinical Neurophysiology*, 1969, Supplement 27, 51-57.

Walter, W. G. Normal rhythms -- their development, distribution and significance. In D. Hill & G. Parr (Eds.), *Electroencephalography, a sumposium on its various aspects*. London: MacDonald, 1950.

Walter, W. G. Intrinsic rhythms of the brain. In J. Field, H. W. Magoun, & V. E. Hall (Eds.), *Handbook of physiology, neurophysiology*. Volume I. Washington, D.C.: American Physiological Society, 1959. Pp. 279-298.

Wittelson, S. F., & Pallie, W. Left hemisphere specialization for language in the newborn: Neuroanatomical evidence of asymmetry. *Brain*, 1973, *96*, 641-646.

Wolff, P. H. The development of attention in young infants. *Annals of the New York Academy of Sciences*, 1965, *118*(21), 815-830.

# PART VIII

# ANATOMICAL ASYMMETRY

# 26.
# Anatomical Asymmetries of Human Cerebral Cortex

*ALAN B. RUBENS*

University of Minnesota Medical School

The history of the study of cerebral dominance begins with the phenomenon of aphasia, the first and most dramatic example of an isolated defect of intellectual function resulting from damage to a particular, lateralized portion of the brain. It has been known for over a century that the cerebral structures most indispensable for normal language function are located in man's left hemisphere, almost entirely within a ring of cortex that forms the upper and lower banks of the sylvian fissure (Broca, 1865; Wernicke, 1874). This includes Broca's area, which is located in the frontal operculum just anterior to the cortical facial motor complex, and Wernicke's area, lying in the posterior-superior portion of the temporal lobe.

Not long after the functional significance of these regions was established, the left sylvian fissure was shown to be longer than its counterpart in a significant majority of adult brains (Cunningham, 1892; Eberstaller, 1890). Subsequent studies demonstrated that this asymmetry occurred posterior to the central sulcus and was therefore accompanied by asymmetries of the parietal and posterior temporal operculi (including the region of the planum temporale), which were longer on the left side (Connolly, 1950; Shellshear, 1937; von Economo & Horn, 1930).

Until quite recently these morphological differences received very little attention. They were generally considered insufficient to account for the known marked hemispheric functional asymmetries, particularly the striking dominance of the left hemisphere for language. For instance, in 1962, von Bonin

summarized the significance of the then known anatomical asymmetries of human cerebral cortex as follows:  "But all these
morphological differences are after all quite small.  How to correlate these with the astonishing differences in function, such
as the speech function on the left side, is an entirely different
question and one that I am unable to answer (p. 6)."

Six years later Geschwind and Levitsky (1968) made a major
contribution toward answering this question when they demonstrated in a large series of normal adult brains that the left planum
temporale, the cortical area that lies within the sylvian fissure
posterior to Heschl's gyrus on the superior surface of the temporal lobe, and which therefore comprises a significant portion
of Wernicke's speech area, is significantly longer on the left in
65% of specimens.  Their report brought to an abrupt end the era
in which the hemispheres were regarded as more or less structurally identical, and generated a great amount of renewed interest in morphological correlates of functional asymmetry in
animals and man.

The following is a brief review of this subject with particular emphasis on asymmetry of the sylvian fissures and perisylvian
structures in man.  Because of certain ambiguities regarding the
terminal portion of the sylvian fissure and consequently the
border between temporal and parietal lobes and the length of the
planum temporale, the methods used by various investigators for
determining the length of sylvian fissure and the planum temporale will be dealt with in some detail.  The reader is also
referred to the excellent reviews of this subject by Geschwind
(1974) and LeMay (1976).


SYLVIAN FISSURE LENGTH AND SLOPE IN MAN

According to Cunningham (1892), Eberstaller (1890) was the
first to make careful measurements of the sylvian fissures and
to report significant inequalities in their lengths.  He was also
one of the first to comment on the difficulty of establishing
reliable anterior and posterior sylvian fissure landmarks.  As
an arbitrary posterior landmark he therefore chose the point
where the horizontal portion of the sylvian fissure, the posterior horizontal ramus (PHR), turns abruptly upward into the parietal lobe to become the posterior ascending ramus (PAR) or downward as the posterior descending ramus (PDR) when the PAR is not
present.  Anteriorly Eberstaller measured from the juncture of
the anterior ascending ramus (AAR) and the PHR.  Eberstaller's
measurements, and those of other authors who subsequently adopted
his posterior point, therefore excluded the lengths of the terminal ascending and/or descending branches and, although frequently referred to in the literature as measurements of sylvian fissure length, applied only to PHR length.  In 170 left hemispheres
he found a mean PHR length of 58.2 mm compared to that of 51.8 mm

in 183 right hemispheres. The mean difference was therefore
6.5 mm. Significantly, the left PHR was longer in 63% of
specimens.

These findings were confirmed 2 years later by Cunningham
(1892) who adopted Eberstaller's posterior landmark but preferred as a more reliable anterior limit the point at which the
sylvian fissure first reaches the outer surface of the hemisphere. In order to minimize differences due to suspected left/
right inequalities in total hemispheric length he expressed his
PHR measurements as a percentage of the total anterior-posterior
hemispheric length. This so called *mean index of the sylvian
fissure* (really PHR index) was found to be 28 in 23 left adult
hemispheres and 24.4 in 28 right adult hemispheres.

Sylvian fissure length asymmetry was also found to be present
before birth. In fetuses ranging from 7 1/2 to 8 1/2 months of
gestation (six left and six right hemispheres) Cunningham found
a mean index on the left of 29 compared to 27 on the right. In
five left and six right neonatal hemispheres the index on the
left was 29.2 compared to 27.8 on the right.

Cunningham also compared the slopes of the sylvian fissures
by measuring the angles they formed with a line drawn perpendicu-
lar to the true anterior-posterior axis of the hemisphere (sylvian angle). This was $4^0$ more acute on the right ($70.3^0$ in 15
left hemispheres; $66.3^0$ in 16 right hemispheres). In other
words, compared to the horizontal the right sylvian fissure
sloped upward $4^0$ more steeply than the left. Although Cunningham
did not state whether the PAR was included in this measurement,
an accompanying illustration (Cunningham, 1892, Figure 32,
p. 132) appears to indicate that it was not.

Because of the greater upward inclination of the right PHR,
Cunningham expected to find the posterior end of the sylvian
fissure to be higher on the right side. He was therefore surprised to find that in 34 adult brains the right sylvian fissure
was actually slightly lower than the left when they were compared
at the cross-sectional level of the postcentral gyrus. He therefore concluded that the inequality of the sylvian fissure slope
was not gradual but took place predominantly in the regions
posterior to the postcentral gyrus.

Again, Cunningham found this slope asymmetry to be present in
the brains of six 7 1/2 to 8 1/2 month fetuses in which the left
sylvian angle averaged $64.8^0$ while that of the right averaged
$57.3^0$ (mean difference $7.5^0$). Cunningham's data therefore
appear to be the first to indicate that asymmetries of sylvian
fissure length and slope are present before birth and thus precede early environmental experience (cf. Turkewitz, this volume).

The significance of sylvian fissure asymmetry was further enhanced by the studies of von Economo and Horn (1930), Shellshear (1937), and Connolly (1950) who convincingly demonstrated
that the inequality of sylvian fissure lengths occurs posterior
to the central sulvus. Von Economo and Horn (1930) demonstrated

in a small series that the planum temporale tended to be longer
on the left side. Based on their cytoarchitectural studies of
seven brains, these authors attributed the increase in the surface area of the planum temporale on the left to an increase in
the surface area of auditory parakoniocortex, TB. However, they
also stressed the great interindividual as well as interhemispheric variability in their material and suggested caution in
interpretation of their findings.

In 1937, Shellshear further documented the fact that the
longer course of the left sylvian fissure posterior to the central fissure was responsible for the inequalities of sylvian fissure length reported by earlier investigators. The distance
from the lower end of the central sulcus to the end of the PHR
was significantly longer on the left in 20 out of 21 Australian
aboriginal brains. On the left this averaged 3.0 cm compared to
2.0 cm on the right, with a mean left-right difference of 1.0 cm.
Shellshear estimated that the difference would be closer to
1.5 cm if allowances were made for fixation shrinkage. The inequalities of PHR length resulted in a characteristic difference
in the courses of left and right sylvian fissures. In 18 of 23
right hemispheres, because of the relative PHR shortness, the
PAR ascended in close proximity to the central sulcus leaving
relatively little cortical surface area between the two. This
pattern occurred in only 2 of 22 left hemispheres. A similar
pattern was found in the brains of southern Chinese. A short
PHR, and hence a reduced anterior-posterior parietal opercular
length, were found in 30 of 50 right hemispheres but only 4 of
50 left hemispheres.

Connolly (1950) confirmed these findings and stressed that
the longer postcentral course of the PHR on the left resulted
not only in a larger surface area of parietal regions above the
left sylvian fissure but also in a reduction of the surface area
and spacing of sulci of parietal regions posterior to it, particularly in the region of the angular gyrus. (See also,
Blinkov & Glezer, 1968.)

Finally, after a period of 18 years in which these studies
were largely forgotten, Geschwind and Levitsky (1968) demonstrated in 100 normal adult brains that the length of the outer
border of the planum temporale (the distance between points
where the posterior margin of Heschl's gyrus and that of the
sylvian fissure meet the outer surface of the brain) was significantly longer on the left in 65% and on the right in only 11%
of specimens. Their method was relatively simple. They exposed
the upper surface of the temporal lobe of each hemisphere by
sectioning through the plane of the sylvian fissure with a
broad-bladed knife, which was advanced along the line of the
sylvian fissure until it reached the posterior wall (Geschwind,
1974). The left planum temporale was found to measure one-
third longer (.9 cm longer) than its right counterpart (left,
$3.6 \pm 1.0$ cm; right, $2.7 \pm 1.2$ cm).

This finding was significant for two major reasons. First, because the planum is comprised largely of auditory parakonio-cortex, gross morphological asymmetry of this region suggests asymmetry in the surface area of this particular type of auditory association cortex. Second, the study documented in a statisti-cally significant number of adult brains that the region of maximum sylvian fissure asymmetry corresponds with the region where left-sided lesions are most likely to result in Wernicke's aphasia, a profound and long-lasting disruption of all elements of language (Zangwill, 1960).

The predominance in dimensions (length and area) of the left planum temporale has since been repeatedly confirmed in adult brains and, more important, in the brains of fetuses and new-borns (Tezner, Tzavaras, Gruner, & Hecaen, 1972; Wada, 1969; Wada, Clarke, & Hamm, 1975; Witelson & Pallie, 1973). Witelson and Pallie view the asymmetry in the brains of neonates as evi-dence for a preprogrammed biological capacity to process speech sounds. Similarly Wada and his associates believe that the presence of morphological asymmetries in this area, found as early as the twenty-ninth gestational week, indicates a prede-termined morphological capacity for the development of later-alized hemispheric speech and language function in humans (see Gardiner & Walter, this volume).

Finally, angiographic correlates of these posterior sylvian asymmetries in adults have been reported by LeMay and Culebras (1972) and Hochberg and LeMay (1975). These authors reported angiographic asymmetries characterized in the frontal view by a lower left angiographic sylvian point accompanied by narrower arches of branches of the left middle cerebral artery as they leave the posterior part of the sylvian fissure in right-handers. They believe that these angiographic differences correspond with differences in the slope of the sylvian fissures that produce a smaller right parietal operculum.

We are thus presented with a variety of isolated measurements of asymmetries of sylvian fissure length and slope, of planum temporale length and area, and of supra- and retrosylvian pari-etal surface area. It is difficult to visualize how these asym-metries relate to one another in the individual brain. For exam-ple: What is the relationship of the length of the planum temporale to sylvian fissure slope and length? How are these variables related to differences in the size of the parietal operculi?

In order to gain a fuller understanding of these various relationships we compared the courses of left and right sylvian fissures by superimposing left lateral and reversed right lateral Polaroid transparencies of each hemisphere and tracing right and left hemispheric outlines and surface features in different colors (Rubens, Mahowald, & Hutton, 1976). In this manner we studied 36 well-fixed adult brains (ages 14-79 years, mean age 57 years) chosen because they were relatively free of distortion and of gross neuropathological abnormalities. The brains were from 23 males and 13 females. Handedness information was available from the families of 26 cases. Twenty-five were right-handed and one was said to have been ambidextrous.

The brains were carefully stripped of their meninges and vessels and the sylvian fissures were gently opened along their entire course so that their terminal branches could be identified with confidence. The upper and lower end of the central sulcus and the termination of the sylvian fissure were marked. In 21 of these brains the intersections of the posterior margins of Heschl's gyri with the outer surface of the temporal lobe were also marked.

Hemispheres were divided by midsagittal section and Polaroid transparencies were made of their lateral surface using the same degree of magnification for each pair of hemsipheres (but not necessarily the same degree of magnification for each brain). The superior surface of each temporal lobe and its parietal extensions were then exposed by horizontal section and these were photographed from above. Left lateral and reversed right lateral transparencies were then superimposed so that the hemispheric outlines matched closely. The outlines of the central sulci and sylvian fissures of each hemisphere were traced in different colors. Measurements were made of the lengths of the postcentral portion of the sylvian fissures and of the planum temporale using the anterior and posterior landmarks of Geschwind and Levitsky.

Figure 1 illustrates our results. The hemispheric outlines and central sulci of right and left hemispheres superimposed well. There were no distinct trends of asymmetry of the central sulci. However, there was a great diversity in the course of right and left sylvian fissures with marked interhemispheric and interindividual variability. Asymmetry ranged along a continuum from near-perfect superimposition to marked divergence.

In 25 of 36 brains (69%) a striking divergence in the posterior courses of the sylvian fissures could be seen. These brains were arbitrarily grouped together and are illustrated in Figure 1A. In this group the right sylvian fissure diverged from the left by angulating upward into the inferior parietal region at a point that averaged to 2.4 + .8 cm posterior to the lower end of the rolandic sulcus. The left sylvian fissure continued posteriorly for another 1.6 + .5 cm before it either turned upward or terminated in a simple bifurcation. There were no right-left reversals of this pattern.

In the remaining 11 brains the divergence was less noticeable. These were arbitrarily placed in the symmetrical group (Figure 1B).

In almost every case the divergence occurred posterior to Heschl's gyrus and was relatively abrupt. Eighteen of the 25 asymmetric brains resembled closely the brains described by Shellshear, with a short PHR joining a well-developed PAR on the

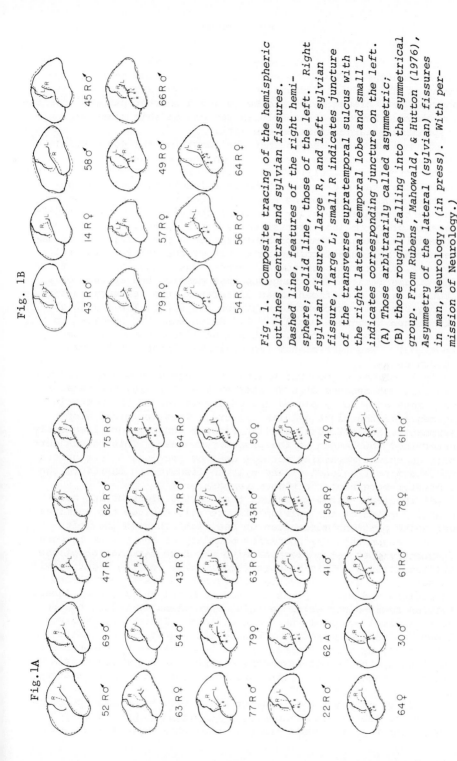

Fig. 1B

Fig.1A

Fig. 1. *Composite tracing of the hemispheric outlines, central and sylvian fissures. Dashed line, features of the right hemisphere; solid line, those of the left. Right sylvian fissure, large R, and left sylvian fissure, large L; small R indicates juncture of the transverse supratemporal sulcus with the right lateral temporal lobe and small L indicates corresponding juncture on the left. (A) Those arbitrarily called asymmetric; (B) those roughly falling into the symmetrical group. From Rubens, Mahowald, & Hutton (1976), Asymmetry of the lateral (sylvian) fissures in man, Neurology, (in press). With permission of Neurology.)*

ALAN B. RUBENS

right.  In fact, in 11 of these brains there was no corresponding PAR on the left.  This more anteriorly placed terminal up-
swing of the sylvian fissure on the right was associated with a
shorter left planum temporale below and a shorter parietal operculum above.  However, retrosylvian regions on this side were correspondingly larger than on the left.

Our measurements showed that the length of the postcentral
portion of the PHR was 4.2 ± .9 cm on the left and 2.8 ± .8 cm
on the right ($p$ < .001).  This portion was longer on the left in
86% of the brains examined.  The mean length of the total postcentral segment (including PAR) was found to be 5.6 ± .9 cm on
the left compared to 5.2 ± 1.5 cm on the right, with a mean difference of .4 cm (not statistically significant).  The lack of
statistical significance probably reflects the difficulty in determining reliable termination points of the sylvian fissure.
However, the total postcentral segment was longer on the left in
75% of specimens.  This suggests that despite the absence of a
statistically significant mean difference, the tendency is for
a longer total postcentral length on the left.  The length of
the planum temporale was 3.1 ± 2.0 cm on the left compared to
1.8 ± 1.3 cm on the right, with a mean difference of 1.2 cm
($p$ = .02).  The left planum temporale was longer in 67% of
specimens.

In 17 of the asymmetric brains the right planum temporale was
shorter, not because of a shorter sylvian fissure, but because
of a more anteriorly placed upward angulation of the posterior
segments of the right sylvian fissure.  Thus, terminal slope
asymmetry, and not total sylvian fissure length, more frequently
determined the length of the planum temporale.  This raises certain questions regarding methods used by previous investigators
to determine the "end" of the sylvian fissure and therefore the
posterior margin of the planum temporale.

It is clear that a knife-cut through the plane of the horizontal portion of the sylvian fissure will exclude the terminal
ascending portions more often on the right than on the left.
We have shown that the posterior boundary of the planum temporale
frequently does not correspond with the true termination of the
sylvian fissure.  This is particularly true for the right sylvian
fissure.  The terminal sylvian fissure bend has been regarded as
an arbitrary dividing point between temporal and parietal lobes.
Sylvian regions posterior to this conventionally belong to the
supramarginal gyrus of the parietal lobe.  Since it is not yet
known how often auditory parakoniocortex, area TB, is limited
posteriorly by this terminal upward bend, it seems reasonable to
question whether gross asymmetry of the planum temporale is a
valid indicator of underlying auditory association cortex asymmetry.

It is of interest that Wada *et al.* (1975) have noted complete
absence of the planum temporale on the right side in 9 of 100
infant and 8 of 100 adult brains.  Does this mean that area TB

was totally lacking in these specimens?  Several illustrations in the paper by von Economo and Horn (1930) appear to indicate that TB may extend posterior to the planum temporale and into the supermarginal region, perhaps somewhat more on the right than on the left.  It would be quite important to study the relationship between the extent of areas TB and TA and the gross morphological asymmetries demonstrated in our study.  Until a cytoarchitectural correlative study of this nature is done, we believe that it is still premature to view planum temporale asymmetry alone as evidence for a preprogrammed biological capacity to process language.

It should also be noted that although these gross asymmetries, taken at face value, support the notion of an inborn anatomical superiority of the left temporal auditory cortical region, at the same time they are inconsistent with the theory that left cerebral language dominance is based on the superior ability of the left hemisphere to make cross-modal associations (Geschwind, 1965).  This theory predicts a greater development of the left posterior parietal region, particularly the angular gyrus.  The retrosylvian parietal region, however, including the angular gyrus, is significantly smaller on the left side.

Szentagothai (1972) has cautioned that gross morphological differences in surface area are difficult to interpret with respect to microscopic structural differences.  For example, a larger area on one side could mean that it contained more cells or larger cells, or that there is a difference in the ratio of cell volume to total tissue volume.  Connectivity, rather than total number of cells, may be more important in certain areas than others.  We therefore conclude that sophisticated cytoarchitectural studies designed to correlate interindividual and interhemispheric differences at microscopic and macroscopic levels are the next logical and necessary steps in the investigation of morphological correlates of functional asymmetry.


THE FRONTAL OPERCULUM IN MAN

The inferior frontal gyrus forms the frontal operculum.  It is subdivided by the two anterior branches of the sylvian fissure, the anterior horizontal ramus (AHR) and the anterior ascending ramus (AAR), into orbital, triangular, and opercular portions.  On the left the triangular and opercular portions are referred to as Broca's area, the so-called cortical center for motor formulation of speech (Truex & Carpenter, 1964).  Eberstaller (1890) defined the relationships between the anterior branches of the sylvian fissure by pointing out that all gradations between a single anterior limb (designated by the letter *I*) and two completely independent lengths (designated by the letter *U*) can be found.  The intermediate types are often referred to as the *Y* and *V* conditions.  These variations result from differential downgrowth of the pars triangularis into a single limb.

Cunningham (1892) found a single limb to be far more common on the right. He reported a single limb in 41% of 46 right hemispheres and in only 15% of 34 left hemispheres. Connolly (1950) confirmed this asymmetry in 60 brains in which he found a single limb to be present in 25% of right hemispheres and in only 3% of left hemispheres. Right-left differences between Y, U, V variations were less significant.

More recently Wada et al. (1975) measured the surface area of the frontal operculum in 100 adult and 85 infant brains. For boundaries they used the prefrontal fissure posteriorly, the inferior frontal fissure superiorly, and the sylvian fissure inferiorly. Anteriorly they were forced to use an arbitrary landmark whose reliability is questionable. This was "a deep sulcus frequently descending from the midpoint of the inferior frontal fissure toward the sylvian fissure [Wada  et al. 1975, p. 242]." The left frontal operculum was found to be slightly smaller in surface area than the right, averaging two-thirds the size of the right frontal operculum. These authors were careful to mention that their surface measurement represented only a portion of the total convolutional surface. It was their impression that there was greater fissuration on the left and that the total cortical surface area might therefore be greater on the left. Because of this possibility, and the ambiguity of their anterior border, their finding of a larger surface area of the right frontal operculum must be interpreted with caution.


SYLVIAN FISSURE ASYMMETRY IN PRIMATES

Recent studies (Gardner & Gardner, 1971; Premack, 1971; Rumbaugh, Glassersfeld, Warner, Pisani, & Gill, 1974) suggest the possibility that the chimpanzee might be capable of acquiring at least a primitive language. In a preliminary report Dewson (this volume; cf. Hamilton; Warren, this volume) has presented data suggesting that in the monkey (Macaca mulatta) the left superior temporal gyrus may be more involved in the mediation of certain complex auditory-dependent activities than the right (cf. Nottebohn, this volume). It is therefore reasonable to ask whether sylvian morphological asymmetries are unique to man or whether they may be found at least in the higher primates.

Early studies on small numbers of animals by Cunningham (1892) suggested a more acute sylvian angle (greater upward slope similar to that in man) on the right in the chimpanzee, oranguatan, and baboon, but not in the macaque. In the brains of two chimpanzees he found a greater sylvian index on the left (31.6 mm on the left compared to 28.8 mm on the right). Wada et al. (1975) reported no asymmetries in the brains of 20 rhesus monkeys and 11 baboons and concluded that morphological asymmetries were unique to man.

LeMay and Geschwind (1975), however, showed that the termination of the right sylvian fissure tended to be higher than the
left in the gorilla, chimpanzee, and orangutan. This asymmetry
was most marked in the orangutan and least marked in the gorilla.
Of 28 great-ape brains, the end of the right sylvian fissure was
higher by more than 3 mm in 16. On the other hand of 41 New
World and Old World monkey brains, only 9 showed such asymmetry
when they were photographically enlarged to the size of the
orangutan brain.

Finally, Yeni-Komshian and Benson (1976) have shown that in
the chimpanzee the left sylvian fissure is longer than the right.
In 25 chimpanzee brains the mean sylvian fissure length on the
left was 45.7 ± 4.6 mm compared to 43.7 ± 4.3 mm on the right.
This difference was highly significant. Their measurements in
25 rhesus brains indicated a slightly longer left sylvian fissure (31.2 ± 2.8 mm left, 30.6 ± 2.0 mm right) but this did not
reach statistical significance. Thus it appears that morphological asymmetries of the sylvian fissures are not unique to man
and are also present at least in the higher primates. (See also,
Webster, this volume.)

CONCLUSIONS

There are some established facts of which we can now be certain. The left sylvian fissure is significantly longer in the
majority of adult and infant human brains. This is particularly
true of the horizontal portion. This is necessarily associated
with a longer left planum temporale below and parietal operculum
above. However, the region of the angular gyrus is definitely
less spacious on the left compared to the right. Similar asymmetries of slope and length have been demonstrated in some of
the higher primates, one of which, the chimpanzee, is thought by
some to be capable of acquiring a rudimentary language.

It is tempting to relate these gross morphological differences
that center around temporal cortical auditory regions to an inborn structural superiority of the left hemisphere for processing
speech sounds and for the development of language. On the other
hand, the smaller left angular gyrus goes against the theory that
language dominance of the left hemisphere is based on its superiority to make cross-modal associations and that this superiority
occurs by virtue of the greater development of the left angular
gyrus. Because of the great interindividual and interhemispheric
variability at microscopic as well as macroscopic levels the significance of gross morphological differences is not yet clear.
Definitive cytoarchitectural and gross morphological correlative
studies are now required.

Finally, those who have studied electrophysiological correlates of functional asymmetry by means of auditory evoked responses to verbal and nonverbal stimuli must now be aware of the

great amount of interindividual and interhemispheric morphological variability in the very region where they have noted the
greatest electrical asymmetries. The region of maximal auditory
evoked response asymmetry has been reported to occur in the temporoparietal region. Electrodes placed midway between temporal
and parietal locations (10-20 system) so that they overlie
Wernicke's area (Matsumiya, Tagliasco, Lombroso, & Goodglass,
1972; Morrell & Salamy, 1971; Gardiner & Walter, this volume) may
be suprasylvian in some left hemispheres but infra- and/or retrosylvian in most right hemispheres. The greater upward inclination of the right posterior sylvian fissure may also affect recordings because a considerable plate of intrasylvian auditory
association cortex assumes an almost vertical orientation in
many right hemispheres. The task is now to determine which of
the reported electrophysiological asymmetries are correlates of
functional asymmetry and which are simply correlates of underlying gross morphological asymmetry.


REFERENCES

Blinkov, S. M., & Glezer, I. I. *Human brain in figures and
tables: A quantitative handbook*. New York: Basic Books,
1968.
Broca, P. Du siège de la faculté du langage articulé. *Bulletins
et Memoires de la Societé D'Anthropologie de Paris*,
1865, *6*, 377-393.
Connolly, C. J. *External morphology of the primate brain*.
Springfield, Illinois: C. C. Thomas, 1950.
Cunningham, D. F. *Contribution to the surface anatomy of the
cerebral hemispheres*. Dublin: Royal Irish Academy, 1892.
Eberstaller, O. *Das Stirnhirn*. Wien and Leipzig: Urban and
Schwarzenberg, 1890.
Gardner, B. T., & Gardner, R. A. Two way communication with an
infant chimpanzee. In A. M. Schrier & F. Stollnitz (Eds.),
*Behavior of non-human primates*. New York: Academic Press,
1971.
Geschwind, N. Disconnection syndromes in animals and man.
Part II. *Brain*, 1965, *88*, 585-644.
Geschwind, N. The anatomical basis of hemispheric differentia-
tion. In S. J. Dimond & J. G. Beaumont (Eds.), *Hemisphere
function in the human brain*. New York: Wiley, 1974.
Geschwind, M., & Levitsky, W. Left-right asymmetries in temporal
speech region. *Science*, 1968, *161*, 186-187.
Hochberg, F. H., & LeMay, M. Arteriographic correlates of
handedness. *Neurology*, 1975, *25*, 218-222.
LeMay, M. Cerebral asymmetries in nonhuman primate, Neanderthal
man, and modern man. In Origins and evolution of language
and speech. *Annals of the New York Academy of Sciences*,
1976, in press.

LeMay, M., & Culebras, A.   Human brain-morphologic differences in the hemispheres demonstrable by carotid arteriography. *New England Journal of Medicine*, 1972, *287*, 168-170.

LeMay, M., & Geschwind, N.   Hemispheric differences in the brains of great apes. *Brain Behavior and Evolution*, 1975, *11*, 48-52.

Matsumiya, T., Tagliasco, V., Lombroso, C. T., & Goodglass, H.   Auditory evoked response:  Meaningfulness of stimuli and interhemispheric asymmetry. *Science*, 1972, *175*, 790-792.

Morrell, L. K., & Salamy, J. G.   Hemsipheric asymmetry of electrocortical responses to speech stimuli. *Science*, 1971, *174*, 164-166.

Premack, D.   On the assessment of language competence in the chimpanzee.   In A. M. Schrier & F. Stollnitz (Eds.), *Behavior of non-human primates*.   New York:   Academic Press, 1971.

Rubens, A. G., Mahowald, M., & Hutton, T.   Asymmetry of the lateral fissures in man. *Neurology*, 1976, in press.

Rumbaugh, D. M., von Glasersfeld, E. C., Warner, H., Pisani, P., & Gill, T. V.   Lana (chimpanzee) learning language:   A progress report. *Brain and Language*, 1974, *1*(2), 205-212.

Shellshear, J. L.   The brain of the aboriginal Australian:   A study in cerebral morphology. *Philosophical Transactions of the Royal Society of London*, Series B., 1937, *227*, 293-409.

Szentagothai, J.   Plasticity in the central nervous system. *Neurosciences Research Progress Bulletin*, 1972, *12*(4), 535.

Teszner, D., Tzavaras, A., Gruner, J., & Hecaen, H.   L'asymetrie droite-gauche du planum temporale; à propos de l'etude anatomique de 100 cerveaux. *Revue Neurologique*, 1972, *126*, 444.

Truex, R., & Carpenter, M. *Strong and Elwyn's human neuroanatomy*.   Baltimore:   Williams and Wilkins, 1964.

von Bonin, G.   Anatomical asymmetries of the cerebral hemispheres.   In V. B. Mountcastle (Ed.), *Interhemispheric relations and cerebral dominance*.   Baltimore:   Johns Hopkins Press, 1962.   Pp. 1-6.

von Economo, C., & Horn, L.   Ueber Windingsrelief, Masse und Rindenarchitektonik der Supratemporalflache, ihre individuellen und ihre Seitenunterschiede. *Zentralblatt Fuer die Gesamte Neurologie und Psychiatrie*, 1930, *130*, 687-757.

Wada, J. A.   Interhemispheric sharing and shift of cerebral speech function. *Excerpta Medica International Congress Series*, 1969, *193*, 296-297.

Wada, J. A., Clarke, R., & Hamm, A.   Cerebral hemispheric asymmetry in humans:   Cortical speech zones in 100 adult and 100 infant brains. *Archives of Neurology*, 1975, *32*, 239-246.

Wernicke, C. *Der Aphasische Symptomen complex*. Breslau:   Max

Cohn and Weigert, 1874.

Witelson, S. F., & Pallie, W.  Left hemisphere specialization for language in the newborn:  Neuroanatomical evidence of asymmetry.  *Brain*, 1973, *96*, 641-646.

Yeni-Komshian, G., & Benson, D.  Anatomical study of cerebral asymmetry in the temporal lobe of humans, chimpanzees and rhesus monkeys.  *Science*, 1976, *192*, 387-389.

Zangwill, O.L.  *Cerebral dominance and its relation to psychological function.*  Springfield, Illinois:  C. C. Thomas, 1960.

# Subject Index

Particularly important principal headings (such as **Asymmetry, Left-right differences**, etc.) which are followed by many sub-entries will appear in **boldface**.

517

and unilateral neglect, 294-296, xxxii
anterior-posterior distribution, 474-477,
486ff, xliv-xlv
as index of hemispheric utilization,
340ff, 368-370, 451-469, 477, 481-495,
xxxvii, xlii-xliv
asymmetries, 262, 343-345, 353ff,
368-370, 416-417, 451-469, 474-477,
482-483, 489-495, xxxviii, xliii-xlv
beta, theta and delta bands, 345ff,
413-414, 486ff
commissurotomized cats, 477
coupling between amplitude and
asymmetry, 463ff, xliii-xliv
desynchronization, 295ff, 457ff, 493-494,
459ff, xliii
drug-effects, 451ff, xliii-xliv
during operant task performance,
457-364, xliii-xliv
during structure vs function matching
task, 368-370, xxxviii
electrode placement, 344, 357-359, 490,
xxxvii
frequency domain (spectral) studies,
341-342, 343-345, 353ff, 368-370,
373-374, 416-417, 451-469, 474-477,
481-495, xxxvii-xxxviii,xlii-xlv
indices of orienting, 294
intrahemispheric measures, 342, 345,
477, xliv
left-right ratios, 357, 409ff, 452ff, 474ff,
484ff, xliii-xlv
methodological critique, see also Event-
Related Potentials 353-359, xxxvii
occipital, 344ff
parietal, 344ff, 452ff, 484ff, xxxviii,
xliii-xlv
relation to Event-related potentials,
347-348, 416-417
resting baselines, 343, 451-452, 455,
474ff, xliii-xliv
reversals of amplitude laterality
relationships, 455ff, 474ff, xliii-xliv
subject and state variables, 343, 356,
xxxvii
survey of asymmetry literature, 341-342,
343-345, 353ff, 416-417, 451-452,
489-495, xxxvii
task difficulty effects, 356, 360ff, 465,
xxxvii-xxxviii, xlii
temporal, 344ff
verbal vs musical input in infants,
481-495, xlv
Eel, 176-177
Electrical stimulation
anterior commissure during learning,

81-86, xxii, xxv
inferior temporal, 389-391
prefrontal, 390-391
striate cortex, 76-79, 85-86, xxi-xxii, xxv
VL (thalamus), 127-129
Electroencephalogram, see EEG
Electrographic correlates of asymmetric
function, see EEG, Evoked potentials,
Event-related potentials, Steady
potential shifts and CNV
Electromyogram, 362
Electrooculoram (EOG), 362, 367, 391ff,
403ff, 430ff, xxxix-xlii
Embryology of asymmetry, 3-18, 173-194,
195-204, xix-xxi, xxvii
oocytic inheritance, 173-175, 196-204,
xxvii
positional information, 173ff, 196ff, xxvii
Embryology of the heart, 175-176
Embryonic inducer for right-left
differentiation, 197ff
Endogenous neurotransmitter
asymmetries, 218ff, 298-299, xxvii-xxix,
xxxi
Engrams, bilateral vs unilateral, 45-62,
75-88, 128-129, xx-xxii, xxv
Environment
biased vs unbiased, 138ff, 198, 243,
251ff, 393-340, xxv-xxvii, xxix-xxxi
effects on asymmetry and laterality,
138-150, 151-172, 184-189, 195-198,
206ff, 243, 251ff, 276, 331ff, xxv-xxvii,
xxix-xxxi
Epilepsy, 92-93, 262, 330, 339
Event-Related Potential (ERP) asymmetries,
see also Evoked potential, CNV,
Steady potential shift, EEG and
Readiness potential
and cognitive lateralization, 349-350,
366-374, 388ff, 429ff, xxxviii, xl-xlii
and linguistic functions, 350-352, 403ff,
429ff, xxxviii, xl-xlii
auditory, 346-347, 351-352, 403ff, xl-xlii
anterior-posterior distribution, 350, 366ff,
388ff, 434ff, xxxviii-xlii
during unimanual response, 360-366,
388ff, 393-401, xxxviii-xl, xlii
effects of task difficulty, 356, 360-361,
366, 369, 374, 445, xxxvii-xxxviii, xlii
endogenous components, 295-296,
348-352, 353ff, 360-368, 370-374, 385ff,
403ff, 429-446, xxxvii-xlii
exogenous components, 295-296,340,
345-348, 391-401, xxxii, xxxvii-xlii
importance of "double dissociation",
355, 366ff, 417, 442-443, 493, xxxvii

lobster claw muscles, 7
magnitude, *see* Degree of asymmetry
maze-learning, 79-80, xxii
motoneuron size, 15-18, xix-xxi
muscle fibre innervation, 11-18, xx
muscle mass, 11-12, 24, 30, xx
neck muscle tonus, 254ff, xxix
neuropil mass, 16-18, 511, xx
nigrostriatal, 213-249, 298-299, xxviii-xxix,
    xxxi-xxxii
number of cells, 11-12, 16-18, 225-229,
    511, xx
paw preference, *see* Handedness
peripheral structures, 4ff, 173ff, 195ff,
    xix-xxi, xxvii
plasticity of, 7, 31, 36-42, 151, 180, 243,
    256, 481ff, xviii-xix, xxiii-xxiv
potentiated by amphetamine, 215-217,
    457ff, xxviii-xxix, xliii-xliv
potentiated by commissurotomy,
    235-236, xxviii-xxix, xxxi
potentiated by task difficulty, 329-331,
    356, 360-361, 366, 369, 374, 457-463,
    xxxv-xxxviii, xliii-xliv
presynaptic and postsynaptic, 218-220,
    225-229, 235-236, 243-245, xxviii
pulvinar, 126-129, 320, xxiv-xxv, xxxiv,
quantitative vs qualitative, 46, 123-124,
    127-129, 137ff, 173ff, 182, 195ff,
    330-331, 333-334, 430, 479, xxiv-xxvii,
    xxxv-xxxvi; *see also* Degree of
    asymmetry
reversal, 4, 36-42, 204, 214, 232-235, 243,
    455ff, 474ff, xviii-xix, xxix, xliii-xliv
sensory thresholds, 252ff, xxix-xxxi
side preferences, 230-245, 251ff, 274ff,
    xxvii-xxxi
susceptibility to neglect, 289, 298-299,
    xxxi-xxxii
sylvian fissure, 503-514, xlv-xlvii
syringeal innervation, 23ff, xviii-xix
syringeal muscle mass, 24, 30
temporal cortex, 63-71, 313-321, 481-495,
    503ff, xxi, xxxiv, xlv-xlvii
tracheosyringealis, 28ff, xviii-xix
underlying global dichotomies, 262, 326,
    xviii, xxx
unilateral parkinsonism, 244
upper and lower axial skeleton, 181
vagus, 25
VL, 124-129, xxiv-xxv
Left-right differentiation, 200
Left-right equipotentiality
    after commissurotomy for seizures, 330,
    xxxv
    canary hypoglossus, 31, xviii-xix
    decapod chelae, 7, xix-xxi

monkey hemispheres, 45-62, 161-171,
    xx-xxii, xxvi
Left-right indifference of genes, 137ff,
    173ff, 189, 195ff, 201-204, xxvii
Left-side advantage in morphogenesis,
    173-194, 201, xxvii
Left-visual-field superiority, 326ff, xxxv
Lesions, *see* Bilateral and unilateral
    effects; *also* Specific structures
Levoisometry, 201, xlvii
Levoratatory protein, 200, xlvii
Limb development, 174-175
Limbic system, 80-81, 86, 291ff, xxii,
    xxxi-xxxii
Lobster *Homarus*, 7
Localization
    of function in canary brain, 23, 28-42,
    xviii-xix
    of function in human brain, 261-263,
    298-299, 313ff, 339ff, 503ff, xxxi-xxxii,
    xxxiv
    and side preference, 242-245, xxviii-xxix
    effects of amphetamine, 95ff, xxiii
    in split-brain kittens, 95ff, xxiii
Locust, 4
Logical-rational/holistic-intuitive
    dichotomy, 262, xviii

# M

Macropotentials, *see* Event-related
    potentials *and* Steady potential shifts
Macroscopic asymmetries, 180ff, xxvii
Magnitude of asymmetry, *see* Degree of
    asymmetry
Major and minor
    chelae, *see* heterochely
    hemispheres, *see* Left hemisphere, Right
    hemisphere *and* specific headings
Male-female differences, *see* Sex
    differences
Manual gestures, 262
Maternal inheritance, 175, 195, 197,
    201-204, 206, xxvii
Maturation
    central nervous system, 92-94, xxiii
    left-right differences, *see* Development
    of asymmetry
    rate, 198
Maze behavior, 79-80, 86, xxii, xxv
    T maze spatial bias, 231ff, xxviii-xxix
MBD, *see* Minimal brain dysfunction
Medial geniculate nucleus, 317-320, xxxiv,
    xxxvi
Memory
    access, 75-79, 80-86, xx-xxii
    and the forebrain commissures, 45-62,